A Clinician's Guide to Alzheimer's Disease

A Clinician's Guide to Alzheimer's Disease

Editor: Trevor Cornfield

AMERICAN
MEDICAL PUBLISHERS
www.americanmedicalpublishers.com

AMERICAN
MEDICAL PUBLISHERS
www.americanmedicalpublishers.com

Cataloging-in-Publication Data

A clinician's guide to alzheimer's disease / edited by Trevor Cornfield.
p. cm.
Includes bibliographical references and index.
ISBN 978-1-63927-432-1
1. Alzheimer's disease. 2. Alzheimer's disease--Patients.
3. Alzheimer's disease--Patients--Care. I. Cornfield, Trevor.
RC523 .A49 2022
616.831--dc23

American Medical Publishers,
41 Flatbush Avenue,
1st Floor, New York,
NY 11217, USA

ISBN 978-1-63927-432-1 (Hardback)

Contents

Preface

Alzheimer's disease (AD) is a progressive condition that causes a continuous decline in thinking, behavioral and social skills. This impairs an individual's ability to function independently. AD mostly affects people over the age of 45 years, although 4-5% of the cases are early-onset Alzheimer's. The cause of Alzheimer's disease is not known. Some of the risk factors for Alzheimer's include a history of depression, hypertension and head injuries. Neuropsychological tests like the mini-mental state examination are used to evaluate the cognitive impairments associated with the disease and diagnose it. The presence of neurological and neuropsychological features of the disease and the absence of alternate conditions is supportive of a diagnosis of AD. This book is a valuable compilation of topics, ranging from the basic to the most complex aspects of Alzheimer's disease. It aims to shed light on some of the unexplored aspects of this disease. The extensive content of this book provides the readers with a thorough understanding of the condition.

This book has been the outcome of endless efforts put in by authors and researchers on various issues and topics within the field. The book is a comprehensive collection of significant researches that are addressed in a variety of chapters. It will surely enhance the knowledge of the field among readers across the globe.

It gives us an immense pleasure to thank our researchers and authors for their efforts to submit their piece of writing before the deadlines. Finally in the end, I would like to thank my family and colleagues who have been a great source of inspiration and support.

Editor

1

Gad67 haploinsufficiency reduces amyloid pathology and rescues olfactory memory deficits in a mouse model of Alzheimer's disease

Yue Wang[1], Zheng Wu[1*], Yu-Ting Bai[1], Gang-Yi Wu[1,2*] and Gong Chen[1*]

Abstract

Background: Alzheimer's disease (AD) is the most common age-related neurodegenerative disorder, affecting millions of people worldwide. Although dysfunction of multiple neurotransmitter systems including cholinergic, glutamatergic and GABAergic systems has been associated with AD progression the underlying mechanisms remain elusive. We and others have recently found that GABA content is elevated in AD brains and linked to cognitive deficits in AD mouse models. The glutamic acid decarboxylase 67 (GAD67) is the major enzyme converting glutamate into GABA and has been implied in a number of neurological disorders such as epilepsy and schizophrenia. However, whether Gad67 is involved in AD pathology has not been well studied. Here, we investigate the functional role of GAD67 in an AD mouse model with *Gad67* haploinsufficiency that is caused by replacing one allele of *Gad67* with green fluorescent protein (*GFP*) gene during generation of GAD67-GFP mice.

Methods: To genetically reduce GAD67 in AD mouse brains, we crossed the *Gad67* haploinsufficient mice (GAD67-GFP$^{+/-}$) with 5xFAD mice (harboring 5 human familial AD mutations in APP and PS1 genes) to generate a new line of bigenic mice. Immunostaining, ELISA, electrophysiology and behavior test were applied to compare the difference between groups.

Results: We found that reduction of GAD67 resulted in a significant decrease of amyloid β production in 5xFAD mice. Concurrently, the abnormal astrocytic GABA and tonic GABA currents, as well as the microglial reactivity were significantly reduced in the 5xFAD mice with *Gad67* haploinsufficiency. Importantly, the olfactory memory deficit of 5xFAD mice was rescued by *Gad67* haploinsufficiency.

Conclusions: Our results demonstrate that GAD67 plays an important role in AD pathology, suggesting that GAD67 may be a potential drug target for modulating the progress of AD.

Keywords: Alzheimer's disease, GAD67, Haploinsufficiency, Amyloid beta, Astrocytic GABA, Tonic inhibition, Neuroinflammation, Microglia, Olfactory memory

* Correspondence: neuronwu@gmail.com; gangyiwu1@gmail.com; gongchen@psu.edu
[1]Department of Biology, Huck Institutes of Life Sciences, Pennsylvania State University, University park, PA 16802, USA
Full list of author information is available at the end of the article

Background

Alzheimer's disease (AD) severely impacts the life quality of millions of people around the world. As the most common aging-related dementia, AD is characterized by accumulation of extracellular amyloid β peptide (Aβ) deposits and declining in cognition and memory [1]. Dysregulation of several neurotransmitter systems have been reported in the disease progress. GABAergic system is the principal inhibitory neurotransmitter system in the brain. Diverse lines of evidence suggest that GABAergic system is altered in AD brains, including GABA [2, 3], GABA synthetase, GABA receptors [4], GABA transporters [3] and GABAergic neurons [5, 6]. For example, the activity of GABAergic neurons in AD mice is significantly reduced [5], and even GABAergic neurons may be lost in AD brains [7, 8]. On the other hand, we and others have discovered that GABA may accumulate in the reactive astrocytes in both human and mouse AD brains [2, 4]. Therefore, GABA system may have a distinct role in AD pathology.

GABA is the major inhibitory neurotransmitter in the adult brain, and is converted from glutamate by glutamic acid decarboxylase (GAD). In mammalian brains, GAD contains two isoforms, GAD65 and GAD67 [9]. GAD65 is mainly localized at the presynaptic nerve terminals, while GAD67 is distributed throughout the cell. Importantly, over 90% of the basal GABA in the brain is synthesized by GAD67 [10, 11]. Accordingly, *Gad67* knockout mice will die within a week after birth, but *Gad67* haploinsufficient mice are viable although with abnormal behaviors [12]. In contrast, *Gad65* knockout mice are largely normal, but exhibiting susceptibility to seizures [13]. Interestingly, dysfunction of GAD67 has been associated with several neurological disorders, including schizophrenia [14], bipolar disorders [15] and Parkinson's disease [16]. In fact, clinical trials targeting at GAD67 for the treatment of Parkinson's disease have achieved some success [17]. For AD, it is reported that GAD67 is not changed in brain tissues of postmortem AD patients, but whether *Gad67* is involved in the progress of AD is largely unknown.

We investigated the functional role of GAD67 in AD by reducing *Gad67* through crossing GAD67-GFP knock-in mice with 5xFAD mice, which carry 5 human familial AD mutations in APP and PS1 genes [18]. Here, we found that the Aβ plaques were significantly reduced by genetic downregulation of GAD67 in 5xFAD brains. Moreover, excessive microglia-mediated neuroinflammation, abnormal astrocytic GABA and excessive GABA tonic inhibition were also largely reduced in 5xFAD brains with *Gad67* haploinsufficiency. Importantly, the olfactory memory deficit in the 5xFAD mice was rescued in the bigenic mice with *Gad67* haploinsufficiency. Therefore, *Gad67* haploinsufficiency in AD mouse model shows significant improvement in both AD pathology and cognitive function. Our results suggest that GAD67 may potentially be a drug target for AD therapy.

Methods

Experimental animals

The GAD67-GFP knock-in mice in a C57BL/6 genetic background were obtained from (Tamamaki et al., 2003). A cDNA encoding *Gfp* was targeted to the *Gad67* promoter locus and the resulting homozygous mice die prenatally but the heterozygous GAD67$^{+/-}$-GFP mice, in which one allele of *Gad67* gene is replaced by *Gfp*, are viable and seem have no global morphological and overt behavioral deficits [19, 20] but see some social behavior changes [12]. The 5xFAD transgenic mice also in a C57BL/6 genetic background, were purchased from the Jackson Lab (stock number: 006554), which harbored two mutations on human PS1 proteins (M146 L and L286 V) and three mutations on human APP [Swedish (K670 N/M671 L)], London (V717I) and Florida (I716V). This transgenic line was crossed with the C57BL/6 for breeding. To assess the effects of reduction of GAD67 in AD mouse model, we generated the compound mouse lines by crossing female GAD67+/−GFP mice with male 5xFAD mice, thus producing the following four genotypes: wild type (AD-GG-), GAD67-GFP$^{+/-}$ (AD-GG+), 5xFAD (AD+GG-) and 5xFAD/GAD67-GFP$^{+/-}$ (AD +GG+, bigenic mice) respectively. Of note, the 5xFAD mice in C57BL/6 J genetic background do not show very early onset. (2–3 month old) amyloid pathology and behavioral deficits as the original line generated by the Vassar group in a B6SJL background [Jackson Lab, https://www.jax.org/strain/006554]; therefore, we assessed the effects of haploinsufficiency of *Gad67* on amyloid pathology and behavioral deficits in 6–10 months old mice, when the 5xFAD mice developed severe Aβ burden and consistent behavioral deficits. The 5xFAD transgene is driven by a Thy-1 promoter, which contains an estrogen responsive element, and is known to display a gender difference in Aβ burden [21]; thus, we kept the female/male ratio comparable cross the 4 genotypes. For immunostaining age- and sex-matched littermates were used. For behavior test, several cohorts with similar age were pooled together for comparison.

The mice were housed in a 12/12-h light-dark cycle with food and water. All experimental procedures were approved by the Pennsylvania State University IACUC, in line with the guidelines of the National Institutes of Health for the Care and Use of Laboratory Animals.

Immunohistochemistry and quantification

Mice were deeply anesthetized by intraperitoneally injected with 2.5% Avertin (10 ml/kg), and then were perfused with ice-cold artificial cerebrospinal fluid (ACSF) to wash off blood in the brain, followed by 4% paraformaldehyde (PFA) fixation in phosphate-buffered saline (PBS). The brain was dissected out and further fixed overnight at 4 °C with 4% PFA. Brain tissue was sliced as sagittal sections at 45 um using the Leica vibratome and stored in 0.1 M PB at 4 °C. For immunostaining, brain slices were rinsed with PBS for three times, 10 min each, and then treated with blocking solution (0.3% Triton-X and 10% normal donkey and goat serum in 0.1 M PBS) for 2 h at room temperature. The brain sections were next incubated with the following primary antibodies at 4 °C overnight [in 5% normal donkey serum (NDS) and 5% normal goat serum (NGS) in 0.1 M PBS]: Monoclonal anti-GAD67 (mouse, 1:500, Millipore, MAB5406); polyclonal anti-GABA (rabbit, 1:1000, Sigma, A2052); Monoclonal anti-Parvalbumin (mouse, 1:2000, Sigma, P3088); Rabbit monoclonal anti-beta Amyloid 1–42 (rabbit, 1:2000, Invitrogen, 700,254); Polyclonal anti-Glial Fibrillary Acidic Protein (chicken, 1:1000, Millipore, AB5541); polyclonal anti-Iba1 (rabbit, 1:500, Wako, 019–19,741); monoclonal anti-iNOS (mouse, 1:500, BD, 610,328). After washing three times with PBS, the brain sections were then incubated with appropriate secondary antibodies conjugated to Alexa Fluor 488 (1:1000, Jackson ImmunoResearch), Cy3(1:500, Jackson ImmunoResearch) or Alexa Fluor 647 (1:1000, Jackson ImmunoResearch) for 2 h at room temperature. After three times of washing using PBS, the brain sections were mounted on slides with the antifading mounting solution with DAPI (Invitrogen by Thermo Fisher Scientific, P36931).

For thioflavin-s staining, the brain slides were firstly treated following the immunohistochemistry protocol described above. After tissue samples were incubated in secondary antibody, the samples were firstly washed by diluted thioflavin-s in PBS (2 μg/ml) for 10 min on the shaker. Then wash the tissue sample with PBS for twice, 10 min each time. Samples were mounted using ProLong Gold antifade reagent (Life Technologies, P36934) on slides.

Fluorescent images were acquired with a Keyence microscope (BIOREVO BZ9000 viewer & analyzer) or an Olympus confocal microscope (FV 1000). The confocal acquisition parameters were set at the same level for each of the individual protein immunostaining (see Additional file 1 Table S1). The mean intensity of each of the immunostaining marker was analyzed by the ImageJ software at the same setting (ImageJ 1.46r, Wayne Rasband, National Institutes of Health, USA).

Human Aβ Elisa

Frontal cortex was isolated from AD+GG- and AD+GG+ littermate mice, and were further lyzed with NP40 cell lysis buffer (Invitrogen, FNN0021) containing protease inhibitor cocktail (Sigma-Aldrich, P2714) and 1 mM PMSF protease inhibitor (Thermo Scientific, 36,978). The lyzed tissue samples were centrifuged at 13,000 rpm at 4 °C. The supernatant was collected for ELISA experiment. Aβ42 and Aβ40 measurement were conducted by using the human Aβ42 ELISA kit (Invitrogen, KHB3441) and human Aβ40 ELISA kit (Invitrogen, KHB3481), and following the protocol of the ELISA kits strictly. Firstly, to bind antigen, load standards and samples to the corresponding wells in the Aβ antibody coated plates (included in the ELISA kit). Secondly, add the human Aβ42 detector antibody (or human Aβ40 detector antibody, respectively), tap the plate to mix thoroughly and then incubate for 3 h at room temperature on a shaker. Next, aspirate the solution and wash the wells with 1× wash buffer for 4 times. Add the HRP-conjugate antibody, incubate the plate at room temperature for 30 min, and then washed the wells 4 times with 1× wash buffer. Then apply the stabilized chromogen in each well, incubate in the dark for 30 min. After adding the stop solution in each well, read the plate within 30 min to get the absorbance at 450 nm and then generate the standard curve (SpectraMax Plus 384 Microplate Reader). With the value of optical density at 450 nm and the known concentration of the standard ladder, the Aβ42 and Aβ40 load of the unknown samples will be analyzed and quantified. Each sample is repeated twice and averaged.

Brain slice electrophysiology

The adult brain slice preparation followed previously described protocols [22]. Briefly, the 12–14 month old adult mice were transcardially perfused with cutting solution (in mM): 93 NMDG, 93 HCl, 2.5 KCl, 1.25 NaH_2PO_4, 30 $NaHCO_3$, 20 HEPES, 15 Glucose, 12 N-Acetyl-L-cysteine, 5 Sodium ascorbate, 2 Thiourea, 3 Sodium pyruvate, 7 $MgSO_4$, 0.5 CaCl2, pH 7.3–7.4, 300 mOsmo, bubbled with 95% O_2/5% CO_2. Then, the mouse brain was removed and cut at 300 μm in the cutting solution at room temperature. Brain slices were collected in the cutting solution and incubated for 12–15 min at 32–34 °C. The slices were kept in the holding solution with continuous 95% O_2/5% CO_2 bubbling (in mM): 92 NaCl, 2.5 KCl, 1.25 NaH_2PO_4, 30 $NaHCO_3$, 20 HEPES, 15 Glucose, 12 N-Acetyl-L-cysteine, 5 Sodium ascorbate, 2 Thiourea, 3 Sodium pyruvate, 2 $MgSO_4$, 2 $CaCl_2$. After 0.5 h recovery in the holding solution, patch-clamp recording was performed in the standard aCSF (in mM): 124 NaCl, 2.5 KCl, 1.25 NaH_2PO_4, 26 $NaHCO_3$, 10 Glucose, 1.3 $MgSO_4$, 2.5 $CaCl_2$.

To record the miniature IPSCs and the tonic GABA currents, 10 μM DNQX, 50 μM AP5 and 1 μM TTX were added into the aCSF. The pipette was filled with high Cl^- internal solution (mM): 135 CsCl, 5 Na-phosphocreatine, 10 HEPES, 5 EGTA, 4 MgATP, and 0.5 Na2GTP (pH 7.3 adjusted with CsOH, 280–290 mOsm). The tonic GABA current was revealed by the change of holding current after local perfusion of 100 μM bicuculline (sigma). The mIPSCs were analyzed by Mini Analysis Program and assisted with visual check. Data were collected with a MultiClamp 700A amplifier and pCLAMP9 software (Molecular Devices).

Olfactory behavior test

Olfactory deficits of mice were tested using the odor habituation and cross dis-habituation test as described previously [23]. Briefly, four neutral odors [Ethyl valerate (#290866), 2-Heptanone (#537683), Isopentyl acetate (#112674), (R)-(+)-Limonene (#183164); Sigma Aldrich, St. Louis, MO] were diluted 1×10^{-3} in mineral oil respectively. For each odor, a cotton applicator stick was firstly dipped in the odor solution and then enclosed inside a plastic tube to prevent a direct contact of liquid odor to the testing chamber. The four odors were randomly presented by inserting the odor stick into a port on the side of the mouse home cage, in 4 successive trials, 20 s each, and separated by 30 s inter-trial intervals. The mouse was caging individually in this odor test to prevent interference from social interaction with other mice. The olfactory behavior test was performed during the light phase of light-dark cycle (12 h/12 h). An observer who was blinded to the genotypes of the animals during test and data analysis recorded the investigation time, which was defined as snout-oriented sniffing time within 1 cm of the odor presentation port [23]. For the measurement of investigation time, the duration time each mouse sniffs the odors presented in different trials were recorded. For investigation time (normalized) were measured by the investigation time (sec) in each trial of odor investigation divided by the sniffing time spent in the mouse's first trial in the same odor presentation. The investigation time and normalized investigation time were then analyzed using two-way ANOVAs followed by Bonferroni post-tests. The cross-habituation index was calculated by the average of subtracting the normalized fourth trial odor investigation value from the following normalized first trial odor investigation value. The cross-habituation index was further analyzed by one-way ANOVAs followed by LSD post hoc test, compare all pairs of columns.

Data analysis

Data were represented as mean ± s.e.m. Student's t-test was used for statistical analysis in two-group comparison. One-way ANOVA or two-way ANOVA analysis was used for comparison among multiple groups. Statistical significance was set at $p < 0.05$. In the olfactory behavior test, for the calculation of F and P value of cross-habituation index, analysis the data using two - way ANOVA with LSD post hoc test via SPSS software. Statistical significance was set at $p < 0.05$, labeled as *. $p < 0.01$, labeled as **. $p < 0.001$, labeled as ***. All behavioral tests and analyses were performed blindly.

Results

GAD67 is reduced in GAD67-GFP knock-in mice

GAD67 is a major enzyme for producing GABA in the brain. Previous study has generated a GAD67-GFP transgenic mouse line [20], where *GFP* gene was knocked into the *Gad67* gene locus so that GABAergic neurons will express GFP under the control of *Gad67* promoter. However, the knock-in of GFP also destroyed the expression of GAD67. Therefore, the heterozygous GAD67-GFP mice had only one copy of *Gad67*, resulting in haploinsufficiency of *Gad67*. The homozygous GAD67-GFP mice were lethal, suggesting that GAD67 is critical for normal brain function. We first confirmed that the GAD67-GFP transgenic mice indeed had reduced GAD67 level. As expected, most of the GFP-positive cells (>95%) were GABA-immunopositive neurons (Fig. 1a). Moreover, a subset of GFP-positive cells were also immunopositive for parvalbumin (PV), a typical marker for a subtype of GABAergic neurons (Fig. 1b). These data demonstrate that GFP is a reliable reporter for GABAergic neurons in the GAD67-GFP mice.

Because one allele of *Gad67* is replaced by *Gfp* in the heterozygotes (haploinsufficiency), we next compared the expression level of GAD67 between GAD67-GFP$^{+/-}$ and wildtype (WT) littermates. Consistent with previous finding that GAD67 was significantly reduced in the heterozygous GAD67-GFP$^{+/-}$ mice [20], we also found that the immunoreactivity of GAD67 was reduced approximately by half in various brain regions in the heterozygotes (Fig. 1c). Thus, GAD67-GFP knock-in mice provide a unique transgenic mouse model for investigating the functional role of GAD67 in neurological disorders.

Gad67 haploinsufficiency alleviates the amyloid β burden in 5xFAD mouse brains

To investigate the effect of genetic reduction of GAD67 on Alzheimer's disease (AD), we crossed the 5xFAD transgenic mice with GAD67-GFP$^{+/-}$ heterozygotes to generate four different genotypes of littermates: wild type (AD-GG-), GAD67-GFP$^{+/-}$ (AD-GG+), 5xFAD (AD+GG-) and 5xFAD/GAD67-GFP$^{+/-}$ (AD+GG+, bigenic mice). We first tested the effect of reducing GAD67 on the amyloid β (Aβ) plaques, the hallmark for AD [24]. Consistent with previous findings [18, 25], we found that 5xFAD mice (AD+GG-) developed severe Aβ42 deposits across many brain regions (Fig. 2a, top). However, the Aβ42 level appeared to be reduced significantly in the bigenic mice (AD+GG+) with *Gad67* haploinsufficiency (Fig. 2a, bottom) (age 10–11 months). For example, Aβ42 immunostaining signal accumulated at a high level in the frontal cortex (FCX) of AD+ mice, and quantitative analysis revealed that both Aβ42 intensity and

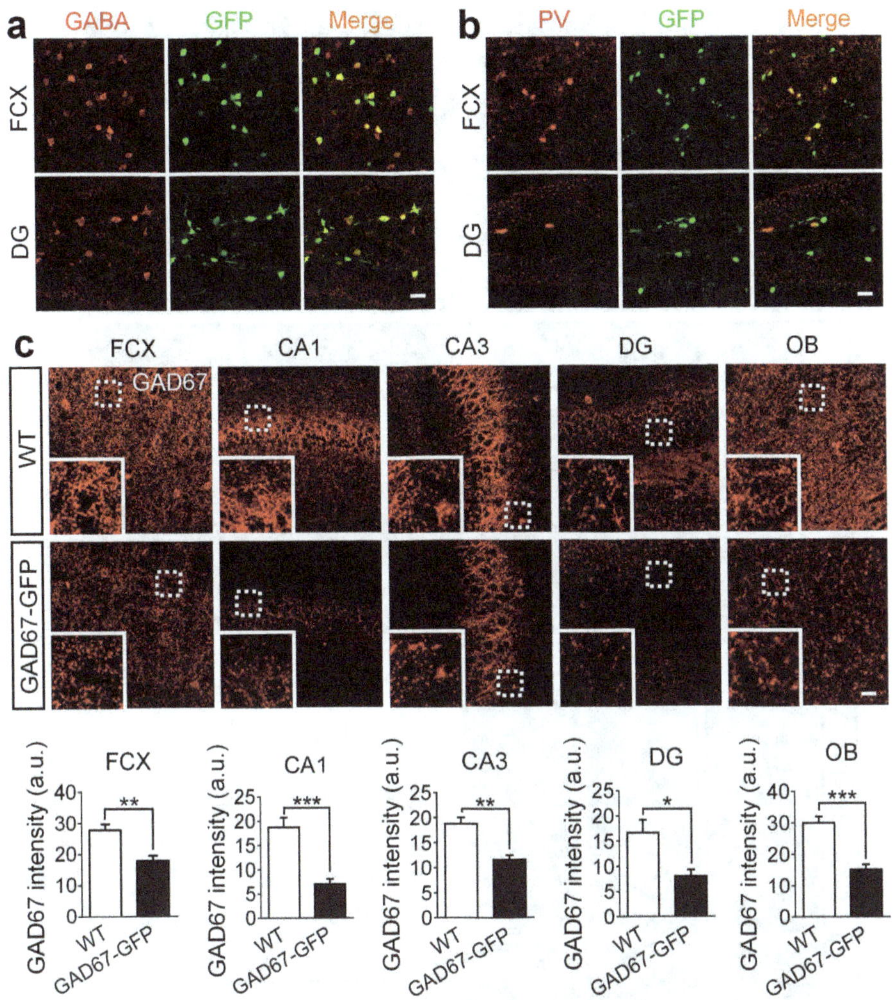

Fig. 1 Characterization of the GAD67-GFP knock-in transgenic mice. **a** Most GABA immunopositive cells (red) are also GFP positive (green) in both frontal cortex (FCX) and dentate gyrus (DG) in hippocampus of the adult GAD67-GFP knock-in mice. **b** In frontal cortex and dentate gyrus of hippocampus, all of the parvalbumin (PV) positive cells (one subtype of GABAergic neurons) (red) are labeled by GFP (green). **c** Representative confocal micrographs display the expression level of GAD67 (red) in GAD67-GFP knock-in mice and GFP-negative mice of 10–11 months old. Dotted line circled regions were zoomed in and were shown in the lower left corner of each micrograph. Quantification data showing GAD67 intensity in frontal cortex (FCX), CA1, CA3, dentate gyrus (DG) and olfactory bulb (OB) of GAD67-GFP knock-in mice is significantly reduced to about half of the GAD67 content level in WT controls. For a-c, scale bars represent 30 μm. $N = 5$ WT mice and 5 GAD67-GFP knock-in mice. Data are presented as mean ± s.e.m., * $p < 0.05$; ** $p < 0.01$; *** $p < 0.001$; Student's t-test

covered area were significantly decreased in AD+GG+ mice compared to the AD+GG- mice (Fig. 2b and c). Besides immunostaining, we further employed an Aβ ELISA kit (Aβ40 and Aβ42) to examine the Aβ production level in 5xFAD mouse brains with *Gad67* haploinsufficiency. Consistent with our Aβ42 immunostaining results, the ELISA test also showed a significant reduction of Aβ42 (Fig. 2d; AD+GG-: 10.32 ± 0.79, $n = 6$; AD+GG+: 7.31 ± 0.55, n = 6, $p < 0.02$, Student's t test), as well as Aβ40 (Fig. 2d; AD+GG-: 9.47 ± 0.91, n = 6; AD+GG+: 5.95 ± 0.80, n = 6, $p < 0.02$; Student's t test) in the AD +GG+ FCX homogenates. Therefore, Aβ production in the 5xFAD mouse brains is downregulated by *Gad67* haploinsufficiency.

We further analyzed the Aβ42 level in the olfactory bulb (OB) and the piriform cortex (PIRC) in mice with different genetic background (Fig. 3). Consistently, the Aβ42 deposit was significantly increased in both OB (Fig. 3a) and PIRC (Fig. 3c) in the AD+ mice compared to AD- mice (age 10–11 months). Interestingly, among AD+ mice, the GG+ mice showed a significant reduction of Aβ42 in the OB and PIRC compared to the GG- mice (Fig. 3a and c, bottom two rows). Quantitative analysis confirmed a significant decrease of Aβ42 in both OB and PIRC of bigenic mice (AD+GG+) compared to the 5xFAD littermates (AD+GG-) (Fig. 3b and d). We have also quantified the Aβ42 level in the hippocampus, which showed slight reduction in AD+GG+ mice (Aβ42: AG+GG-, 2.89 ± 0.80 vs

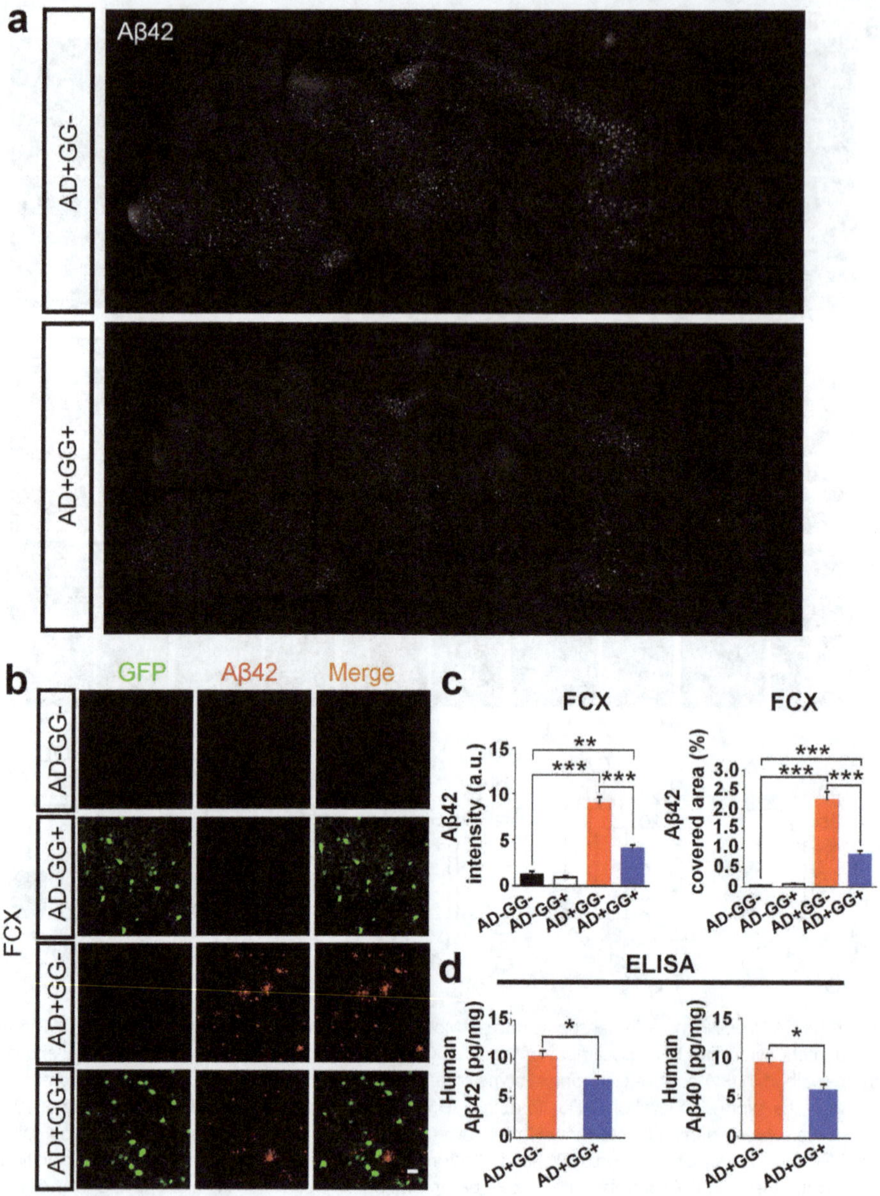

Fig. 2 A significant reduction of amyloid-beta plaques in the *Gad67* haploinsufficiency 5xFAD mouse brains. **a** Images of the sagittal section of whole brain showing decreased Aβ42 deposits (white) in AD+GG- (top) and AD+GG+ (bottom) mice of 10–11 months age. **b** Representative confocal images display the level of Aβ42 deposits (red) in the four genotypes (AD-GG-, AD-GG+, AD+GG-, AD+GG+) generated by crossing of GAD67-GFP knock-in mice with 5xFAD mice. GFP cells showed in green. Scale bar = 30 μm. **c** Quantification analysis showing a remarkable reduction of Aβ42 (left panel and right panel, Aβ42 intensity and Aβ42 covered area percentage, respectively) in the bigenic (AD+GG+) mice brain than 5xFAD mice of similar age. $N = 6$ mice of 10–11 months age in each genotype groups (AD-GG-, AD-GG+, AD+GG-, AD+GG+). **d** Elisa data also showing the Aβ40 and Aβ42 were significantly reduced in 5xFAD mice by Gad67 haploinsufficiency (unpaired Student's *t* test). Data are presented as mean ± s.e.m., * $p < 0.05$; ** $p < 0.01$; *** $p < 0.001$; one-way ANOVA with the Tukey's post-hoc test when comparing multiple groups

AD+GG+, 1.18 ± 0.13, $n = 3$, $p > 0.1$; Student's *t* test), but it's not as significant as in the cortical areas. We noted a significant low level of Aβ42 in the hippocampus compared to that in the frontal cortex in 5xFAD brains. One potential reason for such difference may be due to different GABAergic neuron population in the hippocampus versus the cortical regions, including the total number of GABAergic neurons and the composition of various subtypes.

In addition to Aβ42 immunostaining, we further employed thioflavin-s staining to verify our findings in the bigenic mice. Thioflavin-s is a chemical dye widely used to visualize Aβ aggregates and hyperphosphorylated tau tangles [26]. We observed a significant reduction of

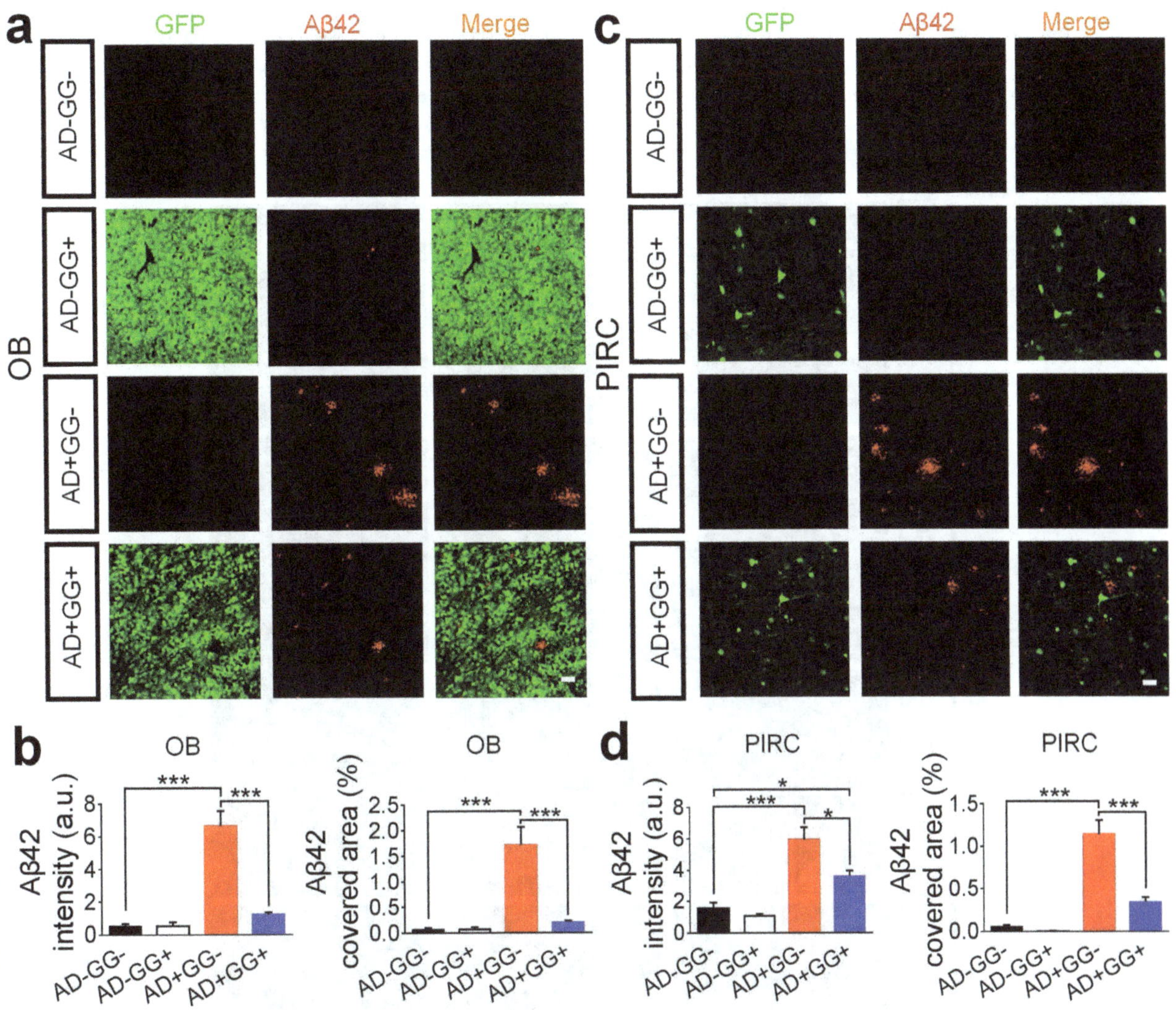

Fig. 3 Changes of amyloid-beta burden in brain regions related olfactory function. **(a-d)** *Gad67* haploinsufficiency 5xFAD mice (AD+GG+) also elicit a reduction of Aβ42 burden (red) in olfactory bulb (OB) (**a-b**) and piriform cortex (PIRC) (**c-d**). GFP positive cells were shown in green. N = 6 mice of 10–11 months age in each genotype groups (AD-GG-, AD-GG+, AD+GG-, AD+GG+). For **a** and **c**, scale bars represent 30 μm. Data are presented as mean ± s.e.m., * $p < 0.05$; ** $p < 0.01$; *** $p < 0.001$; one-way ANOVA with the Tukey's post-hoc test when comparing multiple groups

thioflavin-s labeled plaques in the FCX and PIRC of the bigenic mice (AD+GG+) compared to the AD+GG- mice (Additional file 1: Figures S1). Accompanying the changes of Aβ plaques, we also observed a significant reduction of neuronal density surrounding the Aβ plaques in the FCX of 5xFAD mice (10–11 months old), but such neuronal loss was partially rescued in bigenic mice (AD+GG+) (Additional file 1: Figure S2), suggesting that *Gad67* haploinsufficiency not only reduces amyloid plaques but also preserves surrounding neurons in the 5xFAD mouse model. Taken together, these data demonstrate an unexpected role of *Gad67* haploinsufficiency in alleviating the Aβ deposit and its detrimental effect on neurons in the 5xFAD mouse brains.

Gad67 haploinsufficiency reduces astrocytic GABA in 5xFAD mouse brains

Recently, we and others have found that GABA content is elevated in AD mouse brains and in particular, an abnormal astrocytic GABA has been detected in both AD mouse model and postmortem human AD brain tissue [2, 3]. Since GAD67 is a major enzyme for producing GABA in the brain, we examined whether the astrocytic GABA level in AD mice was altered by *Gad67* haploinsufficiency. Brain sections of all four genotype littermate mice (AD-GG-, AD-GG+, AD+GG-, and AD+GG+; sex- and age-matched for each genotype) at 10–11 months old were double immunostained with GABA and astrocyte marker GFAP. Consistent with previous findings, we found a high level of GABA in the reactive astrocytes of the 5xFAD mice (AD+GG-), but not non-AD mice (AD-GG- and AD-GG+) (Fig. 4a). Interestingly, the abnormal astrocytic GABA was significantly reduced in the bigenic mice with *Gad67* haploinsufficiency (AD+GG+) compared to normal 5xFAD mice (AD+GG-) (Fig. 4a, bottom two rows). Quantitative analyses in the FCX, PIRC, and hippocampal CA1 regions all confirmed a uniform reduction of astrocytic GABA in

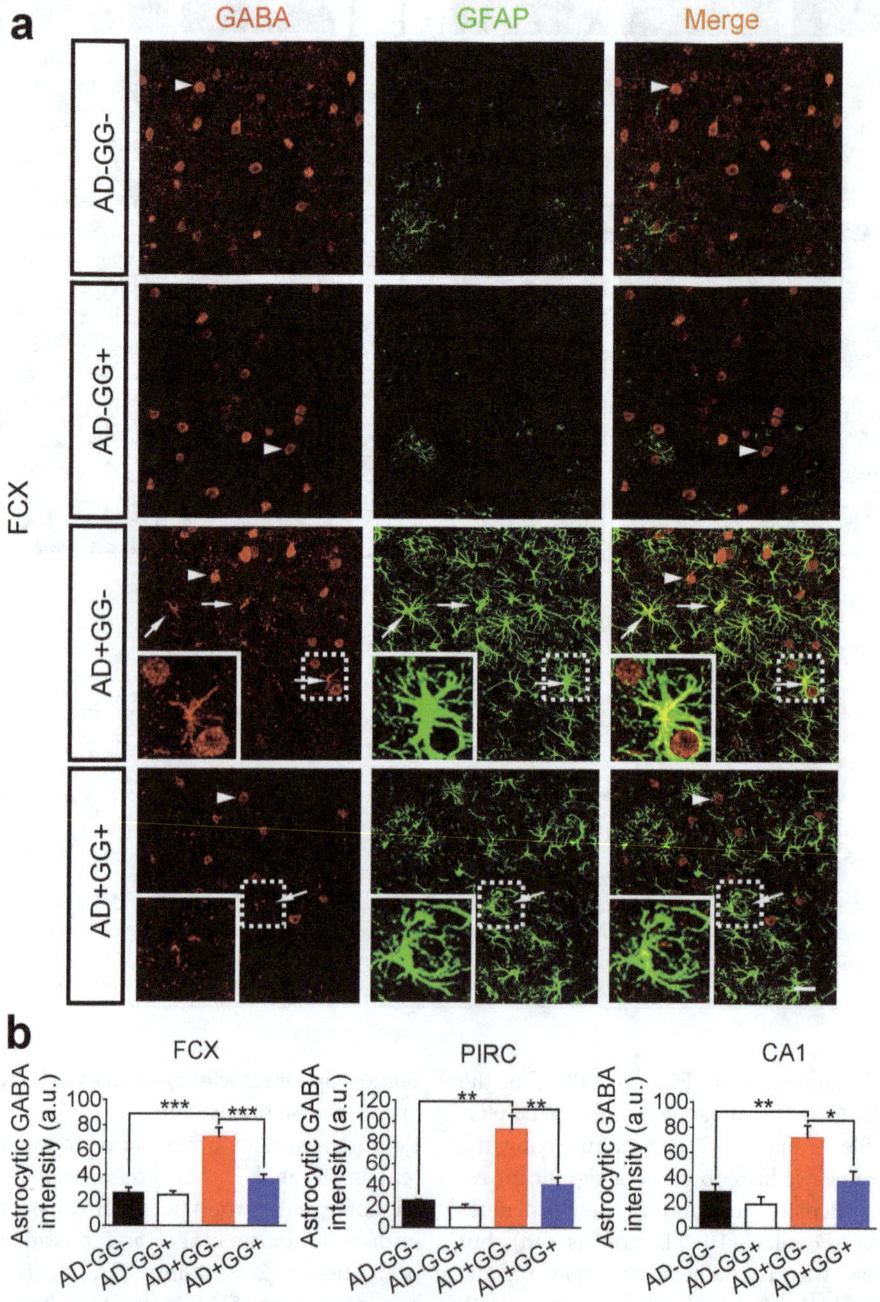

Fig. 4 Mitigation of the abnormal astrocytic GABA in 5xFAD mice with *Gad67* haploinsufficiency. **a** The GABA content level (red) is abnormally enhanced in astrocytes (pseudo colored in green for merge purpose) in 5xFAD mice brain while it is under detectable level in AD-negative mice (the normal condition). Notably, the astrocytic GABA content level is significantly reduced in *Gad67* haploinsufficiency 5xFAD brain. Arrowhead: GABA positive cells (red). Arrow: astrocytic GABA (red). Dotted line circled regions were zoomed in and were shown in the lower left corner of each micrograph. Scale bar represents 30 μm. **b** Quantification data showing the significant reduction of astrocytic GABA in frontal cortex (FCX), piriform cortex (PIRC) and CA1 region of the bigenic (AD+GG+) brain than the 5xFAD mice of similar age. N = 6 mice of 10–11 months age in each genotype groups (AD-GG-, AD-GG+, AD+GG-, AD+GG+). Data are presented as mean ± s.e.m., * $p < 0.05$; ** $p < 0.01$; *** $p < 0.001$; one-way ANOVA with the Tukey's post-hoc test when comparing multiple groups

AD+GG+ mice (Fig. 4b). In contrast to the astrocytic GABA change, we observed no significant change of neuronal GABA level across all four groups of mice (Additional file 1: Figures S3), suggesting that neuronal GABA was not affected by *Gad67* haploinsufficiency in the adult mice, consistent with previous study [20]. Together, our data suggest that the abnormal astrocytic GABA in AD mouse brains can be largely alleviated through genetic reduction of GAD67.

Gad67 haploinsufficiency decreases abnormal tonic GABA currents in 5xFAD mice

Previous studies reported that tonic inhibition is increased in AD mouse brains due to excessive GABA accumulation in the reactive astrocytes [2, 3], or in mouse brains after focal stroke [27]. Since we observed a significant reduction of astrocytic GABA in the 5xFAD brains after genetic reduction of GAD67, we wondered whether tonic GABA currents might also be reduced correspondingly. Whole-cell patch-clamp recordings were performed on the layer IV-VI cortical neurons (Fig. 5a and b). Consistent with our previous findings, tonic GABA currents were significantly increased in the 5xFAD mice (AD+GG-) compared to AD-GG- control littermates (Fig. 5e and f; AD-GG-, 14.4 ± 2.3 pA, n = 9 from 2 mice; AD+GG-, 29.1 ± 6.1 pA, n = 8 from 2 mice; $p < 0.02$; One-way ANOVA). Interestingly, the abnormal tonic GABA currents in 5xFAD mouse brains were significantly reduced by *Gad67* haploinsufficiency (Fig. 5e and f; AD+GG+, 16.6 ± 2.8 pA, n = 15, from 2 mice, $p < 0.03$). On the other hand, there were no obvious differences in the miniature inhibitory postsynaptic currents (mIPSCs) among different groups (Fig. 5c and d). Thus, our results demonstrate that *Gad67* haploinsufficiency results in a reduction of the abnormal GABA tonic currents in cortical neurons of 5xFAD mice.

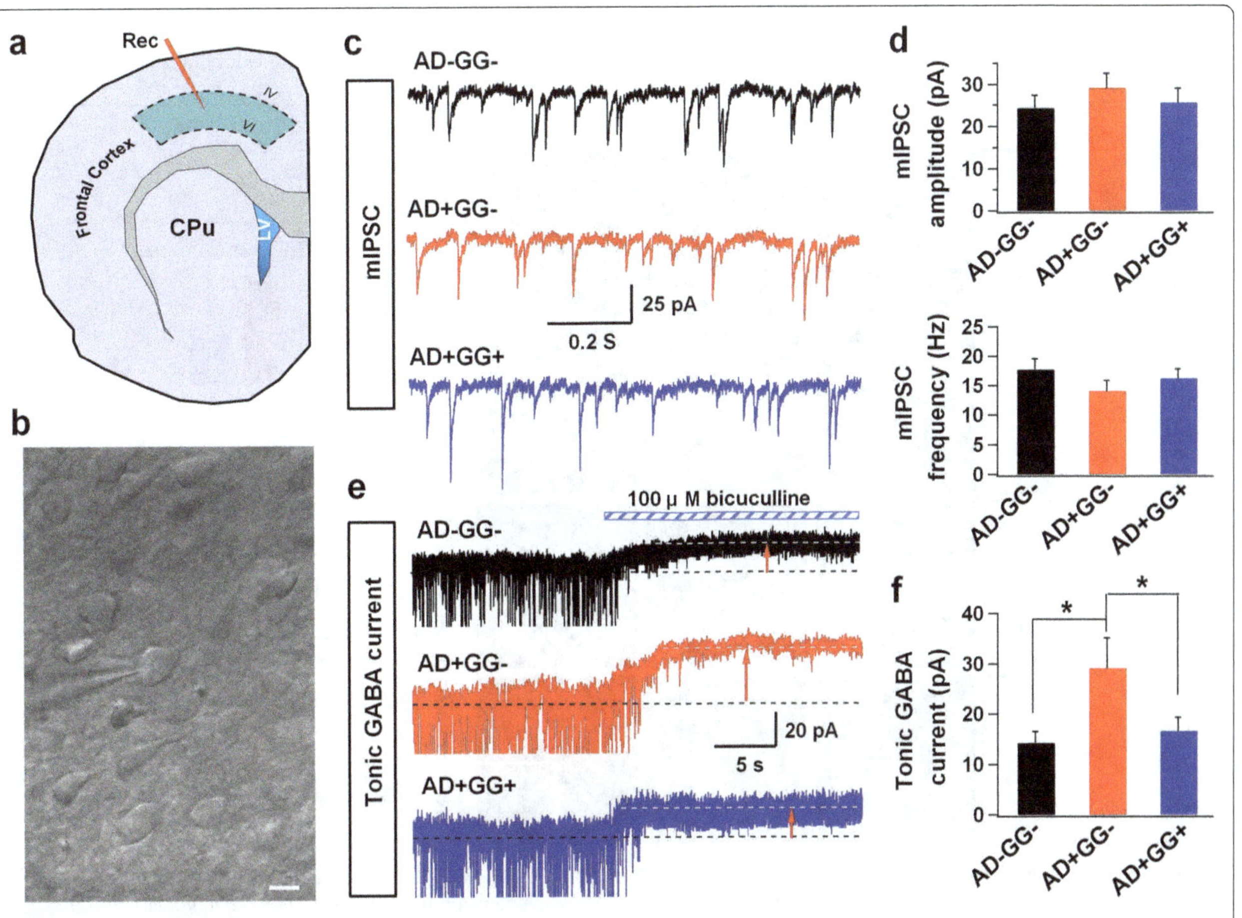

Fig. 5 Abnormal tonic inhibition is decreased in 5xFAD mice with *Gad67* haploinsufficiency. **a** Schematic image illustrate the interesting cortical area for electrophysiology study. **b** A typical phase contrast image showing the whole cell recording in the adult brain slice. Scale bar = 10 μm. **c** Example of the mIPSCs traces in AD-GG-, AD+GG- and AD+GG+ groups. **d** Summary graph of mean amplitude and frequency of mIPSCs. **e** Representative trances of tonic GABA currents. **f** Quantification data showing the abnormal tonic GABA currents in 5xFAD mice are decreased by *Gad67* haploinsufficiency. Data are presented as mean ± s.e.m., * $p < 0.05$; one-way ANOVA with the LSD post-hoc test

Microglia reactivity is ameliorated by *Gad67* haploinsufficiency

Previous study has suggested that microglia activity is regulated by GABA released from astrocytes [28]. Since the astrocytic GABA was dramatically decreased in 5xFAD mice with *Gad67* haploinsufficiency (Fig. 4), we investigated whether microglia activity in 5xFAD mice might also be changed correspondingly. For this purpose, we investigated the inducible nitric oxide synthase (iNOS), a widely used marker for proinflammatory reactive microglia, in 5xFAD mice (Fig. 6a). In non-AD mice (AD-GG- and AD-GG+), iNOS was not detectable in microglia labeled by Iba1; but in AD+GG- mice, strong iNOS immunoreactivity was detected (Fig. 6a). Surprisingly, in AD+GG+ mice, the iNOS immunoreactivity was significantly reduced compared to their AD +GG- littermates (Fig. 6a). Quantitative analysis shows that in both the frontal cortex (Fig. 6b) and piriform cortex (Fig. 6c), the iNOS covered area was significantly reduced in AD+GG+ mice compared to that in AD+GG- mice (Fig. 6b, FCX, AD+GG-: 1.40 ± 0.28%, AD+GG+: 0.68 ± 0.14%, $p < 0.02$, $n = 6$; Fig. 6c, PIRC, AD+GG-: 1.02 ± 0.28%, AD +GG+: 0.27 ± 0.07%, $p < 0.01$, n = 6). Consistent with the iNOS finding, the resting microglia (Iba1+) displayed normal morphology with small soma and ramified processes, and evenly distributed in various brain regions in AD- mice (Fig. 6a). In contrast, in AD+GG- mouse brains, microglia was strongly activated, exhibiting hypertrophic soma with amoeboid-like morphology (Fig. 6a). Notably, in AD+GG+ mice, the microglia became less hypertrophic with more ramified processes compared to those found in AD +GG- mice, suggesting that the microglia reactivity in 5xFAD mice was partially rescued by GAD67 haploinsufficiency (Fig. 6a, Iba1+, green). Together, these results suggest that genetic reduction of GAD67 partially ameliorates microglia reactivity in 5xFAD brains.

Gad67 haploinsufficiency rescues olfactory deficits in 5xFAD mice

We found that several beneficial effects of *Gad67* haploinsufficiency in 5xFAD mice were observed in various brain regions, including the key regions of olfactory circuits and limbic systems as described above. Olfaction sensory impairment has been reported both in AD patients and in mouse models [29, 30]. Therefore, we further investigated whether *Gad67* haploinsufficiency might rescue olfactory deficits in 5xFAD mice. We performed the odor habituation and cross

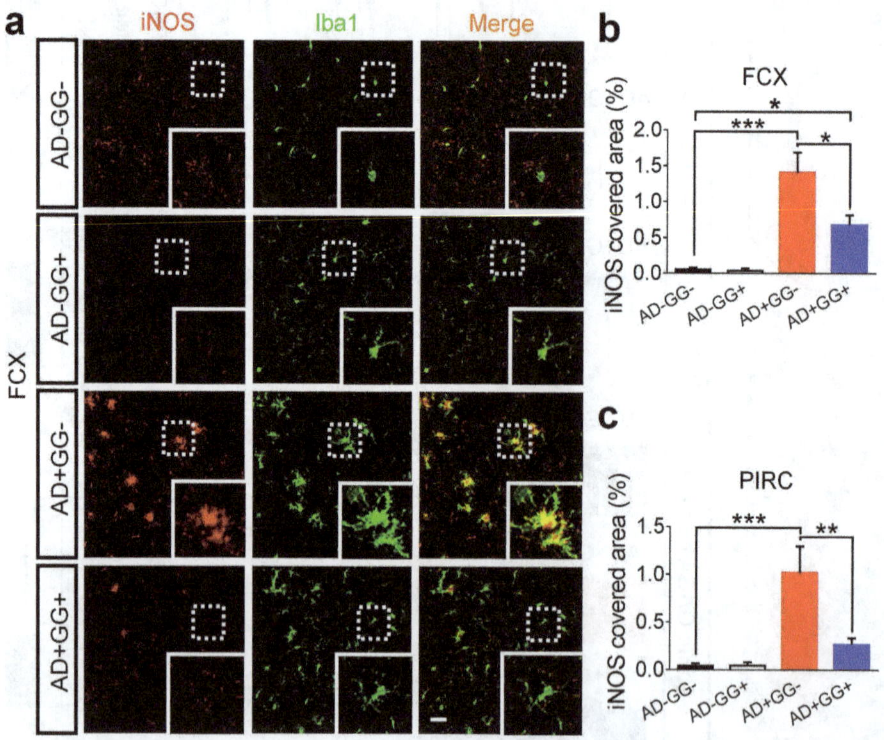

Fig. 6 Neuroinflammation mediated by microglia is alleviated in 5xFAD mice with *Gad67* haploinsufficiency. **a** The iNOS positive immune cells (red), as the pro-inflammatory subtype of microglia (pseudo colored in green for merge purpose), is remarkably reduced in frontal cortex (FCX) and piriform cortex (PIRC) of bigenic brain (AD+GG+), close to the level in AD negative brain (normal condition). Dotted line circled regions were zoomed in and were shown in the lower right corner of each micrograph. Scale bar represents 30 μm. **b-c** Quantification analysis displays a dramatic reduction of iNOS covered area percentage in both frontal cortex and piriform cortex of AD+GG+ than AD+GG- of similar age. N = 6 mice of 10–11 months age in each genotype groups (AD-GG-, AD-GG+, AD+GG-, AD+GG+). Data are presented as mean ± s.e.m., * $p < 0.05$; ** $p < 0.01$; *** $p < 0.001$; one-way ANOVA with the Tukey's post-hoc test when comparing multiple groups

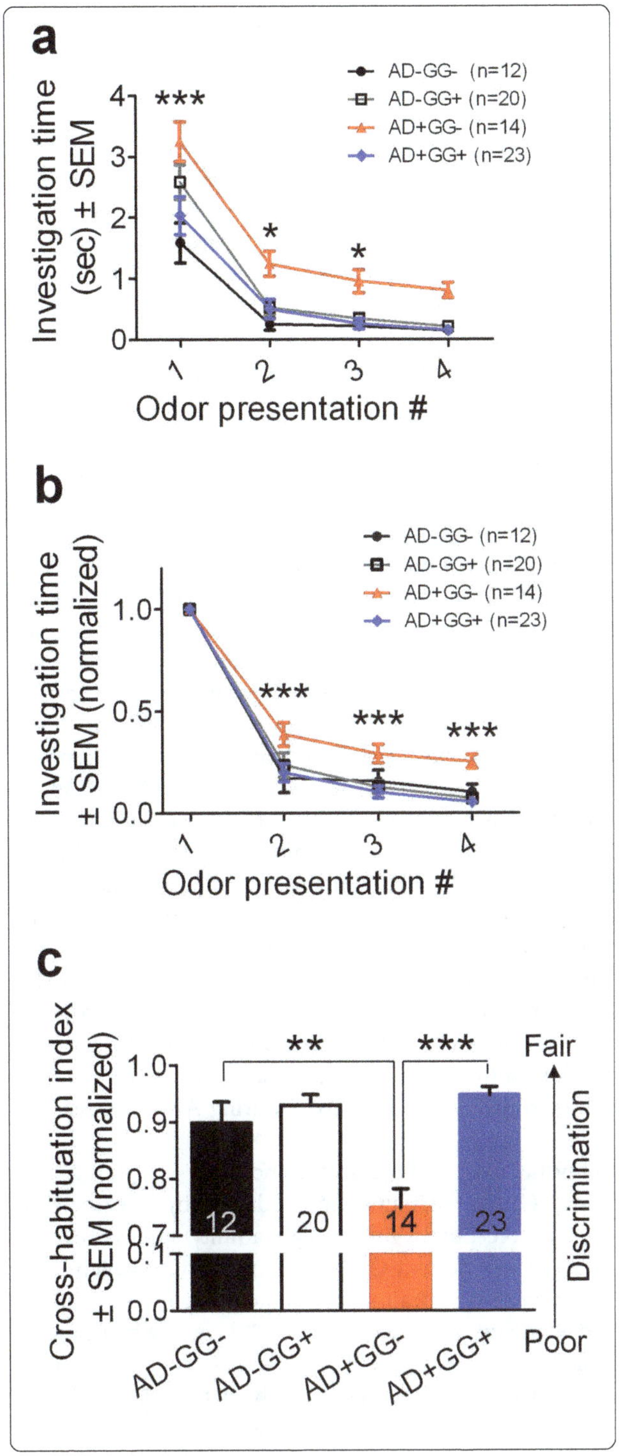

Fig. 7 Rescue of olfactory deficit in 5xFAD mice with *Gad67* haploinsufficiency. Olfactory behavior test is applied to examine the extent of olfactory sensory impairment in the four genotypes of 6–8 months age (AD-GG-, AD-GG+, AD+GG-, AD+GG+). **a** Statistical graph showing the bigenic (AD+GG+) mice displayed a reduction of investigation time in each odor presentation trials than 5xFAD mice (red line). **b** Quantification data showing the AD+GG+ mice displayed a reduction of investigation time (normalized) (blue line) than 5xFAD mice (red line). Notably, AD+GG+ mice displayed almost recovery of the impairment olfactory sensory function (which is a common pathological symptom in 5XFAD), according to the result that the statistic values are very close to that of AD-negative mice (black line: AD-GG-; grey line: AD-GG+). **c** AD+GG+ displayed a recovered cross-habituation index (mean ± s.e.m., normalized). For (A)-(C), n = 12 AD-GG-, 20 AD-GG+, 14 AD+GG-, 23 AD+GG+ mice of 6–8 months age. * $p < 0.05$; ** $p < 0.01$; *** $p < 0.001$; two-way ANOVA followed by LSD post hoc test for comparison among multiple groups for multiple conditions

dis-habituation behavior tests as described in previous studies [23, 31]. Briefly, mice were exposed to four novel neutral odors presented in their home cages, and each odor was delivered across four successive trials. The investigation time for each of the 4 odors across four successive trials was recorded and quantified for olfactory habituation. Typically, when first exposed to an odor stimulus, mice would spend longest investigation time but quickly lost interest when exposed 2nd, 3rd, and 4th time to the same odor (Fig. 7a and b, black line). The 5xFAD mice (AD+GG-) displayed consistent impairments in olfactory habituation, showing prolonged investigation time even after repeated exposure to the same stimulus (Fig. 7a and b, red line). Interestingly, the olfactory deficit of AD+GG- was rescued in 5xFAD mice with *Gad67* haploinsufficiency (AD+GG+) (Fig. 7a and 7b, blue Line), consistent with the reduction of Aβ in the olfactory bulb and piriform cortex of AD+GG+ mice. Similarly, AD+GG- mice exhibited a significant impairment in cross-habituation test, which was also rescued by *Gad67* haploinsufficiency (Fig. 7c, AD-GG-: 0.90 ± 0.04; AD+GG+: 0.95 ± 0.02, $p > 0.05$, n = 12 AD-GG-, 20 AD-GG+, 14 AD+GG-, 23 AD+GG+). Because we did not observe sex differences in olfactory behavioral tests (Additional file 1: Figures S4), data from both sexes were pooled and quantified together (Fig. 7). Two-way ANOVA analysis revealed that both genotypes and successive trials had a significant effect on the investigation time of olfactory habituation (genotype: F (3260) = 12.0; $p < 0.001$; successive trials: F (3260) = 9.0; $p < 0.001$). There was no interaction between genotypes and successive trials (F (9260) = 0.27, $p > 0.05$). Together, our results indicate that *Gad67* haploinsufficiency rescues olfactory deficits in 5xFAD mice.

Discussion

In this study, we unexpectedly found that when 5xFAD mice were crossed with GAD-GFP mice that destroyed one allele of *Gad67*, the Aβ load was significantly decreased throughout many brain regions. Further investigation revealed that accompanying such Aβ reduction, the astrocytic GABA and tonic inhibition were significantly reduced, and microglial reactivity was also alleviated. More importantly, the olfactory memory deficit of AD mice was partially rescued by *Gad67* haploinsufficiency. These results suggest that GAD67 plays an important role in modulating Aβ production and may provide an important drug target for AD treatment.

Aβ reduction in 5xFAD mice with *Gad67* haploinsufficiency

As the principal inhibitory neurotransmitter in the brain, GABA plays a critical role in maintaining excitation/inhibition balance, which is important for information processing in the brain. Imbalance of excitation/inhibition has been implicated in a wide range of neurological and neuropsychiatric disorders including AD [32]. GABA is synthesized from excitatory neurotransmitter glutamate by two distinct but partial redundant glutamic acid decarboxylase isoforms, GAD65 and GAD67. Mice with genetic deletion of *Gad65*, which is mainly localized in the synaptic terminals, are viable and develop normally without obvious changes in the basal GABA transmission and brain GABA content, except an increase in seizure susceptibility [13, 33]. In contrast, GAD67 is largely cytosolic and distributed evenly throughout the cells. Deletion of *Gad67* leads to perinatal death and more than 90% reduction of GABA content [20, 34]. In addition to neuronal GABA function, several recent studies including our own have started to investigate non-neuronal changes of GABA system (review see [35, 36]). In particular, we and others have shown that reactive astrocytes activated by Aβ in 5xFAD mice can accumulate a high amount of GABA, which can lead to exuberant tonic GABA inhibition and contribute to memory deficits [37]. Here, we demonstrate that genetic down-regulation of GAD67 dramatically reduces the reactive astrocytic GABA content, as well as Aβ burden and inflammatory microglia in 5xFAD mice, further suggesting a strong link between astrocytic GABA and AD pathology.

There are now compelling evidences supporting that abnormal astrocytic GABA is associated with disease status such as brain injury and neurodegenerative disorders (for review, see [36]). However, the source(s) and mechanism(s) of astrocytic GABA release are still in debate. Previous reports have shown that human astrocytes have all of the machineries for GABA synthesis, metabolism and release, including GAD67, gamma-aminobutyric acid transaminase (GABAT), glia specific GABA transporter GAT3/4, and functional $GABA_A$ and $GABA_B$ receptors [28, 38]. We found that astrocytic GABA in Alzheimer's brain was synthesized by astrocytic GAD67 and released by astrocyte-specific GABA transporter GAT3/4 [3]. At the same time, another study reported that glial GABA is synthesized through an unconventional pathway by monoamine oxidase B and released via bestrophin 1 (Best1) channel to mediate tonic inhibition [2]. Unfortunately, the clinic trial of MAO-B inhibitor for Alzheimer's treatment has failed in phase IIb clinical trial. Here, we provide in vivo genetic evidence showing that *Gad67* haploinsufficiency can significantly alleviate the abnormal astrocytic GABA in a mouse model of AD, underscoring a major role of GAD67—the conventional GABA biosynthesis pathway—in AD pathology.

While the precise mechanisms of GAD67 in AD require further study, one possible hypothesis based on our results is that genetic reduction of GAD67 reduces astrocytic GABA level in AD brains, corrects abnormal neuronal activity, and reduces Aβ production. Consistent with our hypothesis, knockdown of GAD67 protein level has been reported to normalize neuronal activity in a rat model of Parkinson's disease [39]. In AD mouse models, the generation of Aβ is found coupled with neuronal activity [40, 41], and Aβ pathology can promote neuronal hyperexcitation [5]. Therefore, neuronal activity and Aβ pathology may form a positive feedback loop to boost each other. Disrupt such loop may provide an alternative strategy to delay AD progression. For example, gamma oscillation is a normal rhythmic brain activity important for learning and memory, but it is disrupted in AD mouse brains. Recovery of this rhythmic gamma oscillation not only reduces the Aβ production but also rescues the memory deficits in an AD mouse model [5, 42]. Since >90% GABA is synthesized by GAD67, and GABA is the major inhibitory neurotransmitter, it is possible that *Gad67* haploinsufficiency will regulate GABA production both in neurons and astrocytes, which in turn will modulate neuronal activity during AD progression.

Abnormal tonic GABA currents and AD

Tonic GABA currents are mediated by extrasynaptic $GABA_A$ receptors with a high affinity for GABA and result in a persistent GABAergic inhibition, which is involved in several brain diseases including epilepsy, stroke and Alzheimer's disease [2, 3, 27, 43]. In AD brains, tonic inhibition is upregulated because of the activation of extrasynaptic $GABA_A$ receptors by astrocytic GABA release [2, 3], but synaptic $GABA_A$ receptor-mediated phasic inhibition is not changed significantly [2, 5]. Here, we found that the abnormal GABA accumulation in the reactive astrocytes of 5xFAD mouse brains was remarkably reduced by *Gad67* haploinsufficiency, and the abnormal tonic inhibition was also decreased correspondingly, consistent with the reduction of Aβ production and amelioration of microglial reactivity in the 5xFAD mice with *Gad67* haploinsufficiency. Our finding of GAD67 in regulating AD pathology is also supported by earlier studies demonstrating a strong link between gamma oscillation activity (20–80 Hz) and AD [5, 42] as well as tonic GABA inhibition [44, 45].

Microglia reactivity and AD

The characteristic ramified morphology of microglia and astrocytes and their close relationship with neurons put glial cells in a unique position to sense and maintain a homeostatic microenvironment in the brain (for review see [46]). In recent years, growing evidence has started to unravel an active role of microglia in neuroinflammation, a defense mechanism mediated primarily by reactive microglia and astrocytes [47–49]. However, direct interventions with neuroinflammation have failed in the clinical trials for AD, underscoring the importance of further investigation of the molecular mechanisms of AD pathogenesis. Here, we made an important discovery that aberrant astrocytic GABA may be closely linked to microglia-mediated proinflammatory signaling iNOS and amyloidogenesis. Our findings open a new avenue for therapeutic intervention for AD. Interestingly, consistent with our finding of GAD67 in AD pathology, GABA has been reported to play a pro-neuroinflammatory role in a mouse model for multiple sclerosis [50]. Therefore, this newly discovered link among astrocytic GABA, microglial reactivity, and Aβ production may offer new insight into the complex AD pathology. It is likely that a cocktail approach addressing multiple targets such as neurons, glial cells, and Aβ together, rather than a single drug acting on a single target, will be future solutions to treat complicated syndromes such as AD.

Conclusion

In contrast to the traditional view that GABAergic transmission is relatively well-preserved in AD patients, growing evidences have demonstrated more complex changes of the GABAergic system in AD pathology in recent years [35, 51]. However, direct interventions with either GABA agonists or antagonists have failed in several human studies and clinical trials, raising the pressing needs for a further investigation of the underlying mechanisms and better intervention strategies. Here, by genetically targeting GAD67, an activity-regulated major GABA synthesis enzyme, we show that *Gad67* haploinsufficiency in AD mouse brains has significant beneficial effects on both pathological and behavioral outcomes. Although the precise mechanisms of how aberrant astrocytic GABA is linked to pro-inflammatory microglia and amyloidogenesis still requires further investigation, our study provides a new perspective for understanding the relationship between GABAergic functions and AD pathogenesis. Together with our previous finding of astrocytic GABA in AD brains, our results support the notion that GAD67 may be a potential target for developing a new treatment for AD.

Abbreviations

AD: Alzheimer's disease; Aβ: β-Amyloid; FAD: Familiar Alzheimer's disease; FCX: Frontal cortex; GABA: Gamma-Aminobutyric acid; GAD: Glutamic acid decarboxylase; GFP: Green fluorescent protein; GG: GAD67-GFP$^{+/-}$; iNOS: Inducible nitric oxide synthase; OB: Olfactory bulb; PIRC: Piriform cortex

Acknowledgements

We really appreciate Charles H. Smith Endowment to support our research.

Funding

This work was supported by the National Institutes of Health R01 (AG045656, MH083911), Alzheimer's Association (ZEN-15-321,972) and Charles H. Smith Endowment Fund to G.C.

Authors' contributions

YW played a major role in performing experiments and analyzing the data, as well as writing the initial draft of the manuscript. ZW initiated the study, generated most of the early results, performed the functional analysis, and revised the manuscript. YTB maintained the mouse lines and did genotyping. GYW and GC supervised the entire study, designed the experiments with YW and ZW, participated in data analysis and revised the manuscript. GC provides financial support for the study. All authors have read and approved the final version of the manuscript.

Competing interests

The authors have no competing interests in the manuscript.

Author details

[1]Department of Biology, Huck Institutes of Life Sciences, Pennsylvania State University, University park, PA 16802, USA. [2]School of Life Science, South China Normal University, Guangzhou 510631, China.

References

1. Tanzi RE, Bertram L. Twenty years of the Alzheimer's disease amyloid hypothesis: a genetic perspective. Cell. 2005;120:545–55.
2. Jo S, Yarishkin O, Hwang YJ, Chun YE, Park M, Woo DH, Bae JY, Kim T, Lee J, Chun H, et al. GABA from reactive astrocytes impairs memory in mouse models of Alzheimer's disease. Nat Med. 2014;20:886–96.
3. Wu Z, Guo Z, Gearing M, Chen G. Tonic inhibition in dentate gyrus impairs long-term potentiation and memory in an Alzheimer's [corrected] disease model. Nat Commun. 2014;5:4159.
4. Limon A, Reyes-Ruiz JM, Miledi R. Loss of functional GABA (A) receptors in the Alzheimer diseased brain. Proc Natl Acad Sci U S A. 2012;109:10071–6.
5. Verret L, Mann EO, Hang GB, Barth AM, Cobos I, Ho K, Devidze N, Masliah E, Kreitzer AC, Mody I, et al. Inhibitory interneuron deficit links altered network activity and cognitive dysfunction in Alzheimer model. Cell. 2012;149:708–21.
6. Schmid LC, Mittag M, Poll S, Steffen J, Wagner J, Geis HR, Schwarz I, Schmidt B, Schwarz MK, Remy S, Fuhrmann M. Dysfunction of Somatostatin-Positive Interneurons Associated with Memory Deficits in an Alzheimer's Disease Model. Neuron. 2016;92:114–25.
7. Andrews-Zwilling Y, Bien-Ly N, Xu Q, Li G, Bernardo A, Yoon SY, Zwilling D, Yan TX, Chen L, Huang Y. Apolipoprotein E4 causes age- and Tau-dependent impairment of GABAergic interneurons, leading to learning and memory deficits in mice. J Neurosci. 2010;30:13707–17.
8. Albuquerque MS, Mahar I, Davoli MA, Chabot JG, Mechawar N, Quirion R, Krantic S. Regional and sub-regional differences in hippocampal GABAergic neuronal vulnerability in the TgCRND8 mouse model of Alzheimer's disease. Front Aging Neurosci. 2015;7:30.

9. Erlander MG, Tillakaratne NJ, Feldblum S, Patel N, Tobin AJ. Two genes encode distinct glutamate decarboxylases. Neuron. 1991;7:91–100.
10. Lau CG, Murthy VN. Activity-dependent regulation of inhibition via GAD67. J Neurosci. 2012;32:8521–31.
11. Chattopadhyaya B, Di Cristo G, Wu CZ, Knott G, Kuhlman S, Fu Y, Palmiter RD, Huang ZJ. GAD67-mediated GABA synthesis and signaling regulate inhibitory synaptic innervation in the visual cortex. Neuron. 2007;54:889–903.
12. Sandhu KV, Lang D, Muller B, Nullmeier S, Yanagawa Y, Schwegler H, Stork O. Glutamic acid decarboxylase 67 haplodeficiency impairs social behavior in mice. Genes Brain Behav. 2014;13:439–50.
13. Kash SF, Johnson RS, Tecott LH, Noebels JL, Mayfield RD, Hanahan D, Baekkeskov S. Epilepsy in mice deficient in the 65-kDa isoform of glutamic acid decarboxylase. Proc Natl Acad Sci U S A. 1997;94:14060–5.
14. Kimoto S, Bazmi HH, Lewis DA. Lower expression of glutamic acid decarboxylase 67 in the prefrontal cortex in schizophrenia: contribution of altered regulation by Zif268. Am J Psychiat. 2014;171:969–78.
15. Benes FM, Lim B, Matzilevich D, Walsh JP, Subburaju S, Minns M. Regulation of the GABA cell phenotype in hippocampus of schizophrenics and bipolars. Proc Natl Acad Sci U S A. 2007;104:10164–9.
16. Lanoue AC, Dumitriu A, Myers RH, Soghomonian JJ. Decreased glutamic acid decarboxylase mRNA expression in prefrontal cortex in Parkinson's disease. Exp Neurol. 2010;226:207–17.
17. LeWitt PA, Rezai AR, Leehey MA, Ojemann SG, Flaherty AW, Eskandar EN, Kostyk SK, Thomas K, Sarkar A, Siddiqui MS, et al. AAV2-GAD gene therapy for advanced Parkinson's disease: a double-blind, sham-surgery controlled, randomised trial. Lancet Neurol. 2011;10:309–19.
18. Oakley H, Cole SL, Logan S, Maus E, Shao P, Craft J, Guillozet-Bongaarts A, Ohno M, Disterhoft J, Van Eldik L, et al. Intraneuronal beta-amyloid aggregates, neurodegeneration, and neuron loss in transgenic mice with five familial Alzheimer's disease mutations: potential factors in amyloid plaque formation. J Neurosci. 2006;26:10129–40.
19. Chen L, McKenna JT, Leonard MZ, Yanagawa Y, McCarley RW, Brown RE. GAD67-GFP knock-in mice have normal sleep-wake patterns and sleep homeostasis. Neuroreport. 2010;21:216–20.
20. Tamamaki N, Yanagawa Y, Tomioka R, Miyazaki J, Obata K, Kaneko T. Green fluorescent protein expression and colocalization with calretinin, parvalbumin, and somatostatin in the GAD67-GFP knock-in mouse. J Comp Neurol. 2003;467:60–79.
21. Sadleir KR, Eimer WA, Cole SL, Vassar R. Abeta reduction in BACE1 heterozygous null 5XFAD mice is associated with transgenic APP level. Mol Neurodegener. 2015;10:1.
22. Ting JT, Daigle TL, Chen Q, Feng G. Acute brain slice methods for adult and aging animals: application of targeted patch clamp analysis and optogenetics. Methods Mol Biol. 2014;1183:221–42.
23. Wesson DW, Levy E, Nixon RA, Wilson DA. Olfactory dysfunction correlates with amyloid-beta burden in an Alzheimer's disease mouse model. J Neurosci. 2010;30:505–14.
24. Selkoe DJ. The therapeutics of Alzheimer's disease: where we stand and where we are heading. Ann Neurol. 2013;74:328–36.
25. Eimer WA, Vassar R. Neuron loss in the 5XFAD mouse model of Alzheimer's disease correlates with intraneuronal Abeta42 accumulation and Caspase-3 activation. Mol Neurodegener. 2013;8:2.
26. Zhang Z, Song M, Liu X, Kang SS, Kwon IS, Duong DM, Seyfried NT, Hu WT, Liu Z, Wang JZ, et al. Cleavage of tau by asparagine endopeptidase mediates the neurofibrillary pathology in Alzheimer's disease. Nat Med. 2014;20:1254–62.
27. Clarkson AN, Huang BS, Macisaac SE, Mody I, Carmichael ST. Reducing excessive GABA-mediated tonic inhibition promotes functional recovery after stroke. Nature. 2010;468:305–9.
28. Lee M, Schwab C, McGeer PL. Astrocytes are GABAergic cells that modulate microglial activity. Glia. 2011;59:152–65.
29. Stamps JJ, Bartoshuk LM, Heilman KM. A brief olfactory test for Alzheimer's disease. J Neurol Sci. 2013;333:19–24.
30. Doty RL, Kamath V. The influences of age on olfaction: a review. Front Psychol. 2014;5:20.
31. Cramer PE, Cirrito JR, Wesson DW, Lee CY, Karlo JC, Zinn AE, Casali BT, Restivo JL, Goebel WD, James MJ, et al. ApoE-directed therapeutics rapidly clear beta-amyloid and reverse deficits in AD mouse models. Science. 2012;335:1503–6.
32. Palop JJ, Mucke L. Amyloid-beta-induced neuronal dysfunction in Alzheimer's disease: from synapses toward neural networks. Nat Neurosci. 2010;13:812–8.
33. Asada H, Kawamura Y, Maruyama K, Kume H, Ding R, Ji FY, Kanbara N, Kuzume H, Sanbo M, Yagi T, Obata K. Mice lacking the 65 kDa isoform of glutamic acid decarboxylase (GAD65) maintain normal levels of GAD67 and GABA in their brains but are susceptible to seizures. Biochem Biophys Res Commun. 1996;229:891–5.
34. Asada H, Kawamura Y, Maruyama K, Kume H, Ding RG, Kanbara N, Kuzume H, Sanbo M, Yagi T, Obata K. Cleft palate and decreased brain gamma-aminobutyric acid in mice lacking the 67-kDa isoform of glutamic acid decarboxylase. Proc Natl Acad Sci U S A. 1997;94:6496–9.
35. Li Y, Sun H, Chen Z, Xu H, Bu G, Zheng H. Implications of GABAergic Neurotransmission in Alzheimer's Disease. Front Aging Neurosci. 2016;8:31.
36. Yoon BE, Lee CJ. GABA as a rising gliotransmitter. Front Neural Circuits. 2014;8:141.
37. Mitew S, Kirkcaldie MT, Dickson TC, Vickers JC. Altered synapses and gliotransmission in Alzheimer's disease and AD model mice. Neurobiol Aging. 2013;34:2341–51.
38. Lee M, McGeer EG, McGeer PL. Mechanisms of GABA release from human astrocytes. Glia. 2011;59:1600–11.
39. Horvath L, van Marion I, Tai K, Nielsen TT, Lundberg C. Knockdown of GAD67 protein levels normalizes neuronal activity in a rat model of Parkinson's disease. J Gene Med. 2011;13:188–97.
40. Bero AW, Yan P, Roh JH, Cirrito JR, Stewart FR, Raichle ME, Lee JM, Holtzman DM. Neuronal activity regulates the regional vulnerability to amyloid-beta deposition. Nat Neurosci. 2011;14:750–6.
41. Wu J, Petralia RS, Kurushima H, Patel H, Jung MY, Volk L, Chowdhury S, Shepherd JD, Dehoff M, Li Y, et al. Arc/Arg3.1 regulates an endosomal pathway essential for activity-dependent beta-amyloid generation. Cell. 2011;147:615–28.
42. Iaccarino HF, Singer AC, Martorell AJ, Rudenko A, Gao F, Gillingham TZ, Mathys H, Seo J, Kritskiy O, Abdurrob F, et al. Gamma frequency entrainment attenuates amyloid load and modifies microglia. Nature. 2016;540:230–5.
43. Sun Y, Wu Z, Kong S, Jiang D, Pitre A, Wang Y, Chen G. Regulation of epileptiform activity by two distinct subtypes of extrasynaptic GABAA receptors. Mol Brain. 2013;6:21.
44. Mann EO, Mody I. Control of hippocampal gamma oscillation frequency by tonic inhibition and excitation of interneurons. Nat Neurosci. 2010;13:205–12.
45. Ferando I, Mody I. In vitro gamma oscillations following partial and complete ablation of delta subunit-containing GABAA receptors from parvalbumin interneurons. Neuropharmacology. 2015;88:91–8.
46. Allaman I, Belanger M, Magistretti PJ. Astrocyte-neuron metabolic relationships: for better and for worse. Trends Neurosci. 2011;34:76–87.
47. Akiyama H, Barger S, Barnum S, Bradt B, Bauer J, Cole GM, Cooper NR, Eikelenboom P, Emmerling M, Fiebich BL, et al. Inflammation and Alzheimer's disease. Neurobiol Aging. 2000;21:383–421.
48. Glass CK, Saijo K, Winner B, Marchetto MC, Gage FH. Mechanisms underlying inflammation in neurodegeneration. Cell. 2010;140:918–34.
49. Heppner FL, Ransohoff RM, Becher B. Immune attack: the role of inflammation in Alzheimer disease. Nat Rev Neurosci. 2015;16:358–72.
50. Carmans S, Hendriks JJ, Slaets H, Thewissen K, Stinissen P, Rigo JM, Hellings N. Systemic treatment with the inhibitory neurotransmitter gamma-aminobutyric acid aggravates experimental autoimmune encephalomyelitis by affecting proinflammatory immune responses. J Neuroimmunol. 2013;255:45–53.
51. Limon A, Reyes-Ruiz JM, Miledi R. GABAergic drugs and Alzheimer's disease. Future Med Chem. 2011;3:149–53.

2

Practical considerations for choosing a mouse model of Alzheimer's disease

Joanna L. Jankowsky[1,2,3,4,5*] and Hui Zheng[1,4,5,6*]

Abstract

Alzheimer's disease (AD) is behaviorally identified by progressive memory impairment and pathologically characterized by the triad of β-amyloid plaques, neurofibrillary tangles, and neurodegeneration. Genetic mutations and risk factors have been identified that are either causal or modify the disease progression. These genetic and pathological features serve as basis for the creation and validation of mouse models of AD. Efforts made in the past quarter-century have produced over 100 genetically engineered mouse lines that recapitulate some aspects of AD clinicopathology. These models have been valuable resources for understanding genetic interactions that contribute to disease and cellular reactions that are engaged in response. Here we focus on mouse models that have been widely used stalwarts of the field or that are recently developed bellwethers of the future. Rather than providing a summary of each model, we endeavor to compare and contrast the genetic approaches employed and to discuss their respective advantages and limitations. We offer a critical account of the variables which may contribute to inconsistent findings and the factors that should be considered when choosing a model and interpreting the results. We hope to present an insightful review of current AD mouse models and to provide a practical guide for selecting models best matched to the experimental question at hand.

Keywords: Transgenic mouse, Knockout, Knock-in, Amyloid precursor protein, APP, Aβ, Tau, MAPT, TREM2, Apolipoprotein E, ApoE

Background

Alzheimer's disease (AD) is the most common form of age-associated neurodegenerative disorder clinically characterized by a decline in cognitive function and pathologically defined by the accumulation of extracellular β-amyloid (Aβ) plaques and intracellular neurofibrillary tangles (NFTs). Plaque Aβ peptide of 40 or 42 amino acids is produced by proteolytic cleavage of the amyloid precursor protein (APP) (Fig. 1), while NFTs are composed of hyperphosphorylated and misfolded tau protein. These neuropathological hallmarks are accompanied by profound neuroinflammation marked by astrocytic and microglial activation. A small percentage of AD cases are caused by genetic mutations in APP and presenilins identified in familial AD (FAD), where these mutations alter APP processing in favor of Aβ42 to drive the peptide aggregation thought to initiate disease. These genetic, biochemical, and neuropathological features form the basis for creating and validating animal models of AD. Beyond the autosomal dominant FAD mutations, the apolipoprotein E ε4 allele (APOEε4), along with rare point mutations in the triggering receptor expressed on myeloid cells 2 (TREM2), are strong risk factors for the more common sporadic, late-onset AD (LOAD).

Animal models are critical for understanding disease pathogenesis and also serve as valuable tools for preclinical testing. One of the most important considerations in working with rodent models is matching the mouse (or rat) to the experimental question under study. There are more than 100 different genetically engineered mouse lines reported to capture some aspect of AD - so many that it has become impossible to exhaustively track them all. We focus here on models that have been widely used and which remain available either privately or publically. We also highlight newly created lines that may be useful in modeling LOAD. The unavoidable first step in deciding among them is delineating the experimental question to be asked. Existing mouse models recapitulate amyloid plaques, neurofibrillary tangles, or neurodegeneration,

* Correspondence: jankowsk@bcm.edu; huiz@bcm.edu
[1]Department of Neuroscience, Baylor College of Medicine, Houston, TX 77030, USA
Full list of author information is available at the end of the article

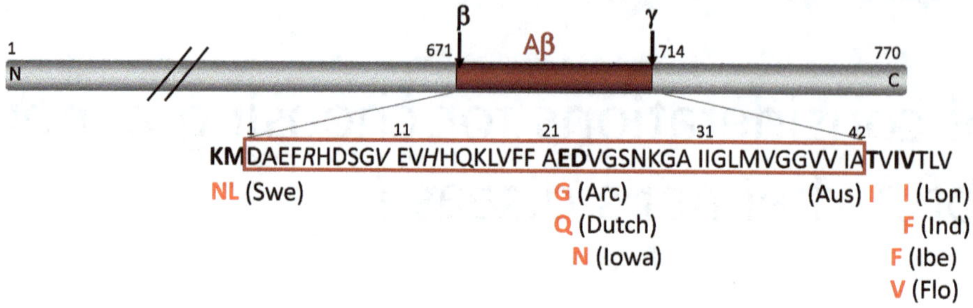

Fig. 1 Diagram of APP illustrating nine FAD mutations that have been incorporated into mouse models. The Aβ domain is highlighted in red, with the β- and γ-cleavage sites identified at residues 671 and 714, respectively, using the numbering convention for full-length 770 amino acid protein. The amino acid sequence of Aβ is outlined in *red*, with the positions of several commonly used FAD mutations and their amino acid substitutions shown (in *bold*) alongside the geographic name identifying each variant. *Italic* residues indicate the three sites at which the Aβ sequence diverges between human and mouse (human is shown). Swe, Swedish; Arc, Arctic; Aus, Austrian; Lon, London; Ind, Indiana; Ibe, Iberian; Flo, Florida

but generally not all in the same mouse. Some models develop these hallmarks rapidly, others more authentically retain the aging facet of the disease. This review will describe key factors to consider when choosing between models, but you must know which features are essential for testing your hypothesis, as well as which are expendable. No mouse model is a faithful reproduction of human AD, but they can be useful tools when appropriately matched to the experimental question of interest.

Matching your model to your experimental question - what is it that you want to study?

A myriad of models is at your fingertips. Most of them were designed to capture some aspect of disease pathology - and primarily plaques or tangles - with degeneration and cognitive decline emerging in some as serendipitous benefits. Choosing among them requires knowing what features of AD are required for your particular experiment, and so we describe below the main strategies that have been used to model these pathologies in genetically engineered mice.

Amyloid plaques and CAA

Amyloid plaques and cerebral amyloid angiopathy (CAA) both arise as insoluble deposits of the amyloid β peptide (Aβ). This peptide is derived by sequential cleavage of the amyloid precursor protein (APP) by the β-APP cleaving enzyme (BACE1) and γ-secretase at N- and C-termini respectively, to release three protein fragments: soluble APP (sAPP) and Aβ into the extracellular space and the amyloid-intracellular domain (AICD) into the cytoplasm. Mutations in APP were the first causes of early-onset FAD to be identified [1]; these autosomal dominant mutations tend to cluster around the β- and γ- processing sites to affect Aβ production. Transgenic expression of familial APP mutations provided the first successful means of reproducing amyloid pathology in mice [2] (Table 1); since then many dozen lines of APP-transgenic and knock-in have been created and characterized. Because amyloid deposition is time- and concentration-dependent, achieving pathology within the mouse lifespan requires that the production of Aβ be dramatically elevated relative to endogenous. This is most often accomplished by overexpressing human APP harboring one or more point mutations identified from FAD (Fig. 1). The Swedish mutation is most commonly used for this purpose (Swe), and is based on a two amino acid substitution adjacent to β-secretase cleavage at the N-terminus of Aβ [3]. The Swe mutation increases APP processing through the β-secretase pathway, thereby elevating production of Aβ relative to wild-type [4].

Additional mutations may also be incorporated at the γ-secretase C-terminus of Aβ to elevate the ratio of Aβ42 relative to the predominant but less aggregation-prone Aβ40. Several familial C-terminal mutations have been used in mouse models including those identified from Indiana (Ind, V717F [5]), London (Lon, V717I [1], Florida (Flo, I716V [6]) and the Iberian Peninsula (Ibe, I716F [7]). By elevating the ratio of Aβ42:40, these C-terminal mutations enhance Aβ aggregation and accelerate the formation of amyloid plaques to produce early onset pathology. Plaque onset can also be accelerated through familial mutations in presenilin 1 (*PSEN1)*, such as M146V [8], M146L [9], L166P [10], L286V [8], or exon 9 deletion (dE9 [11]) (see http://www.alzforum.org/mutations for details). These PSEN1 mutations shift APP processing by γ-secretase to produce longer, more pathogenic Aβ peptides which are useful for accelerating disease in short-lived animal models.

A handful of models also include APP mutations within the central Aβ domain that foster vascular amyloid accumulation. Unlike the β- and γ- cleavage site mutations used to boost Aβ production or shift the 42:40 ratio without affecting the Aβ sequence itself, these internal mutations change the amino acid sequence of Aβ. The mutations most often used in this manner were identified from kindreds in the Netherlands (Dutch, Aβ E22Q [12, 13]), Arctic (Arc, Aβ E22G [14, 15]), and Iowa (Aβ D23N [16]).

In all cases, whether APP modifications are introduced through an over-expressed transgene or via targeted modification of the endogenous allele (knock-in, Table 2),

Table 1 Standard Transgenic Lines for APP, APP + PS1, and Tau

Model	Transgene	Transgenic promoter	Availability	Reference
APP Transgenics				
PDAPP	huAPP$_{770}$ (Ind) minigene (cDNA + introns 6–8)	*PDGFB*	Novartis	[2]
Tg2576	huAPP$_{695}$ (Swe)	hamster *Prnp*	Taconic, Charles River	[95]
C3-3	mo/huAPP$_{695}$ (Swe)	mouse *Prnp*	MMRRC 34828-JAX	[96]
APP23	huAPP$_{751}$ (Swe)	mouse *Thy1*	JAX 030504	[100]
J20	huAPP$_{770}$ (Swe/Ind) minigene (cDNA + introns 6–8)	*PDGFB*	MMRRC 34836-JAX	[54]
TgCRND8	huAPP$_{695}$ (Swe/Ind)	hamster *Prnp*	Peter St. George-Hyslop	[51]
Tg-SwDI	huAPP$_{770}$ (Swe/Dutch/Iowa)	mouse *Thy1*	MMRRC 34843-JAX	[210]
APP/PS1 Transgenics				
APP/PS1 Line 85	mo/huAPP$_{695}$ (Swe); Tg huPSEN1 (ΔE9)	mouse *Prnp*	MMRRC 34832-JAX, 34,829-JAX	[99]
APPPS1	huAPP$_{695}$ (Swe); huPSEN1 (L166P)	mouse *Thy1*	Mathias Jucker	[211]
5XFAD Tg6799	huAPP$_{695}$ (Swe/Flo/Lon); huPSEN1 (M146 L/L286 V)	mouse *Thy1.2*	MMRRC 34840-JAX, 34,848-JAX	[47]
Tau Transgenics				
Tau Tg Line 43	huMAPT$_{3R0N}$ (wt)	mouse *Prnp*	JAX 003741	[212]
JNPL3	huMAPT$_{4R0N}$ (P301L)	mouse *Prnp*	Taconic	[34]
hTau.P301S	huMAPT$_{4R0N}$ (P301S)	mouse *Thy1.2*	Michel Goedert	[213]
PS19	huMAPT$_{4R1N}$ (P301S)	mouse *Prnp*	JAX 008169	[33]
APP/PS1/Tau Transgenic				
3xTg-AD	huAPP$_{695}$ (Swe); MAPT$_{4R0N}$ (P301L); *Psen1*^{M146V} knock-in	mouse *Thy1.2*	MMRRC 34830-JAX	[101]

Tables 1-4: Refer to Fig. 1 for illustration of APP mutations.

the amino acid sequence of Aβ itself is almost always converted from mouse to human by 3 amino acid substitutions at Aβ residues G5R, F10Y and R13H. BACE1 processes murine APP at the +11 rather than +1 site of Aβ [17]. As a result of this shift, mouse Aβ11–40/42 does not aggregate in vivo [18]. Simply humanizing the Aβ sequence yields full-length 1–40/42 peptide which readily aggregates in a time- and concentration-dependent manner to produce amyloid deposits.

The amyloid plaques and CAA produced by genetic modification of APP in mice share many characteristics of the human neuropathology, but important distinctions exist. These distinctions have been recently reviewed and are therefore not covered here in any detail [19]. Generally speaking, most APP modified mice develop both diffuse and fibrillar Aβ deposits that can be distinguished by comparing silver staining or Aβ immunohistochemistry against Congo red or thioflavin-S histology. Fibrillar plaques are often surrounded by reactive astrocytes and microglia and by dystrophic neurites (axonal swellings). Synapse loss can be observed in the zone immediately adjacent to fibrillar deposits and several models display mild neuron loss with age, but none develop the severe atrophy observed in human AD. Some APP models develop modest levels of

Table 2 Lines with physiological expression of APP, PS1, and Tau

Model	Allele	Targeting approach	Availability	Reference
APP^{NLh}	endogenous mouse *App* with Swe mutation and humanized Aβ domain	Knock-in	NA	[89]
APP R1.40	complete human genomic *APP* (Swe)	YAC transgenic	MMRRC 34831-JAX	[86]
APP^{SL}	mouse/human *App* hybrid with humanized Aβ domain (Swe/Lon)	Knock-in	NA	[92]
APP^{DSL}	endogenous mouse *App* with humanized Aβ domain (Swe/Dutch/Lon)	Knock-in	Hui Zheng	[57]
APP^{NL}, APP^{NLF}, and APP^{NLGF}	endogenous mouse *App* with humanized Aβ domain and (Swe (NL), Swe/Ibe (NLF), or Swe/Arc/Ibe (NLGF))	Knock-in	Takaomi Saido	[58]
PS1^{M146V}	endogenous mouse *Psen1* (M146 V)	Knock-in	JAX 004193	[214]
PS1 KI	endogenous mouse *Psen1* (P264L)	Knock-in	NA	[215]
htau	complete human genomic *MAPT* (wt) with targeted disruption of murine *Mapt*	PAC transgenic x *Mapt* KO	JAX 005491	[37]

Tables 1-4: Refer to Fig. 1 for illustration of APP mutations

hyper-phosphorylated tau but none develop true neurofibrillary tangles seen in human AD.

Neurofibrillary tangles

Neurofibrillary tangles (NFTs) composed of aggregated tau protein are a pathological hallmark of AD and more than 20 other neurodegenerative conditions collectively known as tauopathies. The severity of NFTs correlates better than amyloid plaques with cognitive decline and neurodegeneration in AD [20]. Under normal physiological conditions, tau is an unstructured axonal protein that binds and stabilizes microtubules [21]. Hyper-phosphorylation and other aberrant post-translational modifications lead to misfolding and dissociation from microtubules. Redistribution of misfolded tau into the soma and apical dendrites generates NFTs; redistribution to distal dendrites yields neuropil threads [22]. NFT pathology progresses in a hierarchical, stereotyped pattern beginning in the transentorhinal cortex, and gradually extending to hippocampus before ultimately reaching other cortical areas. This pathological spreading through synaptically connected regions is the basis of Braak staging in AD [23]. Mounting evidence from cell culture and mouse models supports the cell-to-cell transfer of tau pathology [24].

In humans, tau is expressed as both three-repeat (3R) or four-repeat (4R) isoforms due to alternative splicing of exon 10 in the microtubule-associated protein tau gene (*MAPT*), however, only 4R tau is expressed in adult mice. Mutations in *MAPT* are not found in AD, but instead cause a subtype of frontotemporal lobar degeneration (FTLD), demonstrating that this pathology is sufficient for neurotoxicity and dementia [25]. Both coding and non-coding mutations have been identified; many of these affect MAPT splicing to favor the 4R isoform arguing that the balance of 3R/4R is important for neuronal health [26, 27]. The genetic imbalance associated with these *MAPT* mutations in FTLD raises the question of whether isoform dysregulation may also underlie sporadic tauopathies such as AD. Based on these genetic findings, multiple transgenic mouse lines have been created to overexpress human 4R tau containing FTLD mutations. Of these, the two models, rTg4510 and PS19, are most commonly used.

rTg4510 is a bigenic line in which the human 4R tau with the P301L mutation is expressed in forebrain neurons under indirect control of the *Camk2a* promoter (described in more detail below under "*Controllable transgenics*"). The mutant tau transgene is expressed at levels ~13-fold higher than endogenous mouse tau and the mice develop aggressive NFT pathology and neurodegeneration [28, 29]. Pathological forms of phospho-tau can be observed at 2–3 months of age followed by mature tangles in the cortex at 4 months and hippocampus at 5.5 months. The model is based on the tetracycline-transactivator expression system and therefore affords the flexibility of turning the transgene on and off (again, see "*Controllable transgenics*" section for details); the tau P301L responder line can also be crossed with other transactivator lines, e.g. EC-tTA [30], to drive expression of mutant tau in other parts of the brain [31, 32]. This flexibility comes with a cost: the system requires two transgenes for expression which complicates further genetic crosses.

The PS19 model is a traditional (non-controllable) transgenic line in which the human 4R tau with the P301S mutation is controlled by the mouse prion promoter, resulting in ~5-fold overexpression compared to the endogenous mouse tau [33]. The tau phenotype is considerably milder than that of rTg4510, with the onset of phospho-tau pathology at ~6 months. Of note, these mice develop hindlimb paralysis due to transgene expression in spinal cord and die between 10 and 12 months of age depending on the genetic background. As a result, mature, thioflavin-S positive NFTs are rare. These same limitations in neuropathology and early lethality are also seen in the JNPL3 line expressing 4R P301L tau under the mouse prion promoter [34].

Generally speaking, overexpression of mutant tau is required for phospho-tau and NFT pathology to manifest. Contrary to most APP/Aβ models and consistent with human clinicopathology, the tau mice exhibit age-dependent neurodegeneration in addition to synaptic and cognitive deficits, suggesting that misfolded and/or aggregated tau is directly neurotoxic. The onset and severity of pathology largely correlate with the level of transgene overexpression and the mutation used. Both the rTg4510 and PS19 mice are suitable models for testing the pathological consequences of tau accumulation. Due to its early onset, rTg4510 serves as a good model to test manipulations expected to ameliorate pathology but not those expected to accelerate; the PS19 model can be used for both purposes. The PS19 mice have also been widely used to model "tau transmission" by inoculating either purified tau fibrils or brain lysates from tauopathy patients or tau transgenic mice, and tracking the appearance of phospho-tau in synaptically connected regions over time [35, 36].

While the tau transgenic models have been successful in modeling NFT pathology and functional impairment, it is important to recognize their shortcomings. First, since no tau mutations have been linked to AD, these mice should be considered models of FTLD, not AD. Second, the transgenic mice express tau cDNA and do not afford modulation of alternative splicing and 3R/4R ratio. Finally, ectopic expression of transgenic tau may not recapitulate the natural evolution of NFT spreading through synaptically connected regions. The htau mice described below overcome these limitations.

Duff, Davies and colleagues created a humanized tau (htau) model by expressing wild-type human *MAPT* genomic DNA on a mouse *Mapt* knockout background [37]. These mice preserve the native human 3R/4R ratio and were initially described to show insoluble, hyperphosphorylated tau by ~9 months of age with spatiotemporal progression resembling early stages of human AD. The htau mice also developed age-dependent synaptic and behavioral deficits as well as neuronal loss [38]. These features make htau an attractive model that is pathophysiology relevant to AD. Nevertheless, some important caveats should be noted. The behavioral and neurodegenerative phenotypes appear to be very mild and may not be readily reproducible [39, 40]. Although not verified, it is suspected that the increasingly delayed and mild phenotypes observed since the model was first introduced may result from shortening of the transgene array over generations of breeding, informally known as 'copy dropping'. The mild phenotype necessitates testing at advanced ages, with the attendant complications in variability, lethality, and cost. Finally, the presence of two alleles (human *MAPT* transgene and mouse *Mapt* deletion) complicates additional genetic manipulation.

Neurodegeneration

The strongest models of AD-related neurodegeneration come from transgenic overexpression of *MAPT* mutations associated with FTLD. In particular, the rTg4510 model expressing P301L tau develops severe forebrain atrophy, losing up to 40% of gross brain weight and >65% of CA1 pyramidal neurons by 5.5 months of age [28, 29, 41]. Significant forebrain atrophy with loss of cortical and hippocampal volumes is also observed in the P301S tau model PS19 at advanced ages [33]. In both of these tau models, neuronal loss outside of the hippocampus also observed. Where quantified for the rTg4510 model, neuron loss in cortex begins later than in hippocampus but still reached >50% by 8.5 months [41]. Even the htau model overexpressing wild-type human *MAPT* was initially described with notable neuronal loss, albeit at much later ages (~17 months) [42], and may have since waned with successive generations of breeding (see *"Neurofibrillary tangles"* section for more detail).

Only four models of amyloid pathology have shown any substantial degree of neuronal loss, and none of the APP mutations produce the same degree of neurodegeneration in mice that is observed in humans. The first APP mutation model described with neuronal loss was APP23, in which the number of hippocampal CA1 pyramidal cells decreased 14–25% by 14–18 months of age, commensurate with plaque load [43]. Neuronal loss was specific for the hippocampus, however, and neuron counts were unchanged in the neocortex of this model [44]. The second model found to develop significant neuronal loss was an intercross between transgenic $APP^{Swe/Lon}$ and $PS1^{M146L}$ lines, which displayed ~25% loss of CA1 pyramidal neurons by 17 months of age [45]. The same group described even greater loss of CA1 neurons in a second APP x PS1 model later that year [46]. This latter model combined 4 FAD mutations (APP Swe + Lon and PS1 M233 T + L235P) to evoke ~ 50% loss of CA1 neurons by 10 months of age. Intriguingly, cell death was again specific to CA1 hippocampal neurons with no net decline in either CA3 or dentate gyrus. The most recent and perhaps most widely used amyloid-based model in which neuronal loss has been described is the 5XFAD line. This mouse is named for its incorporation of 5 distinct AD mutations into a single transgenic line (APP Swe + Flo + Lon and PS1 M146 L + L286 V), which collectively produce rapid amyloid pathology as early as 2 months of age [47]. Neuron loss has been qualitatively described in the subiculum by 9 months of age; in the neocortex, non-biased stereological estimates suggest that 5XFAD mice lose 25–40% of layer 5 pyramidal neurons between 9 and 12 months of age [48, 49]. Neuron loss has not been described in other cortical layers, and despite the marked decrease in layer 5 neurons, the mice show no change in the total number of cortical neurons [48]. This outcome is consistent with the absence of overt brain atrophy in this and other models of Aβ amyloidosis.

Cognitive impairment

A surprising number and variety of mouse AD models develop some form of cognitive impairment. Where they have been tested, nearly all models of Aβ overproduction based on transgenic APP overexpression show deficits in spatial learning and memory (reviewed in [50]). In many but not all APP models, the onset of cognitive decline occurs in close proximity to that of amyloid deposition, such as in the CRND8 model [51], but has been identified both months prior to pathology in the Tg2576 model [52, 53] and months afterwards in the 5XFAD [47] and tet-off APP models (Chiang et al., in press). Of note, the age and disease stage at which cognitive deficits are observed depends in part on the task being used. This is well illustrated by behavioral characterization of the J20 model: this line shows initial plaque onset by 6 months of age [54], but when tested at 12–16 months performed as well as age-matched controls in the Y-maze and contextual fear conditioning despite showing severe impairment in a cheeseboard test of spatial memory [55].

Even knock-in models based on modification of the endogenous *App* sequence alone or in addition to mutation of *Psen1* can develop learning and memory impairment with age (i.e., homozygote $APP^{NLh}/PS1^{P264L}$ [56] or $APP^{NLh}/PS1^{M146V}$ [39, 57]. Perhaps to an even greater extent for knock-in models than for transgenics, both age and task can influence the reproducibility and robustness of cognitive phenotypes. This caveat is especially poignant when considering the newest set of APP knock-in models (i.e., APP^{NL}, APP^{NLF}, and APP^{NLGF}) where behavioral deficits in the same mouse line have varied between laboratories [58]. Using automated IntelliCage testing equipment, Masuda et al. detected only mild deficits in learning, recall, attention, and cognitive flexibility for all but the most aggressive homozygote APP^{NLGF} line [59]. However, a follow up study of the APP^{NLGF} model detected changes in locomotor/exploratory activity, but not learning and memory, despite widespread amyloid deposition [60]. This example serves as a good reminder to check that the model you intend to study has a phenotype in the outcome you intend to measure.

Models of neurofibrillary pathology also show varying degrees of cognitive impairment depending on age, task, and transgene. Like the amyloid models, the tau transgenic lines with more aggressive pathological phenotypes also tend to show more pronounced cognitive changes. The aggressive rTg4510 model develops progressive worsening in spatial memory that parallels the onset of tau hyper-phosphorylation and neuron loss [28, 29]. Similar deficits, although not as clearly progressive in nature, have been reported for the PS19 tau model [61–63]. Learning and memory impairments are less consistent for tau models with milder pathological phenotypes. For example, the htau model expressing human wild-type tau on a mouse tau null background was initially reported to show age-related decline in spatial learning and object recognition memory [38], however, more recent studies have not reproduced these deficits [39, 40, 64]. Variable cognitive impairment has also been reported for the JNPL3 mouse which expresses near-endogenous levels of P301L tau [65, 66]. Our ability to detect progressive learning and memory impairment in mice is limited by both the sensitivity and the range of the behavioral tasks we have available. The take home message may be that the chances of observing consistent and reproducible changes in cognitive function against which to gage effects of therapeutic intervention or genetic manipulation are increased by choosing a model that develops substantial AD pathology, regardless of whether this comes in the form of plaques or tangles.

Yin and yang of mouse models: Deciding between transgenics and knock-ins

After deciding what experimental question you want to address and which phenotype your model must recapitulate to answer that question, you must next decide whether a transgenic mouse line will suffice or if a knock-in model is needed. The central difference between these two approaches is the pattern of protein expression used to induce disease phenotype. In standard transgenic lines, a synthetic cDNA often encoding a disease-associated mutation is controlled by a heterologous promoter that results in an artificial expression pattern of limited spatial and temporal fidelity to the endogenous gene. In knock-in models, the native expression pattern is fully preserved but the protein now contains a disease-associated mutation (i.e., APP^{Swe}) or human-specific variant (i.e., APOEε4). Standard transgenics typically involve biased overexpression of a single splice variant, while knock-ins preserve native splicing at physiological levels. While it is intuitively preferable to use a model that most closely approaches endogenous expression patterns, there are situations where this is not possible or appropriate and where a transgenic model would do better, particularly in driving robust disease pathology. Knowing which compromises can be tolerated is just as important as knowing which may confound your experimental outcome.

There are many cases where the artificial expression of a single disease-associated protein variant may be the most efficient or only way to produce a phenotype in mice. Currently, overexpression of mutant human 4R tau is the only approach that has succeeded in generating thioflavin- and silver-positive neurofibrillary tangles in mice [29, 33]. Interventions to slow tangle formation therefore often accept the compromise between the presence of pathology and the artificial means by which it was produced (for example, [63, 67]). The use of transgenic models is also a reasonable compromise in studies testing cell non-autonomous effects of protein aggregation, where the cells under study are essentially wild-type (for example, [68]).

In contrast, transgenic overexpression can be problematic for studies where the effects of artificial temporal or spatial expression confound the outcome. For example, we found that transgenic APP expression under control of the *Camk2a* promoter caused persistent locomotor hyperactivity that prevented accurate cognitive testing [69]. The effect was traced to a consequence of transgenic APP on circuit development when we found that delaying transgene expression until adulthood was sufficient to abate the locomotor phenotype [70]. The same neurodevelopmental interaction also produced cortical hyper-synchrony in young adult APP mice that could again be abated by delaying transgene onset [71]. Although we found a workaround that met our needs, the emergence of knock-in models preserving the endogenous pattern of APP expression would avoid this confound entirely.

Another factor to bear in mind is that the endogenous proteins overexpressed in transgenic models have physiological functions independent of their role in Alzheimer's pathology. For example, overexpression of APP increases the production of soluble APP (N-terminal) fragments, membrane-associated C-terminal fragments, and the cytoplasmic APP intracellular domain (AICD) in addition to Aβ. Endogenous APP and its fragments contribute to cellular adhesion, neurite outgrowth, synapse formation, neuronal survival, and intracellular signaling [72–75]. Thus it is conceivable and perhaps likely that some of the phenotypes observed in APP transgenic mice arise from over-activation of these innate functions [76]. Along with the differences in spatiotemporal expression, elevated levels of these APP fragments may account for some of the reported distinctions between transgenic and knock-in models. The same concerns will also apply to tau transgenic models, where overexpression of a single isoform also creates an imbalance of the endogenous splice variants.

Reassuringly, several disease-relevant phenotypes identified in APP transgenic animals have been reproduced in knock-in models, including Aβ plaque formation, microglial and astrocytic activation, loss of synaptic markers, impaired hippocampal neurogenesis and diminished gamma frequency oscillations [58, 76–79]. Other features, such as calpain activation, show less agreement between transgenic and knock-in mice [80]. Of note, cognitive impairment that has been described in numerous APP transgenic models [50] has been more variable in knock-in models, albeit far less well studied [56, 58–60]. Phenotypic agreement and discrepancies are also found in the comparison of tau transgenic mice with the htau model which is currently the nearest available to a true knock-in. Admittedly, the comparison between transgenic tau mice expressing mutant variants and htau mice expressing wild-type protein is less apt than for APP models where both transgenics and knock-ins carry FAD mutations. Nevertheless, multiple phenotypes identified in tau transgenic models have also been reported in the htau mouse, including tau hyper-phosphorylation [37, 39, 42, 81–83], diminished neuronal integrity and plasticity [38, 84, 85] and elevated tau kinase activity [42]. Disparities between tau transgenics and the htau model are also observed, most notably in the extent of neurodegeneration, gliosis, and cognitive decline which are quite limited and/or absent even in aged htau animals [39, 40, 81], but see [38, 42].

Taken together, the best approach to mitigate against outcomes arising from the compromises inherent in transgenic models is to test the same outcome in multiple complementary lines. Because the cost of animal studies often renders this impractical, a reasonable alternative might be to choose the model with closest construct validity to the human disease that recapitulates the phenotype under investigation. Perhaps it is easier said than done, but where possible, use models that maintain endogenous protein expression patterns, where not, recognize the caveats that necessarily attend any interpretation of the resulting data.

Factors to bear in mind with knock-in models

While the bulk of early work to model AD in mice was done by standard transgenesis, a parallel thrust in the field sought to build models which avoided ectopic overexpression and maintained native transcript variation. The earliest of these models introduced the entire human *APP* or *MAPT* genes and their regulatory elements into mice via yeast or P1-derived artificial chromosomes (YAC or PAC vectors, respectively) [86–88]. While these models achieved native expression patterns and isoform usage, they shared with traditional transgenic mice the potential for endogenous gene disruption by random chromosomal integration. In addition, the murine *App or Mapt* gene retains expression and may interfere with the human transgene. Evidence for such a cross-species interaction emerged during construction of the htau model where hyper-phosphorylated tau was only observed once the human MAPT PAC mice were placed on a *Mapt* null background [37]. Due to the near-endogenous expression level, the APP YAC mice only develop measurable Aβ pathology when a FAD mutation is included (i.e., Swe) and the transgene is bred to homozygosity. Despite their benefit in construct validity, the mild phenotypes and complicated genetic crosses have limited use of the APP YAC and htau models.

An alternative strategy to achieve physiological expression is the knock-in (KI) approach, which is used to modify selected genes without perturbing off-target genomic perturbations. Multiple *App* and *Psen1* KI lines have been created, but no *Mapt* lines have been reported to date (Table 2). The first APP KI line, APP^{NLh}, reported in 1996 humanized the Aβ sequence and introduced the Swedish mutation into the mouse *App* gene [89]. Despite these modifications, the APP^{NLh} model did not develop Aβ pathology or other overt anomalies until interbred with the $PS1^{P264L}$ knock-in line to produce amyloid deposits, synaptic impairments, and altered hippocampal neurogenesis [79, 90, 91]. Additional *App* knock-in lines have since been created testing various FAD mutations in an effort to promote Aβ pathology. These include APP^{SL} expressing the Swedish and London mutations [92], APP^{DSL} expressing the Swe, Lon, and Dutch mutations [57], and the recent allelic series from Saido and colleagues expressing the Swe (APP^{NL}), Swe and Beyreuther/Ibe (APP^{NLF}), or Swe, Arc, and Ibe mutations (APP^{NLGF}) [58], all with a humanized Aβ domain. Like the original APP^{NLh} model, homozygous APP^{SL} and APP^{DSL} mice failed to develop Aβ pathology unless interbred with *Psen1* mutant mice. However, unlike the APP^{NLh} and APP^{SL} models, addition of the Dutch mutation in the APP^{DSL} mice promoted formation of vascular amyloid characteristic of cerebral amyloid angiopathy (CAA), with cerebral blood flow reduction, late-onset microhemorrhage, and cognitive impairment - but only when intercrossed with a *Psen1* mutant line [57].

Unlike the Lon mutation, the Ibe mutation is sufficient to produce Aβ deposition when combined with the Swe mutation in homozygous APP^{NLF} knock-in mice; addition of the Arctic mutation in APP^{NLGF} mice accelerates this phenotype [58]. These models take advantage of the exceptionally high Aβ42 production afforded by the Beyreuther/Ibe mutation to generate pathology in the absence of *Psen1* mutation. Indeed, the Aβ42/40 ratio was 30-fold higher than under physiological conditions. Similar to other amyloid models, homozygous APP^{NLF} and APP^{NLGF} mice develop age-dependent loss of synaptic markers and reactive gliosis, but show more limited behavioral phenotypes (see *"Cognitive impairment"* section for details) [58, 59].

Overall, the *App* knock-in models provide precise genetic manipulation and faithful physiological expression of target genes. Achieving this physiological fidelity necessitates several genetic compromises for amyloid pathology to manifest. For example, all amyloid-forming knock-in mice carry multiple FAD mutations and in most cases must be bred to homozygosity to elicit Aβ pathology. Additionally, several earlier *App* knock-in lines required homozygous expression of mutant *Psen1* alleles to obtain amyloid deposition (APP^{NLh}, APP^{SL} and APP^{DSL}), while others do so through supra-physiological production of Aβ42 (APP^{NLF} and APP^{NLGF}). It is also important to note that the Dutch and Arctic mutations used in the APP^{DSL} and APP^{NLGF} mice change the primary sequence of Aβ to influence its biophysical properties [15, 93]. These technical and biological issues should be taken into consideration when deciding whether a knock-in model is best for your experimental needs, and if so, which line to use.

Technical considerations for transgenic models

To an even greater degree than for knock-in models, multiple design factors go into creating each transgenic line and should be considered when choosing a model for study. The central disease feature to be examined, be it plaques, tangles, degeneration, or cognitive decline, will determine which class of models to consider, but within that class, the best model may depend on a variety of other factors such as where and when critical features of disease will appear. Simply put, the best model isn't always the one you can get from the lab down the hall.

The transcript itself

Most transgenic constructs are based on artificial cDNAs designed to express a single transcript out of many that are produced by alternative splicing of the endogenous gene. One example of this is the frequent use of the 695 amino acid isoform of APP, the shortest of three alternatively spliced variants (along with 751 and 770 [73]). Because the 695 isoform is predominantly or perhaps exclusively expressed in neurons and accounts for most APP in the brain [94], its use in transgenic constructs intended to increase Aβ production in the brain has been a logical strategy in many cases (i.e., Tg2576 [95], C3–3 [96], and TgCRND8 [51]). Another approach taken in some early transgenic models was to create an APP minigene containing all 18 exons and capable of producing the three main isoforms of 695, 751, and 770 amino acids (i.e., PDAPP [2, 97], and J20 [54]). Both approaches have yielded amyloid pathology in the mouse brain.

Most tau transgenic models have also been constructed using cDNA derived from just one of the six transcripts for human *MAPT*. Several tau models incorporate a familial mutation from FTLD located in the alternatively spliced exon 10 and therefore produce only 4R tau protein rather than a mixture of 3R and 4R tau (i.e., rTg4510 [29] and PS19 [33]). In an effort to overcome the artificial bias introduced by transgenic production of a single tau isoform, Duff and colleagues used a plasmid artificial chromosome (PAC) to introduce the entire human wild-type *MAPT* gene and upstream regulatory sequence into the mouse (i.e., Line 8c [87]). These mice produce all 6 isoforms of human tau at levels several-fold higher than endogenous, but do not develop pathological hyper-phosphorylation unless murine tau is eliminated [37]. In the case of AD, it is known that both 3R and 4R tau protein contribute to pathologic aggregates [98], but the success of 4R transgenic models suggests that this disease phenotype can be reasonably modeled using just one transcript. In other experimental settings, native transcript variation is required. The nature of the experimental question will dictate whether models based on a single transcript are an acceptable substitute in each case.

The transgenic promoter

Historically, the promoter elements used in transgenic constructs were chosen to ensure robust, widespread, life-long expression of ectopic protein. Several common promoter constructs have been used over the years, including prion protein (*Prnp*, i.e., Tg2576 [95], TgCRND8 [51], APP/PS1 Line 85 [99], JNPL3 [34], and PS19 [33]), platelet-derived growth factor B chain (*PDGFB*, i.e., PDAPP [2] and J20 [54]), and thymus cell surface antigen 1 (*Thy1*, i.e., APP23 [100], 5XFAD [47], and 3xTg-AD [101]). While these three promoters induce strong and persistent transgene expression in neurons, *PDGFB* and *Prnp* are also active to a lesser extent in non-neuronal cells of the CNS [102], and all three promoters elicit expression in multiple organs outside of the nervous system including heart and liver [103–105]. All three promoters are active in the embryonic brain [103, 105, 106], and in the adult may be expressed in multiple neuronal subtypes [107–112]. Although these promoters were chosen for strong persistent expression in adult neurons, none of the three is restricted to the CNS and all are active embryonically. If the experimental question at hand requires a more selective temporal or spatial expression pattern, alternative genetic strategies such as the controllable systems described below will be needed to achieve this specificity.

Strain background

In the past, most transgenes were made using hybrid mouse strains such as C3B6 (APP/PS1 Line 85 [99, 113] and PS19 [33]), B6D2 (J20 [54]) or B6SJL (Tg2576 [95]). The push towards congenic strain backgrounds lead to many lines being backcrossed onto a single parental strain, revealing the impact that genetic context could have on transgene-associated phenotypes. Early work on the Tg2576 model revealed that the transgene was well tolerated on the original hybrid background but caused early lethality when backcrossed to C57BL/6 [114]. By the fourth generation, none of transgenic offspring survived past 2.5 months of age. Other APP^{Swe} transgenic lines have since been backcrossed to C57BL/6 for >10 generations without loss (i.e., APP/PS1 Line 85, C3–3, and J20), suggesting that this strain is not inherently problematic for AD models and that the premature lethality of Tg2576 likely arose from a specific interaction between the genomic integration site and genetic modifiers of the background strain. Later work using the YAC transgenic model R1.40 demonstrated that genetic background could influence both APP processing and the age at which amyloid deposits appeared, dramatically delaying onset from 13.5 months on C57BL/6 to >20 months on DBA/2 [115]. These two background strains also influenced phenotype in the APP/PS1 line 85 mice, where the DBA/2 background substantially increased susceptibility to lethal seizures compared to C57BL/6 [116]. Multiple genetic loci may contribute to these strain differences [117], including the kinesin light chain-1 gene identified as a modifier of amyloid onset in the DBA/2 background [118]. As these studies demonstrate, the genetic context in which any transgene acts can significantly influence the resulting phenotype. Several transgenic models are available on multiple inbred and hybrid backgrounds (5XFAD, APP/PS1 Line 85, Tg2576), and it is worth investing some time into weighing the options between experimental needs and known characteristics of each strain (i.e., FVB/N breed well but are blind as adults; C57BL/6 mice breed less well but are a reasonable option for cognitive testing, etc.).

Age of onset

The age at which disease-associated phenotypes first appear in each model results from a complex mixture of the strength of the transgene promoter, the aggressiveness of familial mutations included in the transgene, the number of transgene copies incorporated into the insertion site, the chromosomal location of transgene integration, and the genetic background on which the transgene is expressed. The design of the transgene construct likely has the greatest impact on the level at which the transgene is expressed and thus on the age at which phenotypes appear, however, chromosomal integration site and copy number also have substantial influence and cannot (usually) be controlled. As an example of how these latter factors can affect onset, TgCRND8 and C3–3 models both express APP^{Swe} under control of a prion protein promoter, yet amyloid pathology appears by 2 months of age in TgCRND8 but not until 18 months in C3–3 [51, 119]. If the experimental manipulation is predicted to delay pathogenesis, then an early onset model may be most appropriate. Conversely, if acceleration is anticipated, a late onset model would be better. Bear in mind, however, that while the early onset models may be faster to study, they also create a disconnect between chronological age and pathological condition that does not accurately reflect the aging physiology under which most AD will occur.

Animal source

Although it is easy and inexpensive to obtain transgenic models from a lab down the hall, publically-supported repositories like the Jackson Laboratory (Jax) or the Mutant Mouse Research and Resource Centers (MMRRC) in the US, the RIKEN BioResource Center (BRC) Experimental Animal Division in Japan, and the European Mouse Mutant Archive (EMMA) provide genetic validation of their models that is well worth the added cost. As an example of this, Jax screens all incoming models for the presence of common extraneous alleles (Cre, Flp, neo, tTA, GFP and RFP), often to discover that donating labs have intercrossed the line with another transgenic resulting in mistyped offspring that continue to carry the unrecognized modification. Once identified, these extraneous alleles can be removed before the strain is cryopreserved or expanded for distribution. Moreover, Jax routinely genotypes new mice using a single nucleotide polymorphism (SNP) panel to characterize the strain background and elucidate any uncertainties in the parentage of the donated animals. The stock or strain number of the transgenic line also provides a clear means of identifying which model was tested. Common nomenclature can be muddied by varying abbreviations adopted by different laboratories, therefore the stock number can be a universal identifier easily referenced by other researchers. Finally, by supporting communication with receiving investigators, issues that arise in the field can be verified and shared, as done recently for the 3xTg-AD mice upon learning from the donating investigator that male mice may no longer display the phenotypes initially described for this line, while female animals appear unaffected (https://www.jax.org/strain/004807). Similar reporting from users in the field lead to the identification of transgene copy loss in the J20 strain that was remedied by re-importing the line from the donating laboratory; qPCR is for copy number is now a routine part of colony maintenance for this strain (https://www.jax.org/strain/006293). This type of unpublished information and quality assurance are invaluable in helping to ensure that research effort and resources yield informative and reproducible outcomes. Don't waste your time or funding on mice that aren't what they're meant to be.

Sex as biological variable

In general, female mice are more susceptible to plaques and tangles than their male counterparts. Earlier-onset pathology has been consistently noted in females across multiple APP transgenic models, including Tg2576 [120], APP/PS1 [121, 122], an intercross of APP^{Swe} x $PS1^{A246E}$ [123], and 3xTg-AD [124]. Where tested, transgene expression appears similar in male and female APP mice [125]; instead the accelerated pathology may be attributable to increased β-secretase processing in females [124, 126]. Tau pathology also tends to be more pronounced in female transgenic mice, as noted in the rTg4510 [127] and JNPL3 models [128, 129], albeit not in 3xTg-AD [124, 130]. Perhaps as a result of elevated neuropathology, cognitive impairments are also generally greater in female mice, including Tg2576 [131], APP/PS1 [121], CRND8 [132], APP/TTA [125], 3xTg-AD [130], and rTg4510 models [127]. Females also respond more drastically to environmental stress, developing higher amyloid levels in 5XFAD [133], insoluble and caspase-cleaved tau in a tau P301L model [134]. Not all phenotypes are female-biased, however, as markers of neuroendocrine aging appeared earlier in male than female 3xTg-AD mice [135]. While sex-based differences in pathological phenotypes are not found in every model and are not consistent even for a single feature across all lines, there is accumulating evidence that it can make a difference and should be considered when designing experiments and measuring outcomes. The NIH has made a strong case for greater attention to sex as a biological variable in all basic and translational research, and it is clearly an important factor to consider for AD where gender clearly contributes to risk [136].

Alternative approaches for transgene expression - viral gene delivery

While genetically engineered mice are the most common animal models for AD, viral-mediated gene expression systems have been increasingly used to elicit neuropathology either alone or in conjunction with existing genetic models. Two viral systems have been employed for gene expression in rodent brains: lentivirus and adeno-associated virus (AAV). While both systems deliver localized gene expression when stereotaxically injected to the adult brain, AAV can also be used to achieve widespread gene expression when injected into the neonatal brain. There are at least 13 different AAV serotypes with varying tropism. Of these AAV serotypes 1, 2, 6, 8, 9, and 10 have been demonstrated to drive neuronal expression of target genes. Table 3 summarizes the viral models of Aβ and tau pathology created using wild-type rat and mouse.

Viral expression of APP has not yielded much success in producing robust amyloid pathology. Out of a series of amyloid-based expression vectors injected into the hippocampus of adult rats (Aβ40, Aβ42, and APP^{Swe}), amyloid deposits were only detected in animals receiving Aβ42 virus (i.e., BRI-Aβ42 [137]). By incorporating multiple FAD mutations into APP (Swe/Lon/Aus), Koukouli et al. achieved AD-like amyloid deposits, microgliosis, and reactive astrogliosis 12 months after AAV injection into the prefrontal cortex of adult mice, along with NFT pathology [138].

Compared to the dearth of amyloid viral transgenics displaying AD-like pathology, considerably more tau viral transgenic models have been reported. An exhaustive review of viral tau models has recently been published by Cubinkova et al. and we refer readers to this article for more detailed information [139]. Both lentivirus and AAV have been used to express tau in wild-type mice and rats, and both can generate hyperphosphorylated tau in vivo. Both wild-type and mutant (P301L or P301S) tau have been tested, and both can give rise to pathological hyperphosphorylation, although mutant tau produces a more aggressive phenotype [140]. Mature NFTs have been elusive with viral models unless combined with standard APP transgenics [141] (but see [142]), however, a recent study using neonatal intracerebral ventricular (ICV) injection of AAV1-tau-P301L produced widespread tau hyperphosphorylation in wild-type mice followed by thioflavin-S positive NFTs, suggesting that the onset, duration, or multiplicity of transduction may influence the progression of viral tau pathology [143]. Surprisingly, although the mice exhibited behavioral abnormalities, no neuronal loss was observed.

Viral transgenesis has numerous advantages over traditional transgenic models: 1) it is less expensive and faster to generate than germline manipulations; 2) pathology can be regionally targeted, thus allowing analysis of neuronal projections and avoiding peripheral expression; 3) the same virus can often be used in mice or rats, young or old animals, and any region of interest; and 4) viral injection can be combined with genetic models to test functional interactions more quickly and easily than inter-breeding multiple alleles. However, just as with any other system, these benefits come with a cost. First and foremost is mosaicism: not all cells will be transduced, and those that are transduced may take up different numbers of viral particles and express at different levels. This heterogeneity and inter-animal variability necessitates higher animal numbers for each experiment. Second, surgical injection and/or viral transduction may cause an unintended injury response, thus the observed phenotypes may result from an interaction between the expressed viral transgene and the cellular response to injection or transduction. It is therefore important to include a set of animals injected with a control virus encoding a non-pathogenic protein (i.e., GFP or other marker) to confirm that the observed phenotype is transgene-specific. Finally, both AAV and lentivirus are limited in their packaging capacity which prevents the use of large transgenes. For AAV, the maximal transgene size is approximately 4.5 kb, and is not much larger for lentivirus.

Other tools for specific experimental needs - controllable transgenics

While the first generation transgenic models were useful tools for in vivo studies of protein-protein interactions

Table 3 Viral transgenic lines for APP and Tau

Transgene	Promoter	Viral packaging	Host	Reference
Stereotaxically Targeted APP/Aβ Viral Transgenics				
BRI-Aβ40 BRI-Aβ42	CBA	AAV1	adult rat	[137]
huAPP$_{695}$ (Swe/Lon/Aus)	*(human?) EF1A*	AAV (serotype not stated)	adult mouse	[138]
Stereotaxically Targeted Tau Viral Transgenics				
hu*MAPT*$_{4R2N}$ (P301L)	CAG	AAV2	adult rat	[142]
hu*MAPT*$_{4R0N}$ (P301S)	mouse *Pgk*	lentivirus	adult mouse	[141]
hu*MAPT*$_{4R1N}$ (P301L)	CMV	AAV2	adult mouse	[216]
hu*MAPT*$_{4R2N}$ (P301L) hu*MAPT*$_{4R2N}$ (wt)	human *SYN1*	AAV1	adult mouse	[217]
hu*MAPT*$_{4R1N}$ (P301L) hu*MAPT*$_{4R1N}$ (wt)	CMV	lentivirus	adult rat	[140]
hu*MAPT*$_{4R2N}$ (P301L)	human *SYN1*	AAV9	adult mouse	[218]
hu*MAPT*$_{4R0N}$ (P301S) hu*MAPT*$_{4R0N}$ (wt)	mouse *Pgk1*	AAV6	adult mouse	[219]
Whole-Brain Tau Viral Transgenics				
hu*MAPT* (P301L) (isoform not stated)	CAG	AAV1	neonatal mouse	[143]
hu*MAPT*$_{4R2N}$ (P301L)	CAG	AAV1	neonatal mouse	[220]

CAG cytomegalovirus immediate early enhancer combined with the chicken β actin promoter [209]
CBA chicken β-actin
CMV cytomegalovirus
Tables 1-4: Refer to Fig. 1 for illustration of APP mutations.

and cellular responses implicated in AD, their design was rigid with no way to modify where or when the disease-associated protein was produced. Questions that required more selective patterns of transgene expression - for example, expression in mature neurons but not neural progenitors - or which required the ability to turn off expression - for example, mimicking the effect of Aβ-lowering therapies - lead to the creation of new controllable transgenic models based on the tetracycline-transactivator (tTA) expression system. In this bi-partite system, tTA acts as an artificial transcription which binds selectively to an artificial DNA promoter sequence known as the tetracycline response element (*TRE*), both derived from the *E. coli* operon controlling tetracycline resistance. Co-expression of tTA in mice under a selective promoter (the driver line) with a TRE-dependent transgene (the responder line) produces transcription in a pattern dependent on the transgenic tTA promoter. Because the two transgenes are independent of one another, the same responder line can be mated with various driver lines to produce offspring expressing the same transgene in different cell types. When the tTA protein is exposed to tetracycline or its chemical analogs, it undergoes a conformational change that prevents it from binding DNA. Exposure to tetracycline (or the more commonly used doxycycline (dox)) thus provides temporal control over expression of the responder transgene. Two versions of the tTA have been created and are used under different circumstances. The original tet-off system is based on tTA and as its name implies, is active under basal conditions and arrested upon exposure to dox. The subsequent tet-on system based on the reverse tTA (rtTA) is inactive under basal conditions, and opposite from tTA, causes transcriptional activation upon dox administration.

tTA-expressing driver lines

Transgene expression with the tet-controlled system requires two parts - a driver line expressing tTA and a responder line expressing the gene of interest under control of a *TRE* promoter - interbred to yield offspring carrying both alleles. Multiple versions of the *TRE* promoter have been created (*tetO*, P_{TRE}, P_{TRE3G}, etc.), and all work with the two most common versions of tTA (now known as 'first' and 'second' generation transactivators, but originally named tTA [144] and tTA-2 [145]). Although these tet-off transactivators are now considered legacy products by their commercial vendor in favor of increasing signal-to-noise improvements in tet-on products, it is the older tet-off system that has been most successful for controllable transgene expression in the mouse brain. Lines expressing tTA or tTA-2 under control of the calcium calmodulin kinase type IIα (*Camk2a* [146]), neurofilament heavy chain (*NEFH* [147]), and kallikrein related-peptidase 8 promoters (*Klk8*; also called Prss19 or neuropsin [30]) have been used to direct controllable transgene expression in neuronal subsets of the entorhinal/limbic areas (*Klk8*), the broader forebrain (*Camk2a*), or throughout the CNS (*NEFH*), as needed for the particular experiment (Table 4). The potential for tTA-controlled transgene expression in other cell types was greatly increased by the introduction of two Cre-dependent tTA transgenic lines from Luo, Roos, and colleagues [148, 149]. These 'converter' lines

Table 4 Controllable transgenic lines for APP and Tau

Model	Transgene	Promoter	Availability	Reference
tTA-Dependent Responder Lines				
tetO-APP Lines 102 and 107	mo/huAPP$_{695}$ (Swe/Ind)	TetO (first generation TRE from pTet-Splice)	MMRRC 34845-JAX, 34846-JAX	[69]
rTg4510	huMAPT$_{4R0N}$ (P301L)	TRE (first generation TRE from pTRE)	JAX 015815, 024854	[29]
rTg21221	huMAPT$_{4R0N}$ (wt)	TRE (first generation TRE from pTRE)	Karen Ashe	[156]
rTg9191	huAPP$_{695}$ (Swe/Lon)	TRE (first generation TRE from pTRE)	Karen Ashe	[155]
hTau-A152T Line L1	huMAPT$_{4R1N}$ (A152T)	TRE-Tight (second generation TRE)	JAX 028979	[157]
hTau-WT Line L32	huMAPT$_{4R1N}$ (wt)	TRE-Tight (second generation TRE)	JAX 029269	[157]
tTA-Expressing Driver Lines				
Camk2a-tTA Line B	tTA (first generation)	mo*Camk2a*	JAX 007004, 003010	[146]
EC-tTA	tTA2 (second generation)	*Nop/Klk8*	MMRRC 031779-MU	[30]
NEFH-tTA Line 8	tTA (first generation)	human *NEFH*	JAX 025397	[147]
ROSA:LNL:tTA	optimized/modified tTA (mtTA)	ROSA26-LNL (Cre-dependent)[a]	JAX 011008	[148]
ROSA26-ZtTA	tTA (first generation)	ROSA26-CAG-LβL (Cre-dependent)[b]	JAX 012266 (see also 024107)	[149]

[a]LNL: loxP-(neomycin/poly A)-loxP
[b]LβL: loxP-(β-geo (lacZ-neomycin phosphotransferase fusion)/3x poly A-loxP
Tables 1–4: Refer to Fig. 1 for illustration of APP mutations.

allow tTA-dependent transgene expression in any cell type for which there is a Cre-specific driver, but has the disadvantage of added breeding to combine three independently assorting alleles (Promoter-Cre x Cre-dependent [lox-stop-lox]-tTA x TRE-[gene-of-interest]). The flexibility and strength of this approach was nicely demonstrated by the Allen Institute in recent work showing the expression of TRE-dependent transgenes in a variety of neuronal cell types for which only Cre-expressing driver lines exist [150]. This tripartite system maintained the spatial expression pattern imparted by the Cre driver, while gaining the transcriptional amplification provided by tTA.

A number of tet-on (rtTA) driver lines have also been produced but have been generally less successful than tet-off (tTA) lines for CNS expression. Illustrating the difficulty with the tet-on drivers for brain studies, rtTA expression under control of the ubiquitously expressed *ROSA26* promoter or the artificial *CAGGS* promoter produced strong doxycycline-dependent expression of their respective responder transgenes in peripheral tissue, but neither line achieved transgene expression in the brain [151, 152]. The lack of brain expression was attributed to relatively poor CNS permeability of doxycycline required for transcriptional activation with the tet-on system. Indeed, when rtTA has been used for controllable neuronal transgene expression in the brain, doxycycline concentrations up to 30× higher are needed for transgene expression by the tet-on (rtTA) than for transgene suppression by tet-off (tTA) [153]. More recently, a ubiquitously expressed rtTA controlling PGC1α was shown to diminish the aggregation of mutant huntingtin protein in the brain of transgenic mice, however, the effect may have been peripherally mediated [154].

TRE-controlled responder lines

A number of tet-controlled responder lines relevant to AD have been created, characterized, and made available through public repositories. Multiple responder lines are available to express APP harboring dual FAD mutations (APP$^{Swe/Ind}$ lines 102 and 107 [69] and APP$^{Swe/Lon}$ line rTg9191 [155]), while tau models are available to express either wild-type (huMAPT$_{4R0N}$ line rTg21221 [156] and huMAPT$_{4R1N}$ line L32 [157]) or FTLD-associated variants (huMAPT^{P301L} line rTg4510 [29] and huMAPT^{A152T} line L1 [157]). Similar to their standard transgenic counterparts, the tet-controlled APP and MAPT strains develop either amyloid plaques or hyper-phosphorylated tau, but can do so on an accelerated timeline compared with traditional models. For example, tetO-APP line 102 used with the Camk2a-tTA driver can develop amyloid plaques by 1–2 months of age (JLJ, unpublished data), while the rTg4510 line (also used with the Camk2a-tTA driver) develops argyrophilic tangles by 4 months and gross forebrain atrophy by 10 months [29]. The aggressiveness of these models is likely due to the high level of transgene expression attained with the tet-transactivator system which can exceed 10× that of endogenous APP or tau, but is by no means the case for every controllable line.

Transgene suppression with tet-off models

One of the main reasons for working with the tet-system is the opportunity for temporal control over transgene expression. Doxycycline is commonly used to regulate the system due to better stability than tetracycline; dox has good tissue penetration, is safe for chronic use, and has been well-characterized pharmacologically. Dox can be administered orally via drinking water or chow, with several companies offering standard dox chow formulations in addition to custom compounding. The dose required for transgene suppression via tTA is higher than for veterinary therapeutic use: 50–200 ppm in chow comes to roughly 0.15–0.6 mg per day for an adult mouse, while therapeutic use at 2.5–5 mg/kg PO q12 comes to 0.025–0.05 mg/day [158]. While safe at these doses, doxycycline is not inert: in vitro it can inhibit MMP2 and MMP9 [159, 160] although this effect has not been demonstrated in vivo [161]. More relevant for neurodegeneration studies is the potential anti-inflammatory effect of dox treatment. Where dox has been used as an anti-inflammatory drug, the doses administered are universally higher than used for tTA regulation, in some cases as much as 15× greater [162–165]. The same trend is true in vitro where dox has been found to dampen cytokine responses by cultured microglial cells, but often at concentrations considerably higher than experienced in vivo [164, 166–168]. Minocycline is a stronger anti-inflammatory than doxycycline, and is more commonly used for its anti-inflammatory effect in vivo (for example, see [169–177]). Thus, while there is a potential for inflammatory modulation by dox, it is a considerably weaker agent than minocycline and is usually used in tet-off transgenic models at doses below those shown to suppress microglial function in vivo.

The optimal dose for transgene suppression is influenced by both driver and responder lines and must be determined empirically for each combination. Depending on perdurance of the transgenic protein, maximal suppression is usually attained within days of starting dox treatment [178]. Conversely, the tTA system can be used to activate transgene expression by removing dox from animals reared on the drug [70, 147, 178, 179]. This 'reverse' use of dox treatment comes with the risk of diminished transgene expression in animals removed from dox compared with animals never exposed to the drug, especially when treatment is started before transgene expression begins [180] (JLJ unpublished data). Transgene onset after withdrawing dox can be slower than transgene suppression upon dox exposure, and can require up to 2 weeks to reach maximal levels depending on the model and the dosage [181] (JLJ unpublished data). Even under the best conditions, transgene suppression via dox is good but not complete. The TRE controlling the responder transgene contains not only the tet operator sequence that binds tTA but also a minimal CMV promoter to engage transcription. As a result, early versions of TRE-controlled strains produced low levels of transgenic protein even after dox treatment or in the absence of tTA [69, 178, 179]. Later iterations of the *TRE* have shortened the minimal promoter to reduce transactivator-independent expression (i.e., P_{TRE3G}); complementary improvements in tTA-2 pared the transcriptional activation domain to limit activity in the presence of dox [145](http://www.tetsystems.com/science-technology/scientific-figures/). Nevertheless, be aware that transgene suppression is not the same as the absence of expression.

The value of tTA controls

Finally, know that tTA and rtTA are themselves artificial transgenes that should be controlled for in your experimental design. Most common (r)tTA lines were produced by random insertion into the genome and may have disrupted one or more genes in the process. In most cases the insertion site has not been identified, and the possibility of bystander hemizygosity at the disrupted locus should always be considered. In addition, tTA expression may have phenotypic effects of its own. Several groups have reported neurodegenerative phenotypes in tTA-expressing transgenic models, including the heavily used Camk2a-tTA line [182, 183]. In each case, dox-rearing abrogated cell loss, suggesting that the active conformation of tTA and not genome disruption was to blame. Peripheral expression of tTA or rtTA has been linked to lung abnormalities, cardiomyopathy, and microphthalmia independent of any responder transgene [184–186](P. Overbeek, unpublished observation). Inclusion of a tTA-only control group can therefore provide valuable reassurance that observed phenotypes are due to the transgenic protein under study and not to artifacts of this powerful but highly artificial expression system.

Modeling LOAD - incorporating risk alleles for ApoE and TREM2

Recapitulating amyloid or tau pathology in mice requires the use of dominant mutations identified from rare familial cases of early-onset AD or FTLD. This belies the fact that the vast majority of patients develop late-onset AD (LOAD) and do not carry mutations in *APP, PSEN1* or *PSEN2*, and that *MAPT* mutations are not found in AD. Whether these mutation-based, neuropathology-driven models truly capture the key pathological progression of LOAD is an open question. Studies of LOAD have identified multiple genetic factors that influence the risk of AD but which do not directly cause disease. A quarter century ago, Allen Roses and colleagues established the apolipoprotein E ε4 allele (APOEε4) as a major susceptibility factor for LOAD [187]; to date ApoEε4 remains the most common and significant risk factor for LOAD. Recent genome-wide association studies have uncovered >30 additional risk polymorphisms for LOAD [188]. Collectively, these candidate risk genes suggest that astrocytes, microglia, and immune system dysfunction play a significant role in disease pathogenesis [189]. APOE is normally expressed by astrocytes in the CNS, while another strong modifier, the triggering receptor expressed on myeloid cells 2 (TREM2), is expressed exclusively by microglia in the brain [190, 191]. The effects of these polymorphisms are an area of active investigation, and accordingly, multiple mouse lines of APOE and TREM2 have been created. Modeling of other LOAD genes has been more challenging than for *APOE* and *TREM2* due to weak individual effect sizes and the location of risk-associated polymorphisms in non-coding regions of the gene.

ApoE

APOE is an apolipoprotein that binds cholesterol to facilitate its transport. The three APOE isoforms in humans differ at residues 112 and 158: ε2 (Cys 112, Cys158), ε3 (Cys112, Arg158) and ε4 (Arg112, Arg158). APOEε4 increases AD risk and ε2 mitigates it. Mouse has only one ApoE isoform and it is believed to resemble human APOEε3 in its biophysical properties [192]. Mice deficient in ApoE were created by gene targeting nearly 25 years ago [193, 194]. Homozygous *ApoE* null mice are viable and overtly healthy but develop hypercholesterolemia and atherosclerotic lesions with age (Table 5). Within the CNS, the *ApoE* null mice display none of the characteristic AD pathologies, but do have impaired adult hippocampal neurogenesis [195], however, the relevance of this phenotype is unclear. The *ApoE* knock-out mice have been crossed with various AD models to test how loss-of-function affects pathology relative to animals expressing one of the three human APOE isoforms (described below).

Three sets of human APOE mice have been generated. The Holtzman group produced transgenic mice expressing human APOEε3 or APOEε4 cDNA under control of the human GFAP promoter and then removed murine ApoE from the background by crossing the transgenics onto the *ApoE* null line (line 37 for ε3 and line 22 for ε4) [196]. The resulting mice express human APOE in the brain at a level similar to that of adult human cortex. While the mice are useful in examining the role of astrocytic APOE and for comparing the effects of ε3 and ε4, inherent differences in transgene integration site, copy number, and expression level may confound interpretation of differences between the two isoforms. In addition, the need to maintain each transgene on an *ApoE* null background for "humanization" of the model makes further genetic studies complicated.

Bruce Lamb's group created APOEε2, ε3 and ε4 knock-in mice by targeting human ε2, ε3, and ε4 cDNAs in-frame into the endogenous mouse *ApoE* gene [197]. Because these mice express human APOE under the endogenous mouse promoter, differences between the APOE isoforms can be accurately compared. An added advantage of this strategy is its direct "humanization" by simultaneously inserting the human allele and disrupting

Table 5 APOE and TREM2 Models

Model	Allele	Targeting approach	Availability	Reference
ApoE Lines				
GFAP-ApoE3 Line 37, GFAP-ApoE4, Line 1	hu*APOE3* or *E4* cDNA	Transgenic, hu*GFAP* promoter	JAX 004633, 004631	[196]
ApoE2, E3, E4 KI	hu*APOE2, E3,* or *E4*	Targeted insertion of *APOE* cDNAs	NA	[197]
ApoE KO	*Apoe* deletion (exon 3 replacement)	Targeted neo insertion replacing part of *Apoe* exon 3	JAX 002052; 014556	[193, 221]
APOE*3, E*4 KI	hu*APOE3 or E4*	Targeted replacement of *Apoe* exons 2–4	JAX 027894 (E4) JAX 029018 (E3)	NA
APOE2, E3, E4 Targeted replacement	hu*APOE2, E3, or E4*	Targeted replacement of *Apoe* exons 2–4	Taconic	[199–201]
TREM2 Lines				
TREM2 KO	*Trem2* deletion (exon 2–3 deletion)	Targeted lacZ/neo replacement of TREM2 exons 2–4	UCD/KOMP VG10093	[206]
TREM2$^{-/-}$	*Trem2* deletion (exon 2–3 deletion)	Targeted deletion TREM2 exons 3–4	Marco Colonna	[205]
TREM2 KO	*Trem2* deletion (Q17X)	CRISPR/Cas9 targeted deletion	JAX 027197	NA
TREM2 R47H KI	endogenous mouse *Trem2* (R47H)	CRISPR/Cas9 targeted mutation	JAX 027918	NA
TREM2 Y38C KI	endogenous mouse *Trem2* (Y38C)	CRISPR/Cas9 targeted mutation	JAX 029725	NA
TREM2 p.T66 M	endogenous mouse *Trem2* (T66 M)	CRISPR/Cas9 targeted mutation	Christian Haass	[208]
TREM2 flox	*Trem2*$^{tm1c(EUCOMM)Wtsi}$ loxP-flanked mouse *Trem2* exons 2–3	Targeted insertion	JAX 029853	NA

mouse *ApoE*. Unfortunately, no isoform-specific differences in brain cholesterol or Aβ levels were detected and the utility of the mice is thus limited.

Through a similar gene-targeting approach, Maeda and colleagues created the so-called APOE targeted-replacement mice in which human *APOEε2* [198], *ε3* [199], or *ε4* [200] alleles were inserted into the endogenous mouse *ApoE* locus (Table 5). Unlike the APOE knock-in series, coding exons 2–4 and the associated intronic sequences of each *APOE* gene were used instead of cDNA and mouse *ApoE* gene was deleted instead of disrupted. These mice exhibit allele-specific differences in both the CNS and periphery and are the most popular APOE mice for testing differential effects of APOE isoforms either on their own or in a model of AD pathology. Although the mice can be purchased through Taconic, there are restrictions on use of the animals. To overcome these limitations, a similar set of APOE-targeted humanization mice was recently created and made available through Jax with few restrictions (APOE*4 KI, Stock No. 027894; APOE*3 KI, Stock No. 029018).

Because the focus of the current review is on practical considerations for best using the models rather than their biological or pathological underpinnings, it will suffice to say that APOE mediates diverse functions in the brain, modifying parenchymal and vascular amyloid pathology, tau-mediated neurodegeneration, and neuroinflammation in an isoform-dependent manner [201–203].

TREM2

TREM2 is a type-1 membrane protein expressed in myeloid cells. Autosomal recessive mutations of TREM2 such as Y38C and T66M lead to Nasu-Hakola disease characterized by bone cysts and dementia, believed to arise through loss of function [204]. Rare variants in the TREM2 extracellular domain, particularly R47H, appear to confer LOAD risk in an autosomal dominant manner [190, 191]. The first *Trem2* knock-out strain was created by Colonna and colleagues through targeted deletion of exons 3 and 4 encoding a portion of the transmembrane and cytoplasmic domains [205]. A separate knock-out

Table 6 Quick guide to the pros and cons of commonly used AD mouse models

Model	Main features	Pros	Cons	Examples of use in AD research
Tg2576	mid-life amyloid pathology (10–14 mo)	well-characterized, maintains aging feature of AD	high lethality on C57 background, Tg male aggressive and needs to be single-housed	[222–224]
APP/PS1	early-onset (~6 mo) amyloid pathology	well-characterized, co-integrated transgenes breed as a single allele	like other co-integrated models, cannot control for independent transgene effects	[225–227]
5XFAD	juvenile-onset amyloid pathology (~3 mo)	rapid onset phenotype, co-integrated transgenes breed as a single allele	non-physiological combination of FAD mutations, marked intracellular Aβ accumulation	[228–230]
3xTg-AD	early- to mid-life amyloid pathology plus hyperphosphorylated tau	captures both Aβ and phospho-tau features of AD	variable pathology between colonies and sexes, genetic drift has been observed	[231–233]
rTg4510	early-onset neurofibrillary tangles (~5–6 mo), severe neurodegeneration	temporally controllable, rapid onset phenotype, develops true NFT pathology, well-characterized	breeding complicated by need for two independent transgenes, 13-fold overexpression of tau protein	[67, 234, 235]
PS19	mid-life neurofibrillary tangles (6–9 mo), marked neurodegeneration	single-transgenic model, mid-life on set allows use in experiments expected to either delay or exacerbate pathology	transgene expression in spinal cord causes paralysis by mid-life	[236–238]
APP^{NLF}	mid-life amyloid pathology (~12 mo for homozygote, but note >24 mo for heterozygote allele)	endogenous APP level, native human Aβ sequence	limited cognitive impairment, requires homozygous allele for mid-life onset	[59, 239]
APP^{NLGF}	juvenile-onset amyloid pathology (~3–4 mo for homozygote, ~9 mo for heterozygote)	endogenous APP level, can be used as heterozygote	non-native Aβ sequence, mild cognitive phenotype	[60, 240]
hTau	mid-life hyperphosphorylated tau (~6 mo)	near-endogenous level expression of all 6 human wild-type tau isoforms	complicated breeding of transgene on null background, mild phenotype variable between colonies	[81, 82]
APOE2, E3, E4 Targeted replacement	allele-specific effects on Aβ, tau, brain atrophy, and neuroinflammation; both central and peripheral functions influenced by allele	widely-studied, expressed at endogenous levels, mouse ApoE deleted	cannot distinguish central vs. peripheral effects; available through Taconic but with restrictions on usage	[201, 241]

line was generated by the UC Davis KnockOut Mouse Project (KOMP) through targeted replacement of exons 2, 3, and most of 4 with a lacZ reporter and neomycin resistance cassette [206]. While the KOMP *Trem2* line has proven to be a true loss-of-function allele, the deletion results in upregulation of Treml1 which may complicate interpretation of resulting phenotypes [207]. In contrast, marginal Treml1 upregulation was detected in the Colonna line or in a new knock-out line from Jax made using CRISPR/Cas9 genome editing to delete a 175 base pair fragment and create a stop codon at amino acid 17 (Jax stock #027197). Jax has also created a Cre-conditional allele of *Trem2* by flanking exons 2 and 3 with loxP sites, which will allow peripheral vs. central effects of TREM2 to be dissected (Jax stock #029853). Finally, knock-in lines incorporating the R47H and Y38C (Jax stock #027918 and 029725) or T66M [208] variants have been generated. These mice will be valuable for investigating pathogenic mechanisms of TREM2 in both LOAD and Nasu-Hakola disease.

Conclusions

Although the neuropathology of AD had long been established, it was not until the discovery of familial mutations responsible for early-onset FAD and FTLD that mouse models capturing the hallmark features of AD became possible. Since the first amyloid model was published in 1995, many dozen more genetically engineered lines have been described with select aspects of AD neuropathology and downstream behavioral and degenerative phenotypes. It is our hope that this review presents an insightful and unbiased coverage of the pros and cons of the various AD mouse models as well as the practical considerations for choosing and using these models. To further facilitate the selection process, below we provide a summary for the most commonly used models (Table 6).

Genetics has been and will remain the driving factor in AD mouse model development. While studies of early-onset cases established the importance of neurons in APP/Aβ and tau/NFT pathology, more recent LOAD genes suggest a crucial role for non-neuronal cells, particularly microglia, in disease progression. Future studies would do well to consider changes in the immune system alongside those in neuropathology and cognition. Further, since the vast majority of AD cases arise not from autosomal dominant mutations but through the complex interaction of multiple genetic polymorphisms and environmental risk factors that accrue overtime, future modeling should also shift from single FAD gene targeting to simultaneous manipulation of multiple LOAD genes. With the advent of CRISPR-Cas9 genome editing and with investment from the National Institutes of Health towards resources such as MODEL-AD (https://model-ad.org), we expect major progress in this next phase of AD model development.

Abbreviations

3R/4R: Three-repeat or four-repeat tau protein; AD: Alzheimer's disease; ApoE: Apolipoprotein E; APP: Amyloid precursor protein; Aβ: Amyloid β peptide; Arc: Arctic (familial APP mutation); Aus: Austrian (familial APP mutation); BACE1: β-APP cleaving enzyme; CAA: Cerebral amyloid angiopathy; CAG: Cytomegalovirus immediate early enhancer combined with the chicken β-actin promoter; Camk2a: Calcium calmodulin kinase type IIα; CBA: Chicken β-actin; CMV: Cytomegalovirus; Dox: Doxycycline; FAD: Familial Alzheimer's disease; Flo: Florida (familial APP mutation); FTLD: Frontotemporal lobar degeneration; Ibe: Iberian (familial APP mutation); Ind: Indiana (familial APP mutation); Jax: The Jackson Laboratory; KI: Knock-in; Klk8: Kallikrein related-peptidase 8; KOMP: KnockOut Mouse Project; LOAD: Late-onset Alzheimer's disease; Lon: London (familial APP mutation); MAPT: Microtubule-associated protein tau; NEFH: Neurofilament heavy chain; NFT: Neurofibrillary tangle; PAC: P1-derived artificial chromosome; PDGFB: Platelet-derived growth factor B chain; Prnp: Prion protein; PSEN1 (or PS1): Presenilin 1; rtTA: Reverse tetracycline transactivator; Swe: Swedish (familial APP mutation); Thy1: Thymus cell surface antigen 1; TRE: Tetracycline response element; tTA: Tetracycline transactivator; TREM2: Triggering receptor expressed on myeloid cells 2; YAC: Yeast artificial chromosome

Acknowledgements
NA

Funding
This work was supported by NIH grants AG058188, AG056028, AG054160, and NS092615 (JLJ) and AG020670, AG032051, AG054111, and NS093652 (HZ).

Authors' contributions
JLJ and HZ both wrote, edited, and approved the final version of the manuscript.

Competing interests
The authors declare that they have no competing interests.

Author details
[1]Department of Neuroscience, Baylor College of Medicine, Houston, TX 77030, USA. [2]Department of Neurology, Baylor College of Medicine, Houston, TX 77030, USA. [3]Department of Neurosurgery, Baylor College of Medicine, Houston, TX 77030, USA. [4]Department of Molecular and Cellular Biology, Baylor College of Medicine, Houston, TX 77030, USA. [5]Huffington Center on Aging, Baylor College of Medicine, Houston, TX 77030, USA. [6]Department of Molecular and Human Genetics, Baylor College of Medicine, Houston, TX 77030, USA.

References

1. Goate A, Chartier-Harlin MC, Mullan M, Brown J, Crawford F, Fidani L, Giuffra L, Haynes A, Irving N, James L, et al. Segregation of a missense mutation in the amyloid precursor protein gene with familial Alzheimer's disease. Nature. 1991;349:704–6.
2. Games D, Adams D, Alessandrini R, Barbour R, Berthelette P, Blackwell C, Carr T, Clemens J, Donaldson T, Gillespie F, et al. Alzheimer-type neuropathology in transgenic mice overexpressing V717F beta-amyloid precursor protein. Nature. 1995;373:523–7.

3. Mullan M, Crawford F, Axelman K, Houlden H, Lilius L, Winblad B, Lannfelt L. A pathogenic mutation for probable Alzheimer's disease in the APP gene at the N-terminus of beta-amyloid. Nat Genet. 1992;1:345–7.
4. Citron M, Oltersdorf T, Haass C, McConlogue L, Hung AY, Seubert P, Vigo-Pelfrey C, Lieberburg I, Selkoe DJ. Mutation of the beta-amyloid precursor protein in familial Alzheimer's disease increases beta-protein production. Nature. 1992;360:672–4.
5. Murrell J, Farlow M, Ghett B, Benson MD. A mutation in the amyloid precursor protein associated with heridtary Alzheimer's disease. Science. 1991;254:97–9.
6. Eckman CB, Mehta ND, Crook R, Perez-tur J, Prihar G, Pfeiffer E, Graff-Radford N, Hinder P, Yager D, Zenk B, et al. A new pathogenic mutation in the APP gene (I716V) increases the relative proportion of a beta 42(43). Hum Mol Genet. 1997;6:2087–9.
7. Guerreiro RJ, Baquero M, Blesa R, Boada M, Bras JM, Bullido MJ, Calado A, Crook R, Ferreira C, Frank A, et al. Genetic screening of Alzheimer's disease genes in Iberian and African samples yields novel mutations in presenilins and APP. Neurobiol Aging. 2010;31:725–31.
8. Sherrington R, Rogaev EI, Liang Y, Rogaeva EA, Levesque G, Ikeda M, Chi H, Lin C, Li G, Holman K, et al. Cloning of a gene bearing missense mutations in early-onset familial Alzheimer's disease. Nature. 1995;375:754–60.
9. Alzheimer's Disease Collaborative G. The structure of the presenilin 1 (S182) gene and identification of six novel mutations in early onset AD families. Nat Genet. 1995;11:219–22.
10. Moehlmann T, Winkler E, Xia X, Edbauer D, Murrell J, Capell A, Kaether C, Zheng H, Ghetti B, Haass C, Steiner H. Presenilin-1 mutations of leucine 166 equally affect the generation of the notch and APP intracellular domains independent of their effect on Abeta 42 production. Proc Natl Acad Sci U S A. 2002;99:8025–30.
11. Perez-Tur J, Froelich S, Prihar G, Crook R, Baker M, Duff K, Wragg M, Busfield F, Lendon C, Clark RF, et al. A mutation in Alzheimer's disease destroying a splice acceptor site in the presenilin-1 gene. Neuroreport. 1995;7:297–301.
12. Van Broeckhoven C, Haan J, Bakker E, Hardy JA, Van Hul W, Wehnert A, Vegter-van der Vlis M, Roos RA. Amyloid beta protein precursor gene and hereditary cerebral hemorrhage with amyloidosis (Dutch). Science. 1990;248: 1120–2.
13. Levy E, Carman MD, Fernandez-Madrid IJ, Power MD, Lieberburg I, van Duinen SG, Bots GT, Luyendijk W, Frangione B. Mutation of the Alzheimer's disease amyloid gene in hereditary cerebral hemorrhage, Dutch type. Science. 1990;248:1124–6.
14. Kamino K, Orr HT, Payami H, Wijsman EM, Alonso ME, Pulst SM, Anderson L, O'Dahl S, Nemens E, White JA, et al. Linkage and mutational analysis of familial Alzheimer disease kindreds for the APP gene region. Am J Hum Genet. 1992;51:998–1014.
15. Nilsberth C, Westlind-Danielsson A, Eckman CB, Condron MM, Axelman K, Forsell C, Stenh C, Luthman J, Teplow DB, Younkin SG, et al. The 'Arctic' APP mutation (E693G) causes Alzheimer's disease by enhanced Abeta protofibril formation. Nat Neurosci. 2001;4:887–93.
16. Grabowski TJ, Cho HS, Vonsattel JP, Rebeck GW, Greenberg SM. Novel amyloid precursor protein mutation in an Iowa family with dementia and severe cerebral amyloid angiopathy. Ann Neurol. 2001;49:697–705.
17. Cai H, Wang Y, McCarthy D, Wen H, Borchelt DR, Price DL, Wong PC. BACE1 is the major beta-secretase for generation of Abeta peptides by neurons. Nat Neurosci. 2001;4:233–4.
18. Xu G, Ran Y, Fromholt SE, Fu C, Yachnis AT, Golde TE, Borchelt DR. Murine Abeta over-production produces diffuse and compact Alzheimer-type amyloid deposits. Acta Neuropathol Commun. 2015;3:72.
19. Drummond E, Wisniewski T. Alzheimer's disease: experimental models and reality. Acta Neuropathol. 2017;133:155–75.
20. Giannakopoulos P, Herrmann FR, Bussiere T, Bouras C, Kovari E, Perl DP, Morrison JH, Gold G, Hof PR. Tangle and neuron numbers, but not amyloid load, predict cognitive status in Alzheimer's disease. Neurology. 2003;60: 1495–500.
21. Mandelkow EM, Mandelkow E. Biochemistry and cell biology of tau protein in neurofibrillary degeneration. Cold Spring Harb. Perspect. Med. 2012;2:a006247.
22. Lee VM, Goedert M, Trojanowski JQ. Neurodegenerative tauopathies. Annu Rev Neurosci. 2001;24:1121–59.
23. Braak H, Braak E. Staging of Alzheimer's disease-related neurofibrillary changes. Neurobiol Aging. 1995;16:271–8. discussion 278-284
24. Goedert M, Eisenberg DS, Crowther RA. Propagation of tau aggregates and Neurodegeneration. Annu Rev Neurosci. 2017;40:189–210.
25. Gendron TF, Petrucelli L. The role of tau in neurodegeneration. Mol Neurodegener. 2009;4:13.
26. Hong M, Zhukareva V, Vogelsberg-Ragaglia V, Wszolek Z, Reed L, Miller BI, Geschwind DH, Bird TD, McKeel D, Goate A, et al. Mutation-specific functional impairments in distinct tau isoforms of hereditary FTDP-17. Science. 1998;282:1914–7.
27. Hutton M, Lendon CL, Rizzu P, Baker M, Froelich S, Houlden H, Pickering-Brown S, Chakraverty S, Isaacs A, Grover A, et al. Association of missense and 5′-splice-site mutations in tau with the inherited dementia FTDP-17. Nature. 1998;393:702–5.
28. Ramsden M, Kotilinek L, Forster C, Paulson J, McGowan E, SantaCruz K, Guimaraes A, Yue M, Lewis J, Carlson G, et al. Age-dependent neurofibrillary tangle formation, neuron loss, and memory impairment in a mouse model of human tauopathy (P301L). J Neurosci. 2005;25:10637–47.
29. SantaCruz K, Lewis J, Spires T, Paulson J, Kotilinek L, Ingelsson M, Guimaraes A, DeTure M, Ramsden M, McGowan E, et al. Tau suppression in a neurodegenerative mouse model improves memory function. Science. 2005;309:476–81.
30. Yasuda M, Johnson-Venkatesh EM, Zhang H, Parent JM, Sutton MA, Umemori H. Multiple forms of activity-dependent competition refine hippocampal circuits in vivo. Neuron. 2011;70:1128–42.
31. Liu L, Drouet V, Wu JW, Witter MP, Small SA, Clelland C, Duff K. Trans-synaptic spread of tau pathology in vivo. PLoS One. 2012;7:e31302.
32. de Calignon A, Polydoro M, Suarez-Calvet M, William C, Adamowicz DH, Kopeikina KJ, Pitstick R, Sahara N, Ashe KH, Carlson GA, et al. Propagation of tau pathology in a model of early Alzheimer's disease. Neuron. 2012;73:685–97.
33. Yoshiyama Y, Higuchi M, Zhang B, Huang SM, Iwata N, Saido TC, Maeda J, Suhara T, Trojanowski JQ, Lee VM. Synapse loss and microglial activation precede tangles in a P301S tauopathy mouse model. Neuron. 2007;53:337–51.
34. Lewis J, McGowan E, Rockwood J, Melrose H, Nacharaju P, Van Slegtenhorst M, Gwinn-Hardy K, Paul Murphy M, Baker M, Yu X, et al. Neurofibrillary tangles, amyotrophy and progressive motor disturbance in mice expressing mutant (P301L) tau protein. Nat Genet. 2000;25:402–5.
35. Iba M, Guo JL, McBride JD, Zhang B, Trojanowski JQ, Lee VM. Synthetic tau fibrils mediate transmission of neurofibrillary tangles in a transgenic mouse model of Alzheimer's-like tauopathy. J Neurosci. 2013;33:1024–37.
36. Holmes BB, Furman JL, Mahan TE, Yamasaki TR, Mirbaha H, Eades WC, Belaygorod L, Cairns NJ, Holtzman DM, Diamond MI. Proteopathic tau seeding predicts tauopathy in vivo. Proc Natl Acad Sci U S A. 2014;111:E4376–85.
37. Andorfer C, Kress Y, Espinoza M, de Silva R, Tucker KL, Barde YA, Duff K, Davies P. Hyperphosphorylation and aggregation of tau in mice expressing normal human tau isoforms. J Neurochem. 2003;86:582–90.
38. Polydoro M, Acker CM, Duff K, Castillo PE, Davies P. Age-dependent impairment of cognitive and synaptic function in the htau mouse model of tau pathology. J Neurosci. 2009;29:10741–9.
39. Guo Q, Li H, Cole AL, Hur JY, Li Y, Zheng H. Modeling Alzheimer's disease in mouse without mutant protein Overexpression: cooperative and independent effects of Abeta and tau. PLoS One. 2013;8:e80706.
40. Yetman MJ, Fowler SW, Jankowsky JL. Humanized tau mice with regionalized Amyloid exhibit behavioral deficits but no pathological interaction. PLoS One. 2016;11:e0153724.
41. Spires TL, Orne JD, SantaCruz K, Pitstick R, Carlson GA, Ashe KH, Hyman BT. Region-specific dissociation of neuronal loss and neurofibrillary pathology in a mouse model of tauopathy. Am J Pathol. 2006;168:1598–607.
42. Andorfer C, Acker CM, Kress Y, Hof PR, Duff K, Davies P. Cell-cycle reentry and cell death in transgenic mice expressing nonmutant human tau isoforms. J Neurosci. 2005;25:5446–54.
43. Calhoun ME, Wiederhold KH, Abramowski D, Phinney AL, Probst A, Sturchler-Pierrat C, Staufenbiel M, Sommer B, Jucker M. Neuron loss in APP transgenic mice. Nature. 1998;395:755–6.
44. Bondolfi L, Calhoun M, Ermini F, Kuhn HG, Wiederhold KH, Walker L, Staufenbiel M, Jucker M. Amyloid-associated neuron loss and gliogenesis in the neocortex of amyloid precursor protein transgenic mice. J Neurosci. 2002;22:515–22.
45. Schmitz C, Rutten BP, Pielen A, Schafer S, Wirths O, Tremp G, Czech C, Blanchard V, Multhaup G, Rezaie P, et al. Hippocampal neuron loss exceeds amyloid plaque load in a transgenic mouse model of Alzheimer's disease. Am J Pathol. 2004;164:1495–502.
46. Casas C, Sergeant N, Itier JM, Blanchard V, Wirths O, van der Kolk N, Vingtdeux V, van de Steeg E, Ret G, Canton T, et al. Massive CA1/2 neuronal loss with intraneuronal and N-terminal truncated Abeta42 accumulation in a novel Alzheimer transgenic model. Am J Pathol. 2004;165:1289–300.

47. Oakley H, Cole SL, Logan S, Maus E, Shao P, Craft J, Guillozet-Bongaarts A, Ohno M, Disterhoft J, Van Eldik L, et al. Intraneuronal β-amyloid aggregates, neurodegeneration, and neuron loss in transgenic mice with five famlial alzheimer's disease mutations: potential factors in amyloid plaque formation. J Neurosci. 2006;26:10129–40.
48. Jawhar S, Trawicka A, Jenneckens C, Bayer TA, Wirths O. Motor deficits, neuron loss, and reduced anxiety coinciding with axonal degeneration and intraneuronal Abeta aggregation in the 5XFAD mouse model of Alzheimer's disease. Neurobiol Aging. 2012;33:196 e129–40.
49. Eimer WA, Vassar R. Neuron loss in the 5XFAD mouse model of Alzheimer's disease correlates with intraneuronal Abeta42 accumulation and Caspase-3 activation. Mol Neurodegener. 2013;8:2.
50. Webster SJ, Bachstetter AD, Nelson PT, Schmitt FA, Van Eldik LJ. Using mice to model Alzheimer's dementia: an overview of the clinical disease and the preclinical behavioral changes in 10 mouse models. Front Genet. 2014;5:88.
51. Chishti MA, Yang DS, Janus C, Phinney AL, Horne P, Pearson J, Strome R, Zuker N, Loukides J, French J, et al. Early-onset amyloid deposition and cognitive deficits in transgenic mice expressing a double mutant form of amyloid precursor protein 695. J Biol Chem. 2001;276:21562–70.
52. Lesne S, Koh MT, Kotilinek L, Kayed R, Glabe CG, Yang A, Gallagher M, Ashe KH. A specific amyloid-beta protein assembly in the brain impairs memory. Nature. 2006;440:352–7.
53. Westerman MA, Cooper-Blacketer D, Mariash A, Kotilinek L, Kawarabayashi T, Younkin LH, Carlson GA, Younkin SG, Ashe KH. The relationship between Abeta and memory in the Tg2576 mouse model of Alzheimer's disease. J Neurosci. 2002;22:1858–67.
54. Mucke L, Masliah E, Yu GQ, Mallory M, Rockenstein EM, Tatsuno G, Hu K, Kholodenko D, Johnson-Wood K, McConlogue L. High-level neuronal expression of A-beta 1-42 in wild-type human amyloid protein precursor transgenic mice: synaptotoxicity without plaque formation. J Neurosci. 2000; 20:4050–8.
55. Karl T, Bhatia S, Cheng D, Kim WS, Garner B. Cognitive phenotyping of amyloid precursor protein transgenic J20 mice. Behav Brain Res. 2012;228:392–7.
56. Webster SJ, Bachstetter AD, Van Eldik LJ. Comprehensive behavioral characterization of an APP/PS-1 double knock-in mouse model of Alzheimer's disease. Alzheimers Res Ther. 2013;5:28.
57. Li H, Guo Q, Inoue T, Polito VA, Tabuchi K, Hammer RE, Pautler RG, Taffet GE, Zheng H. Vascular and parenchymal amyloid pathology in an Alzheimer disease knock-in mouse model: interplay with cerebral blood flow. Mol Neurodegener. 2014;9:28.
58. Saito T, Matsuba Y, Mihira N, Takano J, Nilsson P, Itohara S, Iwata N, Saido TC. Single app knock-in mouse models of Alzheimer's disease. Nat Neurosci. 2014; 17:661–3.
59. Masuda A, Kobayashi Y, Kogo N, Saito T, Saido TC, Itohara S. Cognitive deficits in single app knock-in mouse models. Neurobiol Learn Mem. 2016;135:73–82.
60. Whyte LS, Hemsley KM, Lau AA, Hassiotis S, Saito T, Saido TC, Hopwood JJ, Sargeant TJ. Reduction in open field activity in the absence of memory deficits in the AppNL-G-F knock-in mouse model of Alzheimer's disease. Behav Brain Res. 2018;336:177–81.
61. Brunden KR, Zhang B, Carroll J, Yao Y, Potuzak JS, Hogan AM, Iba M, James MJ, Xie SX, Ballatore C, et al. Epothilone D improves microtubule density, axonal integrity, and cognition in a transgenic mouse model of tauopathy. J Neurosci. 2010;30:13861–6.
62. Takeuchi H, Iba M, Inoue H, Higuchi M, Takao K, Tsukita K, Karatsu Y, Iwamoto Y, Miyakawa T, Suhara T, et al. P301S mutant human tau transgenic mice manifest early symptoms of human tauopathies with dementia and altered sensorimotor gating. PLoS One. 2011;6:e21050.
63. Zhang B, Carroll J, Trojanowski JQ, Yao Y, Iba M, Potuzak JS, Hogan AM, Xie SX, Ballatore C, Smith AB 3rd, et al. The microtubule-stabilizing agent, epothilone D, reduces axonal dysfunction, neurotoxicity, cognitive deficits, and Alzheimer-like pathology in an interventional study with aged tau transgenic mice. J Neurosci. 2012;32:3601–11.
64. Geiszler PC, Barron MR, Pardon MC. Impaired burrowing is the most prominent behavioral deficit of aging htau mice. Neuroscience. 2016;329:98–111.
65. Morgan D, Munireddy S, Alamed J, DeLeon J, Diamond DM, Bickford P, Hutton M, Lewis J, McGowan E, Gordon MN. Apparent behavioral benefits of tau overexpression in P301L tau transgenic mice. J. Alzheimers Dis. 2008;15:605–14.
66. Arendash GW, Lewis J, Leighty RE, McGowan E, Cracchiolo JR, Hutton M, Garcia MF. Multi-metric behavioral comparison of APPsw and P301L models for Alzheimer's disease: linkage of poorer cognitive performance to tau pathology in forebrain. Brain Res. 2004;1012:29–41.
67. Polito VA, Li H, Martini-Stoica H, Wang B, Yang L, Xu Y, Swartzlander DB, Palmieri M, di Ronza A, Lee VM, et al. Selective clearance of aberrant tau proteins and rescue of neurotoxicity by transcription factor EB. EMBO Mol. Med. 2014;6:1142–60.
68. Condello C, Yuan P, Schain A, Grutzendler J. Microglia constitute a barrier that prevents neurotoxic protofibrillar Abeta42 hotspots around plaques. Nat Commun. 2015;6:6176.
69. Jankowsky JL, Slunt HH, Gonzales V, Savonenko AV, Wen JC, Jenkins NA, Copeland NG, Younkin LH, Lester HA, Younkin SG, Borchelt DR. Persistent amyloidosis following suppression of Aβ production in a transgenic model of Alzheimer's disease. PLoS medicine. 2005;2:e355.
70. Rodgers SP, Born HA, Das P, Jankowsky JL. Transgenic APP expression during postnatal development causes persistent locomotor hyperactivity in the adult. Mol Neurodegener. 2012;7:28.
71. Born HA, Kim JY, Savjani RR, Das P, Dabaghian YA, Guo Q, Yoo JW, Schuler DR, Cirrito JR, Zheng H, et al. Genetic suppression of transgenic APP rescues hypersynchronous network activity in a mouse model of Alzeimer's disease. J Neurosci. 2014;34:3826–40.
72. van der Kant R, Goldstein LS. Cellular functions of the amyloid precursor protein from development to dementia. Dev Cell. 2015;32:502–15.
73. Zheng H, Koo EH. Biology and pathophysiology of the amyloid precursor protein. Mol Neurodegener. 2011;6:27.
74. Dawkins E, Small DH. Insights into the physiological function of the beta-amyloid precursor protein: beyond Alzheimer's disease. J Neurochem. 2014;129:756–69.
75. Muller UC, Deller T, Korte M. Not just amyloid: physiological functions of the amyloid precursor protein family. Nat Rev Neurosci. 2017;18:281–98.
76. Sasaguri H, Nilsson P, Hashimoto S, Nagata K, Saito T, De Strooper B, Hardy J, Vassar R, Winblad B, Saido TC. APP mouse models for Alzheimer's disease preclinical studies. EMBO J. 2017;36:2473–87.
77. Nakazono T, Lam TN, Patel AY, Kitazawa M, Saito T, Saido TC, Igarashi KM. Impaired in vivo gamma oscillations in the medial Entorhinal cortex of knock-in Alzheimer model. Front Syst Neurosci. 2017;11:48.
78. Malthankar-Phatak G, Poplawski S, Toraskar N, Siman R. Combination therapy prevents amyloid-dependent and -independent structural changes. Neurobiol Aging. 2012;33:1273–83.
79. Zhang C, McNeil E, Dressler L, Siman R. Long-lasting impairment in hippocampal neurogenesis associated with amyloid deposition in a knock-in mouse model of familial Alzheimer's disease. Exp Neurol. 2007;204:77–87.
80. Saito T, Matsuba Y, Yamazaki N, Hashimoto S, Saido TC. Calpain activation in Alzheimer's model mice is an artifact of APP and Presenilin Overexpression. J Neurosci. 2016;36:9933–6.
81. Bhaskar K, Konerth M, Kokiko-Cochran ON, Cardona A, Ransohoff RM, Lamb BT. Regulation of tau pathology by the microglial fractalkine receptor. Neuron. 2010;68:19–31.
82. Maphis N, Xu G, Kokiko-Cochran ON, Jiang S, Cardona A, Ransohoff RM, Lamb BT, Bhaskar K. Reactive microglia drive tau pathology and contribute to the spreading of pathological tau in the brain. Brain. 2015;138:1738–55.
83. Ojo JO, Mouzon B, Greenberg MB, Bachmeier C, Mullan M, Crawford F. Repetitive mild traumatic brain injury augments tau pathology and glial activation in aged hTau mice. J Neuropathol Exp Neurol. 2013;72:137–51.
84. Alldred MJ, Duff KE, Ginsberg SD. Microarray analysis of CA1 pyramidal neurons in a mouse model of tauopathy reveals progressive synaptic dysfunction. Neurobiol Dis. 2012;45:751–62.
85. Dickstein DL, Brautigam H, Stockton SD Jr, Schmeidler J, Hof PR. Changes in dendritic complexity and spine morphology in transgenic mice expressing human wild-type tau. Brain Struct Funct. 2010;214:161–79.
86. Lamb BT, Call LM, Slunt HH, Bardel KA, Lawler AM, Eckman CB, Younkin SG, Holtz G, Wagner SL, Price DL, et al. Altered metabolism of familial Alzheimer's disease-linked amyloid precursor protein variants in yeast artificial chromosome transgenic mice. Hum Mol Genet. 1997;6:1535–41.
87. Duff K, Knight H, Refolo LM, Sanders S, Yu X, Picciano M, Malester B, Hutton M, Adamson J, Goedert M, et al. Characterization of pathology in transgenic mice over-expressing human genomic and cDNA tau transgenes. Neurobiol Dis. 2000;7:87–98.
88. Lamb BT, Sisodia SS, Lawler AM, Slunt HH, Kitt CA, Kearns WG, Pearson PL, Price DL, Gearhart JD. Introduction and expression of the 400 kilobase amyloid precursor protein gene in transgenic mice [corrected]. Nat Genet. 1993;5:22–30.
89. Reaume AG, Howland DS, Trusko SP, Savage MJ, Lang DM, Greenberg BD, Siman R, Scott RW. Enhanced amyloidogenic processing of the beta-amyloid precursor protein in gene-targeted mice bearing the Swedish familial Alzheimer's disease mutations and a "humanized" Abeta sequence. J Biol Chem. 1996;271:23380–8.

90. Flood DG, Reaume AG, Dorfman KS, Lin YG, Lang DM, Trusko SP, Savage MJ, Annaert WG, De Strooper B, Siman R, Scott RW. FAD mutant PS-1 gene-targeted mice: increased a beta 42 and a beta deposition without APP overproduction. Neurobiol Aging. 2002;23:335–48.
91. Chang EH, Savage MJ, Flood DG, Thomas JM, Levy RB, Mahadomrongkul V, Shirao T, Aoki C, Huerta PT. AMPA receptor downscaling at the onset of Alzheimer's disease pathology in double knockin mice. Proc Natl Acad Sci U S A. 2006;103:3410–5.
92. Kohler C, Ebert U, Baumann K, Schroder H. Alzheimer's disease-like neuropathology of gene-targeted APP-SLxPS1mut mice expressing the amyloid precursor protein at endogenous levels. Neurobiol Dis. 2005; 20:528–40.
93. Tsubuki S, Takaki Y, Saido TC. Dutch, Flemish, Italian, and Arctic mutations of APP and resistance of Abeta to physiologically relevant proteolytic degradation. Lancet. 2003;361:1957–8.
94. Sisodia SS, Koo EH, Hoffman PN, Perry G, Price DL. Identification and transport of full-length amyloid precursor proteins in rat peripheral nervous system. J Neurosci. 1993;13:3136–42.
95. Hsiao K, Chapman P, Nilsen S, Eckman C, Harigaya Y, Younkin S, Yang F, Cole G. Correlative memory deficits, Abeta elevation, and amyloid plaques in transgenic mice. Science. 1996;274:99–102.
96. Borchelt DR, Thinakaran G, Eckman CB, Lee MK, Davenport F, Ratovitsky T, Prada CM, Kim G, Seekins S, Yager D, et al. Familial Alzheimer's disease-linked presenilin 1 variants elevate Abeta1-42/1-40 ratio in vitro and in vivo. Neuron. 1996;17:1005–13.
97. Rockenstein EM, McConlogue L, Tan H, Power M, Masliah E, Mucke L. Levels and alternative splicing of amyloid beta protein precursor (APP) transcripts in brains of APP transgenic mice and humans with Alzheimer's disease. J Biol Chem. 1995;270:28257–67.
98. Espinoza M, de Silva R, Dickson DW, Davies P. Differential incorporation of tau isoforms in Alzheimer's disease. J. Alzheimers Dis. 2008;14:1–16.
99. Jankowsky JL, Fadale DJ, Anderson J, Xu GM, Gonzales V, Jenkins NA, Copeland NG, Lee MK, Younkin LH, Wagner SL, et al. Mutant presenilins specifically elevate the levels of the 42 residue β-amyloid peptide in vivo: evidence for augmentation of a 42-specific γ-secretase. Hum Mol Genet. 2004;13:159–70.
100. Sturchler-Pierrat C, Abramowski D, Duke M, Wiederhold KH, Mistl C, Rothacher S, Ledermann B, Burki K, Frey P, Paganetti PA, et al. Two amyloid precursor protein transgenic mouse models with Alzheimer disease-like pathology. Proc Natl Acad Sci U S A. 1997;94:13287–92.
101. Oddo S, Caccamo A, Shepherd JD, Murphy MP, Golde TE, Kayed R, Metherate R, Mattson MP, Akbari Y, LaFerla FM. Triple-transgenic model of Alzheimer's disease with plaques and tangles: intracellular Abeta and synaptic dysfunction. Neuron. 2003;39:409–21.
102. Lesuisse C, Xu G, Anderson J, Wong M, Jankowsky J, Holtz G, Gonzalez V, Wong PC, Price DL, Tang F, et al. Hyper-expression of human apolipoprotein E4 in astroglia and neurons does not enhance amyloid deposition in transgenic mice. Hum Mol Genet. 2001;10:2525–37.
103. Campsall KD, Mazerolle CJ, De Repentingy Y, Kothary R, Wallace VA. Characterization of transgene expression and Cre recombinase activity in a panel of Thy-1 promoter-Cre transgenic mice. Dev. Dyn. 2002;224:135–43.
104. Borchelt DR, Davis J, Fischer M, Lee MK, Slunt HH, Ratovitsky T, Regard J, Copeland NG, Jenkins NA, Sisodia SS, Price DL. A vector for expressing foreign genes in the brains and hearts of transgenic mice. Genet Anal. 1996; 13:159–63.
105. Sasahara M, Fries JW, Raines EW, Gown AM, Westrum LE, Frosch MP, Bonthron DT, Ross R, Collins T. PDGF B-chain in neurons of the central nervous system, posterior pituitary, and in a transgenic model. Cell. 1991;64:217–27.
106. Davis JA, Naruse S, Chen H, Eckman C, Younkin S, Price DL, Borchelt DR, Sisodia SS, Wong PC. An Alzheimer's disease-linked PS1 variant rescues the developmental abnormalities of PS1-deficient embryos. Neuron. 1998;20:603–9.
107. Lee WC, Huang H, Feng G, Sanes JR, Brown EN, So PT, Nedivi E. Dynamic remodeling of dendritic arbors in GABAergic interneurons of adult visual cortex. PLoS Biol. 2006;4:e29.
108. O'Mahony A, Raber J, Montano M, Foehr E, Han V, Lu SM, Kwon H, LeFevour A, Chakraborty-Sett S, Greene WC. NF-kappaB/Rel regulates inhibitory and excitatory neuronal function and synaptic plasticity. Mol Cell Biol. 2006;26:7283–98.
109. van den Pol AN, Ghosh PK, Liu RJ, Li Y, Aghajanian GK, Gao XB. Hypocretin (orexin) enhances neuron activity and cell synchrony in developing mouse GFP-expressing locus coeruleus. J Physiol. 2002;541:169–85.
110. Hantman AW, van den Pol AN, Perl ER. Morphological and physiological features of a set of spinal substantia gelatinosa neurons defined by green fluorescent protein expression. J Neurosci. 2004;24:836–42.
111. Setsuie R, Wang YL, Mochizuki H, Osaka H, Hayakawa H, Ichihara N, Li H, Furuta A, Sano Y, Sun YJ, et al. Dopaminergic neuronal loss in transgenic mice expressing the Parkinson's disease-associated UCH-L1 I93M mutant. Neurochem Int. 2007;50:119–29.
112. Feng G, Mellor RH, Bernstein M, Keller-Peck C, Nguyen QT, Wallace M, Nerbonne JM, Lichtman JW, Sanes JR. Imaging neuronal subsets in transgenic mice expressing multiple spectral variants of GFP. Neuron. 2000;28:41–51.
113. Jankowsky JL, Slunt HH, Ratovitski T, Jenkins NA, Copeland NG, Borchelt DR. Co-expression of multiple transgenes in mouse CNS: a comparison of strategies. Biomol Eng. 2001;17:157–65.
114. Carlson GA, Borchelt DR, Dake A, Turner S, Danielson V, Coffin JD, Eckman C, Meiners J, Nilsen SP, Younkin SG, Hsiao KK. Genetic modification of the phenotypes produced by amyloid precursor protein overexpression in transgenic mice. Hum Mol Genet. 1997;6:1951–9.
115. Lehman EJ, Kulnane LS, Gao Y, Petriello MC, Pimpis KM, Younkin L, Dolios G, Wang R, Younkin SG, Lamb BT. Genetic background regulates beta-amyloid precursor protein processing and beta-amyloid deposition in the mouse. Hum Mol Genet. 2003;12:2949–56.
116. Jackson HM, Onos KD, Pepper KW, Graham LC, Akeson EC, Byers C, Reinholdt LG, Frankel WN, Howell GR. DBA/2J genetic background exacerbates spontaneous lethal seizures but lessens amyloid deposition in a mouse model of Alzheimer's disease. PLoS One. 2015;10:e0125897.
117. Ryman D, Gao Y, Lamb BT. Genetic loci modulating amyloid-beta levels in a mouse model of Alzheimer's disease. Neurobiol Aging. 2008;29:1190–8.
118. Morihara T, Hayashi N, Yokokoji M, Akatsu H, Silverman MA, Kimura N, Sato M, Saito Y, Suzuki T, Yanagida K, et al. Transcriptome analysis of distinct mouse strains reveals kinesin light chain-1 splicing as an amyloid-beta accumulation modifier. Proc Natl Acad Sci U S A. 2014;111:2638–43.
119. Borchelt DR, Ratovitski T, van Lare J, Lee MK, Gonzales V, Jenkins NA, Copeland NG, Price DL, Sisodia SS. Accelerated amyloid deposition in the brains of transgenic mice coexpressing mutant presenilin 1 and amyloid precursor proteins. Neuron. 1997;19:939–45.
120. Callahan MJ, Lipinski WJ, Bian F, Durham RA, Pack A, Walker LC. Augmented senile plaque load in aged female beta-amyloid precursor protein-transgenic mice. Am J Pathol. 2001;158:1173–7.
121. Gallagher JJ, Minogue AM, Lynch MA. Impaired performance of female APP/PS1 mice in the Morris water maze is coupled with increased Abeta accumulation and microglial activation. Neurodegener Dis. 2013;11:33–41.
122. Jiao SS, Bu XL, Liu YH, Zhu C, Wang QH, Shen LL, Liu CH, Wang YR, Yao XQ, Wang YJ. Sex dimorphism profile of Alzheimer's disease-type pathologies in an APP/PS1 mouse model. Neurotox Res. 2016;29:256–66.
123. Wang J, Tanila H, Puolivali J, Kadish I, van Groen T. Gender differences in the amount and deposition of amyloidbeta in APPswe and PS1 double transgenic mice. Neurobiol Dis. 2003;14:318–27.
124. Hirata-Fukae C, Li HF, Hoe HS, Gray AJ, Minami SS, Hamada K, Niikura T, Hua F, Tsukagoshi-Nagai H, Horikoshi-Sakuraba Y, et al. Females exhibit more extensive amyloid, but not tau, pathology in an Alzheimer transgenic model. Brain Res. 2008;1216:92–103.
125. Melnikova T, Fromholt S, Kim H, Lee D, Xu G, Price A, Moore BD, Golde TE, Felsenstein KM, Savonenko A, Borchelt DR. Reversible pathologic and cognitive phenotypes in an inducible model of Alzheimer-amyloidosis. J Neurosci. 2013;33:3765–79.
126. Schafer S, Wirths O, Multhaup G, Bayer TA. Gender dependent APP processing in a transgenic mouse model of Alzheimer's disease. J Neural Transm (Vienna). 2007;114:387–94.
127. Yue M, Hanna A, Wilson J, Roder H, Janus C. Sex difference in pathology and memory decline in rTg4510 mouse model of tauopathy. Neurobiol Aging. 2011;32:590–603.
128. Asuni AA, Boutajangout A, Quartermain D, Sigurdsson EM. Immunotherapy targeting pathological tau conformers in a tangle mouse model reduces brain pathology with associated functional improvements. J Neurosci. 2007; 27:9115–29.
129. Buccarello L, Grignaschi G, Castaldo AM, Di Giancamillo A, Domeneghini C, Melcangi RC, Borsello T. Sex impact on tau-aggregation and postsynaptic protein levels in the P301L mouse model of Tauopathy. J. Alzheimers Dis. 2017;56:1279–92.
130. Clinton LK, Billings LM, Green KN, Caccamo A, Ngo J, Oddo S, McGaugh JL, LaFerla FM. Age-dependent sexual dimorphism in cognition and stress response in the 3xTg-AD mice. Neurobiol Dis. 2007;28:76–82.

131. King DL, Arendash GW, Crawford F, Sterk T, Menendez J, Mullan MJ. Progressive and gender-dependent cognitive impairment in the APP(SW) transgenic mouse model for Alzheimer's disease. Behav Brain Res. 1999;103:145–62.
132. Granger MW, Franko B, Taylor MW, Messier C, George-Hyslop PS, Bennett SA. A TgCRND8 mouse model of Alzheimer's disease exhibits sexual dimorphisms in behavioral indices of cognitive reserve. J. Alzheimers Dis. 2016;51:757–73.
133. Devi L, Alldred MJ, Ginsberg SD, Ohno M. Sex- and brain region-specific acceleration of beta-amyloidogenesis following behavioral stress in a mouse model of Alzheimer's disease. Mol Brain. 2010;3:34.
134. Sotiropoulos I, Silva J, Kimura T, Rodrigues AJ, Costa P, Almeida OF, Sousa N, Takashima A. Female hippocampus vulnerability to environmental stress, a precipitating factor in tau aggregation pathology. J. Alzheimers Dis. 2015;43:763–74.
135. Gimenez-Llort L, Arranz L, Mate I, De la Fuente M. Gender-specific neuroimmunoendocrine aging in a triple-transgenic 3xTg-AD mouse model for Alzheimer's disease and its relation with longevity. Neuroimmunomodulation. 2008;15:331–43.
136. Alzheimer'sAssociation. Alzheimer's disease facts and figures. Alzheimers Dement. 2017;2017(13):325–73.
137. Lawlor PA, Bland RJ, Das P, Price RW, Holloway V, Smithson L, Dicker BL, During MJ, Young D, Golde TE. Novel rat Alzheimer's disease models based on AAV-mediated gene transfer to selectively increase hippocampal Abeta levels. Mol Neurodegener. 2007;2:11.
138. Koukouli F, Rooy M, Maskos U. Early and progressive deficit of neuronal activity patterns in a model of local amyloid pathology in mouse prefrontal cortex. Aging (Albany NY). 2016;8:3430–49.
139. Cubinkova V, Valachova B, Brezovakova V, Szabo R, Zimova I, Kostecka Z, Jadhav S. Next generation tau models in Alzheimer's disease research - virus based gene delivery systems. Acta Virol. 2017;61:13–21.
140. Caillierez R, Begard S, Lecolle K, Deramecourt V, Zommer N, Dujardin S, Loyens A, Dufour N, Auregan G, Winderickx J, et al. Lentiviral delivery of the human wild-type tau protein mediates a slow and progressive neurodegenerative tau pathology in the rat brain. Mol. Ther. 2013;21:1358–68.
141. Osinde M, Clavaguera F, May-Nass R, Tolnay M, Dev KK. Lentivirus tau (P301S) expression in adult amyloid precursor protein (APP)-transgenic mice leads to tangle formation. Neuropathol Appl Neurobiol. 2008;34:523–31.
142. Klein RL, Lin WL, Dickson DW, Lewis J, Hutton M, Duff K, Meyer EM, King MA. Rapid neurofibrillary tangle formation after localized gene transfer of mutated tau. Am J Pathol. 2004;164:347–53.
143. Cook C, Kang SS, Carlomagno Y, Lin WL, Yue M, Kurti A, Shinohara M, Jansen-West K, Perkerson E, Castanedes-Casey M, et al. Tau deposition drives neuropathological, inflammatory and behavioral abnormalities independently of neuronal loss in a novel mouse model. Hum Mol Genet. 2015;24:6198–212.
144. Furth PA, St Onge L, Boger H, Gruss P, Gossen M, Kistner A, Bujard H, Hennighausen L. Temporal control of gene expression in transgenic mice by a tetracycline-responsive promoter. Proc Natl Acad Sci U S A. 1994;91:9302–6.
145. Urlinger S, Baron U, Thellmann M, Hasan MT, Bujard H, Hillen W. Exploring the sequence space for tetracycline-dependent transcriptional activators: novel mutations yield expanded range and sensitivity. Proc Natl Acad Sci U S A. 2000;97:7963–8.
146. Mayford M, Bach ME, Huang YY, Wang L, Hawkins RD, Kandel ER. Control of memory formation through regulated expression of a CaMKII transgene. Science. 1996;274:1678–83.
147. Walker AK, Spiller KJ, Ge G, Zheng A, Xu Y, Zhou M, Tripathy K, Kwong LK, Trojanowski JQ, Lee VM. Functional recovery in new mouse models of ALS/FTLD after clearance of pathological cytoplasmic TDP-43. Acta Neuropathol. 2015;130:643–60.
148. Wang L, Sharma K, Deng HX, Siddique T, Grisotti G, Liu E, Roos RP. Restricted expression of mutant SOD1 in spinal motor neurons and interneurons induces motor neuron pathology. Neurobiol Dis. 2008;29:400–8.
149. Li L, Tasic B, Micheva KD, Ivanov VM, Spletter ML, Smith SJ, Luo L. Visualizing the distribution of synapses from individual neurons in the mouse brain. PLoS One. 2010;5:e11503.
150. Madisen L, Garner AR, Shimaoka D, Chuong AS, Klapoetke NC, Li L, van der Bourg A, Niino Y, Egolf L, Monetti C, et al. Transgenic mice for intersectional targeting of neural sensors and effectors with high specificity and performance. Neuron. 2015;85:942–58.
151. Hochedlinger K, Yamada Y, Beard C, Jaenisch R. Ectopic expression of Oct-4 blocks progenitor-cell differentiation and causes dysplasia in epithelial tissues. Cell. 2005;121:465–77.
152. Premsrirut PK, Dow LE, Kim SY, Camiolo M, Malone CD, Miething C, Scuoppo C, Zuber J, Dickins RA, Kogan SC, et al. A rapid and scalable system for studying gene function in mice using conditional RNA interference. Cell. 2011;145:145–58.
153. Yamamoto M, Wada N, Kitabatake Y, Watanabe D, Anzai M, Yokoyama M, Teranishi Y, Nakanishi S. Reversible suppression of glutamatergic neurotransmission of cerebellar granule cells in vivo by genetically manipulated expression of tetanus neurotoxin light chain. J Neurosci. 2003;23:6759–67.
154. Tsunemi T, Ashe TD, Morrison BE, Soriano KR, Au J, Roque RA, Lazarowski ER, Damian VA, Masliah E, La Spada AR. PGC-1alpha rescues Huntington's disease proteotoxicity by preventing oxidative stress and promoting TFEB function. Sci. Transl. Med. 2012;4:142ra197.
155. Liu P, Paulson JB, Forster CL, Shapiro SL, Ashe KH, Zahs KR. Characterization of a novel mouse model of Alzheimer's disease–Amyloid pathology and unique beta-Amyloid Oligomer profile. PLoS One. 2015;10:e0126317.
156. Hoover BR, Reed MN, Su J, Penrod RD, Kotilinek LA, Grant MK, Pitstick R, Carlson GA, Lanier LM, Yuan LL, et al. Tau mislocalization to dendritic spines mediates synaptic dysfunction independently of neurodegeneration. Neuron. 2010;68:1067–81.
157. Maeda S, Djukic B, Taneja P, Yu GQ, Lo I, Davis A, Craft R, Guo W, Wang X, Kim D, et al. Expression of A152T human tau causes age-dependent neuronal dysfunction and loss in transgenic mice. EMBO Rep. 2016;17:530–51.
158. Carpenter JW, Marion CJ: Exotic animal formulary. 4th edn. St. Louis, Mo.: Elsevier; 2013.
159. Golub LM, Lee HM, Ryan ME, Giannobile WV, Payne J, Sorsa T. Tetracyclines inhibit connective tissue breakdown by multiple non-antimicrobial mechanisms. Adv Dent Res. 1998;12:12–26.
160. Liu J, Xiong W, Baca-Regen L, Nagase H, Baxter BT. Mechanism of inhibition of matrix metalloproteinase-2 expression by doxycycline in human aortic smooth muscle cells. J Vasc Surg. 2003;38:1376–83.
161. Golledge J, Norman PE, Murphy MP, Dalman RL. Challenges and opportunities in limiting abdominal aortic aneurysm growth. J Vasc Surg. 2017;65:225–33.
162. Yrjanheikki J, Keinanen R, Pellikka M, Hokfelt T, Koistinaho J. Tetracyclines inhibit microglial activation and are neuroprotective in global brain ischemia. Proc Natl Acad Sci U S A. 1998;95:15769–74.
163. Lazzarini M, Martin S, Mitkovski M, Vozari RR, Stuhmer W, Bel ED. Doxycycline restrains glia and confers neuroprotection in a 6-OHDA Parkinson model. Glia. 2013;61:1084–100.
164. Cho Y, Son HJ, Kim EM, Choi JH, Kim ST, Ji IJ, Choi DH, Joh TH, Kim YS, Hwang O. Doxycycline is neuroprotective against nigral dopaminergic degeneration by a dual mechanism involving MMP-3. Neurotox Res. 2009;16:361–71.
165. Zhang GB, Feng YH, Wang PQ, Song JH, Wang P, Wang SA. A study on the protective role of doxycycline upon dopaminergic neuron of LPS-PD rat model rat. Eur Rev Med Pharmacol Sci. 2015;19:3468–74.
166. Maezawa I, Zimin PI, Wulff H, Jin LW. Amyloid-beta protein oligomer at low nanomolar concentrations activates microglia and induces microglial neurotoxicity. J Biol Chem. 2011;286:3693–706.
167. Lai AY, Todd KG. Hypoxia-activated microglial mediators of neuronal survival are differentially regulated by tetracyclines. Glia. 2006;53:809–16.
168. Karlsson M, Hammers S, Nilsson-Ehle I, Malmborg AS, Wretlind B. Concentrations of doxycycline and penicillin G in sera and cerebrospinal fluid of patients treated for neuroborreliosis. Antimicrob Agents Chemother. 1996;40:1104–7.
169. Maier K, Merkler D, Gerber J, Taheri N, Kuhnert AV, Williams SK, Neusch C, Bahr M, Diem R. Multiple neuroprotective mechanisms of minocycline in autoimmune CNS inflammation. Neurobiol Dis. 2007;25:514–25.
170. Peng J, Xie L, Stevenson FF, Melov S, Di Monte DA, Andersen JK. Nigrostriatal dopaminergic neurodegeneration in the weaver mouse is mediated via neuroinflammation and alleviated by minocycline administration. J Neurosci. 2006;26:11644–51.
171. Fan LW, Lin S, Pang Y, Rhodes PG, Cai Z. Minocycline attenuates hypoxia-ischemia-induced neurological dysfunction and brain injury in the juvenile rat. Eur J Neurosci. 2006;24:341–50.
172. Hunter CL, Bachman D, Granholm AC. Minocycline prevents cholinergic loss in a mouse model of Down's syndrome. Ann Neurol. 2004;56:675–88.
173. Garwood CJ, Cooper JD, Hanger DP, Noble W. Anti-inflammatory impact of minocycline in a mouse model of tauopathy. Front Psychiatry. 2010;1:136.
174. Hou Y, Ryu CH, Park KY, Kim SM, Jeong CH, Jeun SS. Effective combination of human bone marrow mesenchymal stem cells and minocycline in experimental autoimmune encephalomyelitis mice. Stem Cell Res Ther. 2013;4:77.

175. Aras M, Urfali B, Serarslan Y, Ozgur T, Ulutas KT, Urfali S, Altas M, Yilmaz N. Protective effects of minocycline against short-term ischemia-reperfusion injury in rat brain. Pediatr Neurosurg. 2013;49:172–8.
176. Chen M, Ona VO, Li M, Ferrante RJ, Fink KB, Zhu S, Bian J, Guo L, Farrell LA, Hersch SM, et al. Minocycline inhibits caspase-1 and caspase-3 expression and delays mortality in a transgenic mouse model of Huntington disease. Nat Med. 2000;6:797–801.
177. Yrjanheikki J, Tikka T, Keinanen R, Goldsteins G, Chan PH, Koistinaho J. A tetracycline derivative, minocycline, reduces inflammation and protects against focal cerebral ischemia with a wide therapeutic window. Proc Natl Acad Sci U S A. 1999;96:13496–500.
178. Fowler SW, Chiang AC, Savjani RR, Larson ME, Sherman MA, Schuler DR, Cirrito JR, Lesne SE, Jankowsky JL. Genetic modulation of soluble abeta rescues cognitive and synaptic impairment in a mouse model of Alzheimer's disease. J Neurosci. 2014;34:7871–85.
179. Igaz LM, Kwong LK, Lee EB, Chen-Plotkin A, Swanson E, Unger T, Malunda J, Xu Y, Winton MJ, Trojanowski JQ, Lee VM. Dysregulation of the ALS-associated gene TDP-43 leads to neuronal death and degeneration in mice. J Clin Invest. 2011;121:726–38.
180. Bejar R, Yasuda R, Krugers H, Hood K, Mayford M. Transgenic calmodulin-dependent protein kinase II activation: dose-dependent effects on synaptic plasticity, learning, and memory. J Neurosci. 2002;22:5719–26.
181. Glazewski S, Bejar R, Mayford M, Fox K. The effect of autonomous alpha-CaMKII expression on sensory responses and experience-dependent plasticity in mouse barrel cortex. Neuropharmacology. 2001;41:771–8.
182. Barton MD, Dunlop JW, Psaltis G, Kulik J, DeGennaro L, Kwak SP. Modified GFAP promoter auto-regulates tet-activator expression for increased transactivation and reduced tTA-associated toxicity. Brain Res Mol Brain Res. 2002;101:71–81.
183. Han HJ, Allen CC, Buchovecky CM, Yetman MJ, Born HA, Marin MA, Rodgers SP, Song BJ, Lu HC, Justice MJ, et al. Strain background influences neurotoxicity and behavioral abnormalities in mice expressing the tetracycline transactivator. J Neurosci. 2012;32:10574–86.
184. McCloskey DT, Turnbull L, Swigart PM, Zambon AC, Turcato S, Joho S, Grossman W, Conklin BR, Simpson PC, Baker AJ. Cardiac transgenesis with the tetracycline transactivator changes myocardial function and gene expression. Physiol Genomics. 2005;22:118–26.
185. Morimoto M, Kopan R. rtTA toxicity limits the usefulness of the SP-C-rtTA transgenic mouse. Dev Biol. 2009;325:171–8.
186. Sisson TH, Hansen JM, Shah M, Hanson KE, Du M, Ling T, Simon RH, Christensen PJ. Expression of the reverse tetracycline-transactivator gene causes emphysema-like changes in mice. Am J Respir Cell Mol Biol. 2006;34:552–60.
187. Strittmatter WJ, Saunders AM, Schmechel D, Pericak-Vance M, Enghild J, Salvesen GS, Roses AD. Apolipoprotein E: high-avidity binding to beta-amyloid and increased frequency of type 4 allele in late-onset familial Alzheimer disease. Proc Natl Acad Sci U S A. 1993;90:1977–81.
188. Karch CM, Goate AM. Alzheimer's disease risk genes and mechanisms of disease pathogenesis. Biol Psychiatry. 2015;77:43–51.
189. Efthymiou AG, Goate AM. Late onset Alzheimer's disease genetics implicates microglial pathways in disease risk. Mol Neurodegener. 2017;12:43.
190. Guerreiro R, Wojtas A, Bras J, Carrasquillo M, Rogaeva E, Majounie E, Cruchaga C, Sassi C, Kauwe JS, Younkin S, et al. TREM2 variants in Alzheimer's disease. N Engl J Med. 2013;368:117–27.
191. Jonsson T, Stefansson H, Steinberg S, Jonsdottir I, Jonsson PV, Snaedal J, Bjornsson S, Huttenlocher J, Levey AI, Lah JJ, et al. Variant of TREM2 associated with the risk of Alzheimer's disease. N Engl J Med. 2013;368:107–16.
192. Chen HK, Liu Z, Meyer-Franke A, Brodbeck J, Miranda RD, McGuire JG, Pleiss MA, Ji ZS, Balestra ME, Walker DW, et al. Small molecule structure correctors abolish detrimental effects of apolipoprotein E4 in cultured neurons. J Biol Chem. 2012;287:5253–66.
193. Piedrahita JA, Zhang SH, Hagaman JR, Oliver PM, Maeda N. Generation of mice carrying a mutant apolipoprotein E gene inactivated by gene targeting in embryonic stem cells. Proc Natl Acad Sci U S A. 1992;89:4471–5.
194. Zhang SH, Reddick RL, Piedrahita JA, Maeda N. Spontaneous hypercholesterolemia and arterial lesions in mice lacking apolipoprotein E. Science. 1992;258:468–71.
195. Yang CP, Gilley JA, Zhang G, Kernie SG. ApoE is required for maintenance of the dentate gyrus neural progenitor pool. Development. 2011;138:4351–62.
196. Sun Y, Wu S, Bu G, Onifade MK, Patel SN, LaDu MJ, Fagan AM, Holtzman DM. Glial fibrillary acidic protein-apolipoprotein E (apoE) transgenic mice: astrocyte-specific expression and differing biological effects of astrocyte-secreted apoE3 and apoE4 lipoproteins. J Neurosci. 1998;18:3261–72.
197. Mann KM, Thorngate FE, Katoh-Fukui Y, Hamanaka H, Williams DL, Fujita S, Lamb BT. Independent effects of APOE on cholesterol metabolism and brain Abeta levels in an Alzheimer disease mouse model. Hum Mol Genet. 2004;13:1959–68.
198. Sullivan PM, Mezdour H, Quarfordt SH, Maeda N. Type III hyperlipoproteinemia and spontaneous atherosclerosis in mice resulting from gene replacement of mouse Apoe with human Apoe*2. J Clin Invest. 1998;102:130–5.
199. Sullivan PM, Mezdour H, Aratani Y, Knouff C, Najib J, Reddick RL, Quarfordt SH, Maeda N. Targeted replacement of the mouse apolipoprotein E gene with the common human APOE3 allele enhances diet-induced hypercholesterolemia and atherosclerosis. J Biol Chem. 1997;272:17972–80.
200. Knouff C, Hinsdale ME, Mezdour H, Altenburg MK, Watanabe M, Quarfordt SH, Sullivan PM, Maeda N. Apo E structure determines VLDL clearance and atherosclerosis risk in mice. J Clin Invest. 1999;103:1579–86.
201. Shi Y, Yamada K, Liddelow SA, Smith ST, Zhao L, Luo W, Tsai RM, Spina S, Grinberg LT, Rojas JC, et al. ApoE4 markedly exacerbates tau-mediated neurodegeneration in a mouse model of tauopathy. Nature. 2017;549:523–7.
202. Brendza RP, Bales KR, Paul SM, Holtzman DM. Role of apoE/Abeta interactions in Alzheimer's disease: insights from transgenic mouse models. Mol Psychiatry. 2002;7:132–5.
203. Liu CC, Liu CC, Kanekiyo T, Xu H, Bu G. Apolipoprotein E and Alzheimer disease: risk, mechanisms and therapy. Nat Rev Neurol. 2013;9:106–18.
204. Colonna M. TREMs in the immune system and beyond. Nat Rev Immunol. 2003;3:445–53.
205. Turnbull IR, Gilfillan S, Cella M, Aoshi T, Miller M, Piccio L, Hernandez M, Colonna M. Cutting edge: TREM-2 attenuates macrophage activation. J Immunol. 2006;177:3520–4.
206. Jay TR, Miller CM, Cheng PJ, Graham LC, Bemiller S, Broihier ML, Xu G, Margevicius D, Karlo JC, Sousa GL, et al. TREM2 deficiency eliminates TREM2 + inflammatory macrophages and ameliorates pathology in Alzheimer's disease mouse models. J Exp Med. 2015;212:287–95.
207. Kang SS, Kurti A, Baker KE, Liu CC, Colonna M, Ulrich JD, Holtzman DM, Bu G, Fryer JD. Behavioral and transcriptomic analysis of Trem2-null mice: not all knockout mice are created equal. Hum Mol Genet. 2017;
208. Kleinberger G, Brendel M, Mracsko E, Wefers B, Groeneweg L, Xiang X, Focke C, Deussing M, Suarez-Calvet M, Mazaheri F, et al. The FTD-like syndrome causing TREM2 T66M mutation impairs microglia function, brain perfusion, and glucose metabolism. EMBO J. 2017;36:1837–53.
209. Niwa H, Yamamura K, Miyazaki J. Efficient selection for high-expression transfectants with a novel eukaryotic vector. Gene. 1991;108:193–9.
210. Davis J, Xu F, Deane R, Romanov G, Previti ML, Zeigler K, Zlokovic BV, Van Nostrand WE. Early-onset and robust cerebral microvascular accumulation of amyloid beta-protein in transgenic mice expressing low levels of a vasculotropic Dutch/Iowa mutant form of amyloid beta-protein precursor. J Biol Chem. 2004;279:20296–306.
211. Radde R, Bolmont T, Kaeser SA, Coomaraswamy J, Lindau D, Stoltze L, Calhoun ME, Jaggi F, Wolburg H, Gengler S, et al. Abeta42-driven cerebral amyloidosis in transgenic mice reveals early and robust pathology. EMBO Rep. 2006;7:940–6.
212. Ishihara T, Hong M, Zhang B, Nakagawa Y, Lee MK, Trojanowski JQ, Lee VM. Age-dependent emergence and progression of a tauopathy in transgenic mice overexpressing the shortest human tau isoform. Neuron. 1999;24:751–62.
213. Allen B, Ingram E, Takao M, Smith MJ, Jakes R, Virdee K, Yoshida H, Holzer M, Craxton M, Emson PC, et al. Abundant tau filaments and nonapoptotic neurodegeneration in transgenic mice expressing human P301S tau protein. J Neurosci. 2002;22:9340–51.
214. Guo Q, Fu W, Sopher BL, Miller MW, Ware CB, Martin GM, Mattson MP. Increased vulnerability of hippocampal neurons to excitotoxic necrosis in presenilin-1 mutant knock-in mice. Nat Med. 1999;5:101–6.
215. Siman R, Reaume AG, Savage MJ, Trusko S, Lin YG, Scott RW, Flood DG. Presenilin-1 P264L knock-in mutation: differential effects on abeta production, amyloid deposition, and neuronal vulnerability. J Neurosci. 2000;20:8717–26.
216. Ubhi K, Rockenstein E, Doppler E, Mante M, Adame A, Patrick C, Trejo M, Crews L, Paulino A, Moessler H, Masliah E. Neurofibrillary and neurodegenerative pathology in APP-transgenic mice injected with AAV2-mutant TAU: neuroprotective effects of Cerebrolysin. Acta Neuropathol. 2009;117:699–712.
217. Jaworski T, Dewachter I, Lechat B, Croes S, Termont A, Demedts D, Borghgraef P, Devijver H, Filipkowski RK, Kaczmarek L, et al. AAV-tau mediates pyramidal neurodegeneration by cell-cycle re-entry without neurofibrillary tangle formation in wild-type mice. PLoS One. 2009;4:e7280.

218. Siman R, Lin YG, Malthankar-Phatak G, Dong Y. A rapid gene delivery-based mouse model for early-stage Alzheimer disease-type tauopathy. J Neuropathol Exp Neurol. 2013;72:1062–71.
219. Yang S, Cacquevel M, Saksida LM, Bussey TJ, Schneider BL, Aebischer P, Melani R, Pizzorusso T, Fawcett JW, Spillantini MG. Perineuronal net digestion with chondroitinase restores memory in mice with tau pathology. Exp Neurol. 2015;265:48–58.
220. Platt TL, Beckett TL, Kohler K, Niedowicz DM, Murphy MP. Obesity, diabetes, and leptin resistance promote tau pathology in a mouse model of disease. Neuroscience. 2016;315:162–74.
221. Maeda N, Johnson L, Kim S, Hagaman J, Friedman M, Reddick R. Anatomical differences and atherosclerosis in apolipoprotein E-deficient mice with 129/SvEv and C57BL/6 genetic backgrounds. Atherosclerosis. 2007;195:75–82.
222. Bero AW, Yan P, Roh JH, Cirrito JR, Stewart FR, Raichle ME, Lee JM, Holtzman DM. Neuronal activity regulates the regional vulnerability to amyloid-beta deposition. Nat Neurosci. 2011;14:750–6.
223. Sevigny J, Chiao P, Bussiere T, Weinreb PH, Williams L, Maier M, Dunstan R, Salloway S, Chen T, Ling Y, et al. The antibody aducanumab reduces Abeta plaques in Alzheimer's disease. Nature. 2016;537:50–6.
224. Amar F, Sherman MA, Rush T, Larson M, Boyle G, Chang L, Gotz J, Buisson A, Lesne SE. The amyloid-beta oligomer Abeta*56 induces specific alterations in neuronal signaling that lead to tau phosphorylation and aggregation. Sci Signal. 2017;10
225. Liu CC, Zhao N, Yamaguchi Y, Cirrito JR, Kanekiyo T, Holtzman DM, Bu G. Neuronal heparan sulfates promote amyloid pathology by modulating brain amyloid-beta clearance and aggregation in Alzheimer's disease. Sci. Transl. Med. 2016;8:332ra344.
226. Ofengeim D, Mazzitelli S, Ito Y, DeWitt JP, Mifflin L, Zou C, Das S, Adiconis X, Chen H, Zhu H, et al. RIPK1 mediates a disease-associated microglial response in Alzheimer's disease. Proc Natl Acad Sci U S A. 2017;114:E8788–97.
227. Wojtas AM, Kang SS, Olley BM, Gatherer M, Shinohara M, Lozano PA, Liu CC, Kurti A, Baker KE, Dickson DW, et al. Loss of clusterin shifts amyloid deposition to the cerebrovasculature via disruption of perivascular drainage pathways. Proc Natl Acad Sci U S A. 2017;114:E6962–71.
228. Fu AK, Hung KW, Yuen MY, Zhou X, Mak DS, Chan IC, Cheung TH, Zhang B, Fu WY, Liew FY, Ip NY. IL-33 ameliorates Alzheimer's disease-like pathology and cognitive decline. Proc Natl Acad Sci U S A. 2016;113:E2705–13.
229. Iaccarino HF, Singer AC, Martorell AJ, Rudenko A, Gao F, Gillingham TZ, Mathys H, Seo J, Kritskiy O, Abdurrob F, et al. Gamma frequency entrainment attenuates amyloid load and modifies microglia. Nature. 2016;540:230–5.
230. Andrew RJ, Fernandez CG, Stanley M, Jiang H, Nguyen P, Rice RC, Buggia-Prevot V, De Rossi P, Vetrivel KS, Lamb R, et al. Lack of BACE1 S-palmitoylation reduces amyloid burden and mitigates memory deficits in transgenic mouse models of Alzheimer's disease. Proc Natl Acad Sci U S A. 2017;114:E9665–74.
231. Caccamo A, Branca C, Talboom JS, Shaw DM, Turner D, Ma L, Messina A, Huang Z, Wu J, Oddo S. Reducing ribosomal protein S6 Kinase 1 expression improves spatial memory and synaptic plasticity in a mouse model of Alzheimer's disease. J Neurosci. 2015;35:14042–56.
232. Mably AJ, Gereke BJ, Jones DT, Colgin LL. Impairments in spatial representations and rhythmic coordination of place cells in the 3xTg mouse model of Alzheimer's disease. Hippocampus. 2017;27:378–92.
233. Zenaro E, Pietronigro E, Della Bianca V, Piacentino G, Marongiu L, Budui S, Turano E, Rossi B, Angiari S, Dusi S, et al. Neutrophils promote Alzheimer's disease-like pathology and cognitive decline via LFA-1 integrin. Nat Med. 2015;21:880–6.
234. Sherman MA, LaCroix M, Amar F, Larson ME, Forster C, Aguzzi A, Bennett DA, Ramsden M, Lesne SE. Soluble conformers of Abeta and tau Alter selective proteins governing axonal transport. J Neurosci. 2016;36:9647–58.
235. Cheng J, Ji D. Rigid firing sequences undermine spatial memory codes in a neurodegenerative mouse model. elife. 2013;2:e00647.
236. Min SW, Chen X, Tracy TE, Li Y, Zhou Y, Wang C, Shirakawa K, Minami SS, Defensor E, Mok SA, et al. Critical role of acetylation in tau-mediated neurodegeneration and cognitive deficits. Nat Med. 2015;21:1154–62.
237. Kaufman SK, Sanders DW, Thomas TL, Ruchinskas AJ, Vaquer-Alicea J, Sharma AM, Miller TM, Diamond MI. Tau Prion strains dictate patterns of cell pathology, progression rate, and regional vulnerability in vivo. Neuron. 2016;92:796–812.
238. Boluda S, Iba M, Zhang B, Raible KM, Lee VM, Trojanowski JQ. Differential induction and spread of tau pathology in young PS19 tau transgenic mice following intracerebral injections of pathological tau from Alzheimer's disease or corticobasal degeneration brains. Acta Neuropathol. 2015;129:221–37.
239. Zhang H, Wu L, Pchitskaya E, Zakharova O, Saito T, Saido T, Bezprozvanny I. Neuronal store-operated calcium entry and mushroom spine loss in Amyloid precursor protein knock-in mouse model of Alzheimer's disease. J Neurosci. 2015;35:13275–86.
240. Hernandez AL, Shah D, Craessaerts K, Saido T, Saito T, De Strooper B, Van der Linden A, D'Hooge R. Subtle behavioral changes and increased prefrontal-hippocampal network synchronicity in APP(NL-G-F) mice before prominent plaque deposition. Behav Brain Res. 2017;
241. Zhao N, Liu CC, Van Ingelgom AJ, Martens YA, Linares C, Knight JA, Painter MM, Sullivan PM, Bu G. Apolipoprotein E4 impairs neuronal insulin signaling by trapping insulin receptor in the Endosomes. Neuron. 2017;96:115–29. e115

3

Early long-term administration of the CSF1R inhibitor PLX3397 ablates microglia and reduces accumulation of intraneuronal amyloid, neuritic plaque deposition and pre-fibrillar oligomers in 5XFAD mouse model of Alzheimer's disease

Justyna Sosna[1], Stephan Philipp[1], Ricardo Albay III[1], Jorge Mauricio Reyes-Ruiz[1], David Baglietto-Vargas[3], Frank M. LaFerla[3] and Charles G. Glabe[1,2*]

Abstract

Background: Besides the two main classical features of amyloid beta aggregation and tau-containing neurofibrillary tangle deposition, neuroinflammation plays an important yet unclear role in the pathophysiology of Alzheimer's disease (AD). Microglia are believed to be key mediators of neuroinflammation during AD and responsible for the regulation of brain homeostasis by balancing neurotoxicity and neuroprotective events. We have previously reported evidence that neuritic plaques are derived from dead neurons that have accumulated intraneuronal amyloid and further recruit Iba1-positive cells, which play a role in either neuronal demise or neuritic plaque maturation or both.

Methods: To study the impact of microglia on neuritic plaque development, we treated two-month-old 5XFAD mice with a selective colony stimulation factor 1 receptor (CSF1R) inhibitor, PLX3397, for a period of 3 months, resulting in a significant ablation of microglia. Directly after this treatment, we analyzed the amount of intraneuronal amyloid and neuritic plaques and performed behavioral studies including Y-maze, fear conditioning and elevated plus maze.

Results: We found that early long-term PLX3397 administration results in a dramatic reduction of both intraneuronal amyloid as well as neuritic plaque deposition. PLX3397 treated young 5XFAD mice also displayed a significant decrease of soluble fibrillar amyloid oligomers in brain lysates, a depletion of soluble pre-fibrillar oligomers in plasma and an improvement in cognitive function measured by fear conditioning tests.

Conclusions: Our findings demonstrate that CSF1R signaling, either directly on neurons or mediated by microglia, is crucial for the accumulation of intraneuronal amyloid and formation of neuritic plaques, suggesting that these two events are serially linked in a causal pathway leading to neurodegeneration and neuritic plaque formation. CSF1R inhibitors represent potential preventative or therapeutic approach that target the very earliest stages of the formation of intraneuronal amyloid and neuritic plaques.

Keywords: Alzheimer's disease, Amyloid beta, Plaques, Intraneuronal amyloid, Microglia, Neuroinflammation

* Correspondence: cglabe@uci.edu
[1]Department of Molecular Biology and Biochemistry, University of California, Irvine, USA
[2]Biochemistry Department, Faculty of Science and Experimental Biochemistry Unit, King Fahd Medical Research Center, King Abdulaziz University, Jeddah 21589, Saudi Arabia
Full list of author information is available at the end of the article

Background

AD is classically characterized by the presence of neurofibrillary tangles (NFTs), containing aggregates of the microtubule binding protein tau and plaque deposits composed of aggregates of the amyloid beta peptide (Aβ) [1, 2]. The amyloid cascade hypothesis has evolved over the past 30 years as one of the leading theories of disease, which states that the secretion of Aβ leads to the formation of toxic oligomers that play a causal role in AD [3]. However, the cellular and molecular mechanism by which Aβ aggregates induce these pathological damages and cause dementia remains unclear. Semagacestat, an inhibitor of γ-secretase which creates the carboxyl terminus of Aβ accelerated the decline in cognitive function in clinical trials [4]. We have proposed an alternative formulation of the amyloid hypothesis, based on the observations that FAD PS mutations interfere with the carboxyl-terminal trimming of the initial "long" Aβ cleavage products leading to their aggregation and accumulation in neurons as intraneuronal amyloid [5]. Several transgenic animal models of Aβ deposition that contain FAD PS mutations demonstrate robust intraneuronal amyloid aggregates that occur prior to plaque deposition and in human brain is associated with early stages of AD [6, 7]. The intraneuronal amyloid is aggregated in an amyloid-like structure because it reacts with aggregation-specific antibodies and or thioflavin S [5, 6, 8]. We hypothesized that the intraneuronal amyloid forms the core of the neuritic plaque after the death of the neuron [5]. The evidence for this includes the observation that the core of neuritic plaques contains the same intraneuronal aggregated amyloid immunoreactivity and stains with dyes specific for DNA [5]. Some of the neuritic plaques also contain NeuN immunoreactivity, providing further evidence of their neuronal origin [5]. Since neuritic plaques are typically surrounded by a halo of microglia, we also have hypothesized that neuritic plaques and cored plaques are developmentally related with microglia removing neuronal debris to produce cored plaques [5]. In order to test critical aspects of these hypotheses, we examined the effect of early ablation of microglia in the 5XFAD mouse model that exhibits widespread and robust intraneuronal amyloid immunoreactivity beginning at 1.5 months, prior to neuritic plaque deposition that begins at 2 months and is robust at 5 months [6]. We pharmacologically ablated microglia with PLX3397, a previously described orally-administered selective CSF1R/c-kit inhibitor that is able to cross the blood-brain barrier [9, 10]. Previous studies have determined the optimal dosing and the time-window for PLX3397-induced microglial ablation and it was reported that a 2 month treatment with PLX3397 was reversible in a short period of 3–14 days and had no effect on cognition and behavior of 5xFAD mice [9]. Microglia repopulation was shown to depend on the internal pool of remaining microglia, which in turn is dependent on IL-1 receptor signaling [11]. In contrast to previous studies starting treatment in ten-month-old 5XFAD mice with no effect on Aβ levels or plaque load [10], we started PLX3397 treatment in mice with an age of 2 months. We found that this early treatment with PLX3397 profoundly inhibited not only neuritic plaque formation but also intraneuronal amyloid accumulation. This observation indicates that CSF1R signaling or the presence of microglia is necessary for neuritic plaque formation and that intraneuronal amyloid accumulation and neuritic plaque formation are developmentally linked in a causal series with intraneuronal amyloid upstream of neuritic plaques, consistent with the hypothesis that intraneuronal amyloid is the penultimate source for the amyloid in the center of neuritic plaques.

Methods

Animal studies

All mouse experiments were performed according to animal protocols approved by the Institutional Animal Care and Use Committee at the University of California, Irvine. The 5XFAD (B6SJL-Tg(APPSwFlLon,PSEN1*M146 L*L286 V)6799Vas/Mmjax) mice were obtained from The Jackson Laboratory [6]. Mice were housed in groups of 2 to 5 or single-housed for aggressive males, under a 12-h light/12-h dark cycle at 21 °C, with food and water ad libitum. All transgenic animals were genotyped by qPCR (automated genotyping using human APP and PS1 primers, TransnetYX, Cordova, TN) and only animals expressing comparable levels of the human APP and PS1 were chosen for the study. To pharmacologically ablate microglia, six males and nine females of two-month-old 5XFAD mice were treated with PLX3397 (290 mg/kg formulated in standard chow) [9, 10]. Age-matched control groups, ten males and eight females, were fed same standard chow without PLX3397. Previous studies have tested the effects of PLX3397 on wild-type animals and performed the necessary controls [9, 10]. Wild-type littermates were fed with the same PLX3397 chow (two males and two females) or without drug (three males and three females). After 3 months of controlled chow administration, the behavior of treated mice (12 5XFAD animals (five males and seven females) with drug and 11 5XFAD animals (six males and five females) without drug) as well as age-matched controls was analyzed prior to euthanasia. At 5 months, 5XFAD mice display extensive amyloid pathology, manifested predominantly by the presence of intraneuronal amyloid and neuritic plaque accumulation. After behavioral testing, mice were euthanized, blood samples collected intracardiacally with a 21 G needle in a 1 mL syringe and mixed with 0.1 mM EDTA solution to prevent clotting. Each blood sample was centrifuged for 15 min at 2500×g to obtain the plasma fraction. Further, mice were intracardially perfused using a peristaltic pump with approximately 120 ml of phosphate buffered saline over 10 min. Brains were isolated and one hemisphere was fixed in 4% (*w*/*v*) paraformaldehyde while the other half was microdissected to isolate cortex and hippocampus and snap frozen in liquid nitrogen for further analysis.

Immunohistochemistry and confocal microscopy

Paraformaldehyde-fixed brain tissues from 5XFAD mice and age-matched controls were sectioned with a Vibratome Series 1000 vibrating microtome (The Vibratome Co., St. Louis, section thickness 50 μm). Free-floating sections were collected in PBS containing 0.02% (*w*/*v*) NaN_3, pH 7.4 and stored at 4 °C prior to staining. Sections were washed with PHEM buffer (60 mM Pipes, 25 mM Hepes, 10 mM EGTA, 2 mM $MgCl_2$ pH 6.9), permeabilized in 0.1% (*v*/*v*) Triton X-100 in PHEM buffer for 30 min and blocked by 1 h incubation in PHEM containing 2% (*w*/*v*) BSA, 1.5% (v/v) goat serum and mouse-on-mouse polymer basic kit according to manufacturer's protocol (BMK-2202, Vectashield) in order to block non-specific binding to endogenous mouse IgG in the mouse tissue.

Tissue slices were probed with primary antibodies against Iba1 (ionized calcium-binding adapter molecule 1) (1 μg / ml of 019–19,741, Wako Pure Chemicals) in combination with purified anti-β-amyloid, 1–16 antibody (5 μg / ml of 6E10, 803,003, BioLegend) in PHEM buffer overnight at room temperature. After rinsing 3 times with PHEM buffer, sections were blocked in PHEM with 2% (*w*/*v*) BSA for 1 h and incubated with highly cross-absorbed goat-anti-rabbit or goat-anti-mouse, respectively, secondary antibodies (1:250) coupled to Alexa Fluor 488 or 647 dyes (A-11034 or A32728, Invitrogen, Thermo Fisher Scientific). Total Iba1 positive cells, the area fraction of plaques and intraneuronal amyloid were quantified by imaging whole sections of comparable regions of the brain from each animal with a Leica TCS SP8 confocal microscope using a 63× objective. Neuritic plaques were determined by a presence of a diffuse DAPI-positive core surrounded by 6E10-positive dystrophic neurites [5]. Immunofluorescence data were analyzed by Volocity 6.3 high-performance 3D imaging software (PerkinElmer) in which objects were counted automatically based on the threshold of cellular size and intensity. Quantification was followed by statistical analyses applying two-tailed unpaired t-test or *one-way ANOVA* with post-hoc *Tukey* HSD (Honestly Significant Difference) by IBM SPSS Statistics Version 24 software. Data are shown as mean ± SEM. p values are as follows: $^{*}p < 0.05$, $^{**}p < 0.01$, $^{***}p < 0.001$ $^{****}p < 0.0001$, $^{*****}p < 0.00001$ and $^{******}p < 0.000001$.

Dot blot analyses

The flash-frozen cortex and hippocampus from each brain hemisphere were ground with a bullet blender and lysis beads (Pink, Next Advance, Eppendorf), in TNE total lysis buffer (20 mM Tris (pH 7.5), 150 mM NaCl, 1% (*v*/v) Triton X-100, 1:10 complete protease inhibitors (Roche)). The mixture was centrifuged (20,000×g, 15 min, 4 °C) and the total protein concentration of the supernatant was assessed by the BCA protein assay (Pierce, ThermoScientific). Afterwards, an equal amount of protein (6 μg) was spotted on a nitrocellulose membrane (0.2 μm). Similarly, an equal amount of plasma (1 μg) for each animal was spotted on the nitrocellulose membrane (0.2 μm) and followed the same procedure. Membranes were blocked with 2% (*w*/*v*) non-fat milk for 1 h followed by an overnight incubation at room temperature with respective antibodies: rabbit monoclonal antibody mA11–204 and mA11–118 [8] detecting pre-fibrillar oligomers or rabbit monoclonal antibodies mOC23 and mOC78 [12], detecting fibrillar oligomers. Membranes were washed three times with PBS/0.1% (*v*/v) Triton X-100 and incubated for 1 h at room temperature with goat-anti-rabbit secondary IgG (H + L) coupled to horseradish peroxidase (111–035-144, Jackson ImmunoResearch). Dot blots were incubated with ECL substrate (Clarity Western, 170–5061, Biorad) and the chemiluminescent signal was detected by a digital imaging using a CCD camera. The densitometric analyses of dot blots were performed by the quantitation of total integrated density after automated light background subtraction and uniform adjustment of the background using ImageJ 1.51j8 (Wayne Rasband, NIH).

Behavioral tests

Elevated plus maze

Animals were tested for anxiety-like behavior on an elevated plus maze, based on a previously described protocol [13]. Under normal conditions, rodents enter significantly fewer times into the open arms as well as spend significantly less time in open arms (avoidance of heights/open spaces) when compared to the closed arms (approach toward dark, enclosed spaces). The elevated plus maze consists of 4 intersecting arms (5 × 30 cm), two of which have walls ("closed", 15 cm in height) and the other two of which have no walls ("open"). The entire maze is elevated 40 cm above the ground and placed in the center of a room with lighting adjusted to 15 lx. Animals were placed at the junction of these arms and allowed to freely explore the maze for 5 min. Video footage was captured and later analyzed by a blinded investigator for the time spent in open and closed arms, and the total number of arm entries. An animal was considered in an arm whenever the body (not including the tail) was entirely in the arm. The maze was thoroughly cleaned with 70% ethanol in between trials.

Y-maze

Y-maze spontaneous alternation was conducted to measure the willingness of rodents to explore new environments. Mice typically prefer to explore a new arm/region rather than returning to the region previously visited within the maze [14]. The Y maze consisted of a central arm with two sides arms positioned perpendicular to the main arm. Each arm was 21 cm long and the maze width was 13.5 cm. The walls of the maze were made of transparent acrylic and were 20 cm tall. Each mouse was placed at the end of one arm and allowed to move freely through the maze during an 8-min session. The series of arms entries was recorded visually. An arm entry was considered when the mouse has completely entered in the arm. Alternation was defined as successive entries into the three arms on overlapping triplet sets.

Contextual fear conditioning

The fear conditioning test is based on the Pavlovian fear conditioning paradigm, in which a previously neutral (conditioned) stimulus is paired with an aversive (unconditioned) stimulus, which results in a measurable state of fear [15]. Studies have demonstrated that induced fear responses like freezing are dependent on the integrity of the amygdala complex [16]. However, the nature by which a specific stimulus produces fear-eliciting properties remains unclear [17]. During training, mice were placed in the fear-conditioning chamber (San Diego Instruments, San Diego, CA) and allowed to explore for 2 min and 30 s before receiving one electric foot shocks (duration, 2 s; intensity, 0.2 mA). Animals were returned to the home cage 30 s after the foot shock. Twenty-four hours later, behavior in the conditioning chamber was video recorded for 5 min and subsequently analyzed for freezing, which was defined as the absence of all movement except for respiration.

Results

Early, long-term administration of PLX3397 inhibits the accumulation of intraneuronal amyloid and formation of neuritic plaques

Two-month-old 5XFAD mice were selected for this study as they exhibit robust intraneuronal aggregated amyloid at 1.5 months, prior to neuritic plaque formation that begins at 2 months and is robust by 5 months, and display memory deficits starting by 4 months of age [18]. From earlier experiments we observed, that after at the age of 5 months non-treated 5XFAD mice showed both intraneuronal amyloid accumulation and excessive amyloid pathology (Fig. 1). We have observed in 5XFAD mice that the majority of extracellular amyloid deposits in the cortex, hippocampus and amygdala were a neuritic type of plaque with DAPI-positive center of the plaque surrounded by 6E10-positive rim and Iba1-positive cells and only a small fraction of all amyloid deposits were other than neuritic plaques (Fig. 1). During the 3 months treatment with PLX3397, no behavior or health problems were observed in mice, which is in line with previous findings by Kim Green and coworkers using short (21 days) and long term (2 months) PLX3397 treatment reported no such negative effects [9]. Surprisingly, we found that early treatment of two-month-old 5XFAD mice with PLX3397 for 3 months significantly reduced both the amount of intraneuronal amyloid and amyloid plaques when compared with non-treated 5XFAD mice (Fig. 2). Consistent with previous studies, treatment with PLX3397 significantly reduced (~ 70–80%) the number of Iba1-positive cells and reduced approximately 99% of the area fraction occupied by Iba1-positive cells in five-month-old 5XFAD mice (Fig. 3a) [9]. Compared with control animals, in 5XFAD mice treated with PLX3397, Iba1-positive cells appeared altered: they are much smaller and possess a few short and residual ramifications (Fig. 2). This is probably due to programmed apoptotic cell death triggered by inhibition of CSF1R by PLX3397 in Iba1-positive cells such as microglia and macrophages, which both express CSF1R [19].

PLX3397 treatment also led to a decrease in the accumulation of intraneuronal amyloid and extracellular amyloid deposits (Fig. 2). The decrease of intraneuronal amyloid and plaques is evident in all regions of the brain and is highly statistically significant (Fig. 3b, c). In this and our previous study [5] we have observed that the majority of extracellular amyloid deposits in the cortex, hippocampus and amygdala of 5XFAD mice are neuritic plaques with a DAPI-positive center of the plaque and a 6E10-positive rim of dystrophic neurites surrounded by Iba1-positive microglia. The treatment with PLX3397 removed ~ 90% of the neuritic plaques in all analyzed regions of the brains (Fig. 3c). The plaques that accumulate in PLX3397 treated brain are significantly smaller and more compact than the neuritic plaques in control mice (Fig. 3d) even though the plaques in PLX3397 treated mice are associated with the remaining microglia (Fig. 2). This indicates that the drug treatment not only decreases the number of amyloid plaques but also alters the process of plaque formation. Collectively, these data indicate that treatment of 5XFAD mice with PLX3397 leads to a reduction in both intraneuronal amyloid and neuritic plaque accumulation.

PLX3397 administration improves behavioral phenotype

Since PLX3397 treatment significantly reduces the amount of intraneuronal amyloid and neuritic plaques

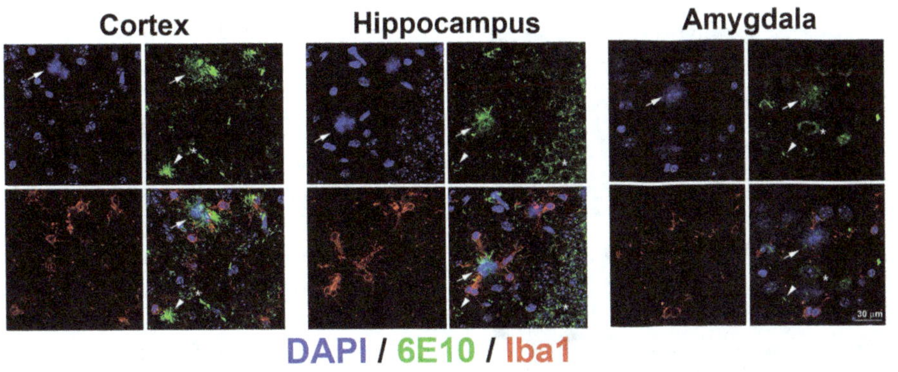

Fig. 1 Intraneuronal amyloid and neuritic plaques are present in 5 mo 5XFAD mice. Representative 63× images of intraneuronal amyloid (asterisk), neuritic plaques (arrows) with DAPI-positive core (blue) surrounded by a 6E10-positive amyloid rim (green) and Iba1-positive cells (red) in cortex, hippocampus and amygdala. Arrowheads point to non-neuritic 6E10-positive plaques without a DAPI-positive center. The confocal acquisition was applied and a total z-plane of 10 µm was merged into single overlay images. Bar = 30 µm

accumulation, we examined whether this effect on amyloid pathology would result in an improvement in the behavioral phenotype of 5XFAD mice. Thus, mice were tested in two hippocampal tests, the Y-maze and contextual fear condition, allowing us to determine whether PLX3397 treatment mitigate the spatial and emotional memory deficits observed in these mice. Our data demonstrate that PLX3397 treatment reverses the emotional and contextual memory as 5XFAD mice showed an improvement of a fear-associated memory when treated with PLX3397 (Fig. 4a). However, no changes were observed in spatial hippocampal memory (Fig. 4b). It is not clear why some measures of hippocampal function respond to drug treatment and others do not, but it seems to indicate that some measures of AD-related behavioral deficits can be dissociated by drug treatment. In addition, the animals did not show any differences in exploratory and anxiety-like behavior in an elevated plus maze test, as no differences in the numbers of entries in the open versus closed arms, the overall exploration of the middle part of the platform and manifestation of a risky behavior is observed between groups (Fig. 4c). Taken together, our findings implicate a strong relationship between amyloid pathology, microglia and amygdala and hippocampus-related behaviors in 5XFAD mice that are reversed by a treatment with CSF1R inhibitor and microglia reduction.

Treatment with PLX3397 lowers the levels of pre-fibrillar oligomers in plasma and fibrillar amyloid in the brain

Based on our observation that PLX3397 treatment inhibited intraneuronal amyloid accumulation and neuritic plaque deposition, we were interested in determining how the levels of pre-fibrillar oligomers and soluble fibrillar amyloid oligomers change in response to treatment. In total brain lysates, pre-fibrillar oligomers were not detected in any of the cohorts, however, the level of soluble fibrillar amyloid, detected by monoclonal antibodies mOC23 and mOC78, is significantly reduced by drug treatment (Fig. 5a-b). Consistent with the increase in amyloid plaques observed by immunofluorescence, we found that the level of soluble fibrillar amyloid was increased in 5XFAD mice in both cortex and hippocampus. The levels of fibrillar amyloid were significantly reduced by the treatment with PLX3397 (Fig. 5b).

In contrast to the results obtained with brain lysates, we have shown that pre-fibrillar oligomers, but not fibrillar oligomers were detected in plasma (Fig. 5c). Interestingly, the level of mA11–204-positive amyloid oligomers was significantly increased in the 5XFAD mice when compared with the wild-type littermates, whereas treatment with PLX3397 significantly decreased the levels of those amyloid oligomers (Fig. 5d). Together, these data support the findings that treatment with PLX3397 reduces the level of soluble fibrillar oligomers in the brain and the level of pre-fibrillar, toxic oligomers in plasma.

Discussion

A rapidly growing body of evidence indicates that microglia play an important role in brain homeostasis, neuroinflammation and neurodegenerative disorders such as AD (reviewed in [20, 21]). We and others have suggested that intraneuronal amyloid might play a crucial role in the pathophysiology of AD, especially as neuritic plaques are believed to originate from dying neurons with intraneuronal amyloid [5, 22–24]. Here we demonstrate early long-term administration of PLX3397 dramatically reduces microglia levels and inhibits both intraneuronal amyloid and neuritic plaque accumulation and ameliorates emotional and contextual memory deficits. Thus, early long-term administration seems to be crucial to significantly reduce amyloid pathology, since other investigators have reported that PLX3397 and other

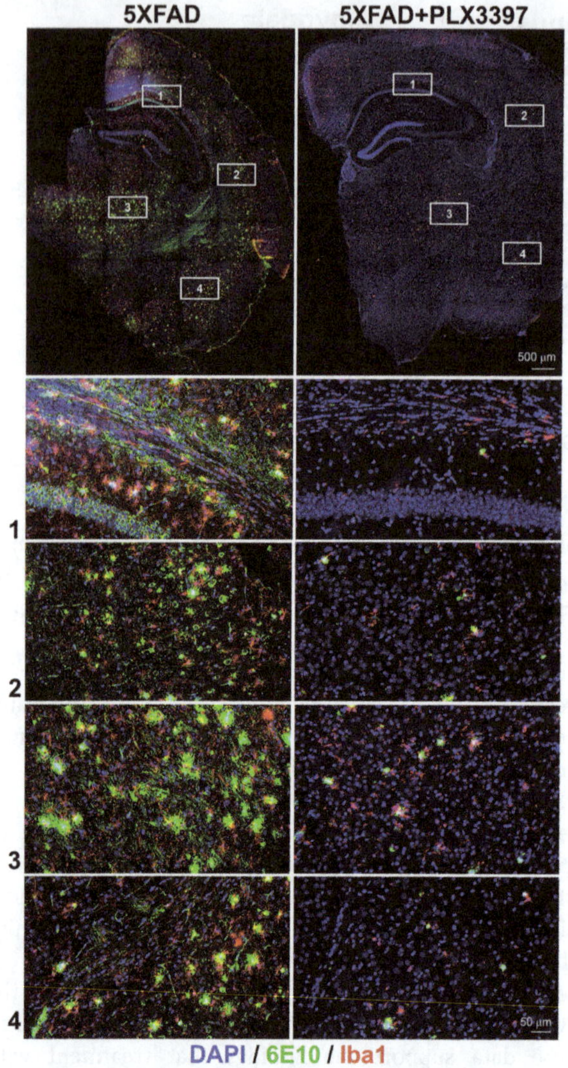

Fig. 2 Long-term administration of PLX3397 ablates microglia and reduces neuritic plaque formation in 5XFAD mice. Top panels: representative 20× images of coronal brain sections with immunolabeling of microglia (Iba1, red) and staining for amyloid Aβ (6E10, green) in five-month-old 5XFAD mice kept on a standard diet or fed for 3 months with PLX3397 (290 mg/kg). Bottom panels: representative images of magnified regions of (1) hippocampus, (2) cortex, (3) thalamus and (4) amygdalar nucleus. The confocal acquisition was applied and a total z-plane of 30 µm was scanned across all regions and merged into single overlay images

CSF1R inhibitor-induced ablation of microglia does not cause a reduction in amyloid plaque load when treatment is initiated at later times after robust amyloid plaque deposition in 5XFAD mice [10]. The simplest interpretation for this difference is that CSF1R inhibition and microglia ablation prevent the formation of neuritic plaques, but do not have an impact after plaques have already formed. The fact that intraneuronal amyloid precedes neuritic plaque formation and both types of deposits are dramatically reduced by PLX3397 treatment suggests that intraneuronal amyloid deposits and neuritic plaque amyloid are linked in a causal series. If instead intraneuronal amyloid accumulation and neuritic plaque deposition were coincidental but independent events, it would be unlikely that the drug would inhibit both pathways independently because the drug has been shown to have no effect on Aβ production in 5XFAD mice [10]. While inhibition of neuritic plaque formation could be easily explained as a consequence of the necessity of microglial phagocytosis for plaque formation, the effect of CSF1R inhibition and microglia ablation on intraneuronal amyloid is more surprising and puzzling. It implies that either microglial signaling to neurons or CSF1R signaling on neurons is necessary for intraneuronal amyloid accumulation. Using lineage-tracing experiments, Wyss-Coray and coworkers reported that a small number of neurons in the hippocampus and cortex express CSF1R under physiological conditions [25]. Thus, it is possible that CSF1R signaling in neurons is responsible for promoting the accumulation of intraneuronal amyloid. An alternate explanation is that microglia might regulate the accumulation of intraneuronal amyloid by producing inflammatory cytokines and chemokines that promote intraneuronal amyloid accumulation [26, 27]. Both hypotheses require further investigation.

If intraneuronal amyloid leads to neuronal death and initiates neuritic plaques, then the inhibition of CSF1R signaling or CSF1R-dependent microglial signaling would be protective for AD according to this model. This is the opposite of the more widely held view that CSF1R signaling is neuroprotective. A study by Luo and coworkers reported that CSF1 ameliorated memory deficits in the hAPP mouse model and CSF1 and IL34 administration strongly reduced excitotoxic neuronal loss, while deletion of CSF1R in neurons exacerbated excitotoxic neuronal death [25]. Although the reason for this difference is not yet clear, the simplest interpretations is that it is due to the differences between the specific genetic ablation in a subset of neurons while pharmacological inhibition hits more targets in more cell types. It may also suggest that amyloid pathogenesis is regulated in a different CSF1R-dependent mechanism than excitotoxicity. In contrast to the neuroprotective functions, CSF1R signaling during amyloid pathogenesis might instead activate pro-inflammatory processes. A similar pro-inflammatory function of CSF1R signaling has been described in an animal model of arthritis, where antibody blockade of CSF1R signaling significantly reduced the inflammatory response and ameliorated disease-related symptoms [28]. Our results also indicate that microglia are closely associated with Aβ deposition because the remaining plaques after drug treatment are still surrounded by the remaining microglia, even though both are strongly reduced in number. The remaining

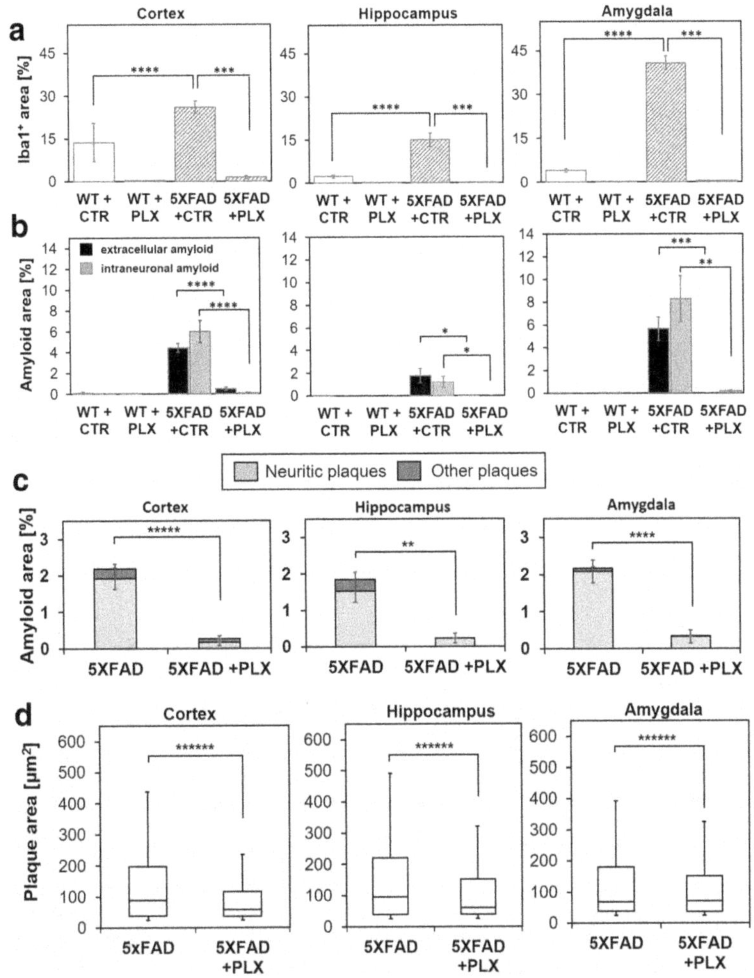

Fig. 3 PLX3397 treatment reduces microglia, accumulation of intraneuronal amyloid and extracellular amyloid deposits in 5XFAD mice. **a** Area occupied by Iba1-positive microglia in the analyzed brains is increased by ~ 40%–90% in the regions of cortex, hippocampus and amygdala in 5XFAD mice compared to wild-type ($p < 0.0001$ denoted by ****). PLX3397 treatment eliminates ~ 99% of microglia in both wild-type and 5XFAD mice ($p < 0.001$ denoted by ***). Graph bars indicate mean ± SEM ($n = 9$/group). **b** Area fraction occupied by intraneuronal amyloid and extracellular amyloid deposits was quantified for the regions of cortex, hippocampus and amygdala independently. Long-term treatment with PLX3397 significantly prevented accumulation of the intraneuronal amyloid and nearly completely aborted formation of amyloid plaques in the cortex ($p <$ 0.0001 denoted by ****). In the hippocampus, the accumulation of intraneuronal amyloid was significantly reduced ($p < 0.024$ denoted by *) as the formation of extracellular amyloid plaques ($p < 0.05$ denoted by *). In the amygdala region of the brains intraneuronal amyloid was reduced ($p < 0.0002$ denoted by ***) and formation of amyloid plaques was prevented ($p < 0.003$ denoted by **). Graph bars indicate mean ± SEM ($n = 9$/group). **c** Based on morphology and presence or absence of DAPI-positive core, extracellular amyloid was divided into neuritic or other types of plaques and quantified in brains. Treatment with PLX3397 significantly reduced area fraction occupied by neuritic plaques and other types of plaques (non-neuritic) in the cortex ($p < 0.000005$ denoted by *****), hippocampus ($p < 0.005$ denoted by **) and amygdala ($p < 0.00001$ denoted by ****). Graph bars indicate mean ± SEM ($n = 12$/group). **d** Size of amyloid plaques was quantified in three regions of brains. Treatment with PLX3397 significantly reduced the size of amyloid plaques in the cortex, hippocampus and amygdala ($p < 0.000001$, denoted by ******). Graph bars indicate mean ± SEM ($n = 12$/group and the total size of > 300 plaques/group were analyzed)

plaques in drug-treated animals are smaller, which indicates that the process of plaque formation is also altered by drug treatment. Whatever the explanation is for the role of CSF1R signaling on intraneuronal amyloid accumulation, the fact that neuritic plaque formation is prevented suggests that inhibition of CSF1R signaling may be a preventative approach, or therapeutic when applied at the very earliest stages of amyloid deposition during AD.

Amyloid oligomers are widely believed to be a primary toxic species of Aβ. Amyloid oligomers are structurally polymorphic and can be classified as prefibrillar oligomers (A11+/OC-) or fibrillar (A11-/OC+) oligomers on the basis of their differential immunoreactivity with conformation-dependent antibodies [29–32]. We present a novel finding that treatment with PLX3397 lead to a significant reduction of mA11–204 positive prefibrillar oligomers in plasma of 5XFAD mice. This result may

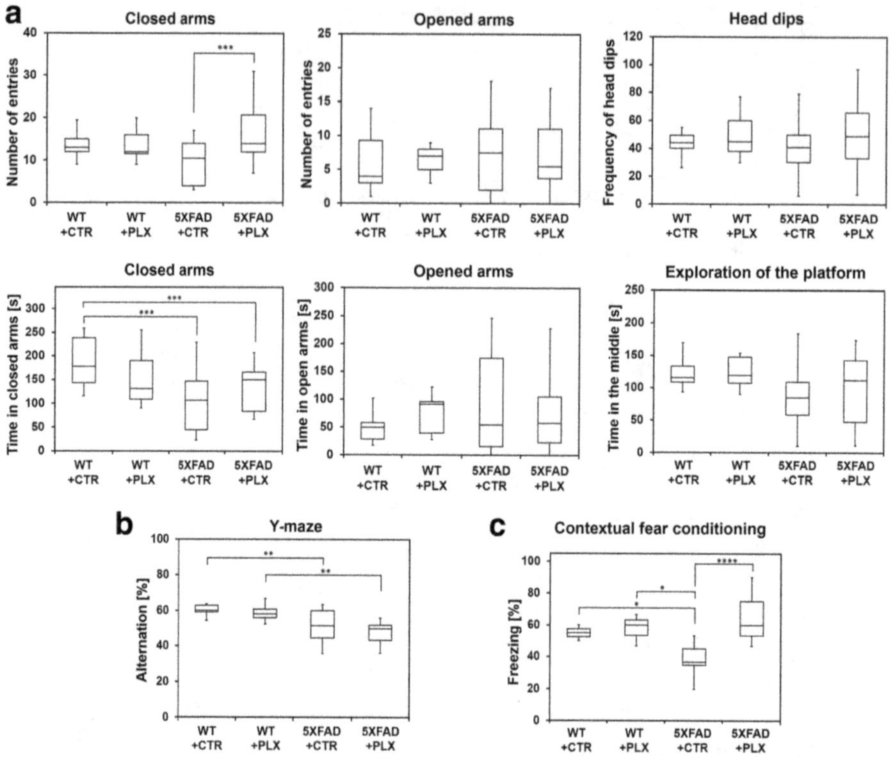

Fig. 4 PLX3397 treatment improves behavioral phenotype. Contextual fear conditioning (**a**), Y-maze (**b**) and elevated plus maze (**c**) tests were performed. **a** In the contextual fear conditioning test, 5XFAD mice show significantly lower levels of contextual freezing than wild-type controls ($p < 0.02$, denoted by *). However, treatment with PLX3397 significantly reversed the impaired fear behavior to the level of a normal reconsolidation of the contextual fear memory ($p < 0.00008$ with Tukey correction test, denoted by ****). **b** The total number of arm entries was significantly changed in the group of 5XFAD mice regardless the treatment ($p < 0.005$ with Tukey correction test, denoted by **), indicating lower levels of motor and exploratory activity in the group of AD mice. **c** In the elevated plus maze test, although the number of entries into closed arms was increased in the 5XFAD mice treated with PLX3397 ($p < 0.001$ denoted by ***), the number of entries into opened arms was not significantly different among all four groups. Neither another behavioral parameter such as head dips, which is a complementary parameter to assess risky and or an exploratory behavior in the evaluation of anxiety, was not changed between groups. Whereas, 5XFAD mice spend less time in the closed arms ($p < 0.0002$, denoted by ***), regardless the treatment, there was no difference in the time spent in the opened arms or exploring the center zone of the platform. Box plots show median with interquartile lower and upper range and the minimum and maximum values. Total number of wild-type animals in the behavioral study was four animals (two males and two females) with drug and six animals without drug (three males and three females), respectively. The total number of animals in the behavioral study was 12 5XFAD animals (five males and seven females) with drug and 11 5XFAD animals without drug (six males and five females), respectively

reflect a neuroprotective activity of drug treatment as studies have shown that prefibrillar oligomers are neurotoxic [33]. We have detected prefibrillar oligomers only in plasma, but not in brain lysates of 5XFAD mice, perhaps due to their preferential secretion or transport into the bloodstream. We have also observed low levels of prefibrilar oligomers, detected by A11–204 monoclonal antibody, in wilde-type mice. The presence of A11–204 pre-fibrilar oligomers might represent kind of "background noise" since oligomer-specific A11–204 also recognizes soluble oligomers from various proteins, such as α-synuclein, islet amyloid polypeptide, polyglutamine (PolyQ), lysozyme, human insulin and prion peptide [8, 29]. Importantly, treatment with PLX3397 reduced level of toxic prefibrillar A11-positive oligomers to the level of "background noise" of healthy individuals.

Finally, our behavioral studies showed that long-term administration of PLX3397 in young 5XFAD mice improved associative learning (contextual fear conditioning), which had also been reported for shorter administration in older ten-month-old 5XFAD mice [10]. The contextual fear conditioning test investigates the involvement of both amygdala and hippocampus [34], in which atrophy can be detected in the earliest clinical stages of AD [35]. Other behavioral tests on spatial memory (Y-maze test) or anxiety (elevated plus-maze test) showed only a beneficial trend, but none of them was statistically significant, suggesting that a longer treatment may be necessary to recover these behavioral tests. Taken together, we

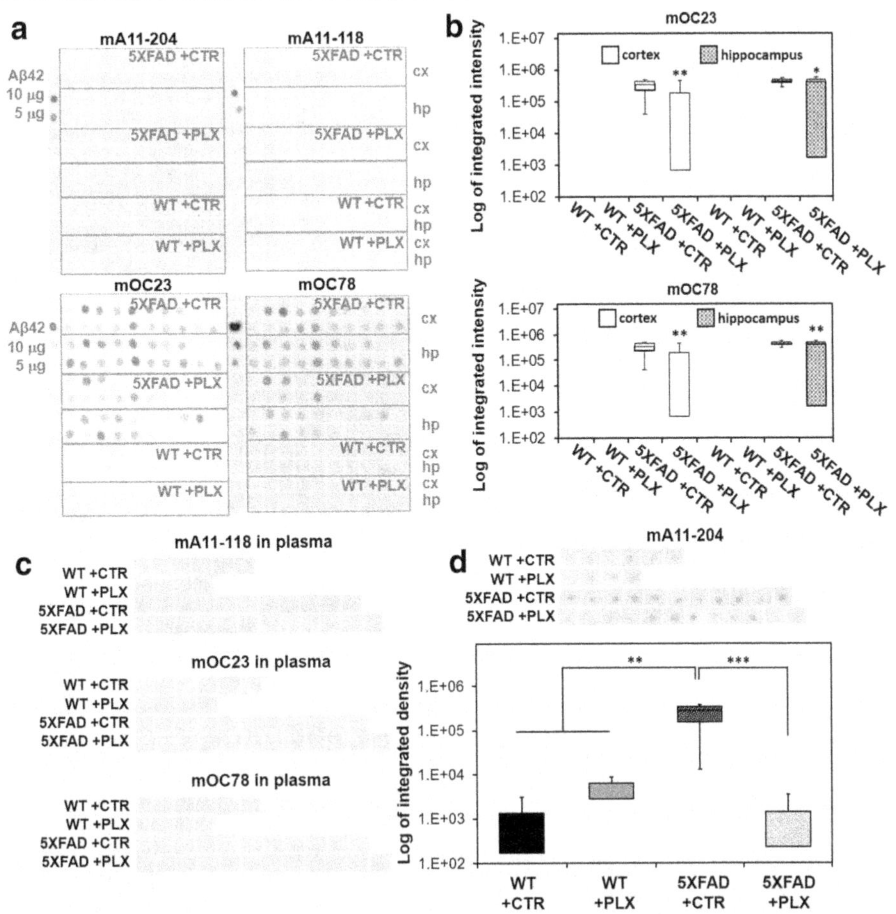

Fig. 5 Treatment with PLX3397 reduces the level of fibrillar amyloid in the total brain lysates and pre-fibrillar oligomers in the blood plasma of 5XFAD mice. **a** An equal amount (6 μg) of total lysate from the cortex (cx) or hippocampus (hp) of each group of mice (male and female) were spotted on the membrane and incubated with antibodies specifically detecting pre-fibrillar oligomers (mA11) or fibrillar aggregates (mOC). 5 μM of oligomerized for 3 days Aβ42 was spotted as a control for antibodies to confirm the ability of the antibodies to distinguish between oligomeric vs. fibrillar conformation. Additionally, 5/10 μg of rabbit IgG were spotted as a positive control for the secondary anti-rabbit antibody. **b** The dot blot analyses were quantified for the mOC23 and mOC78. Whereas wild-type brains were free of amyloid, the fibrillar soluble amyloid was increased in the cortex and hippocampal lysates. However, long-term treatment with PLX3397 (290 mg/kg) decreased significantly the amount of soluble fibrillar mOC23 amyloid in the cortex ($p < 0.004$ with Tukey test, denoted by **) and in the hippocampus ($p < 0.05$ with Tukey test, denoted by *) and soluble fibrillar mOC78 amyloid in the cortex ($p < 0.0018$ with Tukey test, denoted by **) and in the hippocampus ($p < 0.0012$, denoted by **) when compared with the control-chow treated 5XFAD mice. **c** An equal amount of blood plasma (1 μg) of each group (male and female) was spotted on the membrane and incubated as in (**a**). Neither the antibodies against fibrillar mOC23, mOC78 nor mA11–118 against pre-prefibrillar oligomers detected a soluble amyloid in blood plasma. However, antibody mA11–204 has detected pre-fibrillar amyloid in the blood plasma of analyzed cohorts. **d** Quantification of the dot blot for mA11–204 presence in blood plasma. Some endogenous pre-fibrillar amyloid was detected in the wild-type animals, however, the amount of mA11-204-positive amyloid increased significantly in the plasma of 5XFAD animals ($p < 0.0011$ with Tukey test, denoted by **). Long-term administration of PLX3397 in young 5XFAD decreased the amount of pre-fibrillar oligomers (mA11–204) in blood plasma ($p < 0.00082$ with Tukey test, denoted by ***). A-D each assay was performed once for each individual animal due to non-significant inter-assay variability

demonstrated that early long-term treatment with the CSF1R inhibitor, PLX3397 significantly reduced intraneuronal amyloid, neuritic plaque formation, a reduced amount of toxic prefibrillar oligomers and improved cognitive function in particular associative learning in the contextual fear conditioning of 5XFAD mice. These data show that CSF1R signaling, either through microglia or directly on neurons profoundly contributes to amyloid pathogenesis.

Conclusions

CSF1R signaling significantly contributes to the accumulation of intraneuronal amyloid and formation of neuritic plaques in 5XFAD model. Long-term treatment of young 5XFAD mice with PLX3397 lead to an ablation of microglia, a reduction of intraneuronal amyloid and neuritic plaque accumulation. Moreover, the level of soluble fibrillar amyloid in the brain and pre-fibrillar oligomers in blood plasma was significantly reduced. Overall, treatment with PLX3397 improved hippocampal contextual memory. These results suggest that inhibition of CSF1R signaling may be a preventative approach, or therapeutic when applied at the very earliest stages of amyloid deposition during AD.

Abbreviations

5XFAD: Transgenic mouse model carrying five familial Alzheimer's disease mutations (B6SJL-Tg(APPSwFlLon,PSEN1*M146 L*L286 V)6799Vas/Mmjax); AD: Alzheimer's disease; APP: Amyloid precursor protein; Aβ: Amyloid β; CSF1R: Colony stimulation factor 1 receptor; FAD: Familial Alzheimer's disease; Iba1: Ionized calcium binding adaptor molecule 1; IL34: Interleukin 34; NeuN: Neuronal nuclear protein; NFTs: Neurofibrillary tangles; PS: Presenilin

Acknowledgements

This research was supported/partially supported by NIH grants AG00538 (GC and FML), AG056507 (GC), AG027544 (FML), the Cure Alzheimer Fund (GC) and the Alzheimer's Association NIRG-15-363477 (DBV). We are thankful to our colleagues Ms. Mariam Mansour, Ms. Pan Gao, Mr. Marc Farah, Mr. John Farah, Mr. Andre Ksajikan and Mr. Justin Ong who provided technical support in the preparation of mouse tissue.

Funding

This work was supported by NIH grants AG00538 (CG and FML), AG056507 (GC), AG027544 (FML), the Cure Alzheimer Fund (GC) and the Alzheimer's Association NIRG-15-363477 (DBV).

Authors' contributions

CG, JS, SP, and JMRR designed the experiments and JS, SP, and JMRR did the practical work. JS, SP, and RA analyzed the data. DBV performed behavioral tests. JS, SP, FML and CG wrote the manuscript. All authors read and approved the final manuscript.

Competing interests

The authors declare that they have no competing interests.

Author details

[1]Department of Molecular Biology and Biochemistry, University of California, Irvine, USA. [2]Biochemistry Department, Faculty of Science and Experimental Biochemistry Unit, King Fahd Medical Research Center, King Abdulaziz University, Jeddah 21589, Saudi Arabia. [3]Institute for Memory Impairments and Neurological Disorders (UCIMIND), University of California, Irvine, USA.

References

1. Ramirez-Bermudez J. Alzheimer's disease: critical notes on the history of a medical concept. Arch Med Res. 2012;43(8):595–9.
2. Alzheimer A. Über eine eigenartige Erkrankung der Hirnrinde. Allg Z Psychiatrie Psychisch-gerichtl Med. 1907;64:146–8.
3. Barage SH, Sonawane KD. Amyloid cascade hypothesis: pathogenesis and therapeutic strategies in Alzheimer's disease. Neuropeptides. 2015;52:1–18.
4. Doody RS, Raman R, Farlow M, Iwatsubo T, Vellas B, Joffe S, Kieburtz K, He F, Sun X, Thomas RG, et al. A phase 3 trial of semagacestat for treatment of Alzheimer's disease. N Engl J Med. 2013;369(4):341–50.
5. Pensalfini A, Albay R, 3rd, Rasool S, Wu JW, Hatami A, Arai H, Margol L, Milton S, Poon WW, Corrada MM et al: Intracellular amyloid and the neuronal origin of Alzheimer neuritic plaques. Neurobiol Dis 2014, 71:53–61.
6. Oakley H, Cole SL, Logan S, Maus E, Shao P, Craft J, Guillozet-Bongaarts A, Ohno M, Disterhoft J, Van Eldik L, et al. Intraneuronal beta-amyloid aggregates, neurodegeneration, and neuron loss in transgenic mice with five familial Alzheimer's disease mutations: potential factors in amyloid plaque formation. J Neurosci. 2006;26(40):10129–40.
7. Oddo S, Caccamo A, Shepherd JD, Murphy MP, Golde TE, Kayed R, Metherate R, Mattson MP, Akbari Y, LaFerla FM. Triple-transgenic model of Alzheimer's disease with plaques and tangles: intracellular Abeta and synaptic dysfunction. Neuron. 2003;39(3):409–21.
8. Kayed R, Canto I, Breydo L, Rasool S, Lukacsovich T, Wu J, Albay R, 3rd, Pensalfini A, Yeung S, Head E et al. Conformation dependent monoclonal antibodies distinguish different replicating strains or conformers of prefibrillar Abeta oligomers. Mol Neurodegener. 2010;5:57.
9. Elmore MRP, Najafi AR, Koike MA, Dagher NN, Spangenberg EE, Rice RA, Kitazawa M, Matusow B, Nguyen H, West BL, et al. Colony-stimulating factor 1 receptor signaling is necessary for microglia viability, unmasking a microglia progenitor cell in the adult brain. Neuron. 2014;82(2):380–97.
10. Spangenberg EE, Lee RJ, Najafi AR, Rice RA, Elmore MRP, Blurton-Jones M, West BL, Green KN. Eliminating microglia in Alzheimer's mice prevents neuronal loss without modulating amyloid-beta pathology. Brain. 2016;139:1265–81.
11. Bruttger J, Karram K, Wortge S, Regen T, Marini F, Hoppmann N, Klein M, Blank T, Yona S, Wolf Y, et al. Genetic cell ablation reveals clusters of local self-renewing microglia in the mammalian central nervous system. Immunity. 2015;43(1):92–106.
12. Hatami A, Albay R 3rd, Monjazeb S, Milton S, Glabe C. Monoclonal antibodies against Abeta42 fibrils distinguish multiple aggregation state polymorphisms in vitro and in Alzheimer disease brain. J Biol Chem. 2014;289(46):32131–43.
13. Walf AA, Frye CA. The use of the elevated plus maze as an assay of anxiety-related behavior in rodents. Nat Protoc. 2007;2(2):322–8.
14. Sarnyai Z, Sibille EL, Pavlides C, Fenster RJ, McEwen BS, Toth M. Impaired hippocampal-dependent learning and functional abnormalities in the hippocampus in mice lacking serotonin(1A) receptors. Proc Natl Acad Sci U S A. 2000;97(26):14731–6.
15. McAllister WR, McAllister DE. Behavioral measurements of conditioned fear. In: Brush FR, editor. Aversive conditioning and learning. New York: Academic Press; 1971. p. 105–79.
16. Fendt M. Injections of the NMDA receptor antagonist aminophosphonopentanoic acid into the lateral nucleus of the amygdala block the expression of fear-potentiated startle and freezing. J Neurosci. 2001;21(11):4111–5.
17. Jones SV, Heldt SA, Davis M, Ressler KJ. Olfactory-mediated fear conditioning in mice: simultaneous measurements of fear-potentiated startle and freezing. Behav Neurosci. 2005;119(1):329–35.
18. Eimer WA, Vassar R. Neuron loss in the 5XFAD mouse model of Alzheimer's disease correlates with intraneuronal Abeta42 accumulation and Caspase-3 activation. Mol Neurodegener. 2013;8:2.
19. Szalay G, Martinecz B, Lenart N, Kornyei Z, Orsolits B, Judak L, Csaszar E, Fekete R, West BL, Katona G, et al. Microglia protect against brain injury and their selective elimination dysregulates neuronal network activity after stroke. Nat Commun. 2016;7:11499.
20. Salter MW, Stevens B. Microglia emerge as central players in brain disease. Nat Med. 2017;23(9):1018–27.
21. Sarlus H, Heneka MT. Microglia in Alzheimer's disease. J Clin Invest. 2017;127(9):3240–9.
22. Glabe C. Intracellular mechanisms of amyloid accumulation and pathogenesis in Alzheimer's disease. J Mol Neurosci. 2001;17(2):137–45.
23. Friedrich RP, Tepper K, Ronicke R, Soom M, Westermann M, Reymann K, Kaether C, Fandrich M. Mechanism of amyloid plaque formation suggests an intracellular basis of Abeta pathogenicity. Proc Natl Acad Sci U S A. 2010;107(5):1942–7.
24. LaFerla FM, Green KN, Oddo S. Intracellular amyloid-beta in Alzheimer's disease. Nat Rev Neurosci. 2007;8(7):499–509.
25. Luo J, Elwood F, Britschgi M, Villeda S, Zhang H, Ding Z, Zhu L, Alabsi H, Getachew R, Narasimhan R, et al. Colony-stimulating factor 1 receptor (CSF1R) signaling in injured neurons facilitates protection and survival. J Exp Med. 2013;210(1):157–72.
26. Wang WY, Tan MS, Yu JT, Tan L. Role of pro-inflammatory cytokines released from microglia in Alzheimer's disease. Ann Transl Med. 2015;3(10):136.

27. Domingues C, da Cruz ESOAB, Henriques AG. Impact of cytokines and chemokines on Alzheimer's disease neuropathological hallmarks. Curr Alzheimer Res. 2017;14(8):870–82.
28. Garcia S, Hartkamp LM, Malvar-Fernandez B, van Es IE, Lin H, Wong J, Long L, Zanghi JA, Rankin AL, Masteller EL, et al. Colony-stimulating factor (CSF) 1 receptor blockade reduces inflammation in human and murine models of rheumatoid arthritis. Arthritis Res Ther. 2016;18:75.
29. Kayed R, Head E, Thompson JL, McIntire TM, Milton SC, Cotman CW, Glabe CG. Common structure of soluble amyloid oligomers implies common mechanism of pathogenesis. Science. 2003;300(5618):486–9.
30. Kayed R, Head E, Sarsoza F, Saing T, Cotman CW, Necula M, Margol L, Wu J, Breydo L, Thompson JL, et al. Fibril specific, conformation dependent antibodies recognize a generic epitope common to amyloid fibrils and fibrillar oligomers that is absent in prefibrillar oligomers. Mol Neurodegener. 2007;2:18.
31. Breydo L, Kurouski D, Rasool S, Milton S, Wu JW, Uversky VN, Lednev IK, Glabe CG. Structural differences between amyloid beta oligomers. Biochem Bioph Res Co. 2016;477(4):700–5.
32. Knight EM, Kim SH, Kottwitz JC, Hatami A, Albay R, Suzuki A, Lublin A, Alberini CM, Klein WL, Szabo P, et al. Effective anti-Alzheimer a beta therapy involves depletion of specific a beta oligomer subtypes. Neurol Neuroimmunol Neuroinflamm. 2016;3:e237.
33. Diociaiuti M, Macchia G, Paradisi S, Frank C, Camerini S, Chistolini P, Gaudiano MC, Petrucci TC, Malchiodi-Albedi F. Native metastable prefibrillar oligomers are the most neurotoxic species among amyloid aggregates. Biochim Biophys Acta. 2014;1842(9):1622–9.
34. Puzzo D, Lee L, Palmeri A, Calabrese G, Arancio O. Behavioral assays with mouse models of Alzheimer's disease: practical considerations and guidelines. Biochem Pharmacol. 2014;88(4):450–67.
35. Poulin SP, Dautoff R, Morris JC, Barrett LF, Dickerson BC. Alzheimer's disease neuroimaging I: amygdala atrophy is prominent in early Alzheimer's disease and relates to symptom severity. Psychiatry Res. 2011;194(1):7–13.

4

Peripheral immune system in aging and Alzheimer's disease

Wei Cao* and Hui Zheng*

Abstract

Alzheimer's disease (AD) represents an urgent public health mandate. AD is no longer considered a neural-centric disease; rather, a plethora of recent studies strongly implicate a critical role played by neuroinflammation in the pathogeneses of AD and other neurodegenerative conditions. A close functional connection between the immune system and central nervous system is increasingly recognized. In late-onset AD, aging represents the most significant risk factor. Here, from an immunological perspective, we summarize the prominent molecular and cellular changes in the periphery of aging individuals and AD patients. Moreover, we review the knowledge gained in the past several years that implicate specific arms of the peripheral immune system and other types of immune responses in modulating AD progression. Taken together, these findings collectively emphasize a dynamic role of a concert of brain-extrinsic, peripheral signals in the aging and degenerative processes in the CNS. We believe that a systematic view synthesizing the vast amounts of existing results will help guide the development of next-generation therapeutics and inform future directions of AD investigation.

Keywords: Alzheimer's disease, Aging, Senescence, Peripheral immune response, Adaptive immune response, Humoral immune response, T cells, T regulatory cells, Immunosignature

Background

Alzheimer's disease (AD), the most common form of age-associated dementia and neurodegenerative disorder, is a major public health predicament and represents a fundamental scientific challenge. Traditionally, AD has been viewed as a brain-specific disease. Pathologically, AD brains harbor amyloid plaques that contain extracellularly deposited amyloid β (Aβ) from cleaved amyloid precursor protein, and neurofibrillary tangles formed by intracellular accumulation of hyperphosphorylated and misfolded tau protein. These characteristic entities inspired a leading theory that centers on the loss of proteostasis within the brain, which instigates the pathogenic course of AD. The Amyloid Cascade Hypothesis [1–3] has guided numerous studies in the past two decades, which helped reveal insights of the neuronal properties and pathological events initiated by Aβ and subsequently by tau aggregation. However, it is clear that late-onset Alzheimer's disease (LOAD) is collectively modified by numerous genetic factors that govern diverse cellular and molecular pathways, including many genes involved in the immune responses [4–6]. Consequently, The Neuroinflammation Hypothesis emphasizes the dysregulation of central nervous system (CNS) immune response as a key factor in the etiology of neurodegenerative diseases. In recent years, neuroinflammation is increasingly recognized as an integral and critical contributor in AD pathogenesis [7–9].

The role played by the immune system in AD pathogenesis is prominent but is by no means limited to the brain. Copious evidence from clinical and experimental research suggests an influential, yet largely underappreciated, force in AD pathogenesis: systemic immune signals originating outside the brain. This review will primarily focus on the changes and involvement of the peripheral immune system in aging and AD. Readers interested in the functions of microglia, brain-resident macrophage-like immune cells at the center of neuroinflammation, in aging and AD can refer to other recent publications [10–15]. Here we summarize the current understanding of the profound effects of aging on the systemic components of the host. We further review how different elements of the peripheral immune system

* Correspondence: wei.cao@bcm.edu; huiz@bcm.edu
Department of Molecular and Human Genetics, Baylor College of Medicine, Huffington Center on Aging, Houston, TX 77030, USA

and diverse responses modulate the functions of the brain, influence neuroinflammation, and participate in AD pathogenesis with a focus on Aβ-associated events, and discuss implications in the therapeutic development for AD. By uniting multiple influential processes and bridging cross-disciplinary studies, we present a unique systematic perspective to broaden the comprehension on the molecular and cellular players involved in AD pathogenesis.

Systemic changes associated with aging

Inflammaging

As the most significant risk factor for AD, aging itself exerts profound impacts on the immune system and the peripheral tissues (Fig. 1). Innate immunity protects the host by detecting pathogen-associated pattern molecules and activating signaling pathways that result in rapid secretion of cytokines and chemokines, the key soluble immune effector molecules. It has been shown that aging alters the components of innate immunity ranging from the expression of signaling molecules to the behavior of neutrophils, monocytes, dendritic cells, NK cells, etc. [16]. The phenomenon of inflammaging is characterized by chronic low-grade inflammation and functional decline in an aging host [17, 18]. Inflammasomes are intracellular multicomponent structures that enable the secretion of IL-1β and IL-18, important proinflammatory cytokines [19, 20]. The expression of specific inflammasome gene modules in older individuals is associated with higher incidence of elevated blood pressure, arterial stiffness, metabolic dysfunction, oxidative stress and shortened life span [21]. Accordingly, age-related increase in circulating IL-18 is significantly reduced in mice lacking Nlrp3 inflammasome or inflammasome adaptor Asc [22]. Other cytokines and proinflammatory factors have also been associated with age-related decline in physical and cognitive function [23, 24].

Immune cell skewing

Aging is associated with increased cell-to-cell transcriptional variability in different tissues, including cells of the hematopoietic lineage [25–28]. Accordingly, aged peripheral immune cells contain highly heterogeneous epigenetic modifications between individuals and from cell to cell, as revealed by single-cell chromatin modification profiling [28]. In addition, substantial alteration in the populations of cells mediating adaptive immunity is well-documented: naïve T cells and circulating B cells are reduced while terminally differentiated T cells are increased in aged individuals [16, 29]. The age-dependent loss of T cell homeostasis has been linked to thymus involution, which is mediated by Nlrp3 inflammasome [22]. Aged naïve T cells possess a less diverse T cell receptor (TCR) repertoire and may switch to a dysfunctional "virtual memory" cell phenotype, which is accompanied by profound epigenetic changes [28–34]. Furthermore, both aged $CD4^{+}$ and $CD8^{+}$ T cells display features of cellular senescence (see below). In aging, B cell receptor repertoire diversity and switched memory B cells are significantly reduced, which is accompanied by a diminished antibody response to antigen challenge. On the other hand, a distinct subset of mature B cells, termed age-associated B cells, accumulates in aged mice and older humans, which may promote inflammation and autoimmunity while inhibiting B cell lymphopoiesis [35, 36]. Beyond blood, aging shifts the functional balance between self-renewal and differentiation in hematopoietic stem cells in the bone marrow and favors the generation of myeloid lineage cells [37]. Overall, an aged immune system renders the host susceptible to infections and

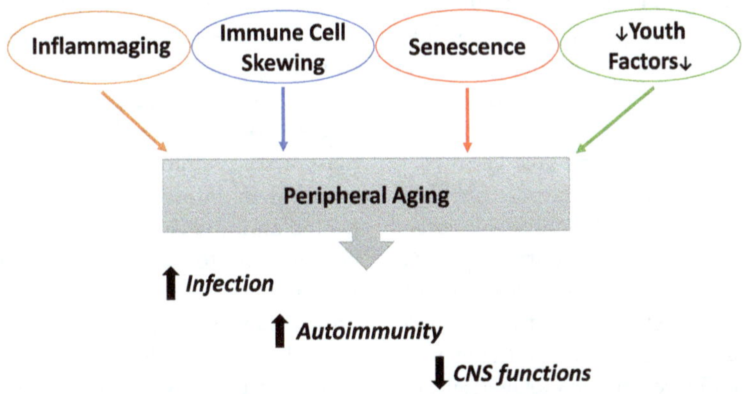

Fig. 1 Multifactorial systemic changes are associated with chronological aging and linked to diminished health status. Peripheral aging is promoted by inflammaging, immune cell skewing, senescence, and depletion of youth protective factors. The broad outcome of aging includes increased incidences of infection, autoimmune diseases, and decline of memory and cognitive functions.

increases the incidences of autoimmune and other diseases, which is accompanied by the decline of cognitive functions (Fig. 1).

Senescence

During aging, senescent cells accumulate in the body by entering a long-lasting form of cell-cycle arrest triggered by various molecular stressors. Breakthrough studies in recent years have revealed a complex mechanism underlying the biogenesis of these cells and their roles in diverse physiological and pathological conditions (reviewed in [38–40]). The involvement of senescent cells in host immunity is closely linked to their acquired ability to secrete proinflammatory cytokines, a phenomenon termed the senescence-associated secretory phenotype (SASP) [18]. SASP is induced primarily by NF-κB in response to DNA damage, oncogenic stress and developmental cues, which initiates the transcription of a host of genes including IL-6, IL-1β, TNF-α, IL-8, etc. [41, 42]. Given the proinflammatory nature of SASP, cellular senescence in multiple organs and tissues significantly promotes inflammaging in the elderly [18, 43]. As mentioned earlier, naïve T cell senescence is associated with a loss of immune diversity. Concomitantly, terminally differentiated senescent T cells expand and over-express cytotoxins and proinflammatory cytokines, contributing to the hyperinflammatory status of the host. Several groups recently demonstrated a remarkable functional restoration in multiple tissues and organs of the mice after selective ablation of senescent cells by genetic manipulation or treatment with senolytic compounds [44]. The classical senescent cells have not been widely identified in aging CNS beyond the description of SASP+ astrocytes [45]. The impact of senescent cell ablation on brain function is yet to be demonstrated.

Diminished youth factors

Aging not only induces the generation of harmful products, it also depletes the molecules that keep the host young [46]. Shared circulation between young and old mice by way of parabiosis has demonstrated the ability of old blood to transfer aging phenotypes to peripheral tissues and the brain of young mice, and vice versa [47]. Immune factors enriched in aged plasma, such as CCL11 and B2M, have been shown to negatively affect neurogenesis and memory [47, 48]. In contrast, growth and differentiation factor 11 (GDF-11) supplementation to aged mice was shown to benefit the heart and muscle and increase neurogenesis [49–51]. However, the expression and function of GDF-11 remains controversial and further studies are needed to confirm its role in host rejuvenation [52, 53]. Nevertheless, a proof-of-concept study demonstrated a near complete restoration of synaptic and neuronal proteins in aged amyloid precursor protein (APP)-expressing mice after exposure to circulating young blood or receiving plasma transfusion [54]. Improved working and associative memory occurred after young plasma administration in the absence of changes in amyloid load [54]. A renewed search for systemic brain rejuvenating factors led to the recent identification of tissue inhibitor of metalloproteases 2 (TIMP2), which is present at highest levels in the human umbilical cord blood, over young and old adult blood [55]. As reported, TIMP2 not only promotes neuronal plasticity inside the brain likely through modulating extracellular matrix, but also affects hippocampal synaptic plasticity from systemic circulation. Although direct translation of the findings to human diseases is uncertain at this point, these studies illustrate a dynamic, complex, and powerful crosstalk between the periphery and the brain.

Molecular alterations in the circulation of AD patients

Early observational studies and meta-analyses detected an association between elevated levels of inflammatory factors and increased risk for AD development [56, 57]. In the past decade, many proteomic surveys have been performed mostly on human plasma and occasionally on serum samples, using diverse technical platforms, ranging from filter-based arrayed sandwich ELISA, 2D-gel electrophoresis coupled with liquid chromatography and mass spectrometry, Luminex xMAP, Myriad RBM, to SOMAscan multiplexed protein technology (reviewed in [51, 58]). Although the list of top altered proteins overlapped and differed between individual studies, a consensus pathway analysis revealed significant changes of multiple immunological processes, among which Complement and Coagulation Cascades and Cytokine-Cytokine Receptor Interaction are ominously affected [58]. Noteworthy is that both are centrally involved in the neuroinflammation inside the brains of AD patients and AD animal models [59, 60].

Although over 20% of people diagnosed with mild cognitive impairment (MCI) develop dementia over the subsequent 3 to 10 years, it remains difficult to predict the disease course for individual patients. By examining the plasma communicome, *i.e.* a group of signaling proteins involved in intracellular communication, *Ray et al* reported an initial success in identifying MCI patients who are *en route* to develop AD based on a panel of 18 affected proteins consisting primarily of chemokines and growth factors [61]. Subsequent studies using more advanced detection technologies and analyzing a larger cohort of patients established a subset of 10-13 plasma proteins, including several apolipoproteins, chemokines and growth factors, whose abundance is associated with disease severity and progression of AD [62, 63]. More recently, a simple combination of two plasma markers (Apo A-II and cortisol) and four cerebrospinal fluid (CSF) proteins (fibroblast growth factor 4, calcitonin, heart-type fatty acid binding protein, and TRAIL-R3) was shown to be valuable in predicting midterm progression from MCI to AD dementia [64]. Hence, molecular changes in the blood may be useful to probe the ongoing neurodegeneration in the brain. Before any of these markers are adopted as blood biomarkers for clinical prognosis, their robustness, accuracy, and reproducibility need to be firmly established.

Involvement of peripheral immune cells in brain homeostasis and aging

Like other organs, the CNS is under regular immune surveillance. While microglia cells reside inside the parenchyma, small but significant numbers of T cells, B cells, NK cells, and dendritic cells migrate into and populate the meninges and choroid plexus (CP) that form a direct interface with the brain parenchyma [65]. A series of studies have established an indispensable role played by $CD4^+$ T cells in maintaining the cognitive and behavioral capacity of naive mice [66–68]. In particular, $CD4^+$ T helper cells and their secreted cytokines after undergoing polarization facilitate memory function and social behaviors. Both IFNγ-producing (T_H1) and IL-4-producing (T_H2) $CD4^+$ T cells reside in the meninges under steady-state conditions. IFNγ supports neuronal circuits that are important for social behavior [69] and IL-4 facilitates learning by regulating meningeal dendritic cells and stimulating BDNF expression in astrocytes [70]. Therefore, T cells and their secreted cytokines are critically involved in preserving the homeostatic functions of the brain (Table 1).

CP is an epithelial tissue located within the ventricles of the brain [71, 72]. As the site of the blood-CSF barrier, CP plays indispensable roles in maintaining brain homeostasis by secreting neurotropic factors into CSF, clearing toxic molecules including Aβ from CSF, and facilitating immune surveillance and leukocyte trafficking [71, 72]. In naïve mice, more than 50% of $CD4^+$ and $CD8^+$ T cells in the brain reside in the stroma of the CP. Most of these T cells have an effector memory phenotype, including T_H1, T_H2 and Tregs, and recognize CNS antigens [73]. However in aged CP, a distorted T_H1: T_H2 balance arises, which results in increased chemokine CCL11 expression, decreased permeability to leukocytes owing to the differential effects of IL-4 and IFNγ on CP epithelial cells, and compromised cognition [73–75] (Table 1). Type I interferon (IFN-I) is a major innate immune cytokine commonly involved in host defense as well as autoimmune conditions. Interestingly, aged CP of both human and mouse display strong IFN-I signaling, which was shown to counter the function of IFNγ (i.e. type II interferon), disrupt the infiltration of monocytes, and hamper cognitive functions and hippocampal neurogenesis [76]. Hence, aging disrupts the balance of brain-homing peripheral immune cells, which negatively impacts essential CNS functions.

Involvement of peripheral immune cells in AD pathogenesis

Innate immune cells

Inside the brain, ongoing AD pathology leads to the differentiation of microglia into a novel type associated with neurodegenerative diseases with altered molecular expression profile and limited phagocytic capacity [77, 78]. The precise origin of plaque-surrounding amoeboid myeloid cells has long been debated, owing to the technical challenge of distinguishing infiltrating myeloid cells from locally-activated microglia. Nevertheless, recent evidence suggests that peripherally-derived macrophages can engraft the brain and maintain a unique functional and transcriptional identity in CNS [79]. Infiltrating peripheral myeloid cells have been demonstrated to participate in Aβ clearance, leading to the notion that monocytes are superior phagocytes when traversed inside the AD brain [80, 81]. However, such a conclusion is challenged by studies showing that infiltrating peripheral myeloid cells, in replacing ablated microglia, adopt a microglia-like phenotype in the brain, *i.e.* with limited phagocytic capacity, likely influenced by local molecular cues [82, 83]. Whether additional signals are needed to boost their phagocytic function *in situ* requires further investigation.

Rare variants in Triggering Receptor Expressed on Myeloid cells 2 (TREM2) increase the risk of developing AD by 2~3 fold. Significant TREM2-dependent

Table 1 T cell subsets maintain homeostatic brain functions

Subset/ Cytokine	Location	Effects on brain function	Specificity	Mechanism	Reference
T_H1/IFNγ	Meninges	↑ Social behavior	bulk	IFNγ signaling activation in inhibitory neurons increases GABAergic currents	[69]
T_H2/IL-4	Meninges	↑ Learning and memory	bulk	Restricts meningeal myeloid cell activation and promotes neutrophic factor expression	[70]
↑T_H2:T_H1 ratio	CP of Aged Mice	↓ Cognitive capacity	CNS antigens	IL-4 induces while IFNγ inhibits CCL11 expression by epithelia cells	[73]

phenotypes in mouse models of AD shed light on the role of TREM2 in regulating neuroinflammation during AD pathogenesis [84]. Besides CNS upregulation, expression of TREM2 mRNA and protein are increased in the peripheral leukocytes of AD patients and correlated with cognitive deficits and hippocampal atrophy [85–88]. It is unclear if elevated peripheral TREM2 expression has functional impact on disease pathogenesis or merely reflects the ongoing systemic inflammation of AD.

Neutrophils are the most abundant myeloid cells in human peripheral blood and participate critically in protective innate immunity. Neutrophils have been detected in the brain parenchyma of 5xFAD and 3xTg-AD mice and were shown to promote amyloid plaques and tau tangles as well as cognitive decline [89]. Yet, a separate study showed that long term treatment of 3xTg-AD mice with a TNF-α modulator led to increased neutrophil infiltration in the brain, which coincided with improved learning and memory, and reduced tau and amyloid pathology [90]. Thus, the functional features of infiltrating neutrophils remain to be fully elucidated.

Adaptive immune cells

Distinct from innate immunity, adaptive immune responses protect the host in a manner that is long-lasting and antigen-specific. Although innate immune responses at the site of brain inflammation are well-established, the role played by adaptive immunity in AD remains vague, primarily due to the scarcity of T cells or B cells inside the parenchyma. Nevertheless, a recent large-scale genome-wide association study strongly implicated the involvement of both adaptive and innate immunity in AD [91]. In addition, the association of a single-nucleotide polymorphism (SNP) of MHC class II HLA-DRB5 with AD implies a potential T cell-mediated process [92]. To assess the overall function of the adaptive immunity, two groups analyzed severely immunocompromised transgenic mice expressing human mutant APP and obtained conflicting results. PSAPP:Rag2$^{-/-}$ mice lacking B and T cells showed reduced Aβ pathology accompanied by highly phagocytic microglia [93], whereas 5xFAD:Rag2$^{-/-}$:Il2rg$^{-/-}$ mice lacking B, T and NK cells displayed exaggerated Aβ plaque deposition and increased neuroinflammation [94]. While the two mouse models do differ in several aspects, the primary reason for the discrepant observations is unclear. Given the memory and behavior impairment in Rag2$^{-/-}$ mice [68, 95, 96], how this may confound Aβ-associated functional decline was not addressed.

B cells in adaptive immunity

Humoral immune response (*i.e.* antibody production) by B cells to amyloid β has been studied for over 20 years. It was first discovered that immortalized B cells from the peripheral blood of an AD patient secreted antibodies that specifically recognize Aβ peptide [97]. Circulating anti-Aβ antibody at various levels has since been detected in the blood of human subjects with or without AD [98–101]. The groundbreaking study by Schenk et al, in which Aβ immunization prevented the development of amyloid plaques, neuritic dystrophy and gliosis in PDAPP mice, demonstrated the therapeutic potential of B cell-mediated immune response [102]. However, human vaccination trial AN1792 based on the same principle had to be halted due to life-threatening encephalitis, which was later attributed largely to the pathogenic autoimmune T_H1 response stimulated by active immunization (see next section). Subsequent studies in animal models demonstrated the ability of individual Aβ-specific antibody clones to attenuate AD pathogenesis without the involvement of T cells, lending support for the clinical trials to passively immunize AD patients with anti-Aβ antibodies. However, such a strategy has yielded mixed outcomes with several trials still ongoing (reviewed by [103–105]; also see section *Passive Immunotherapy*)).

Besides the humoral response specific to proteins associated with AD pathology, the peripheral immunoglobulin repertoire is dysregulated in AD. Spontaneously secreted by B cells without exogenous stimulation, natural antibodies are abundant in normal sera, typically poly- or self-reactive, and fulfill important functions of targeting pathogens and removing cellular and molecular waste in the body [106]. The levels of natural IgG recognizing self-antigens was shown to be influenced by age, sex and disease [107]. Significant reduction of the number of autoantibodies was detected in the sera from patients with AD, Parkinson's disease (PD), and multiple sclerosis, a neuroinflammatory condition [107]. The cause and functional significance of such a decrease is unclear. Unexpectedly, a recent time-course global proteomic analysis of APP^{NL-F} mice reported an inverse correlation between Aβ burden in the brain and IgM levels in the blood [108]. Again, the implication of this finding remains to be seen. Nevertheless using a panel of autoantibodies as biomarkers, DeMarshall et al. were able to differentiate mild-moderate AD patients from age-matched controls, MCI, and other neurological disorders with high confidence [109].

Another insight on the role of immunoglobulin in AD came from the study by Marsh et al. [94]. Increased mouse IgGs were detected in association with microglia in the brains of 5xFAD mice. Lacking specificity for Aβ, these proteins were shown to engage with microglia Fc receptor, induce an activating signaling pathway, and stimulate phagocytosis of Aβ, which lead to a decreased plaque load. Although the antigen-specificity of the infiltrating IgG was not studied in this study, the protective effect of mouse IgG is reminiscent of the beneficial influence previously reported with intravenous Immunoglobulin (IVIg), a pooled human IgG product [110–112]. Whether any specific subset of the natural IgGs confers enhanced neuroprotection remains to be investigated.

T cells in adaptive immunity

Inside the post-mortem brains of AD patients, both $CD4^+$ and $CD8^+$ T cells were detected, occasionally next to the neuritic plaques or microglia [113–115]. Similarly, increased numbers of T cells have been found infiltrating the brain parenchyma of multiple transgenic mice expressing mutant human APP [116, 117]. In one study, significant fractions of infiltrating T cells were found to produce IFNγ and IL-17 in APP/PS1 brain [117]. However, Ferretti et al. reported that infiltrating T cells consistently display an inactivated phenotype with reduced IFNγ production and lack of local proliferation and do not co-localize with amyloid plaques in three AD models (ArcAβ, APP/PS1 and Tg2576) [116]. In line with this, peripheral $CD4^+$ T cells were found hyporesponsive to Aβ peptides in Tg2576 mice, which resulted in a defective Aβ-specific antibody response [118]. In humans, an early study reported unresponsiveness to Aβ40 peptide by peripheral lymphocytes from AD patients [119]. However, peripheral T cells reactive to Aβ42 peptide, which is more immunogenic than Aβ40, was later found significantly increased in AD patients and older adults over middle-aged healthy controls [120]. T regulatory cells (Tregs) are a crucial T cell subset that suppresses effector immune responses and maintains immune tolerance. AD and Down syndrome patients both display Aβ plaque accumulation and similarly have increased Aβ-specific IL-10-producing Treg cells in their blood [121]. Elevated Treg levels and suppressive activities in the periphery of AD patients were reported by other groups [122–124], which is affirmed by the increased $FoxP3^+$ Tregs in the spleens of 5xFAD mice [125].

Given the distinct and powerful roles played by T helper subsets in numerous diseases, it would be vital to dissect how different T_H cell populations specifically modulate AD. In the APP/PS1 model, adoptive transfer of Aβ-specific T_H1 cells, but not T_H2 or T_H17 cells, led to their homing to the brain and worsened AD pathology along with impaired cognitive function and exaggerated microglia activation [117]. The pathogenic and plaque clearing roles of T_H1 cells were demonstrated in an earlier study, in which, post-Aβ vaccination, Aβ-specific IFNγ-producing T cells infiltrated the brain of J20 mice to clear amyloid plaques but induced meningoencephalitis, mirroring the pathogenic events of the failed human vaccination trial AN1792 [126]. However, direct cerebrospinal injection of Aβ-specific T_H1 cells led to amyloid plaque clearance and increased neurogenesis in the absence of autoimmunity, implying an added impact of peripheral T_H1 cells in APP/PS1 model [127]. On the other hand, adoptively transferred Aβ-specific T_H2 cells, while with no evidence of brain filtration, improved working memory of APP/PS1 mice in conjunction with reduced systemic inflammation and vascular amyloidosis [128]. Therefore, Aβ-specific T_H1 and T_H2 effector subsets seemingly alter the Aβ pathology in distinct ways (Table 2).

Substantial yet contradictory impacts of Tregs on AD pathogenesis have been demonstrated by recent studies in several experimental models (Table 3). By way of antibody-mediated depletion, adoptive transfer of purified cells, and low-dose IL-2-induced peripheral expansion, multiple groups independently provided experimental evidence that collectively suggested an overall protective role of Tregs in restoring memory deficits, reducing plaque load and decreasing microglia activation as well as inflammation in several APP transgenic models [129–132]. These results are consistent with the impaired learning and memory in $IL\text{-}2^{-/-}$ mice, which lack functional Tregs [133]. Whether Tregs convey neuroprotection in an antigen-specific manner is not clear at this time.

On the other hand, two consecutive reports from Michal Schwartz's group strongly argued for detrimental effects of Tregs in AD pathogenesis [125, 134]. They first demonstrated that 5xFAD mice

Table 2 Aβ-specific T cell subsets regulate AD pathogenesis in experimental models

Subset	Location	AD Model	Specificity	Effects on pathogenesis	Reference
T_H1	Parenchyma	APP/PS1	Aβ	Adoptively transferred cells increased microglia activation and Aβ deposition	[117]
T_H1	Parenchyma	J20 with Aβ peptide vaccination	Aβ	Migrated to Aβ plaques with increased clearance, while inducing transient meningoencephalitis	[126]
T_H1	Parenchyma	APP/PS1	Aβ	Cells injected to cerebrospinal ventricle migrated to Aβ plaques, increased Aβ clearance and promote neurogenesis	[127]
T_H2	Outside the brain	APP/PS1	Aβ	Adoptively transferred cells improved working memory, decreased microgliosis and reduced plasma cytokines. No effect on plaque load inside the parenchyma but reduced vascular amyloidosis	[128]

Table 3. Treg cells regulate AD pathogenesis in experimental models

Subset	Location	AD model	Specificity	Effects on pathogenesis	Reference
T_{reg}	Systemic	APP/PS1	bulk	Transient depletion of Treg accelerated cognitive decline; increased Treg with low-dose IL-2 treatment restored cognitive functions	[129]
T_{reg}	Systemic	3xTg	bulk	Adoptively transferred cells improved cognitive functions and reduced Aβ deposition; long-term Treg depletion resulted in exacerbated spatial learning deficits, Aβ plaque load and microgliosis	[130]
T_{reg}	Systemic and Parenchyma	App/PS1 ΔE9	bulk	AAV-IL-2 expression within the brain induced Treg expansion and astrocyte activation, reduced Aβ plaque and improved synaptic plasticity and spine density	[131]
T_{reg}	Systemic	AβPPswe/PS1 Δ E9	bulk	Adoptively transferred cells improved cognitive function, while reducing Aβ deposition, microgliosis and systematic inflammation	[132]
T_{reg}	Systemic	5xFAD APP/PS1	bulk	Transient depletion or pharmacological inhibition of Treg lead to Aβ plaque clearance, reduced neuroinflammation and reversal of cognitive decline. It affected CP with increased recruitment of peripheral monocytes and Tregs to Aβ plaque	[125]
T_{reg}	Systemic	5xFAD	bulk	Anti-PD1 treatment stimulated IFNγ-dependent systematic immune response, which resulted in the recruitment of peripheral monocytes and Tregs to Aβ plaque, clearance of plaque, and improvement of cognitive performance. Repeated treatments maintained a long-lasting beneficial effects	[134]
T_{reg}		$ThyAPP/PS1_{m146L}$ $ThyAPP/PS1_{A246E}$ PD-APP	bulk	Anti-PD1 treatments had no effect on amyloid pathology nor induced infiltration of peripheral monocyte into the brain	[135]

have reduced expression in choroid plexus of molecules critical for transepithelial migration, which correlated with the loss of IFNγ signaling, a condition similar to brain aging [125]. This led to a hypothesis that a dysregulated CP exacerbates AD pathogenesis by blocking protective immune cell infiltration. Since Tregs are the primary suppressor of IFNγ-producing T_H1 cells, depleting or disabling Treg function was shown to restore IFNγ signaling in CP, increase the number of peripheral immune cells in the parenchyma, clear amyloid plaques, and rescue memory and behavior defects in 5xFAD mice [125, 134]. In more detail, Baruch et al. perturbed the Treg population by various experimental schemes, which included selective depletion in 5xFAD:FoxP3-DTR mice with diphtheria toxin, chemical treatments to boost or diminish the functionality of Tregs or stimulate their induction, and administrating antibody against PD1 to break Treg suppression in 5xFAD and/or APP/PS1 models (Table 3).

At this time, it is unclear whether these directly opposing results reported on Tregs are affected by the genetic background of the AD models or other factors. Nevertheless, a T cell-based intervention with anti-PD1 antibody, which is largely analogous to the cancer checkpoint immunotherapy, was proposed as a translatable approach of AD therapeutics based on the findings by Baruch et al. [135]. However most recently, a joint study by three pharmaceutical companies questioned the effectiveness of systemic PD-1 blockade in modifying amyloid burden in several AD mouse models, where the authors also failed to detect monocyte infiltration into the brain ([136]; Table 3). Hence, the mechanism of how Tregs modulate Aβ pathology remains to be fully elucidated and the pre-clinical support for PD-1 blockade approach in AD patients is weak at this time.

Peripheral immune responses modify AD pathogenesis

Pathogens

The brain can readily respond to inflammatory signals originated from the periphery. For example, peripheral administration of microbial mimetics, such as LPS and polyI:C, that induce strong systemic inflammatory response, exacerbates neurodegeneration [137, 138]. Microglia are shown to be highly receptive to these treatments and the resulting enhanced neuroinflammation compels the disease pathogenesis [139]. Living in a bustling world, humans are exposed to exogenous infectious agents, cohabit with a complex microbiome, and are afflicted increasingly by chronic ailments as we age. Immune system is the frontline protection against microbial infections. When the infectious agents are not well controlled, HIV patients develop dementia that is highly analogous to AD, West Nile Virus infection leads to long term cognitive impairment, and periodontitis exacerbates the cognitive decline in AD patients, etc. [140–142].

Microbiota

Mammals host trillions of microbes that reside in the barrier tissues such as gut, skin, and lung. Research in recent years have revealed a dynamic interaction between the microbiome and the immune system and the pathogenic outcomes of dysbiosis [143, 144]. Microbes in the gut profoundly affect the development of microglia [145] and effectively prime microglia in the brain via secreted short-chain fatty acids [146], highlighting an eminent gut-brain axis [147]. Several studies have suggested that gut microbiota plays a vital role in the pathogenesis of PD via modulating neuroinflammation [148, 149]. To understand its potential relevance to AD, two groups surveyed the gut microbe taxa in elderly individuals. AD patients have reduced microbial diversity and harbor a distinct bacteria genera, which is correlated with changes in CSF biomarkers [150]. A similar association was made between inflammatory bacteria and pro-inflammatory circulating cytokines in patients with cognitive impairment [151]. Consistent with this, a shift in the gut microbiota was detected in APP/PS1 mice compared with non-transgenic controls. Depletion of microbiota by antibiotic treatments or germ-free host re-derivation resulted in reduced Aβ plaque load in conjunction with altered microglia morphology [152, 153]. Intriguingly, transient perturbation of microbial diversity in APP/PS1 mice shortly after birth can result in long-lasting alteration of brain Aβ pathology [154]. Although microbiota can modulate CNS profiles in mice [155], whether and how gut microbiota affect cognition and memory in AD models has yet to be fully revealed. This area of research is being actively pursued and will surely help illuminate how such key environmental factor modulate AD risk and progression.

Chronic inflammation

A recent prospective survey of 1,633 participants revealed a positive association between midlife peripheral inflammation and shrinkage of brain volume in late-life [156]. Not unexpectedly, a genetic epidemiology study identified SNPs that are shared between LOAD and common chronic inflammatory diseases, such as psoriasis, type 1 diabetes and Crohn disease [92]. Chronic conditions with inflammatory traits, such as vascular diseases and diabetes, are well-known comorbidities of AD. Aging is also associated with higher incidents of autoinflammatory diseases, such as rheumatoid arthritis (RA) and psoriasis, two diseases also co-morbid with AD [157, 158]. RA patients receiving anti-inflammatory treatments have overall reduced risk of developing AD, and peripheral neutralization of TNF-α, a key cytokine driving RA pathogenesis, was shown effective in AD animal models [159]. Therefore, diverse systemic inflammatory responses play a crucial role in modulating AD pathogenesis.

Therapeutic applications in AD by harnessing the immune system

Deemed the greatest global challenge for health and social care in the 21st century, dementia affected an estimated 47 million people globally in 2015, a number which may increase to 131 million by 2050 as the world's population ages. The task to develop effective treatments for AD is exceedingly daunting, due to the multifaceted nature of the disease, lack of sensitive and definitive biomarkers, incomplete understanding of the pathogenic and regulatory pathways, dearth of disease stage-specific molecular targets, and technical difficulties for effective CNS drug delivery. Nevertheless, a range of strategies harnessing our knowledge of immune responses and aging/AD pathogenesis are being actively pursued.

Passive immunotherapy

Despite the strong implication of Aβ peptide in AD, strategies targeting monomeric Aβ failed in late stage AD populations [104, 160]. Along the protein misfolding pathway, soluble oligomeric assemblies are recognized as the primary pathogenic species of misfolded proteins [161, 162]. Although antibodies against different forms of aggregated Aβ are detected in the peripheral blood of healthy individuals, the levels of these antibodies decrease with normal aging and decline further with progression from mild to severe AD [163, 164]. Inoculation of antibodies recognizing aggregated Aβ effectively modified amyloid plaque pathology and rescued cognitive decline in AD animal models [165–167]. Given the protective humoral response in the host, a "reverse translational medicine" approach was devised. A fully humanized IgG1 mAb reactive to aggregated but not monomeric Aβ, aducanumab, was obtained from a screen of healthy advanced-age donors with normal cognition who presumably harbor naturally developed protective mAbs against Aβ. Preliminary results from a double-blind, placebo-controlled phase 1b trial with aducanumab showed reduced brain Aβ plaques in a dose- and time-dependent manner and a trend of slowing clinical decline in AD patients [167]. Two large-scale phase 3 trials with aducanumab are ongoing and will be completed in 2022. In addition to Aβ, antibodies specific to tau protein are also being actively evaluated for their clinical potentials [160].

One significant impediment for the success of passive immunotherapy for AD is the insufficient entry of antibodies into the CNS. It was estimated that only approximately 0.1% of peripherally-administered antibody can enter the brain in the presence of an intact blood brain barrier (BBB), a network of vascular endothelial cells, pericytes and astrocytes, which significantly blunted the drug availability inside the brain [168, 169]. Different strategies are being devised to improve CNS delivery of therapeutic antibodies. A bispecific antibody design with one arm recognizing transferrin receptor, a surface molecule highly expressed by BBB endothelial cells, greatly enhanced transcytosis of the antibody across the BBB and increased the antibody levels inside the brain [170, 171]. On the other hand, transient opening of the BBB can be achieved by focused ultrasound treatment, which was shown to result in the reduction of amyloid burden in AD models and enhanced the protective effect of a tau-specific antibody *in vivo* recently [172–175].

Targeting immune molecules

Consistent with the notion of a pathogenic influence of inflammation, early epidemiological studies suggested that long term use of anti-inflammatory drugs was associated with reduced risk of developing AD [176, 177]. This led to multiple clinical trials designed to suppress general inflammation, which included using nonsteroidal anti-inflammatory drugs, statins, low dose-prednisone, and NF-κB blocker, etc.; however, no clinical benefit has been demonstrated in AD patients (reviewed in [178, 179]). Intravenous immunoglobulins have been used clinically for treating various autoimmune and infectious diseases and exhibited protective effects in AD animal models, as discussed earlier [110, 111]. Yet, clinical trials with IVIg failed to show positive effect [180–182].

Given the complex role played by immune cells and responses inside and outside the brain, a deeper understanding of the molecular mechanisms is a prerequisite for translational success. Therapies targeting specific immune molecules that are crucial in AD pathogenesis or protection presumably offer improvement over non-specific interventions. TNF-α is a proinflammatory cytokine highly implicated in many peripheral inflammatory diseases as well as AD. Peripheral TNF-α neutralization was effective in reducing Aβ plaques and neuronal dysfunction in an AD model [159]. A small, double-blind, placebo-controlled phase 2 trial with Etanercept, a decoy receptor for TNF-α, reported a tolerated response [183]. Yet, future trial with large patient cohort is necessary to establish the effectiveness of this strategy. On the other hand, administration of the cytokine Granulocyte-Macrophage Colony-Stimulating Factor (GM-CSF) was shown effective in improving memory in aged mice, reducing brain amyloidosis and reversing the cognitive impairment in AD mice, and associated with improved cognition in cancer patients [55, 184, 185]. A small number of AD patients treated with Leukine®, recombinant human GM-CSF, reported rapid improvement of cognitive functions in a double-blind, placebo-controlled phase 2 trial [186].

Anti-aging strategies

Besides disease-specific targeting, slowing down the clock of age-related systemic decline should be beneficial for a wide spectrum of diseases, including AD. Although most studies were carried out in rodents, the exciting findings on the power of young blood and molecules with capacity to rejuvenate the old offer a novel prospect of therapeutics [46]. An ongoing phase I Plasma for Alzheimer's Symptom Amelioration (PLASMA) trial examines the safety, tolerability and feasibility of infused blood plasma from young donors to patients with mild to moderate Alzheimer's disease [187]. Alternatively, via selective destruction of senescent cells, senolytics have emerged recently as a novel class of anti-aging agents in animal studies. In the coming years, therapeutic potential to target senescence in humans will surely be explored (reviewed in [44]).

Conclusions

We have summarized the knowledge gained in recent years on the changes of the periphery in aging and Alzheimer's disease and the emerging significance of the peripheral immune system and their responses in modulating AD pathogenesis. It is thus apparent that the prevailing neuro-immune connection is not limited to localized neuroinflammation inside the brain. Here we emphasize the importance of diverse signals from the periphery to modify the course of AD pathogenesis (Fig. 2). The systemic influences comprise a multitude of age-dependent organismal changes, protective and pathogenic immune cell surveillance, and ongoing immune responses to environmental factors and self-derived molecules. These elements operate jointly and dynamically with the ongoing brain-intrinsic aging and degenerative processes. We believe such

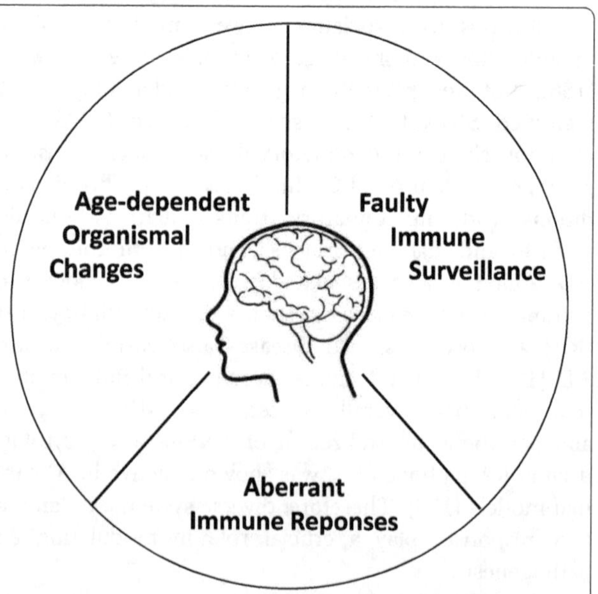

Fig. 2 AD pathogenesis is influenced by multiple systemic factors. Aging-induced systemic changes, surveillance by various immune cell populations, and influence of altered systemic immune responses all influence the onset and progression of AD. Understanding the interplay between these elements and AD pathogenesis is crucial for the successful intervention of the disease.

understanding helps comprehend the vast amount of existing literature and expand our perspectives in AD research.

Despite the latest immense interest in understanding the role of immune system modulation in AD, some major knowledge gaps remain. Below we identify six key areas that the field should address in the future:

Contribution of aging to AD

Given the importance of aging in LOAD, it is not surprising that AD pathology *in vivo* is modulated highly by immune responses in an age- and disease-state dependent manner [188, 189]. This poses a significant problem since the development of AD has been mostly studied in adult, but not necessarily advanced-age, animals so far. With the advent of increasingly refined knock-in and transgenic AD animal models [190, 191], analysis of properly aged hosts will offer opportunity to evaluate the physiologically relevant contributing factors in AD pathogenesis and to test the efficacy of targeted regimen for translational potential. In the coming years, it would also be critical to establish and dissect how senescence within and outside CNS partakes in AD pathogenesis.

A systematic understanding of LOAD

Genetic studies of LOAD have identified numerous immune-related risk factors [4–6]. The involvement of implicated genes and related pathways in AD has been investigated in genetically engineered mouse models in recent years [84, 189, 192–195]. It is important to note that these genes and pathways are expressed at elevated levels both inside the brain and in the periphery in aging and/or AD, such as TREM2, inflammasome, and complement cascade as discussed earlier. Since the in vivo studies focused primarily on events within CNS, the contribution of simultaneously altered peripheral immune compartment is largely ignored. Recently identified as genetic risk factors in the Chinese population, risk variants of both GCH1 and KCNJ15 have altered expression in the peripheral immune cells of AD subjects, suggesting apparent functional effects through the immune system [196]. Examination of the peripheral leukocytes and their alterations together with the cells inside the brain should provide further insights on how the immune system comprehensively influences AD pathogenesis. With the same goal, it would also be necessary to examine the effects of lineage-specific gene knockouts to thoroughly dissect the immune compartments critical for the assigned gene function.

Adaptive immune system in AD pathogenesis

Despite genetic evidence implicating adaptive immunity in AD [91, 92], it remains ill-defined how adaptive immune cells with limited presence inside the parenchyma exert their effects on AD pathologies and cognitive functions. Nevertheless, T cells have been shown to participate in other neurodegenerative diseases, such as PD and amyotrophic lateral sclerosis [197, 198]. As reviewed earlier, many inconsistent results have been reported on the impacts of T cell subsets on CNS pathogenesis in Aβ-based experimental models. Thus, it is critical in the future to reconcile the main findings and differentiate the neuro-protective molecules, cells, and responses from the pathogenic ones, while elucidating the context-dependent functions influenced by specific host factors. Noticeably missing at this time is the examination of tau-specific T cells and the possible involvement of Treg cells in tau pathology, a major gap in understanding the participation of the adaptive immune arm in AD pathogenesis. Despite the technical challenge to study rare cells, new technologies such as high-dimensional single-cell analysis should significantly improve the quantification and classification of diverse immune cell populations in the AD brain. Whether T and B cells, self-reactive or bystanders, afford protective immune surveillance or pathogenic immune attack requires thorough delineation.

Peripheral immune responses in modulating AD

Despite strong clinical implications, how peripheral immune responses influence AD progression remains enigmatic. Though useful and informative, current animal models of AD, however, have severe limitations in their capacity to facilitate immunological inquiries. The animals are usually analyzed after life-long housing in the absence of natural microbial pathogens, which may result in reduced host fitness and poor disease resistance [143]. Given the importance of gut microbiota, alternative experimental modeling that incorporates the elements of peripheral conditioning is imperative for dissecting the immune responses in AD. One fundamental question is whether peripheral responses alone are sufficient to initiate the process of neuroinflammation and eventually drive neuropathology under any circumstances. Equally important is to understand whether peripheral events can imprint CNS with long-lasting alterations, a notion highlighted by the detected microglia memory formed upon peripheral LPS administrations [199]. On the other hand, high-dimensional and functional peripheral immune profiling of AD patients may reveal much needed insights into ongoing peripheral responses, which may help stratify the patients for targeted therapeutic interventions.

Neurovascular interface in AD

The brain is dynamically circulated not only by blood vessels, but also via a perivascular network and meningeal lymphatic vessels [200, 201]. In AD, it yet has to be revealed how peripheral immune cell populations traverse through these neurovascular networks to enter, remain in, and exit the brain, and more importantly, the functional outcome of such events. It is equally unclear how specific components of the neurovascular barrier is differentially regulated by the inflammatory milieu of AD. Understanding the selectivity of gateway trafficking for leukocytes and the associated regulatory mechanism is critical not only for dissecting the crosstalk between the periphery and CNS, but also for devising therapeutic strategies to modify such interactions.

Neuro-immune feedback mechanism in AD

The immune system and the nervous system share several key features: both regulate physiological homeostasis and protect the host from threats; both are composed of heterogeneous cell populations with extensive functional specialization; and both use synapses and soluble factors for cell-to-cell communication and memory formation [202, 203]. With expression of receptors for cytokines and neural transmitters, immune cells and nerve cells crosstalk and cooperate to maintain the homeostasis of the host. Although we have focused on the effects of peripheral inflammation on CNS, it is known that CNS can exert control of peripheral immune responses through spinal sympathetic and brain stem vagus nerve efferent signaling [204, 205]. For example, the vagus-nerve-based circuit inhibits TNF-α production in the spleen via the splenic nerve, acetylcholine-synthesizing T cells, and response by macrophage to acetylcholine [206]. Among the brain regions that integrate and regulate neuro-immune reflex, both thalamus and hypothalamus harbor pathological changes in AD patients [207, 208]. Therefore, it would be interesting to investigate whether the CNS regulatory circuit is compromised in AD, which may result in dysregulated peripheral immune responses and consequently a feedforward loop for systemic inflammation.

Overall, a new era of discovery compels us to fully grasp the many molecular and cellular players that partake the neuro-immune communications in AD and other neurodegenerative diseases under aging conditions. Better deciphering the influence of the immune system on the brain will surely provide further insights and guidance for the development of next-generation therapeutics.

Abbreviations

AD: Alzheimer's disease; APP: Amyloid precursor protein; Aβ: Amyloid β; BBB: Blood brain barrier; CNS: Central nervous system; CSF: Cerebrospinal fluid; GDF-11: Growth and differentiation factor 11; IFN-I: Type I interferon; IVIg: Intravenous Immunoglobulin; LOAD: Late-onset Alzheimer's disease; SASP: Senescence-associated secretory phenotype; SNP: Single-nucleotide polymorphism; TCR: T cell receptor; Tregs: T regulatory cells; TREM2: Triggering Receptor Expressed on Myeloid cells 2

Acknowledgements

The authors would like to thank Ethan Roy for assistance in editing the manuscript.

Funding

This work was supported by NIH grants AG057587 (WC), AG020670, AG032051 and AG054111 (HZ).

Authors' contributions

WC proposed the topic of the paper, reviewed the literature, drafted and revised the manuscript, and constructed the figures. HZ critically revised the manuscript. All authors read and approved the final manuscript.

Competing interests

The authors declare that they have no competing interests.

References

1. Hardy J, Selkoe DJ. The amyloid hypothesis of Alzheimer's disease: progress and problems on the road to therapeutics. Science. 2002;297.
2. Selkoe DJ, Hardy J. The amyloid hypothesis of Alzheimer's disease at 25 years. EMBO Molecular Medicine. 2016.
3. Walsh DM, Selkoe DJ. A critical appraisal of the pathogenic protein spread hypothesis of neurodegeneration. Nat Rev Neurosci. 2016;17:251–60.
4. Lambert JC, Ibrahim-Verbaas CA, Harold D, Naj AC, Sims R, et al. Meta-analysis of 74,046 individuals identifies 11 new susceptibility loci for Alzheimer's disease. Nat Genet. 2013;45:1452–8.
5. Sims R, van der Lee SJ, Naj AC, Bellenguez C, Badarinarayan N, et al. Rare coding variants in PLCG2, ABI3, and TREM2 implicate microglial-mediated innate immunity in Alzheimer's disease. Nat Genet. 2017; advance online publication.
6. Efthymiou AG, Goate AM. Late onset Alzheimer's disease genetics implicates microglial pathways in disease risk. Mol Neurodegener. 2017;12:43.
7. Heneka MT, Carson MJ, El Khoury J, Landreth GE, Brosseron F, Feinstein DL, Jacobs AH, Wyss-Coray T, Vitorica J, Ransohoff RM, Herrup K, Frautschy SA, Finsen B, Brown GC, Verkhratsky A, Yamanaka K, Koistinaho J, Latz E, Halle A, Petzold GC, Town T, Morgan D, Shinohara ML, Perry VH, Holmes C, Bazan NG, Brooks DJ, Hunot S, Joseph B, Deigendesch N, Garaschuk O, Boddeke E, Dinarello CA, Breitner JC, Cole GM, Golenbock DT, Kummer MP. Neuroinflammation in Alzheimer's disease. Lancet Neurol. 2015;14:388–405.
8. Ransohoff RM. How neuroinflammation contributes to neurodegeneration. Science. 2016;353:777–83.
9. Heppner FL, Ransohoff RM, Becher B. Immune attack: the role of inflammation in Alzheimer disease. Nat Rev Neurosci. 2015;16:358–72.
10. Hickman SE, Kingery ND, Ohsumi TK, Borowsky ML, Wang LC, Means TK, El Khoury J. The microglial sensome revealed by direct RNA sequencing. Nat Neurosci. 2013;16:1896–905.
11. Galatro TF, Holtman IR, Lerario AM, Vainchtein ID, Brouwer N, Sola PR, Veras MM, Pereira TF, Leite REP, Moller T, Wes PD, Sogayar MC, Laman JD, den Dunnen W, Pasqualucci CA, Oba-Shinjo SM, Boddeke EWGM, Marie SKN, Eggen BJL. Transcriptomic analysis of purified human cortical microglia reveals age-associated changes. Nat Neurosci. 2017; advance online publication.
12. Soreq L, Consortium UKBE, North American Brain Expression C, Rose J, Soreq E, Hardy J, Trabzuni D, Cookson MR, Smith C, Ryten M, Patani R, Ule J. Major Shifts in Glial Regional Identity Are a Transcriptional Hallmark of Human Brain Aging. Cell Rep. 2017;18:557–70.
13. Salter MW, Stevens B. Microglia emerge as central players in brain disease. Nat Med. 2017;23:1018–27.

14. Sarlus H, Heneka MT. Microglia in Alzheimer's disease. J Clin Invest. 2017; 127:3240–9.
15. Biber K, Moller T, Boddeke E, Prinz M. Central nervous system myeloid cells as drug targets: current status and translational challenges. Nat Rev Drug Discov. 2016;15:110–24.
16. Pinti M, Appay V, Campisi J, Frasca D, Fulop T, Sauce D, Larbi A, Weinberger B, Cossarizza A. Aging of the immune system: Focus on inflammation and vaccination. Eur J Immunol. 2016;46:2286–301.
17. Goldberg EL, Dixit VD. Drivers of age-related inflammation and strategies for healthspan extension. Immunol Rev. 2015;265:63–74.
18. Franceschi C, Campisi J. Chronic inflammation (inflammaging) and its potential contribution to age-associated diseases. J Gerontol A Biol Sci Med Sci. 2014;69(Suppl 1):S4–9.
19. Netea MG, van de Veerdonk FL, van der Meer JWM, Dinarello CA, Joosten LAB. Inflammasome-Independent Regulation of IL-1-Family Cytokines. Annual Review of Immunology. 2015;33:49–77.
20. Latz E, Xiao TS, Stutz A. Activation and regulation of the inflammasomes. Nat Rev Immunol. 2013;13:397–411.
21. Furman D, Chang J, Lartigue L, Bolen CR, Haddad F, Gaudilliere B, Ganio EA, Fragiadakis GK, Spitzer MH, Douchet I, Daburon S, Moreau J-F, Nolan GP, Blanco P, Dechanet-Merville J, Dekker CL, Jojic V, Kuo CJ, Davis MM, Faustin B. Expression of specific inflammasome gene modules stratifies older individuals into two extreme clinical and immunological states. Nat Med. 2017;23:174–84.
22. Youm YH, Grant RW, McCabe LR, Albarado DC, Nguyen KY, Ravussin A, Pistell P, Newman S, Carter R, Laque A, Munzberg H, Rosen CJ, Ingram DK, Salbaum JM, Dixit VD. Canonical Nlrp3 inflammasome links systemic low-grade inflammation to functional decline in aging. Cell Metab. 2013;18:519–32.
23. Newman AB, Sanders JL, Kizer JR, Boudreau RM, Odden MC, Zeki Al Hazzouri A, Arnold AM. Trajectories of function and biomarkers with age: the CHS All Stars Study. Int J Epidemiol. 2016;45:1135–45.
24. Varadhan R, Yao W, Matteini A, Beamer BA, Xue QL, Yang H, Manwani B, Reiner A, Jenny N, Parekh N, Fallin MD, Newman A, Bandeen-Roche K, Tracy R, Ferrucci L, Walston J. Simple biologically informed inflammatory index of two serum cytokines predicts 10 year all-cause mortality in older adults. J Gerontol A Biol Sci Med Sci. 2014;69:165–73.
25. Martinez-Jimenez CP, Eling N, Chen H-C, Vallejos CA, Kolodziejczyk AA, Connor F, Stojic L, Rayner TF, Stubbington MJT, Teichmann SA, de la Roche M, Marioni JC, Odom DT. Aging increases cell-to-cell transcriptional variability upon immune stimulation. Science. 2017;355:1433–6.
26. Bahar R, Hartmann CH, Rodriguez KA, Denny AD, Busuttil RA, Dolle ME, Calder RB, Chisholm GB, Pollock BH, Klein CA, Vijg J. Increased cell-to-cell variation in gene expression in ageing mouse heart. Nature. 2006;441:1011–4.
27. Enge M, Arda HE, Mignardi M, Beausang J, Bottino R, Kim SK, Quake SR. Single-Cell Analysis of Human Pancreas Reveals Transcriptional Signatures of Aging and Somatic Mutation Patterns. Cell. 2017;171:321–30.e14.
28. Cheung P, Vallania F, Warsinske HC, Donato M, Schaffert S, Chang SE, Dvorak M, Dekker CL, Davis MM, Utz PJ, Khatri P, Kuo AJ. Single-Cell Chromatin Modification Profiling Reveals Increased Epigenetic Variations with Aging. Cell 173. 2018;e14:1385–97.
29. Nikolich-Žugich J. The twilight of immunity: emerging concepts in aging of the immune system. Nature Immunology. 2018;19:10–9.
30. Ucar D, Marquez EJ, Chung CH, Marches R, Rossi RJ, Uyar A, Wu TC, George J, Stitzel ML, Palucka AK, Kuchel GA, Banchereau J. The chromatin accessibility signature of human immune aging stems from CD8(+) T cells. J Exp Med. 2017;214:3123–44.
31. Rudd BD, Venturi V, Li G, Samadder P, Ertelt JM, Way SS, Davenport MP, Nikolich-Zugich J. Nonrandom attrition of the naive CD8+ T-cell pool with aging governed by T-cell receptor:pMHC interactions. Proc Natl Acad Sci U S A. 2011;108:13694–9.
32. Pulko V, Davies JS, Martinez C, Lanteri MC, Busch MP, Diamond MS, Knox K, Bush EC, Sims PA, Sinari S, Billheimer D, Haddad EK, Murray KO, Wertheimer AM, Nikolich-Zugich J. Human memory T cells with a naive phenotype accumulate with aging and respond to persistent viruses. Nat Immunol. 2016;17:966–75.
33. Chiu BC, Martin BE, Stolberg VR, Chensue SW. Central memory CD8 T cells in aged mice are virtual memory cells. J Immunol. 2013;191:5793–6.
34. Moskowitz DM, Zhang DW, Hu B, Le Saux S, Yanes RE, Ye Z, Buenrostro JD, Weyand CM, Greenleaf WJ, Goronzy JJ. Epigenomics of human CD8 T cell differentiation and aging. Sci Immunol. 2017;2:eaag0192.
35. Naradikian MS, Hao Y, Cancro MP. Age-associated B cells: key mediators of both protective and autoreactive humoral responses. Immunol Rev. 2016; 269:118–29.
36. Riley RL, Khomtchouk K, Blomberg BB. Age-associated B cells (ABC) inhibit B lymphopoiesis and alter antibody repertoires in old age. Cell Immunol. 2017;321:61–7.
37. Geiger H, de Haan G, Florian MC. The ageing haematopoietic stem cell compartment. Nat Rev Immunol. 2013;13:376–89.
38. He S, Sharpless NE. Senescence in Health and Disease. Cell. 2017;169:1000–11.
39. Ito Y, Hoare M, Narita M. Spatial and Temporal Control of Senescence. Trends Cell Biol. 2017.
40. Munoz-Espin D, Serrano M. Cellular senescence: from physiology to pathology. Nat Rev Mol Cell Biol. 2014;15:482–96.
41. Coppé J-P, Patil CK, Rodier F, Sun Y, Muñoz DP, Goldstein J, Nelson PS, Desprez P-Y, Campisi J. Senescence-Associated Secretory Phenotypes Reveal Cell-Nonautonomous Functions of Oncogenic RAS and the p53 Tumor Suppressor. PLoS Biol. 2008;6:e301.
42. Martinez-Zamudio RI, Robinson L, Roux PF, Bischof O. SnapShot: Cellular Senescence Pathways. Cell. 2017:170, 816–816.e1.
43. Campisi J. Aging, cellular senescence, and cancer. Annu Rev Physiol. 2013; 75:685–705.
44. Childs BG, Gluscevic M, Baker DJ, Laberge RM, Marquess D, Dananberg J, van Deursen JM. Senescent cells: an emerging target for diseases of ageing. Nat Rev Drug Discov. 2017;16:718–35.
45. Salminen A, Ojala J, Kaarniranta K, Haapasalo A, Hiltunen M, Soininen H. Astrocytes in the aging brain express characteristics of senescence-associated secretory phenotype. Eur J Neurosci. 2011;34:3–11.
46. Wyss-Coray T. Ageing, neurodegeneration and brain rejuvenation. Nature. 2016;539:180–6.
47. Villeda SA, Luo J, Mosher KI, Zou B, Britschgi M, Bieri G, Stan TM, Fainberg N, Ding Z, Eggel A, Lucin KM, Czirr E, Park J-S, Couillard-Despres S, Aigner L, Li G, Peskind ER, Kaye JA, Quinn JF, Galasko DR, Xie XS, Rando TA, Wyss-Coray T. The ageing systemic milieu negatively regulates neurogenesis and cognitive function. Nature. 2011;477:90–4.
48. Smith LK, He Y, Park JS, Bieri G, Snethlage CE, Lin K, Gontier G, Wabl R, Plambeck KE, Udeochu J, Wheatley EG, Bouchard J, Eggel A, Narasimha R, Grant JL, Luo J, Wyss-Coray T, Villeda SA. beta2-microglobulin is a systemic pro-aging factor that impairs cognitive function and neurogenesis. Nat Med. 2015;21:932–7.
49. Sinha M, Jang YC, Oh J, Khong D, Wu EY, Manohar R, Miller C, Regalado SG, Loffredo FS, Pancoast JR, Hirshman MF, Lebowitz J, Shadrach JL, Cerletti M, Kim M-J, Serwold T, Goodyear LJ, Rosner B, Lee RT, Wagers AJ. Restoring Systemic GDF11 Levels Reverses Age-Related Dysfunction in Mouse Skeletal Muscle. Science. 2014;344:649–52.
50. Katsimpardi L, Litterman NK, Schein PA, Miller CM, Loffredo FS, Wojtkiewicz GR, Chen JW, Lee RT, Wagers AJ, Rubin LL. Vascular and neurogenic rejuvenation of the aging mouse brain by young systemic factors. Science. 2014;344:630–4.
51. Chiam JT, Dobson RJ, Kiddle SJ, Sattlecker M. Are blood-based protein biomarkers for Alzheimer's disease also involved in other brain disorders? A systematic review. J Alzheimers Dis. 2015;43:303–14.
52. Walker RG, Poggioli T, Katsimpardi L, Buchanan SM, Oh J, Wattrus S, Heidecker B, Fong YW, Rubin LL, Ganz P, Thompson TB, Wagers AJ, Lee RT. Biochemistry and Biology of GDF11 and Myostatin: Similarities, Differences, and Questions for Future Investigation. Circ Res. 2016;118:1125–41 discussion 42.
53. Schafer MJ, Atkinson EJ, Vanderboom PM, Kotajarvi B, White TA, Moore MM, Bruce CJ, Greason KL, Suri RM, Khosla S, Miller JD, Bergen HR 3rd, LeBrasseur NK. Quantification of GDF11 and Myostatin in Human Aging and Cardiovascular Disease. Cell Metab. 2016;23:1207–15.
54. Middeldorp J, Lehallier B, Villeda SA, Miedema SS, Evans E, Czirr E, Zhang H, Luo J, Stan T, Mosher KI, Masliah E, Wyss-Coray T. Preclinical Assessment of Young Blood Plasma for Alzheimer Disease. JAMA Neurol. 2016;73:1325–33.
55. Castellano JM, Mosher KI, Abbey RJ, McBride AA, James ML, Berdnik D, Shen JC, Zou B, Xie XS, Tingle M, Hinkson IV, Angst MS, Wyss-Coray T. Human umbilical cord plasma proteins revitalize hippocampal function in aged mice. Nature. 2017;544:488–92.
56. Laurin D, David Curb J, Masaki KH, White LR, Launer LJ. Midlife C-reactive protein and risk of cognitive decline: a 31-year follow-up. Neurobiol Aging. 2009;30:1724–7.

57. Koyama A, O'Brien J, Weuve J, Blacker D, Metti AL, Yaffe K. The role of peripheral inflammatory markers in dementia and Alzheimer's disease: a meta-analysis. J Gerontol A Biol Sci Med Sci. 2013;68:433–40.
58. Kiddle SJ, Sattlecker M, Proitsi P, Simmons A, Westman E, Bazenet C, Nelson SK, Williams S, Hodges A, Johnston C, Soininen H, Kloszewska I, Mecocci P, Tsolaki M, Vellas B, Newhouse S, Lovestone S, Dobson RJ. Candidate blood proteome markers of Alzheimer's disease onset and progression: a systematic review and replication study. J Alzheimers Dis. 2014;38:515–31.
59. Becher B, Spath S, Goverman J. Cytokine networks in neuroinflammation. Nat Rev Immunol. 2017;17:49–59.
60. Rogers J, Cooper NR, Webster S, Schultz J, McGeer PL, Styren SD, Civin WH, Brachova L, Bradt B, Ward P, et al. Complement activation by beta-amyloid in Alzheimer disease. Proc Natl Acad Sci U S A. 1992;89:10016–20.
61. Ray S, Britschgi M, Herbert C, Takeda-Uchimura Y, Boxer A, Blennow K, Friedman LF, Galasko DR, Jutel M, Karydas A, Kaye JA, Leszek J, Miller BL, Minthon L, Quinn JF, Rabinovici GD, Robinson WH, Sabbagh MN, So YT, Sparks DL, Tabaton M, Tinklenberg J, Yesavage JA, Tibshirani R, Wyss-Coray T. Classification and prediction of clinical Alzheimer's diagnosis based on plasma signaling proteins. Nat Med. 2007;13:1359–62.
62. Sattlecker M, Kiddle SJ, Newhouse S, Proitsi P, Nelson S, Williams S, Johnston C, Killick R, Simmons A, Westman E, Hodges A, Soininen H, Kloszewska I, Mecocci P, Tsolaki M, Vellas B, Lovestone S, Dobson RJ. Alzheimer's disease biomarker discovery using SOMAscan multiplexed protein technology. Alzheimers Dement. 2014;10:724–34.
63. Hye A, Riddoch-Contreras J, Baird AL, Ashton NJ, Bazenet C, Leung R, Westman E, Simmons A, Dobson R, Sattlecker M, Lupton M, Lunnon K, Keohane A, Ward M, Pike I, Zucht HD, Pepin D, Zheng W, Tunnicliffe A, Richardson J, Gauthier S, Soininen H, Kloszewska I, Mecocci P, Tsolaki M, Vellas B, Lovestone S. Plasma proteins predict conversion to dementia from prodromal disease. Alzheimers Dement. 2014;10:799–807.e2.
64. Lehallier B, Essioux L, Gayan J, Alexandridis R, Nikolcheva T, Wyss-Coray T, Britschgi M. Combined Plasma and Cerebrospinal Fluid Signature for the Prediction of Midterm Progression From Mild Cognitive Impairment to Alzheimer Disease. JAMA Neurol. 2016;73:203–12.
65. Korin B, Ben-Shaanan TL, Schiller M, Dubovik T, Azulay-Debby H, Boshnak NT, Koren T, Rolls A. High-dimensional, single-cell characterization of the brain's immune compartment. Nat Neurosci. 2017; advance online publication.
66. Ziv Y, Ron N, Butovsky O, Landa G, Sudai E, Greenberg N, Cohen H, Kipnis J, Schwartz M. Immune cells contribute to the maintenance of neurogenesis and spatial learning abilities in adulthood. Nat Neurosci. 2006;9:268–75.
67. Ron-Harel N, Segev Y, Lewitus GM, Cardon M, Ziv Y, Netanely D, Jacob-Hirsch J, Amariglio N, Rechavi G, Domany E, Schwartz M. Age-dependent spatial memory loss can be partially restored by immune activation. Rejuvenation Res. 2008;11:903–13.
68. Kipnis J, Cohen H, Cardon M, Ziv Y, Schwartz M. T cell deficiency leads to cognitive dysfunction: implications for therapeutic vaccination for schizophrenia and other psychiatric conditions. Proc Natl Acad Sci U S A. 2004;101:8180–5.
69. Filiano AJ, Xu Y, Tustison NJ, Marsh RL, Baker W, Smirnov I, Overall CC, Gadani SP, Turner SD, Weng Z, Peerzade SN, Chen H, Lee KS, Scott MM, Beenhakker MP, Litvak V, Kipnis J. Unexpected role of interferon-gamma in regulating neuronal connectivity and social behaviour. Nature. 2016;535: 425–9.
70. Derecki NC, Cardani AN, Yang CH, Quinnies KM, Crihfield A, Lynch KR, Kipnis J. Regulation of learning and memory by meningeal immunity: a key role for IL-4. J Exp Med. 2010;207:1067–80.
71. Schwartz M, Deczkowska A. Neurological Disease as a Failure of Brain-Immune Crosstalk: The Multiple Faces of Neuroinflammation. Trends Immunol. 2016;37:668–79.
72. Balusu S, Brkic M, Libert C, Vandenbroucke RE. The choroid plexus-cerebrospinal fluid interface in Alzheimer's disease: more than just a barrier. Neural Regen Res. 2016;11:534–7.
73. Baruch K, Ron-Harel N, Gal H, Deczkowska A, Shifrut E, Ndifon W, Mirlas-Neisberg N, Cardon M, Vaknin I, Cahalon L, Berkutzki T, Mattson MP, Gomez-Pinilla F, Friedman N, Schwartz M. CNS-specific immunity at the choroid plexus shifts toward destructive Th2 inflammation in brain aging. Proc Natl Acad Sci U S A. 2013;110:2264–9.
74. Kunis G, Baruch K, Rosenzweig N, Kertser A, Miller O, Berkutzki T, Schwartz M. IFN-gamma-dependent activation of the brain's choroid plexus for CNS immune surveillance and repair. Brain. 2013;136:3427–40.
75. Deczkowska A, Baruch K, Schwartz M. Type I/II Interferon Balance in the Regulation of Brain Physiology and Pathology. Trends Immunol. 2016;37: 181–92.
76. Baruch K, Deczkowska A, David E, Castellano JM, Miller O, Kertser A, Berkutzki T, Barnett-Itzhaki Z, Bezalel D, Wyss-Coray T, Amit I, Schwartz M. Aging-induced type I interferon response at the choroid plexus negatively affects brain function. Science. 2014;346:89–93.
77. Keren-Shaul H, Spinrad A, Weiner A, Matcovitch-Natan O, Dvir-Szternfeld R, Ulland TK, David E, Baruch K, Lara-Astaiso D, Toth B, Itzkovitz S, Colonna M, Schwartz M, Amit I. A Unique Microglia Type Associated with Restricting Development of Alzheimer's Disease. Cell 169. 2017;e17:1276–90.
78. Tarasoff-Conway JM, Carare RO, Osorio RS, Glodzik L, Butler T, Fieremans E, Axel L, Rusinek H, Nicholson C, Zlokovic BV, Frangione B, Blennow K, Menard J, Zetterberg H, Wisniewski T, de Leon MJ. Clearance systems in the brain-implications for Alzheimer disease. Nat Rev Neurol. 2015;11:457–70.
79. Cronk JC, Filiano AJ, Louveau A, Marin I, Marsh R, Ji E, Goldman DH, Smirnov I, Geraci N, Acton S, Overall CC, Kipnis J. Peripherally derived macrophages can engraft the brain independent of irradiation and maintain an identity distinct from microglia. J Exp Med. 2018;215:1627.
80. Simard AR, Soulet D, Gowing G, Julien JP, Rivest S. Bone marrow-derived microglia play a critical role in restricting senile plaque formation in Alzheimer's disease. Neuron. 2006;49:489–502.
81. Butovsky O, Kunis G, Koronyo-Hamaoui M, Schwartz M. Selective ablation of bone marrow-derived dendritic cells increases amyloid plaques in a mouse Alzheimer's disease model. Eur J Neurosci. 2007;26:413–6.
82. Prokop S, Miller KR, Drost N, Handrick S, Mathur V, Luo J, Wegner A, Wyss-Coray T, Heppner FL. Impact of peripheral myeloid cells on amyloid-beta pathology in Alzheimer's disease-like mice. J Exp Med. 2015;212:1811–8.
83. Varvel NH, Grathwohl SA, Degenhardt K, Resch C, Bosch A, Jucker M, Neher JJ. Replacement of brain-resident myeloid cells does not alter cerebral amyloid-beta deposition in mouse models of Alzheimer's disease. J Exp Med. 2015;212:1803–9.
84. Ulrich JD, Ulland TK, Colonna M, Holtzman DM. Elucidating the Role of TREM2 in Alzheimer's Disease. Neuron. 2017;94:237–48.
85. Hu N, Tan MS, Yu JT, Sun L, Tan L, Wang YL, Jiang T, Tan L. Increased expression of TREM2 in peripheral blood of Alzheimer's disease patients. J Alzheimers Dis. 2014;38:497–501.
86. Mori Y, Yoshino Y, Ochi S, Yamazaki K, Kawabe K, Abe M, Kitano T, Ozaki Y, Yoshida T, Numata S, Mori T, Iga J, Kuroda N, Ohmori T, S-i U. TREM2 mRNA Expression in Leukocytes Is Increased in Alzheimer's Disease and Schizophrenia. PloS One. 2015;10:e0136835.
87. Ozaki Y, Yoshino Y, Yamazaki K, Sao T, Mori Y, Ochi S, Yoshida T, Mori T, J-i I, S-i U. DNA methylation changes at TREM2 intron 1 and TREM2 mRNA expression in patients with Alzheimer's disease. J Psychiatr Res. 2017;92: 74–80.
88. Tan YJ, Ng ASL, Vipin A, Lim JKW, Chander RJ, Ji F, Qiu Y, Ting SKS, Hameed S, Lee TS, Zeng L, Kandiah N, Zhou J. Higher Peripheral TREM2 mRNA Levels Relate to Cognitive Deficits and Hippocampal Atrophy in Alzheimer's Disease and Amnestic Mild Cognitive Impairment. J Alzheimers Dis. 2017;58: 413–23.
89. Zenaro E, Pietronigro E, Della Bianca V, Piacentino G, Marongiu L, Budui S, Turano E, Rossi B, Angiari S, Dusi S, Montresor A, Carlucci T, Nani S, Tosadori G, Calciano L, Catalucci D, Berton G, Bonetti B, Constantin G. Neutrophils promote Alzheimer's disease-like pathology and cognitive decline via LFA-1 integrin. Nat Med. 2015;21:880–6.
90. Gabbita SP, Johnson MF, Kobritz N, Eslami P, Poteshkina A, Varadarajan S, Turman J, Zemlan F, Harris-White ME. Oral TNFalpha Modulation Alters Neutrophil Infiltration, Improves Cognition and Diminishes Tau and Amyloid Pathology in the 3xTgAD Mouse Model. PLoS One. 2015;10:e0137305.
91. Gagliano SA, Pouget JG, Hardy J, Knight J, Barnes MR, Ryten M, Weale ME. Genomics implicates adaptive and innate immunity in Alzheimer's and Parkinson's diseases. Ann Clin Transl Neurol. 2016;3:924–33.
92. Yokoyama JS, Wang Y, Schork AJ, Thompson WK, Karch CM, Cruchaga C, McEvoy LK, Witoelar A, Chen CH, Holland D, Brewer JB, Franke A, Dillon WP, Wilson DM, Mukherjee P, Hess CP, Miller Z, Bonham LW, Shen J, Rabinovici GD, Rosen HJ, Miller BL, Hyman BT, Schellenberg GD, Karlsen TH, Andreassen OA, Dale AM, Desikan RS, Alzheimer's Disease Neuroimaging I. Association Between Genetic Traits for Immune-Mediated Diseases and Alzheimer Disease. JAMA Neurol. 2016;73:691–7.
93. Spani C, Suter T, Derungs R, Ferretti MT, Welt T, Wirth F, Gericke C, Nitsch RM, Kulic L. Reduced beta-amyloid pathology in an APP transgenic mouse

model of Alzheimer's disease lacking functional B and T cells. Acta Neuropathol Commun. 2015;3:71.
94. Marsh SE, Abud EM, Lakatos A, Karimzadeh A, Yeung ST, Davtyan H, Fote GM, Lau L, Weinger JG, Lane TE, Inlay MA, Poon WW, Blurton-Jones M. The adaptive immune system restrains Alzheimer's disease pathogenesis by modulating microglial function. Proc Natl Acad Sci U S A. 2016;113:E1316–25.
95. Brynskikh A, Warren T, Zhu J, Kipnis J. Adaptive immunity affects learning behavior in mice. Brain Behav Immun. 2008;22:861–9.
96. Wolf SA, Steiner B, Akpinarli A, Kammertoens T, Nassenstein C, Braun A, Blankenstein T, Kempermann G. CD4-positive T lymphocytes provide a neuroimmunological link in the control of adult hippocampal neurogenesis. J Immunol. 2009;182:3979–84.
97. Gaskin F, Finley J, Fang Q, Xu S, Fu SM. Human antibodies reactive with beta-amyloid protein in Alzheimer's disease. J Exp Med. 1993;177:1181–6.
98. Hyman BT, Smith C, Buldyrev I, Whelan C, Brown H, Tang MX, Mayeux R. Autoantibodies to amyloid-beta and Alzheimer's disease. Ann Neurol. 2001; 49:808–10.
99. Du Y, Dodel R, Hampel H, Buerger K, Lin S, Eastwood B, Bales K, Gao F, Moeller HJ, Oertel W, Farlow M, Paul S. Reduced levels of amyloid beta-peptide antibody in Alzheimer disease. Neurology. 2001;57:801–5.
100. Weksler ME, Relkin N, Turkenich R, LaRusse S, Zhou L, Szabo P. Patients with Alzheimer disease have lower levels of serum anti-amyloid peptide antibodies than healthy elderly individuals. Exp Gerontol. 2002;37:943–8.
101. Nath A, Hall E, Tuzova M, Dobbs M, Jons M, Anderson C, Woodward J, Guo Z, Fu W, Kryscio R, Wekstein D, Smith C, Markesbery WR, Mattson MP. Autoantibodies to amyloid beta-peptide (Abeta) are increased in Alzheimer's disease patients and Abeta antibodies can enhance Abeta neurotoxicity: implications for disease pathogenesis and vaccine development. Neuromolecular Med. 2003;3:29–39.
102. Schenk D, Barbour R, Dunn W, Gordon G, Grajeda H, Guido T, Hu K, Huang J, Johnson-Wood K, Khan K, Kholodenko D, Lee M, Liao Z, Lieberburg I, Motter R, Mutter L, Soriano F, Shopp G, Vasquez N, Vandevert C, Walker S, Wogulis M, Yednock T, Games D, Seubert P. Immunization with amyloid-[beta] attenuates Alzheimer-disease-like pathology in the PDAPP mouse. Nature. 1999;400:173–7.
103. Lemere CA, Masliah E. Can Alzheimer disease be prevented by amyloid-beta immunotherapy? Nat Rev Neurol. 2010;6:108–19.
104. Wang YJ. Alzheimer disease: Lessons from immunotherapy for Alzheimer disease. Nat Rev Neurol. 2014;10:188–9.
105. Graham WV, Bonito-Oliva A, Sakmar TP. Update on Alzheimer's Disease Therapy and Prevention Strategies. Annu Rev Med. 2017;68:413–30.
106. Acharya NK, Nagele EP, Han M, Nagele RG. Autoantibodies: Double Agents in Human Disease. Sci Transl Med. 2013;5:186fs19.
107. Nagele EP, Han M, Acharya NK, DeMarshall C, Kosciuk MC, Nagele RG. Natural IgG autoantibodies are abundant and ubiquitous in human sera, and their number is influenced by age, gender, and disease. PLoS One. 2013;8:e60726.
108. Wang H, Williams D, Griffin J, Saito T, Saido TC, Fraser PE, Rogaeva E, Schmitt-Ulms G. Time-course global proteome analyses reveal an inverse correlation between Abeta burden and immunoglobulin M levels in the APPNL-F mouse model of Alzheimer disease. PLoS One. 2017;12:e0182844.
109. DeMarshall CA, Nagele EP, Sarkar A, Acharya NK, Godsey G, Goldwaser EL, Kosciuk M, Thayasivam U, Han M, Belinka B, Nagele RG. Detection of Alzheimer's disease at mild cognitive impairment and disease progression using autoantibodies as blood-based biomarkers. Alzheimers Dement (Amst). 2016;3:51–62.
110. Sudduth TL, Greenstein A, Wilcock DM. Intracranial injection of Gammagard, a human IVIg, modulates the inflammatory response of the brain and lowers Abeta in APP/PS1 mice along a different time course than anti-Abeta antibodies. J Neurosci. 2013;33:9684–92.
111. Counts SE, Ray B, Mufson EJ, Perez SE, He B, Lahiri DK. Intravenous immunoglobulin (IVIG) treatment exerts antioxidant and neuropreservatory effects in preclinical models of Alzheimer's disease. J Clin Immunol. 2014; 34(Suppl 1):S80–5.
112. Du Y, Wei X, Dodel R, Sommer N, Hampel H, Gao F, Ma Z, Zhao L, Oertel WH, Farlow M. Human anti-beta-amyloid antibodies block beta-amyloid fibril formation and prevent beta-amyloid-induced neurotoxicity. Brain. 2003;126:1935–9.
113. Togo T, Akiyama H, Iseki E, Kondo H, Ikeda K, Kato M, Oda T, Tsuchiya K, Kosaka K. Occurrence of T cells in the brain of Alzheimer's disease and other neurological diseases. J Neuroimmunol. 2002;124:83–92.
114. Rogers J, Luber-Narod J, Styren SD, Civin WH. Expression of immune system-associated antigens by cells of the human central nervous system: relationship to the pathology of Alzheimer's disease. Neurobiol Aging. 1988; 9:339–49.
115. Itagaki S, McGeer PL, Akiyama H. Presence of T-cytotoxic suppressor and leucocyte common antigen positive cells in Alzheimer's disease brain tissue. Neurosci Lett. 1988;91:259–64.
116. Ferretti MT, Merlini M, Späni C, Gericke C, Schweizer N, Enzmann G, Engelhardt B, Kulic L, Suter T, Nitsch RM. T-cell brain infiltration and immature antigen-presenting cells in transgenic models of Alzheimer's disease-like cerebral amyloidosis. Brain Behav Immuni. 2016;54:211–25.
117. Browne TC, McQuillan K, McManus RM, O'Reilly JA, Mills KH, Lynch MA. IFN-gamma Production by amyloid beta-specific Th1 cells promotes microglial activation and increases plaque burden in a mouse model of Alzheimer's disease. J Immunol. 2013;190:2241–51.
118. Monsonego A, Maron R, Zota V, Selkoe DJ, Weiner HL. Immune hyporesponsiveness to amyloid beta-peptide in amyloid precursor protein transgenic mice: implications for the pathogenesis and treatment of Alzheimer's disease. Proc Natl Acad Sci U S A. 2001;98:10273–8.
119. Trieb K, Ransmayr G, Sgonc R, Lassmann H, Grubeck-Loebenstein B. APP peptides stimulate lymphocyte proliferation in normals, but not in patients with Alzheimer's disease. Neurobiol Aging. 1996;17:541–7.
120. Monsonego A, Zota V, Karni A, Krieger JI, Bar-Or A, Bitan G, Budson AE, Sperling R, Selkoe DJ, Weiner HL. Increased T cell reactivity to amyloid beta protein in older humans and patients with Alzheimer disease. J Clin Invest. 2003;112:415–22.
121. Loewenbrueck KF, Tigno-Aranjuez JT, Boehm BO, Lehmann PV, Tary-Lehmann M. Th1 responses to beta-amyloid in young humans convert to regulatory IL-10 responses in Down syndrome and Alzheimer's disease. Neurobiol Aging. 2010;31:1732–42.
122. Rosenkranz D, Weyer S, Tolosa E, Gaenslen A, Berg D, Leyhe T, Gasser T, Stoltze L. Higher frequency of regulatory T cells in the elderly and increased suppressive activity in neurodegeneration. J Neuroimmunol. 2007; 188:117–27.
123. Saresella M, Calabrese E, Marventano I, Piancone F, Gatti A, Calvo MG, Nemni R, Clerici M. PD1 negative and PD1 positive CD4+ T regulatory cells in mild cognitive impairment and Alzheimer's disease. J Alzheimers Dis. 2010;21:927–38.
124. Torres KC, Araujo Pereira P, Lima GS, Bozzi IC, Rezende VB, Bicalho MA, Moraes EN, Miranda DM, Romano-Silva MA. Increased frequency of T cells expressing IL-10 in Alzheimer disease but not in late-onset depression patients. Prog Neuropsychopharmacol Biol Psychiatry. 2013;47:40–5.
125. Baruch K, Rosenzweig N, Kertser A, Deczkowska A, Sharif AM, Spinrad A, Tsitsou-Kampeli A, Sarel A, Cahalon L, Schwartz M. Breaking immune tolerance by targeting Foxp3(+) regulatory T cells mitigates Alzheimer's disease pathology. Nat Commun. 2015;6:7967.
126. Monsonego A, Imitola J, Petrovic S, Zota V, Nemirovsky A, Baron R, Fisher Y, Owens T, Weiner HL. Abeta-induced meningoencephalitis is IFN-gamma-dependent and is associated with T cell-dependent clearance of Abeta in a mouse model of Alzheimer's disease. Proc Natl Acad Sci U S A. 2006;103: 5048–53.
127. Fisher Y, Strominger I, Biton S, Nemirovsky A, Baron R, Monsonego A. Th1 polarization of T cells injected into the cerebrospinal fluid induces brain immunosurveillance. J Immunol. 2014;192:92–102.
128. Cao C, Arendash GW, Dickson A, Mamcarz MB, Lin X, Ethell DW. Abeta-specific Th2 cells provide cognitive and pathological benefits to Alzheimer's mice without infiltrating the CNS. Neurobiol Dis. 2009;34:63–70.
129. Dansokho C, Ait Ahmed D, Aid S, Toly-Ndour C, Chaigneau T, Calle V, Cagnard N, Holzenberger M, Piaggio E, Aucouturier P, Dorothee G. Regulatory T cells delay disease progression in Alzheimer-like pathology. Brain. 2016;139:1237–51.
130. Baek H, Ye M, Kang GH, Lee C, Lee G, Choi DB, Jung J, Kim H, Lee S, Kim JS, Lee HJ, Shim I, Lee JH, Bae H. Neuroprotective effects of CD4+CD25+Foxp3 + regulatory T cells in a 3xTg-AD Alzheimer's disease model. Oncotarget. 2016;7:69347–57.
131. Alves S, Churlaud G, Audrain M, Michaelsen-Preusse K, Fol R, Souchet B, Braudeau J, Korte M, Klatzmann D, Cartier N. Interleukin-2 improves amyloid pathology, synaptic failure and memory in Alzheimer's disease mice. Brain. 2017;140:826–42.
132. Yang H, Yang H, Xie Z, Wei L, Bi J. Systemic transplantation of human umbilical cord derived mesenchymal stem cells-educated T regulatory cells

improved the impaired cognition in AbetaPPswe/PS1dE9 transgenic mice. PLoS One. 2013;8:e69129.
133. Petitto JM, Cushman JD, Huang Z. Effects of Brain-Derived IL-2 Deficiency and the Development of Autoimmunity on Spatial Learning and Fear Conditioning. J Neurol Disord. 2015;3:196.
134. Baruch K, Deczkowska A, Rosenzweig N, Tsitsou-Kampeli A, Sharif AM, Matcovitch-Natan O, Kertser A, David E, Amit I, Schwartz M. PD-1 immune checkpoint blockade reduces pathology and improves memory in mouse models of Alzheimer's disease. Nat Med. 2016;22:135–7.
135. Schwartz M. Can immunotherapy treat neurodegeneration? Science. 2017; 357:254–5.
136. Latta-Mahieu M, Elmer B, Bretteville A, Wang Y, Lopez-Grancha M, Goniot P, Moindrot N, Ferrari P, Blanc V, Schussler N, Brault E, Roudieres V, Blanchard V, Yang ZY, Barneoud P, Bertrand P, Roucourt B, Carmans S, Bottelbergs A, Mertens L, Wintmolders C, Larsen P, Hersley C, McGathey T, Racke MM, Liu L, Lu J, O'Neill MJ, Riddell DR, Ebneth A, Nabel GJ, Pradier L. Systemic immune-checkpoint blockade with anti-PD1 antibodies does not alter cerebral amyloid-beta burden in several amyloid transgenic mouse models. Glia. 2018;66:492-504.
137. Field R, Campion S, Warren C, Murray C, Cunningham C. Systemic challenge with the TLR3 agonist poly I:C induces amplified IFNalpha/beta and IL-1beta responses in the diseased brain and exacerbates chronic neurodegeneration. Brain Behav Immun. 2010;24:996–1007.
138. Krstic D, Madhusudan A, Doehner J, Vogel P, Notter T, Imhof C, Manalastas A, Hilfiker M, Pfister S, Schwerdel C, Riether C, Meyer U, Knuesel I. Systemic immune challenges trigger and drive Alzheimer-like neuropathology in mice. J Neuroinflammation. 2012;9:151.
139. Perry VH, Holmes C. Microglial priming in neurodegenerative disease. Nat Rev Neurol. 2014;10:217–24.
140. Ide M, Harris M, Stevens A, Sussams R, Hopkins V, Culliford D, Fuller J, Ibbett P, Raybould R, Thomas R, Puenter U, Teeling J, Perry VH, Holmes C. Periodontitis and Cognitive Decline in Alzheimer's Disease. PLoS One. 2016; 11:e0151081.
141. Vasek MJ, Garber C, Dorsey D, Durrant DM, Bollman B, Soung A, Yu J, Perez-Torres C, Frouin A, Wilton DK, Funk K, DeMasters BK, Jiang X, Bowen JR, Mennerick S, Robinson JK, Garbow JR, Tyler KL, Suthar MS, Schmidt RE, Stevens B, Klein RS. A complement-microglial axis drives synapse loss during virus-induced memory impairment. Nature. 2016; 534:538–43.
142. Gray F, Scaravilli F, Everall I, Chretien F, An S, Boche D, Adle-Biassette H, Wingertsmann L, Durigon M, Hurtrel B, Chiodi F, Bell J, Lantos P. Neuropathology of early HIV-1 infection. Brain Pathol. 1996;6(1):15.
143. Rosshart SP, Vassallo BG, Angeletti D, Hutchinson DS, Morgan AP, Takeda K, Hickman HD, McCulloch JA, Badger JH, Ajami NJ, Trinchieri G, Pardo-Manuel de Villena F, Yewdell JW, Rehermann B. Wild Mouse Gut Microbiota Promotes Host Fitness and Improves Disease Resistance. Cell. 2017;171:1015–28.
144. Schroeder BO, Backhed F. Signals from the gut microbiota to distant organs in physiology and disease. Nat Med. 2016;22:1079–89.
145. Thion MS, Low D, Silvin A, Chen J, Grisel P, Schulte-Schrepping J, Blecher R, Ulas T, Squarzoni P, Hoeffel G, Coulpier F, Siopi E, David FS, Scholz C, Shihui F, Lum J, Amoyo AA, Larbi A, Poidinger M, Buttgereit A, Lledo PM, Greter M, Chan JKY, Amit I, Beyer M, Schultze JL, Schlitzer A, Pettersson S, Ginhoux F, Garel S. Microbiome Influences Prenatal and Adult Microglia in a Sex-Specific Manner. Cell. 2018;172:500–16.
146. Erny D, Hrabe de Angelis AL, Jaitin D, Wieghofer P, Staszewski O, David E, Keren-Shaul H, Mahlakoiv T, Jakobshagen K, Buch T, Schwierzeck V, Utermohlen O, Chun E, Garrett WS, McCoy KD, Diefenbach A, Staeheli P, Stecher B, Amit I, Prinz M. Host microbiota constantly control maturation and function of microglia in the CNS. Nat Neurosci. 2015;18:965–77.
147. Fung TC, Olson CA, Hsiao EY. Interactions between the microbiota, immune and nervous systems in health and disease. Nat Neurosci. 2017;20:145–55.
148. Sampson TR, Debelius JW, Thron T, Janssen S, Shastri GG, Ilhan ZE, Challis C, Schretter CE, Rocha S, Gradinaru V, Chesselet MF, Keshavarzian A, Shannon KM, Krajmalnik-Brown R, Wittung-Stafshede P, Knight R, Mazmanian SK. Gut Microbiota Regulate Motor Deficits and Neuroinflammation in a Model of Parkinson's Disease. Cell. 2016;167:1469–80 e12.
149. Bedarf JR, Hildebrand F, Coelho LP, Sunagawa S, Bahram M, Goeser F, Bork P, Wullner U. Functional implications of microbial and viral gut metagenome changes in early stage L-DOPA-naive Parkinson's disease patients. Genome Med. 2017;9:39.
150. Vogt NM, Kerby RL, Dill-McFarland KA, Harding SJ, Merluzzi AP, Johnson SC, Carlsson CM, Asthana S, Zetterberg H, Blennow K, Bendlin BB, Rey FE. 2017. Gut microbiome alterations in Alzheimer's disease. Sci Rep 7: 13537
151. Cattaneo A, Cattane N, Galluzzi S, Provasi S, Lopizzo N, Festari C, Ferrari C, Guerra UP, Paghera B, Muscio C, Bianchetti A, Volta GD, Turla M, Cotelli MS, Gennuso M, Prelle A, Zanetti O, Lussignoli G, Mirabile D, Bellandi D, Gentile S, Belotti G, Villani D, Harach T, Bolmont T, Padovani A, Boccardi M, Frisoni GB, Group I-F. Association of brain amyloidosis with pro-inflammatory gut bacterial taxa and peripheral inflammation markers in cognitively impaired elderly. Neurobiol Aging. 2017;49:60–8.
152. Minter MR, Zhang C, Leone V, Ringus DL, Zhang X, Oyler-Castrillo P, Musch MW, Liao F, Ward JF, Holtzman DM, Chang EB, Tanzi RE, Sisodia SS. Antibiotic-induced perturbations in gut microbial diversity influences neuro-inflammation and amyloidosis in a murine model of Alzheimer's disease. Sci Rep. 2016;6:30028.
153. Harach T, Marungruang N, Duthilleul N, Cheatham V, Mc Coy KD, Frisoni G, Neher JJ, Fak F, Jucker M, Lasser T, Bolmont T. Reduction of Abeta amyloid pathology in APPPS1 transgenic mice in the absence of gut microbiota. Sci Rep. 2017;7:41802.
154. Minter MR, Hinterleitner R, Meisel M, Zhang C, Leone V, Zhang X, Oyler-Castrillo P, Zhang X, Musch MW, Shen X, Jabri B, Chang EB, Tanzi RE, Sisodia SS. Antibiotic-induced perturbations in microbial diversity during post-natal development alters amyloid pathology in an aged APPSWE/PS1DeltaE9 murine model of Alzheimer's disease. Sci Rep. 2017;7:10411.
155. Sharon G, Sampson TR, Geschwind DH, Mazmanian SK. The Central Nervous System and the Gut Microbiome. Cell. 2016;167:915–32.
156. Walker KA, Hoogeveen RC, Folsom AR, Ballantyne CM, Knopman DS, Windham BG, Jack CR Jr, Gottesman RF. Midlife systemic inflammatory markers are associated with late-life brain volume: The ARIC study. Neurology. 2017;89:2262–70.
157. Abuabara K, Azfar RS, Shin DB, Neimann AL, Troxel AB, Gelfand JM. Cause-specific mortality in patients with severe psoriasis: a population-based cohort study in the U.K. Br J Dermatol. 2010;163:586–92.
158. Gisondi P, Sala F, Alessandrini F, Avesani V, Zoccatelli G, Beltramello A, Moretto G, Gambina G, Girolomoni G. Mild cognitive impairment in patients with moderate to severe chronic plaque psoriasis. Dermatology. 2014; 228:78–85.
159. MacPherson KP, Sompol P, Kannarkat GT, Chang J, Sniffen L, Wildner ME, Norris CM, Tansey MG. Peripheral administration of the soluble TNF inhibitor XPro1595 modifies brain immune cell profiles, decreases beta-amyloid plaque load, and rescues impaired long-term potentiation in 5xFAD mice. Neurobiol Dis. 2017;102:81–95.
160. Gallardo G, Holtzman DM. Antibody Therapeutics Targeting Aβ and Tau. Cold Spring Harb Perspect Med. 2017;7:a024331.
161. Kayed R, Head E, Thompson JL, McIntire TM, Milton SC, Cotman CW, Glabe CG. Common Structure of Soluble Amyloid Oligomers Implies Common Mechanism of Pathogenesis. Science. 2003;300:486–9.
162. Lesne S, Koh MT, Kotilinek L, Kayed R, Glabe CG, Yang A, Gallagher M, Ashe KH. A specific amyloid-beta protein assembly in the brain impairs memory. Nature. 2006;440:352–7.
163. Britschgi M, Olin CE, Johns HT, Takeda-Uchimura Y, LeMieux MC, Rufibach K, Rajadas J, Zhang H, Tomooka B, Robinson WH, Clark CM, Fagan AM, Galasko DR, Holtzman DM, Jutel M, Kaye JA, Lemere CA, Leszek J, Li G, Peskind ER, Quinn JF, Yesavage JA, Ghiso JA, Wyss-Coray T. Neuroprotective natural antibodies to assemblies of amyloidogenic peptides decrease with normal aging and advancing Alzheimer's disease. Proc Natl Acad Sci U S A. 2009; 106:12145–50.
164. Moir RD, Tseitlin KA, Soscia S, Hyman BT, Irizarry MC, Tanzi RE. Autoantibodies to redox-modified oligomeric Abeta are attenuated in the plasma of Alzheimer's disease patients. J Biol Chem. 2005;280:17458–63.
165. Lee EB, Leng LZ, Zhang B, Kwong L, Trojanowski JQ, Abel T, Lee VM. Targeting amyloid-beta peptide (Abeta) oligomers by passive immunization with a conformation-selective monoclonal antibody improves learning and memory in Abeta precursor protein (APP) transgenic mice. J Biol Chem. 2006;281:4292–9.
166. Hillen H, Barghorn S, Striebinger A, Labkovsky B, Muller R, Nimmrich V, Nolte MW, Perez-Cruz C, van der Auwera I, van Leuven F, van Gaalen M, Bespalov AY, Schoemaker H, Sullivan JP, Ebert U. Generation and therapeutic efficacy of highly oligomer-specific beta-amyloid antibodies. J Neurosci. 2010;30: 10369–79.

167. Sevigny J, Chiao P, Bussiere T, Weinreb PH, Williams L, Maier M, Dunstan R, Salloway S, Chen T, Ling Y, O'Gorman J, Qian F, Arastu M, Li M, Chollate S, Brennan MS, Quintero-Monzon O, Scannevin RH, Arnold HM, Engber T, Rhodes K, Ferrero J, Hang Y, Mikulskis A, Grimm J, Hock C, Nitsch RM, Sandrock A. The antibody aducanumab reduces Abeta plaques in Alzheimer's disease. Nature. 2016;537:50–6.
168. Bacher M, Depboylu C, Du Y, Noelker C, Oertel WH, Behr T, Henriksen G, Behe M, Dodel R. Peripheral and central biodistribution of (111)In-labeled anti-beta-amyloid autoantibodies in a transgenic mouse model of Alzheimer's disease. Neurosci Lett. 2009;449:240–5.
169. Poduslo JF, Curran GL, Berg CT. Macromolecular permeability across the blood-nerve and blood-brain barriers. Proc Natl Acad Sci U S A. 1994;91:5705–9.
170. Watts RJ, Dennis MS. Bispecific antibodies for delivery into the brain. Curr Opin Chem Biol. 2013;17:393–9.
171. Yu YJ, Atwal JK, Zhang Y, Tong RK, Wildsmith KR, Tan C, Bien-Ly N, Hersom M, Maloney JA, Meilandt WJ, Bumbaca D, Gadkar K, Hoyte K, Luk W, Lu Y, Ernst JA, Scearce-Levie K, Couch JA, Dennis MS, Watts RJ. Therapeutic bispecific antibodies cross the blood-brain barrier in nonhuman primates. Sci Transl Med. 2014;6:261ra154.
172. Nisbet RM, Van der Jeugd A, Leinenga G, Evans HT, Janowicz PW, Gotz J. Combined effects of scanning ultrasound and a tau-specific single chain antibody in a tau transgenic mouse model. Brain. 2017;140:1220–30.
173. Burgess A, Dubey S, Yeung S, Hough O, Eterman N, Aubert I, Hynynen K. Alzheimer disease in a mouse model: MR imaging-guided focused ultrasound targeted to the hippocampus opens the blood-brain barrier and improves pathologic abnormalities and behavior. Radiology. 2014;273:736–45.
174. Jordao JF, Thevenot E, Markham-Coultes K, Scarcelli T, Weng YQ, Xhima K, O'Reilly M, Huang Y, McLaurin J, Hynynen K, Aubert I. Amyloid-beta plaque reduction, endogenous antibody delivery and glial activation by brain-targeted, transcranial focused ultrasound. Exp Neurol. 2013;248:16–29.
175. Alonso A. Ultrasound-induced blood-brain barrier opening for drug delivery. Front Neurol Neurosci. 2015;36:106–15.
176. McGeer PL, Rogers J, McGeer EG. Inflammation, anti-inflammatory agents and Alzheimer disease: the last 12 years. J Alzheimers Dis. 2006;9:271–6.
177. Int'Veld BA, Ruitenberg A, Hofman A, Launer LJ, van Duijn CM, Stijnen T, Breteler MM, Stricker BH. Nonsteroidal antiinflammatory drugs and the risk of Alzheimer's disease. N Engl J Med. 2001;345:1515–21.
178. Group A-FR. Follow-up evaluation of cognitive function in the randomized Alzheimer's Disease Anti-inflammatory Prevention Trial and its Follow-up Study. Alzheimers Dement. 2015;11:216–25 e1.
179. Andrieu S, Coley N, Lovestone S, Aisen PS, Vellas B. Prevention of sporadic Alzheimer's disease: lessons learned from clinical trials and future directions. Lancet Neurol. 2015;14:926–44.
180. Loeffler DA. Intravenous immunoglobulin and Alzheimer's disease: what now? J Neuroinflammation. 2013;10:70.
181. Dodel R, Rominger A, Bartenstein P, Barkhof F, Blennow K, Forster S, Winter Y, Bach JP, Popp J, Alferink J, Wiltfang J, Buerger K, Otto M, Antuono P, Jacoby M, Richter R, Stevens J, Melamed I, Goldstein J, Haag S, Wietek S, Farlow M, Jessen F. Intravenous immunoglobulin for treatment of mild-to-moderate Alzheimer's disease: a phase 2, randomised, double-blind, placebo-controlled, dose-finding trial. Lancet Neurol. 2013;12:233–43.
182. Relkin N. Clinical trials of intravenous immunoglobulin for Alzheimer's disease. J Clin Immunol. 2014;34(Suppl 1):S74–9.
183. Butchart J, Brook L, Hopkins V, Teeling J, Puntener U, Culliford D, Sharples R, Sharif S, McFarlane B, Raybould R, Thomas R, Passmore P, Perry VH, Holmes C. Etanercept in Alzheimer disease: A randomized, placebo-controlled, double-blind, phase 2 trial. Neurology. 2015;84:2161–8.
184. Boyd TD, Bennett SP, Mori T, Governatori N, Runfeldt M, Norden M, Padmanabhan J, Neame P, Wefes I, Sanchez-Ramos J, Arendash GW, Potter H. GM-CSF upregulated in rheumatoid arthritis reverses cognitive impairment and amyloidosis in Alzheimer mice. J Alzheimers Dis. 2010;21:507–18.
185. Jim HS, Boyd TD, Booth-Jones M, Pidala J, Potter H. Granulocyte Macrophage Colony Stimulating Factor Treatment is Associated with Improved Cognition in Cancer Patients. Brain Disord Ther. 2012:1.
186. Potter H, Woodcock JH, Boyd T, Sillau SH, Bettcher BM, Daniels J, Heffernan K, Gray H. Safety and Efficacy Results from Phase 2 pilot trial of GM-CSF/ Leukine® in mild-tomoderate AD. AAIC. 2017;2017:P38.
187. The Plasma for Alzheimer Symptom Amelioration (PLASMA) Study: Intravenously-Administered Plasma From Young Donors for Treatment of Mild-To-Moderate Alzheimer's Disease (2014-2017). https://clinicaltrials.gov/ct2/show/NCT02256306.
188. Jay TR, Hirsch AM, Broihier ML, Miller CM, Neilson LE, Ransohoff RM, Lamb BT, Landreth GE. Disease Progression-Dependent Effects of TREM2 Deficiency in a Mouse Model of Alzheimer's Disease. J Neurosci. 2017;37:637–47.
189. Shi Q, Chowdhury S, Ma R, Le KX, Hong S, Caldarone BJ, Stevens B, Lemere CA. Complement C3 deficiency protects against neurodegeneration in aged plaque-rich APP/PS1 mice. Sci Transl Med. 2017;9:eaaf6295.
190. Fu H, Rodriguez GA, Herman M, Emrani S, Nahmani E, Barrett G, Figueroa HY, Goldberg E, Hussaini SA, Duff KE. Tau Pathology Induces Excitatory Neuron Loss, Grid Cell Dysfunction, and Spatial Memory Deficits Reminiscent of Early Alzheimer's Disease. Neuron 93. 2017;e5:533–41.
191. Saito T, Matsuba Y, Mihira N, Takano J, Nilsson P, Itohara S, Iwata N, Saido TC. Single App knock-in mouse models of Alzheimer's disease. Nat Neurosci. 2014;17:661–3.
192. Hong S, Beja-Glasser VF, Nfonoyim BM, Frouin A, Li S, Ramakrishnan S, Merry KM, Shi Q, Rosenthal A, Barres BA, Lemere CA, Selkoe DJ, Stevens B. Complement and microglia mediate early synapse loss in Alzheimer mouse models. Science. 2016;352:712–6.
193. Griciuc A, Serrano-Pozo A, Parrado Antonio R, Lesinski Andrea N, Asselin Caroline N, Mullin K, Hooli B, Choi Se H, Hyman Bradley T, Tanzi Rudolph E. Alzheimer's Disease Risk Gene CD33 Inhibits Microglial Uptake of Amyloid Beta. Neuron. 2013;78:631–43.
194. Venegas C, Kumar S, Franklin BS, Dierkes T, Brinkschulte R, Tejera D, Vieira-Saecker A, Schwartz S, Santarelli F, Kummer MP, Griep A, Gelpi E, Beilharz M, Riedel D, Golenbock DT, Geyer M, Walter J, Latz E, Heneka MT. Microglia-derived ASC specks cross-seed amyloid-β in Alzheimer's disease. Nature. 2017;552:355.
195. Heneka MT, Kummer MP, Stutz A, Delekate A, Schwartz S, Vieira-Saecker A, Griep A, Axt D, Remus A, Tzeng T-C, Gelpi E, Halle A, Korte M, Latz E, Golenbock DT. NLRP3 is activated in Alzheimer/'s disease and contributes to pathology in APP/PS1 mice. Nature. 2013;493:674–8.
196. Zhou X, Chen Y, Mok KY, Zhao Q, Chen K, Chen Y, Hardy J, Li Y, Fu AKY, Guo Q, Ip NY, Alzheimer's Disease Neuroimaging I. Identification of genetic risk factors in the Chinese population implicates a role of immune system in Alzheimer's disease pathogenesis. Proc Natl Acad Sci U S A. 2018;115:1697–706.
197. Sheean RK, McKay FC, Cretney E, Bye CR, Perera ND, Tomas D, Weston RA, Scheller KJ, Djouma E, Menon P, Schibeci SD, Marmash N, Yerbury JJ, Nutt SL, Booth DR, Stewart GJ, Kiernan MC, Vucic S, Turner BJ. Association of Regulatory T-Cell Expansion With Progression of Amyotrophic Lateral Sclerosis: A Study of Humans and a Transgenic Mouse Model. JAMA Neurol. 2018;75:681–9.
198. Sulzer D, Alcalay RN, Garretti F, Cote L, Kanter E, Agin-Liebes J, Liong C, McMurtrey C, Hildebrand WH, Mao X, Dawson VL, Dawson TM, Oseroff C, Pham J, Sidney J, Dillon MB, Carpenter C, Weiskopf D, Phillips E, Mallal S, Peters B, Frazier A, Lindestam Arlehamn CS, Sette A. T cells from patients with Parkinson's disease recognize α-synuclein peptides. Nature. 2017;546: 656–61.
199. Wendeln AC, Degenhardt K, Kaurani L, Gertig M, Ulas T, Jain G, Wagner J, Hasler LM, Wild K, Skodras A, Blank T, Staszewski O, Datta M, Centeno TP, Capece V, Islam MR, Kerimoglu C, Staufenbiel M, Schultze JL, Beyer M, Prinz M, Jucker M, Fischer A, Neher JJ. Innate immune memory in the brain shapes neurological disease hallmarks. Nature. 2018;556:332–8.
200. Louveau A, Smirnov I, Keyes TJ, Eccles JD, Rouhani SJ, Peske JD, Derecki NC, Castle D, Mandell JW, Lee KS, Harris TH, Kipnis J. Structural and functional features of central nervous system lymphatic vessels. Nature. 2015;523:337–41.
201. Iliff JJ, Wang M, Liao Y, Plogg BA, Peng W, Gundersen GA, Benveniste H, Vates GE, Deane R, Goldman SA, Nagelhus EA, Nedergaard M. A paravascular pathway facilitates CSF flow through the brain parenchyma and the clearance of interstitial solutes, including amyloid beta. Sci Transl Med. 2012;4:147ra11.
202. Talbot S, Foster SL, Woolf CJ. Neuroimmunity: Physiology and Pathology. Annu Rev Immunol. 2016;34:421–47.
203. Kipnis J. Immune system: The "seventh sense". J Exp Med. 2018;215:397–8.
204. Pavlov VA, Chavan SS, Tracey KJ. Molecular and Functional Neuroscience in Immunity. Ann Rev Immunol. 2018;36:783–812.
205. Pavlov VA, Tracey KJ. Neural regulation of immunity: molecular mechanisms and clinical translation. Nat Neurosci. 2017;20:156–66.

Advances in developing novel therapeutic strategies for Alzheimer's disease

Jiqing Cao[1,2,3], Jianwei Hou[1,2], Jing Ping[3] and Dongming Cai[1,2,3*]

Abstract

Alzheimer's Disease (AD), the most prevalent neurodegenerative disease of aging, affects one in eight older Americans. Nearly all drug treatments tested for AD today have failed to show any efficacy. There is a great need for therapies to prevent and/or slow the progression of AD. The major challenge in AD drug development is lack of clarity about the mechanisms underlying AD pathogenesis and pathophysiology. Several studies support the notion that AD is a multifactorial disease. While there is abundant evidence that amyloid plays a role in AD pathogenesis, other mechanisms have been implicated in AD such as tangle formation and spread, dysregulated protein degradation pathways, neuroinflammation, and loss of support by neurotrophic factors. Therefore, current paradigms of AD drug design have been shifted from single target approach (primarily amyloid-centric) to developing drugs targeted at multiple disease aspects, and from treating AD at later stages of disease progression to focusing on preventive strategies at early stages of disease development. Here, we summarize current strategies and new trends of AD drug development, including pre-clinical and clinical trials that target different aspects of disease (mechanism-based versus non-mechanism based, e.g. symptomatic treatments, lifestyle modifications and risk factor management).

Keywords: Alzheimer's disease, Novel therapies, Pre-clinical and clinical trials, Drug development

Background

Alzheimer's disease (AD) is the most prevalent neurodegenerative disease of aging, and it affects over 26 million people worldwide with this number continuously increasing [1–3]. Nearly all drug treatments tested for AD today have failed to show any efficacy. There is a great need for therapies to prevent and/or slow the progression of AD.

AD is a complex disease with multifactorial etiology. Early-onset AD, a rare form of disease, follows an autosomal-dominant pattern in a majority of cases with mutations identified in amyloid precursor protein (APP), presenilin (PS) 1 and 2. Late-onset AD, a sporadic form of disease, affects over 90% of patients with several genetic loci and risk factors identified by a combination of genetic studies and bioinformatic approaches. These discoveries have shaped our current understanding of AD pathogenesis, as well as the development of therapeutic targets and design of clinical trials. While some of identified genetic risk factors can be linked to the most popular amyloid cascade hypothesis and the Tau theory [3], several commonly shared pathways have been implicated in AD such as immune system dysfunction, lipid and cholesterol dyshomeostasis, and vesicle trafficking and protein degradation pathway dysregulation [4–6]. Other theories have also been suggested such as mitochondrial dysfunction, lack of intrinsic support of neurotrophic factors, pre-existing comorbid medical conditions including cerebrovascular diseases, diabetes and hypertension, as well as environmental exposure such as virus infection [7–10].

Here we focus on current AD therapeutic strategies which comprise of mechanism-based approaches including amyloid-beta (Aβ) clearance, tau protein deposits, apolipoprotein-E (ApoE) function, neuroprotection and neuroinflammation, as well as non-mechanism based approaches including symptomatic cognitive stimulation, AD prevention, lifestyle modifications and risk factor management including non-pharmacological interventions (Table 1: a summary list of therapeutic strategies discussed in this paper).

* Correspondence: dongming.cai@mssm.edu
[1]James J Peters VA Medical Center, Research & Development, Bronx, NY 10468, USA
[2]Department of Neurology, Alzheimer Disease Research Center, Icahn School of Medicine at Mount Sinai, New York, NY 10029, USA
Full list of author information is available at the end of the article

Table 1 A summary of therapeutic approaches discussed in the paper

AD therapeutic strategies
Mechanism-based Approaches
1. Therapies Targeted at Amyloid
1.1 Inhibiting Aβ Production
1.2 Accelerating Aβ Clearance
1.3 Preventing Aβ Aggregation
2. Therapies Targeted at Tau
2.1 Tau Stabilizers and Aggregation Inhibitors
2.2 Therapies Targeted at Tau Post-translational Modifications
2.3 Anti-tau Immunotherapy
3. Therapies Targeted at ApoE
4. Neuroprotective Therapies
4.1 Neurotrophins and Their Receptor-based Therapies
4.2 Therapies Targeted at Neuroinflammation and Oxidative Stress
Non-mechanism Based Approaches
1. Symptomatic Cognitive Enhancers
2. Therapies and Interventions for AD Prevention
2.1 Secondary Prevention Interventions
2.2 Primary Prevention Interventions

Mechanism-based approaches

Therapies targeted at amyloid

According to the amyloid cascade hypothesis, AD-related pathology typically begins with asymptomatic cerebral amyloidosis many years before the onset of clinical symptoms [11]. Accumulation of Aβ in the brain starts with monomeric Aβ leaving its reservoir in the cerebrospinal fluid (CSF) to form toxic aggregates followed by deposition on neuronal surface and synaptic terminals. Therefore, the majority of AD treatment strategies targeted at the amyloid cascade in the past 30 years or so has been focused on reducing Aβ generation through development of β- and γ-secretase inhibitors, accelerating Aβ clearance through active and passive immunotherapies, as well as preventing formation of toxic amyloid aggregates.

Reducing Aβ generation

Amyloid Aβ is derived from APP cleaved by two membrane-bound enzymes, β-secretase and γ-secretase complex. Therefore, modulation of these enzymes to inhibit Aβ production has been a major focus in developing AD therapies. The development of β-site APP cleaving enzyme 1 (BACE1) inhibitors was limited at the beginning due to difficulties in drug delivery. Later brain-penetrant BACE1 inhibitors have been developed with data showing promising efficacy at reducing Aβ in animal models [12, 13]. However, most BACE1 inhibitors tested today failed to survive beyond phase II/III clinical trials due to either lack of efficacy, or undesirable long-term side effects (Table 2: a summary list of AD drugs tested in clinical trials). For example, Merck halted its ongoing clinical trials of verubecestat (MK-8931) in mild to moderate AD patients [14–16], and most recently in people with prodromal AD (the APECS: β amyloid Production and Effects on Cognition Study; NCT01953601). However, despite the disappointing results from current clinical trials of BACE1 inhibitors, a recent study demonstrated that conditional knockout of BACE1 was capable of completely reversing pre-formed amyloid deposition and improving cognitive function in a mouse model with 5× Familial AD (FAD) transgenic background, suggesting sequential and gradual inhibition of BACE1 could be beneficial for AD patients [17]. It was pointed out that BACE1 is necessary to maintain optimal cognitive function and that the BACE1 inhibition is not without concerns [17]. More studies are needed to clarify the mechanism(s) of BACE inhibitors in AD, to determine optimal timing for BACE1 inhibition in adult AD patients, and to search for drug candidates without unwanted and off-target toxicities.

The γ-secretase complex is comprised of four subunits [18, 19], with presenilin (PS) exhibiting catalytic activities of γ -secretase [20–28]. There is a long list of γ-secretase substrates with APP and Notch among the most well-known due to their implications in AD and cancer [18, 29]. Substantial effort has been invested into developing small-molecule inhibitors of γ-secretase for AD therapies. Non-selective γ-secretase inhibitors led to a decrease in brain Aβ [30, 31], and reduced Notch signaling at the same time causing gastrointestinal (GI) symptoms and compromised immune system [32, 33]. Despite the concerns, non-selective γ-secretase inhibitors such as semagacestat were tested in clinical trials (see in Table 2; NCT00762411, NCT00594568, NCT01035138), but discontinued at Phase III stage because of lack of efficacy or even worsened cognitive performance, and patient intolerance due to severe off-target side effects like GI irritation and skin cancer [15, 18, 19, 34–37]. Selective γ-secretase inhibitors include Notch-sparing γ-secretase inhibitors and γ-secretase modulators. Gleevec, the abl kinase inhibitor was found to reduce Aβ production but spare Notch cleavage by γ-secretase in primary neuronal cells and animals [38]. Avagacestat was reported to inhibit APP processing more preferably than Notch cleavage [39]. However, Phase II clinical trial of Avagacestat was discontinued due to adverse side effects suggesting possible Notch inhibition just like Semagacestat ([35]; NCT00890890). A recently developed Notch-sparing γ-secretase inhibitor pinitol (NIC5–15) was derived from natural product and reported to have insulin sensitization property. It is currently in Phase II trial for the treatment of AD ([15, 40]; NCT01928420). Non-steroidal anti-inflammatory drugs (NSAIDs) were the first γ-secretase modulators shown to shift Aβ production from the aggregable form ($A\beta_{42}$) to a more soluble form ($A\beta_{38}$) [41]. One of these NSAIDs, R-flurbiprofen [42] failed to exhibit any efficacy in Phase III trial of mild AD subjects (NCT00105547, NCT00322036).

Table 2 A summary list of AD drugs and therapies tested in clinical trials

AD drugs tested in clinical trials					
Drug	Phase	Subject	NCT	Summary	Reference
1.Therapies Targeted at Amyloid					
1.1 Reducing Aβ Generation					
MK-8931 (BACE inh.)	III	Prodromal AD	NCT01953601	lack of efficacy	14-16
LY450139 (γ-secretase inh.)	III	Mild to moderate AD	NCT00762411; NCT00594568 NCT01035138	lack of efficacy	15,18, 19, 34, 36, 37
Avagacestat	II	Prodromal AD	NCT00890890	no efficacy	35
NIC5-15	II	Probable AD	NCT01928420	completed	15,40
R-flurbiprofen	III	Probable AD	NCT00105547; NCT00322036	lack of efficacy	42
EVP-0962	II	Healthy, MCI or early AD	NCT01661673	terminated	15
1.2 Accelerating Aβ Clearance					
AN-1792	II	Mild-to-moderate AD	NCT00021723	severe meningoencephalitis	44
Affitope AD02	II	Early AD	NCT02008513; NCT01117818	no efficacy	46
CAD106	II/III	Mild AD	NCT02565511	ongoing	15, 47
Bapineuzumab	III	Mild-to-moderate AD	NCT00667810; NCT00575055 NCT00574132	no efficacy	43, 48
Solanezumab	III	Mild-to-moderate AD probable AD	NCT00905372; NCT00904683 NCT01900665	no efficacy	43, 49
BAN2401	II	MCI due to AD and mild AD	NCT01767311	positive results	50
Crenezumab	III	Probable AD or prodromal AD	NCT03114657; NCT02670083	ongoing	
Gantenerumab	III	Probable AD or prodromal AD	NCT03443973; NCT03444870	ongoing	
Aducanumab	I	Prodromal or Mild AD	NCT01677572	positive results but ARIA	51
	III	MCI due to AD or mild AD	NCT02484547; NCT02477800	ongoing	
1.3 Other Anti-amyloidogenic Compounds with Diverse Mechanisms of Action					
ALZT-OP1	III	Early AD	NCT02547818	ongoing	43
GV-971	III	Mild-to-moderate AD	NCT02293915	completed	43
Posiphen	I	MCI or probably AD	NCT02925650	ongoing	52
ELND005	II/III	Mild-to-severe AD		ongoing	53
ALZ801	III	Mild AD (ApoE4 carriers)		ongoing	43
2. Therapies Targeted at Tau					
2.1 Tau Stabilizers and Aggregation Inhibitors					
TPI 287	I	Probable AD	NCT01966666	ongoing	
Rember™	II	Mild or moderate AD	NCT00684944; NCT00515333	no efficacy	62, 63
TRx0237	III	Mild-to-moderate AD/BvFTD	NCT01689233; NCT01689246 NCT02245568	no efficacy	64
TauRx	II/III	Mild or moderate AD	NCT03539380	ongoing	
2.2 Therapies Targeted at Tau Post-translational Modifications					
Lithium and Valproate	II	AD	NCT00088387	no efficacy	67, 68
NP-12	IIb	Mild-to-moderate AD	NCT01350362	no efficacy	69-71
2.3 Anti-tau Immunotherapy					
AADvac1	II	Mild-to-moderate AD	NCT02579252	ongoing	94
ACI-35	I	Mild-to-moderate AD	ISRCTN13033912	completed	61
ABBV-8E12	II	PSP; MCI or probable AD	NCT03391765; NCT02880956	ongoing	
RO7105705	I	Healthy	NCT02820896	ongoing	
3. Therapies Targeted at ApoE					
Bexarotene	II	Probable AD	NCT01782742	no efficacy	142

Table 2 A summary list of AD drugs and therapies tested in clinical trials *(Continued)*

AD drugs tested in clinical trials					
4. Neuroprotective Therapies					
4.1 Neurotrophins and Their Receptor-based Therapies					
NGF	I	Probable early AD	NCT00017940	positive results	170
AAV2-NGF	II	Mild-to-moderate AD	NCT00876863	no efficacy	173
LM11A-31 (p75 inh.)	I/II	Mild-to-moderate AD	NCT03069014	ongoing	
4.2 Therapies Targeted at Neuroinflammation and Oxidative Stress					
Dimebon	III	AD	NCT00912288	no efficacy	209
valacyclovir	II	Probable AD	NCT03282916	ongoing	
5. Symptomatic Cognitive Enhancers					
Idalopirdine	II	Probable AD	NCT01019421	positive results	233
(5-HT6 antag.)	III	Mild-to-moderate AD	NCT01955161; NCT02006641 NCT02006654	no efficacy	234
GSK239512 (H3R antag.)	II	Probable AD	NCT01009255	no efficacy	235
ABT288 (H3R antag.)	II	Mild-to-moderate AD	NCT01018875	no efficacy	236
Rasagiline (MAOB inh.)	II	Probable AD	NCT02359552	ongoing	237
Ladostigil (combined)	II	MCI or Mild-to-moderate AD	NCT01429623; NCT01354691	no efficacy	238-241
AZD0530	Ib	Mild-to-moderate AD	NCT01864655	safety and tolerance	252
(Fyn kinase inh.)	II	Mild AD	NCT02167256	ongoing	
Cilostazol	II	MCI	NCT02491268	positive results	255-257
(PDE3 inh.)	IV	Mild-to-moderate AD	NCT01409564	ongoing	
HT-0712 (PDE4 inh.)	II	Age-associated memory impairment	NCT02013310	completed	253, 254
Roflumilast (PDE4 inh.)	I	Scopolamine-induced CI	NCT02051335	no efficacy	253, 254
	II	Healthy	NCT01433666	positive results	253, 254
		Age-associated memory impairment	ISRCTN96013814	completed	253, 254
BPN14770 (PDE4 inh.)	I	Healthy	NCT02648672; NCT02840279	positive results	253, 254
BI 409306 (PDE9 inh.)	I	Healthy	NCT01343706	safety and tolerance	253
	II	MCI due to AD and mild AD	NCT02337907	ongoing	253, 254
PF044467943	I	Mild-to-moderate AD	NCT00988598	safety and tolerance	253
(PDE9 inh.)	II	Mild-to-moderate AD		no efficacy	253
6. Therapies and Interventions for AD Prevention					
PROSPER (statin)	II	High risk (with AD parents)	NCT00939822	no efficacy	265
ACCORD-MIND	III	DM2	NCT00182910	no efficacy	268
SNIFF (i.n. insulin)	II; II/III	MCI or AD or probable AD	NCT00438568; NCT01767909	ongoing	271-273
Metformin	IV	Age >60 years with IGT	NCT02432287	completed	274
Pioglitazone	II	Mild-to-moderate AD	NCT00982202	safety and tolerance	275
MIND (diet)		BMI≥25 non-demented	NCT02817074	ongoing	277, 278
FABS (fitness)		Non-demented	ACTRN12605000136606	positive results	280
ACTIVE (cog. training)	II/III	MCI	NCT00298558	positive results	282
Vit. E + Memantine	III	Mild to moderate AD	NCT00235716	positive results	284, 285
Ginkgo biloba	III	Non-demented and MCI	NCT00010803	no efficacy	286, 287
EGb 761®	IV	Subjects with memory complaints	NCT00276510	no efficacy	288
MIDAS		Age-associated memory impairment	NCT00278135	positive results	290
FINGER		High risk	NCT01041989	positive results	291
MIND-ADMINI		Prodromal AD	NCT03249688	ongoing	

A γ-secretase modulator EVP-0962 showed potency in preclinical stage but no efficacy in Phase II trial of mild cognitive impairment (MCI) or early AD subjects [15] (NCT01661673).

Accelerating Aβ clearance

On the other hand, immunotherapy via active and passive vaccines against Aβ has been utilized as a therapeutic approach in AD [43]. The clinical trials of active immunotherapy targeted at Aβ failed until now due to autoimmune responses. The first active immunization clinical study in mild to moderate AD patients was discontinued in Phase II because a small portion of cohort developed severe meningoencephalitis with the AN-1792 vaccine targeting full-length $A\beta_{1-42}$ peptide (NCT0 0021723) [44]. Subsequent development of vaccines was tailored to target specific Aβ epitopes such as ACC-001 which targets an N-terminal $A\beta_{1-7}$ peptide fragment [15, 45]. Currently 2 s-generation active immunotherapy vaccines have been progressed into clinical trials (Affitope AD02 terminated in Phase II study [46], NCT02008513; CAD106 [15, 47] still in Phase II/III study, NCT02565511).

Comparing to active vaccination, passive anti-Aβ immunization may be a more promising strategy for treating AD. Unfortunately, most currently available data in clinical trials fail to meet the primary endpoints. Bapineuzumab is an antibody targeted at the N-terminus of Aβ peptide acting on soluble Aβ. However, no beneficial effect was found with Bapineuzumab in Phase III clinical studies of mild-to-moderate AD subjects [43, 48] (NCT00667810; NCT00575055; NCT00574132). Similarly, Solanezumab targeted at $A\beta_{16-24}$ epitope, which was reported to only recognize soluble instead of fibrillary Aβ, failed in Phase III trial of mild AD patients [43, 49] (NCT00905372; NCT00904683; NCT01900665). BAN2401 targeted at soluble Aβ protofibrils, recently completed a Phase II trial of 856 MCI or mild AD subjects with confirmed brain amyloid pathology [50] (NCT01767311) with positive results from the highest dosage treatment group (10 mg/kg bi-weekly). It was reported that the statistical significance was achieved on key efficacy endpoints after 18 months of high dose treatment on slowing clinical progression measured by the Alzheimer's Disease Composite Score (ADCOMS) and the Alzheimer's Disease Assessment Scale-Cognitive Subscale (ADAS-Cog) score, as well as on reducing brain amyloid accumulation determined by amyloid-PET. However, those who interpret these results must be cautious as most of the $ApoE4^{+}$ carriers were removed from the high-dose treatment group due to concerns of developing amyloid-related imaging abnormalities-edema (ARIA-E; based on AAIC 2018 Conference news). The full data set including the detailed demographic information of treatment versus placebo groups has yet to be shared with the scientific community.

Crenezumab (NCT03114657; NCT02670083), Gantenerumab (NCT03443973; NCT03444870), and Aducanumab (NCT02484547; NCT02477800) targeted both soluble and aggregated Aβ species (both oligomeric and fibrillar Aβ), are currently in Phase III trials in patients with prodromal, mild, and early AD, respectively. The results from preclinical and Phase 1b clinical trial studies regarding Aducanumab demonstrated that treatment reduced amyloid plaque levels in prodromal and mild AD patients in a dose-dependent manner. Additionally, cognitive results from clinical dementia rating-sum of the boxes scale (CDR-SB) and mini-mental status examination (MMSE) taken at the 54th week of treatment demonstrated that Aducanumab confers delayed cognitive decline. The main safety and tolerability concerns were ARIA [51] (NCT01677572).

Other anti-amyloidogenic compounds with diverse mechanisms of action

In addition to enzyme inhibitors and vaccines, there are other compounds developed with diverse mechanisms of action. ALZT-OP1, a combination therapy of two drugs with efficacy at preventing Aβ aggregation and neuroinflammation, is currently in Phase III clinical trial [43] (NCT02547818). GV-971, an oral sodium oligomannurarate with the ability to reduce Aβ toxicity in vitro, is in Phase III clinical trial of mild-to-moderate AD patients [43] (NCT02293915). Several low-molecular-weight anti-amyloidogenic drugs are currently in clinical investigations, e.g. Posiphen in Phase I/II trial for the treatment of MCI, AD and Parkinson's disease (PD) [52] (NCT02925650), ELND005 in Phase II/III trial for treatment of AD type dementia [53] (NCT00934050), and ALZ-801 in Phase III clinical trial for AD [43].

The current belief in the field about the failure of anti-Aβ therapies indicates that late stage of interventions failed to provide full effects. Ongoing clinical trials of passive immunotherapy are focusing on targeting prodromal AD study cohorts with the goal to test anti-amyloid treatments in "correct" populations. This will be discussed in detail in the following section of "Therapies and Interventions for AD Prevention". On the other hand, active Aβ immunotherapy as an effective way to prevent AD remains to be tested, and many safety concerns such as the severity of immune responses against the vaccine need to be investigated further.

Therapies targeted at tau

Tau is a microtubule-binding protein which forms neurofibrillary tangles (NFTs), another neuropathological hallmark of AD [54, 55]. Interestingly, previous reports suggest that tau deposit correlates better with cognitive decline than amyloid plaque does [56], and that Aβ-induced neuro-toxicity is mediated by tau hyper-phosphorylation through a toxic gain-of-function effect [57–60]. Because of many recent failures in anti-Aβ drug trials, therapies targeted at tau have come into focus in AD drug development field. Current therapeutic strategies are categorized into inhibiting tau aggregation, reducing hyper-phosphorylation or other toxic post-translational modifications of tau, as well as promoting tau clearance and preventing tau spread [61].

Tau stabilizers and aggregation inhibitors

Most tau stabilizing agents manifested undesirable toxic side effects, e.g. paclitaxel and epothilone D [15]. A recent Phase I clinical trial study of a tau stabilizer TPI 287 in mild-to-moderate AD, progressive supranuclear palsy (PSP), and corticobasal syndrome (CBS) patients, conveyed encouraging results with beneficial effects of TP1 287 on cognitive performance and/or nerve cells activity (based on CTAD 2017 conference news). The trial is still ongoing with more safety and exploratory clinical effects to be analyzed (NCT01966666).

In parallel, several tau aggregation inhibitors tested have failed in clinical trials due to either unwanted side effects or lack of efficacy, e.g. Rember™ in Phase II [62, 63] (NCT00684944; NCT00515333), and TRx0237 (LMTM) in three Phase III trials of patients with mild-to-moderate AD and behavioral variant frontotemporal dementia [64] (NCT01689246; NCT01689233; NCT02245568). An ongoing Phase II/III trial by TauRx, aiming to enroll people with all-cause dementia and AD from multiple sites, will compare a 6-month course of 4 mg of LMTM twice daily to a different kind of placebo. Primary outcomes include ^{18}F- fludeoxyglucose positron emission tomography (FDG-PET) imaging and safety; secondary outcomes include structural magnetic resonance imaging (MRI), as well as measures of cognition and activities of daily living (ADL; NCT03539380).

Therapies targeted at tau post-translational modifications

Another aspect of tau targeted therapies focuses on toxic post-translational modifications of tau: 1) inhibiting tau hyper-phosphorylation kinases such as glycogen synthase kinase 3 beta (GSK3) and cyclin dependent kinase 5 (CDK5); 2) promoting the activity of tau dephosphorylation enzyme protein phosphate 2A (PP2A) [65]; 3) modulating tau acetylation and cis-transformation [66].

There have been no success in clinical trial studies of GSK3 inhibitors, e.g. lithium and valproate in Phase II trial of AD patients [67, 68] (NCT00088387), and NP-031112 (NP-12) in Phase IIb trial [69–71] (NCT01350362). Development of other GSK3 inhibitors like paullone has not progressed past the preclinical trials due to concerns with cytotoxic effects [72, 73]. Unfortunately, there are no tau kinase inhibitors other than GSK3 inhibitors that have entered clinical trials due to several limiting factors such as kinase specificities and unclear safety profiles. Most selective inhibitors of CDK5 with preclinical efficacy [74, 75] have yet to be tested in clinical trials due to uncertainty of how selective these inhibitors are over other CDK family members as well as poor understanding of safety risks associated with CDK5 inhibition in humans. The results of other inhibitors of tau kinases like JNK and DYRKIA were disappointing with either negative clinical outcome measures or severe adverse side effects [66].

Besides tau hyperphosphorylation, other tau post-translational modifications such as acetylation have been implicated in AD and related tauopathies [76–78]. Therapeutic approaches such as limiting tau K280/K281 acetylation [79] or reducing tau acetylation by protein deacetylase SIRT1 [80] could restore microtubule stability and/or ameliorate tau-associated neurodegeneration in animal models. Whether targeting tau acetylation could be a feasible therapeutic approach for AD or other tauopathies is yet to be tested in clinical studies. Furthermore, studies by Lu and colleagues demonstrated that cis-p-tau transformation causes gain-of-toxic conformational changes of tau leading to aggregation, and that a monoclonal antibody against cis-p-tau can block this phenomenon [81–83]. Another strategy is to inhibit O-GlcNAcase, an enzyme that strips sugars from tau. It is believed that O-GlcNAcylation either competes with phosphorylation for the same serine/threonine residues, or simply prevents tau molecules from cozying up to one another. In animal studies, O-GlcNAcase inhibitors suppress tau phosphorylation, prevent tangles, and boost neuronal survival [84, 85]. Further studies are needed to determine the clinical efficacy of these strategies.

Anti-tau immunotherapy

The basis for anti-tau immunotherapy stems upon the discovery of trans-cellular tau spread with evidence supported by studies in mouse models as well as in clinical settings [86–89]. The rationale behind the application of immunization against pathologic tau variants is to interrupt the uptake and propagation processes of abnormal tau [90]. Using high-affinity antibody against phosphorylated tau is an approach that hopefully would not disturb the function of physical tau from active immunization of phosphorylated tau [91].

Several studies using active immunization against phospho-tau peptides modulating tau pathology showed positive results in tauopathy or AD mouse models [92, 93]. Currently, two active vaccines (AADvac1 and ACI-35) are being tested in clinical trials with AD patients [15]. AADvac-1 is a synthetic peptide derived from tau for active immunization which is going into Phase II trials [94] (NCT02579252). ACI-35 is a liposome-based 16-amino acid, tetra-palmitoylated phospho-tau peptide being tested in people with mild to moderate AD during Phase I study [61] (ISRCTN13033912). However, several concerns about active immunization of tau remain to be addressed such as the development of immune responses to other regions of tau epitope also known as epitope spread, and the likelihood of irreversible active immunization processes [64].

Tau-targeted passive immunization is an exciting development in AD because it offers the possibility of halting the spread of tau pathology through the extracellular space. In some tauopathy mouse models, certain tau antibodies halt the progression of NFT pathology even after onset of tangle formation [95–98]. Currently, ABBV-8E12, an antibody against aggregated, extracellular tau, is in two Phase II trials targeting PSP patients and MCI subjects with positive amyloid scan (NCT03391765; NCT02880956). RO7105705, a pan-tau antibody targeted at N-terminus of all six isoforms of human tau, is now in Phase I trial which evaluates once weekly 8400 mg doses of the antibody in healthy controls and AD patients (NCT02820896; AAIC 2017 Conference News). Several other tau antibody candidates are heading toward Phase I trials. However, concerns of autoimmunity against endogenous tau just like Aβ immunotherapy remain to be addressed.

The link between tau pathology and cognitive dysfunction raises the hope that cognitive decline can be slowed or even halted by therapies targeted at tau. Strategies discussed in this section include stabilizing microtubules, reducing tau aggregation, inhibiting hyperphosphorylation or other toxic modifications of tau, as well as active and passive immunization against tau to promote clearance and interrupt transcellular spread. Other approaches that upregulate the clearance and degradation of tau through the ubiquitin/proteasome system and the autophagy/lysosome pathway would likely have favorable effects as well, which are not discussed in this section.

Therapies targeted at ApoE

The ApoE4 genotype is one of the strongest genetic risk factors for developing sporadic AD [99]. On the other hand, those with ApoE2 genotype demonstrate a lower risk of developing AD and a delayed age of onset regarding AD symptoms. Several Aβ-dependent [100–102] and Aβ-independent mechanisms [103, 104] have been proposed for ApoE in AD pathogenesis. Different therapeutic strategies targeted at ApoE were tested in vitro and/or in vivo preclinical animal models including blocking Aβ-ApoE interaction by small peptide fragments [105–108], manipulating ApoE levels (drug treatments to stimulate ApoE expression [109], or decrease ApoE expression [110]), viral delivery of ApoE2 [111, 112], ApoE antibodies [113, 114], structural modifiers [115–117], lipidation promoting compounds [118–121] and ApoE mimetic peptides [122–125].

Blocking the interaction between ApoE and Aβ by a peptide fragment of Aβ reduced brain amyloid accumulation, ameliorated memory deficits [105, 107], and reduced brain insoluble tau levels [126] in AD transgenic mouse models. Interestingly, ApoE immunotherapy can achieve similar effects on decreasing amyloid burden [113, 114]. One possible mechanism of action is blocking the ApoE-Aβ interaction by anti-ApoE antibodies. When given at pre-plaque stage [113] or after plaque deposition [114], an anti-mouse ApoE antibody decreased amyloid plaque load and improved brain functional connectivity and cognition in an APP transgenic mouse model. No overt adverse side effects such as changes in total cholesterol or cerebral amyloid angiopathy load were observed with anti-ApoE therapy in mice [113, 114]. It should be noted that severe dyslipidemia associated with ApoE deficiency [127] needs to be carefully examined before moving forward into clinical applications.

Regulation of ApoE quantity is one of the main therapeutic approaches tested for AD. However, conflicting results have been reported from clinical studies for AD biomarkers comparing ApoE levels of AD patients with normal individuals [128–131]. Interestingly in animal models, decreasing expression of ApoE3 or ApoE4, or increasing expression of ApoE2 lowered brain amyloid deposition [111, 112]. Numerous animal studies have also been performed to evaluate the therapeutic potential of compounds that increase brain ApoE levels [109, 118, 120, 121, 132–141]. For example, oral administration of bexarotene, an agonist of retinoid X receptors (RXRs) which positively regulates ApoE transcription, was found to increase brain ApoE, reduce Aβ deposition and improve cognitive function in an AD transgenic mouse model [109]. However, a later report failed to replicate the beneficial effects of bexarotene in mouse models [137]. When juxtaposed with the adverse side effects of bexarotene including hepatic failure and lack of efficacy in reducing brain amyloid load from a Phase II clinical trial of AD patients (NCT01782742), the enthusiasm for this drug diminished [142].

On the other hand, effects of viral delivery of human ApoE assessed in APP transgenic mice showed reduced amyloid plaque load by ApoE2 and increased plaque load by ApoE4 [111, 112]. Similar effects on mouse Aβ levels were observed in ApoE4 targeted replacement (TR) mice without human APP transgenic background [143]. Overall, results from animal studies suggest that gene therapy increasing ApoE2 expression might be beneficial [144]. Further studies are critical to determine gene therapy strategies for ApoE4 conditions, e.g. gene silencing versus increasing expression [144].

Another line of approach targeted at ApoE in AD is through the modification of ApoE properties such as ApoE structural modifiers and lipidation-promoting agents. It was reported that the interaction between residues Arg61 and Glu255 of ApoE4 confers abnormal structural conformation associated with ApoE4-induced neurotoxicity [145, 146]. Therefore, a potential therapeutic approach is to modify the pathological structure of ApoE4. For example, a recent report using human neurons derived from induced pluripotent stem cells of ApoE4 subjects, demonstrated that treatment with a small-molecule structure corrector of ApoE4 reduced levels of ApoE4 fragments, increased numbers of GABAergic neurons, as well as reduced production and/or secretion of p-tau, $A\beta_{40}$ and $A\beta_{42}$ [117].

Moreover, lipidation of ApoE significantly affects its function [147] and differential properties of lipidation between ApoE isoforms have been reported. ApoE4 is found to be poorly lipidated in humans [148] and in ApoE mice [149, 150], and promoting ApoE4 lipidation through activation of nuclear receptor pathways (the LXR/RXR-ABCA1 axis) could be a therapeutic strategy [140, 151, 152]. However, one potential concern is the likelihood of increasing ApoE4 levels and exacerbating the detrimental effects of ApoE4 [104]. Future work is needed to explore how ApoE lipidation and function are regulated by brain lipid homeostasis [153].

It should be noted that the ApoE4 genotype is an important determinant of therapeutic responses in AD clinical trials [154]. For example, Phase III trials of bapinuezumab showed significant differences in treatment responses between ApoE4$^+$ and ApoE4$^-$ AD patients [155]. Similarly, data from the Cardiovascular Health Cognition Study indicated that protective effects of nonsteroidal anti-inflammatory drugs (NSAIDs) against AD development, can only be seen in 65 years or older ApoE4$^+$ individuals [156]. More importantly, the risk for developing AD was significantly higher in ApoE4$^+$ women than in ApoE4$^+$ men [157–159]. Collectively, the potential impact of ApoE4 genotype and its interaction with sex need to be carefully considered when designing clinical trials to evaluate therapeutic efficacy in AD.

Neuroprotective therapies

In AD, synaptic dysfunction caused by a combination of factors including accumulation of toxic aggregates, age-related processes, and neuroinflammation is one of disease's hallmarks. While the majority of AD therapeutic efforts advanced in clinical trials have been focused on targeting amyloid and tau, neuroprotective strategies are developed to target at degenerative mechanisms triggered by or involving factors mentioned above.

Neurotrophins and their receptor-based therapies

Neurotrophins (NTs) and their receptor-based therapies in AD have been explored for years because of the pleiotropic actions of NTs and receptor signaling [160–166]. However, suboptimal pharmacological profiles of NTs such as short plasma half-lives, poor oral bioavailability and BBB permeability, as well as limited brain tissue diffusion, limit their clinical application [167–169]. Alternatively, gene transfer technology has been utilized in developing NTs-based AD therapy.

A phase I clinical trial of implantation of genetically modified autologous fibroblasts expressing nerve growth factor (NGF) into the basal forebrain area of eight mild AD patients demonstrated efficacy at improving the cognitive decline rate and increasing brain metabolic activity measured by serial 18-fluorodeoxyglucose PET scans [170] (NCT00017940). Autopsied brains confirmed sustained expression and activity of viral-delivered NGF [171]. In addition, it was observed that axons sprouted toward the local source of NGF and cell hypertrophy [172]. Subsequent Phase II trial recruited 49 mild to moderate AD subjects who were randomly assigned to receive intracerebral injections of AAV2-NGF or sham surgery. While AAV2-NGF delivery was well-tolerated, it did not affect clinical outcomes, or selected AD biomarkers 2 years after NGF delivery [173] (NCT0 0876863). It was argued that these results were inconclusive due to a small sample size. In addition, whether viral delivery achieved the targeted expression of NGF in treatment group needs to be evaluated.

NT receptor-based therapies focus on targeting p75, Tropomyosin Receptor Kinase A (TrkA) and TrkB receptors. The goal of p75-targeted therapeutic strategies is to develop small molecules that can inhibit degenerative signaling of p75 [174, 175], and promote survival even in the absence of NTs [175, 176]. A brain-penetrant small molecule, called LMA11A-31, counteracts the toxicity of Aβ and tau to prevent synaptic dysfunction, spine loss, neurite degeneration, microglia activation, and cognitive deficits in animal models [177, 178]. This compound reversed degeneration in 12-month-old AD mice [179], and repaired age-related loss of cholinergic neurons in wild-type mice (CTAD 2017 meeting report). In a Phase I trial, single or multiple doses of LM11A-31 were well tolerated by young or old volunteers with no adverse events reported. An ongoing Phase IIa trial targeted at mild to moderate AD patients will evaluate the effects of LM11A-31 at two dosages (NCT03069014).

Previous conflicting reports implicate the complexity of targeting TrkA for AD therapies, e.g. results showing positive effects of TrkA activation in cellular and mouse models of AD [180, 181] versus data showing beneficial effects of TrkA inhibition [182, 183]. A series of small-molecule ligands have been developed that either bind to and activate TrkB alone, or both TrkB and TrkC as well as downstream effectors of the signaling pathways, demonstrating some beneficial effects in vitro and in wildtype animals [175, 184, 185]. Systemic injection of a TrkB agonist 7,8-dihydroxyflavone (7,8-DHF) reduced brain amyloid load, prevented synaptic loss, and rescued cognitive deficits in 5XFAD mice [186–188]. However, later work failed to show efficacy at reducing pathology or improving cognitive deficits in the APP/PS1 transgenic mouse model with concerns regarding limited bioavailability of 7,8-DHF [189]. Together, NTs and receptor-based therapies have some potential for synergistic intracellular signaling [190], and the feasibility to combat multifaceted pathological mechanisms of AD but these strategies needs to be carefully evaluated before clinical applications.

Therapies targeted at Neuroinflammation and oxidative stress

The role of neuroinflammation and involvement of microglia in AD pathogenesis have been increasingly recognized and supported by a large amount of evidence including genetic studies, data mining and multiscale network analysis [191–194]. The microglial priming model proposes that during pre-symptomatic stage of AD, microglia is activated by proinflammatory mediators [192], and subsequently astrocytes acquire a proinflammatory phenotype amplifying neuronal damage [195–199]. The glial dysfunction may be independent from the presence of Aβ and tau at early stages of disease, leading to synaptic dysfunction and neuronal death [200, 201]. Therefore, molecules that restore physiological function of microglia and astrocytes may offer new directions for AD therapy.

Different strategies are developed at modulating immune cell function in neuroinflammation such as reducing gene expression of cytokines, inhibiting cytokine release and preventing cytokines binding to their receptors [202]. Molecules such as minocycline with anti-inflammatory properties have been shown to reduce cytokine release from astrocytes, and thereby rescue cognitive deficits in AD mouse models [203, 204]. Interestingly, it was found that inhibiting tau phosphorylation kinases such as GSK3β could also achieve satisfactory results of modulating neuroinflammation in animal models [205]. Reduced oxidative injury is another neuroprotective approach. For example, inhibition of cyclooxygenase-2 and inducible nitric oxide synthase has positive outcomes based on in vitro and in vivo animal studies [206–208]. While mitochondrial enhancers like Dimebon (latrepirdine) failed to show efficacy in clinical trials [209] (NCT 00912288), effort continues at searching for more effective agents targeted mitochondrial dysfunction with the hope to restore synaptic and neuronal function [210, 211].

Another strategy targeted at microglial function is through experimental manipulations to promote microglial encapsulation of amyloid plaques and reduce axonal dystrophy [212]. Several groups have shown that passive immunization of anti-Aβ antibody [51, 212, 213], or anti-ApoE antibody [113] increases recruitment of microglia around amyloid plaques in AD mouse models. Genetic deletion of the chemokine receptor CX3CR1 in microglia can also enhance formation of microglial barrier around amyloid plaques [212], and thereby reduce plaque load [214, 215]. Other strategies of neutralizing CX3CR1 include antibodies targeted at the receptor or its ligand, or small molecule antagonists such as AZD8797 [216]. However, therapies targeted at CX3CR1 are not without concerns. The likelihood of exacerbating tau hyperphosphorylation [217, 218], as well as disrupting bacterial clearance by peripheral immune system with systemic suppression of CX3CR1 signaling [219], suggest the importance of searching for approaches to target CX3CR1 signaling specifically in plaque-associated microglia and to minimize potential systemic side effects [220]. Intriguingly, recent reports described that LED-based light flicker stimuli at 40 Hz could promote microglial recruitment, thereby reducing brain amyloid levels in AD transgenic mouse models [221–223].

Studies have linked viral infection with an antimicrobial innate immune response [224, 225], and regulation of AD risk genes [226]. In alignment with these studies, a Phase II trial has been initiated to investigate the efficacy of treating mild AD patients who test positive for serum antibodies for herpes simplex virus 1 or 2, with an anti-viral drug valacyclovir (NCT03282916). The ApoE genotype was taken into consideration during this trial design. The outcome measures include ADAS-cog and ADCS-ADL scores, as well as Aβ and tau burden measured by PET and CSF studies. In addition, changes in cortical thinning on structural MRI, olfactory identification deficits, and antiviral antibody titers from baseline to 78 weeks, will be evaluated. This study will directly address whether virus infections may be etiologic or contribute to the pathology of AD.

Non-mechanism based approaches

Symptomatic cognitive enhancers

Symptomatic therapies aiming at cognitive enhancement have been focused on modulating cholinergic and glutamatergic function: the cholinesterase inhibitors (ACHEIs) and a N-methyl-D-aspartate (NMDA) receptor antagonist (memantine). ACHEIs decrease the degradation of acetylcholine released from cholinergic neurons, thereby increasing synaptic transmission. Evidence suggests that ACHEIs moderately improve cognitive and global function status of mild to moderate AD patients [227]. However, the efficacy wanes with long-term treatment due to side effects such as weight loss and syncope [227]. Memantine blocks over-excited NMDA receptors to prevent glutamate release, thereby inhibiting neurotoxicity [228]. It also inhibits and reverses tau hyper-phosphorylation with only mild adverse effects [229]. A combination therapy of memantine with ACHEIs (Namzaric) has been approved for treatment of moderate to severe AD patients [230].

Therapies targeted at other neurotransmitter systems are currently under study. Phase II trials of two compounds: the alpha-7 nicotinic acid agonist, encenicline [231, 232], and the serotonin 5-HT6 antagonist, idalopirdine [233] showed positive results on primary outcome measures (NCT01019421). However, a recent review of results from three Phase III trials of idalopiridine (NCT01955161, NCT02006641, and NCT02006654) suggests no benefit on cognitive function with treatment [234]. Clinical trial of histamine H3 receptor antagonists failed to show consistent benefits [235, 236] (GSK239512, NCT01009255; ABT288, NCT01018875). A Phase II clinical trial of monoamine oxidase (MAO) B inhibitor rasagiline in people with mild to moderate AD is currently ongoing to evaluate its effects on brain metabolism [237] (NCT02359552). Two Phase II clinical trials of ladostigil, a combination of a cholinesterase inhibitor and a MAO B inhibitor, failed to achieve beneficial effects on primary endpoint measures [238–241] (NCT01429623; NCT01354691). However, one trial that targeted delaying MCI conversion to AD, showed a trend towards benefits on selective cognitive tests and brain MRI measure (NCT00000173).

Therapies targeted at synaptic function have also been tested including protein kinase C epsilon (PKCξ) activators, Fyn kinase inhibitors and phosphodiesterase (PDE) inhibitors. Agents activating PKCξ like bryostatin have been tested based on results showing that reduced PKCξ activity is correlated with impaired synaptic and cognitive functions in AD animal models [242]. Moreover, Fyn kinase has been linked to synaptic function and AD pathogenesis. Fyn plays an important role in synaptic plasticity by regulating trafficking of the NMDA glutamate receptor subunits NR2A and NR2B [243–246]. Fyn deficiency mice presented blunted long-term potentiation (LTP) and impaired contextual fear memory function [243, 247]. On the other hand, Fyn has been found to mediate Aβ toxicity through interaction between oligomeric Aβ and the metabotropic glutamate receptor mGluR5 at the post-synaptic plasma membrane [248–250]. Fyn also phosphorylates dendritic tau [249–251]. A preclinical study reported that saracatinib (AZD0530), a Src family kinase inhibitor with high potency for Fyn and Src kinase, rescued synaptic dysfunction and spatial memory impairment in AD transgenic mice [248]. A Phase Ib study of AZD0530 in 24 subjects of mild to moderate AD indicated a reasonable safety and tolerance profile, as well as good BBB penetration [252] (NCT01864655). A Phase II study is currently ongoing in patients of mild AD diagnosis confirmed by amyloid imaging to compare two doses of AZD0530 (100 mg and 125 mg daily for 12 months) versus placebo and the influence of ApoE genotype was taken into consideration during trial design (NCT02167256).

The therapeutic implications of PDE inhibitors as cognitive enhancers in AD have been explored. As key enzymes hydrolyzing secondary messenger cyclic adenosine monophosphate (cAMP) and cyclic guanosine monophosphate (cGMP), PDEs play important roles in regulating signaling pathways critical in brain function. The major challenges of developing PDE inhibitors for AD therapy are narrow dose-response ranges and selection of isoform specific inhibitors. Out of 11 family members, inhibitors targeted at PDE3, 4, 5 and 9 have been tested in clinical trials for AD [253, 254]. Several clinical trial studies of a PDE3 inhibitor cilostazol demonstrated beneficial effects on cognitive function in MCI and AD patients [255–257] (NCT02491268). An ongoing Phase IV trial is studying the effects of cilostazol on subcortical white matter hyperintensities in AD subjects (NCT01409564). For inhibitors of PDE4: HT-0712 (NCT02013310), roflumilast (NCT02051335; NCT0 1433666; ISRCTN96013814), and BPN 14770 (NCT0 2648672; NCT02840279), and inhibitors of PDE9: BI 409306 (NCT01343706; NCT02337907) and PF-0044 47943 (NCT00988598), available results are limited to determine their clinical efficacy at this point [253, 254].

Therapies and interventions for AD prevention

Similar to stroke prevention, AD prevention becomes the second major wave of effort in the field of neurology. In the paper, we divide the effort on AD prevention into secondary and primary prevention interventions. The key concept of secondary prevention is to initiate the mechanism-based interventions with the hope to treat underlying pathophysiology in order to prevent cognitive symptoms from ever developing [258]. Different from secondary prevention trials, primary prevention trials seek to decrease modifiable risks for AD [259] with strategies including lifestyle interventions, co-morbidity treatments, supplemental and multi-domain interventions.

Secondary prevention interventions

Since 2011, global collaborative efforts have embarked on secondary prevention trials. The five large trials include: 1) the API Autosomal-Dominant AD (ADAD), 2) API APOE4 Trial, 3) the DIAN-Trials Unit (DIAN-TU), 4) the Anti-Amyloid Treatment in Asymptomatic Alzheimer's Disease (A4) trial, and 5) the TOMMORROW Trial. API,

DIAN, and A4 have already formed an umbrella group called the Collaboration for Alzheimer's Prevention (CAP) to maintain regular dialogue about study design and outcome validation. Four of the five trials above have agreed to continue testing the amyloid hypothesis and are actively working together to make sure that the cognitive outcomes are comparable and meaningful [260]. The questions to be addressed include guidelines for safe monitoring of subjects for ARIA [261], timing of interventions for maximal benefit of prevention [260], and innovative cognitive outcomes for approval of investigational drugs for early AD with post-approval monitoring [262].

Primary prevention interventions

Primary prevention targeted at specific lifestyle interventions often includes management of cardiovascular disease or metabolic risk factors, changes in diet and exercise, cognitive stimulation or training, and social engagement [260].

Hypertension and hyperlipidemia were two major cardiovascular risk factors targeted in AD and dementia prevention. The Systolic Hypertension in Europe (Syst-Eur) trial, also called vascular dementia project, demonstrated a significant benefit for stroke with reduction of systolic blood pressure by at least 20 mmHg to a goal of below 150 mmHg [263]. The intervention was found to reduce the incidence of dementia by 50%, with AD dementia included as a subcategory. It was calculated that out of 1000 persons treated for hypertension for 5 years, 19 cases of dementia could be prevented. A recent study of participants in the Framingham Heart Study indicates that the incidence of dementia has declined over the course of three decades, which paralleled with observed improvement in cardiovascular health over time [264]. On the other hand, hyperlipidemia as a potential risk factor for AD remains controversial. Several trials have carried out to evaluate the effects of statins in AD. Two trials considered to meet inclusion criteria by the Cochrane review were the Heart Protection Study (HPS) trial and the Prospective Study of Pravastatin in the Elderly at Risk (PROSPER) trial [265] (NCT00939822). However, neither of these two studies demonstrated any beneficial effects of statins on AD prevention or cognitive decline [266, 267].

Diabetes has been another focus of AD prevention. The most prominent trial was the multi-site randomized study called the Action to Control Cardiovascular Risk in Diabetes Trial with Memory in Diabetes (ACCORD--MIND) sub-study, which showed that the group underwent intensive glycemic control of hemoglobin A1c less than 6%, had greater total brain volume measured by MRI, but no differences in the cognitive scores compared to the group of standard of care with hemoglobin A1c at the range between 7 and 7.9% [268] (NCT00182910).

On the other hand, the observation of insulin resistance in AD forms the foundation of evaluating effects of insulin and insulin-sensitizing agents [269, 270]. Early pilot studies of insulin treatment in MCI and AD subjects showed beneficial effects on cognitive function [271–273] (NCT00438568). An ongoing Phase II/III clinical trial in amnestic MCI and mild AD subjects (SNIFF: Study of Nasal Insulin to Fight Forgetfulness) will determine the effects of intranasal insulin on cognitive decline, brain volume loss, and changes in CSF biomarkers (NCT01767909). Insulin-sensitizing agents such as metformin [274] and peroxisome proliferator-activated receptor gamma (PPARγ) agonists like pioglitazone [275], have been advanced into clinical trials of AD (NCT02432287; NCT00982202). Future follow up evaluations of clinical efficacy are needed.

Non-pharmacological interventions like diet, exercise, cognitive training, and vitamin supplement have also been studied in AD prevention trials. The most promising diet intervention has been the Mediterranean diet, rich in fruits and vegetables, combined with olive oil and fish. The Three-City (3C) Study suggests that participants who adhered to the Mediterranean diet had a slower rate of decline on the mini-mental status examination (MMSE), but not the other cognitive tests [276]. Studies have also shown that the Mediterranean-DASH Intervention for Neurodegenerative Delay (MIND) diet may reduce the risk of Alzheimer's by up to 50%, and the protective effects persist till later time points even when diet recommendations were not followed rigorously [277, 278]. An ongoing preventive trial targeted at 65 years or older overweight individuals without cognitive impairment but with suboptimal diet habits will determine the effects of the MIND diet on cognitive decline and brain neurodegeneration over a 3-year period (NCT02817074).

There have been many studies investigating the association between physical activity and AD. An inverse association has been implicated despite moderate quality of evidence based on literature review of prospective observational and intervention studies [279]. However, current evidence is insufficient to provide detailed recommendations regarding specific physical exercise linked to AD prevention, e.g. type, frequency, intensity and duration of exercise [279]. Overall, it is indicated that physical activities combined with social and cognitive stimulation or diet modification may be more beneficial at reducing risks of AD [279]. For example, in a recent randomized controlled trial known as Fitness for the Aging Brain Study (FABS), subjects with memory complaints but no dementia, who underwent a 6-month exercise program had modest cognitive improvement at 18 months (0.26 points increase on the ADAS-cog score), whereas the control group declined 1.04 points [280] (ACTRN12605000136606). When combined with the Mediterranean diet, physical activity was associated with a significant reduction of AD incidence. For those with a high score for both healthy diet and physical activity, the hazard ratio for AD was 0.65 [281]. Besides physical activity, the effects of cognitive training have also been evaluated. The most robust study to date is the Advanced Cognitive Training for Independent and Vital Elderly (ACTIVE) trial, which provided the strongest evidence for beneficial effects of cognitive intervention in the prevention of cognitive impairment [282] (NCT00298558).

In the past decade or so, more attention has been brought to the use of supplements such as vitamin E, Gingko biloba and omega-3 fatty acids for AD prevention. Based on a recent systematic review, there is no evidence suggesting any beneficial effects of vitamin E on preventing MCI conversion into AD, or improving cognitive function of MCI or AD patient [283]. However, results from a single study of combined vitamin E and memantine therapy in AD subjects suggest that vitamin E may delay functional decline in these patients by 19% per year over the 4-year time period [284, 285] (NCT00235716).

The clinical studies of *Ginkgo biloba* extract, also known as EGb 761, showed no beneficial effects in AD prevention. The Ginkgo Evaluation of Memory (GEM) study of 3069 cognitively normal subjects aged 75 or older and 482 subjects with MCI showed that *Ginkgo biloba* did not prevent cognitive decline in normal aging or MCI subjects during 6 years of follow up [286, 287] (NCT00010803). Another trial called GuidAge had the same results in a group of 2854 subjects with subjective memory complaints who were given the same *Ginkgo biloba* extract for 5 years [288] (NCT00276510).

Omega-3 fatty acids have a complex association with AD, as noted in a recent systematic review, which found that seven out of the 11 observational studies had positive findings, but none of the four clinical trials had any benefit for prevention or treatment of dementia [289]. An example of a clinical trial that has shown the benefits of omega-3 fatty acids is the Memory Improvement with Docasahexaenoic Acid Study (MIDAS) [290] (NCTO 0278135). Future studies are needed to determine the effects of omega-3 fatty acids in larger clinical trials, and possible multimodal interventions for AD prevention.

Finally, multidomain interventions targeting vascular and lifestyle risk factors as previously described have been tested in AD prevention trials: 1) the Prevention of Dementia by Intensive Vascular Care study (PreDIVA), 2) the Finnish Geriatric Intervention Study to Prevent Cognitive Impairment and Disability (FINGER; NCT01041989) [291], 3) the Multidomain Alzheimer Preventive Trial (MAPT), and 4) the Multimodal Preventive trial for AD (MIND-ADMINI; NCT03249688). These ongoing multi-centered trials emphasize the importance of international collaboration and standardization of study design. They are unique in AD clinical research because these are the first randomized, controlled trials looking into a combination of treatments.

Future directions for AD drug development

As research in AD progresses, knowledge of underlying AD pathogenesis will guide future drug development effort. In the past two decades or so, we have learned that amyloid may not be the only critical step or the only mechanism of action to be targeted in AD. Tau-modifying agents have been developed, as well as many other agents discussed in this article as summarized in Table 2, which open the door for combination therapy like the case in cancer, cardiovascular and infectious disease treatment [260] Table 2.

The importance of utilizing biomarkers to help diagnosis of preclinical AD has been increasingly recognized in the field [292]. AD biomarkers include key proteins that reflect AD pathology such as amyloid and tau, as well as biomarkers of neuronal injury and regional patterns of abnormalities detected by various imaging modalities that provide indirect evidence of disease development and progression [293, 294]. AD clinical trials may incorporate biomarkers, so that in trial design precise timing of interventions can be elucidated, as well as subgroups of patients for intervention be determined and outcome measures be monitored. For example, Tau PET imaging is now emerging on the scene and could help further refine the preclinical stages of AD, as well as serve as an important outcome measure in AD prevention trials. The ultimate goal is to develop an algorithm of utilizing multiple biomarkers to predict the probability of conversion or progression to dementia in at-risk individuals [293].

Recent failures of several AD clinical trials make us realize that when AD progresses to certain point, excessive neurodegeneration becomes irreversible and aberrant neural networks cannot be repaired by simply reducing amyloid burden or oxidative stress. Current effort has been shifted to AD prevention in the early stages of disease [260, 295]. The recent report of beneficial effects on slowing down disease progression by anti-Aβ antibody BAN2401 in prodromal AD subjects suggests the feasibility of initiating disease-modifying treatments as early as possible. Many other preventative measures as discussed in this article, such as neuroprotection, cognitive enhancement and lifestyle modifications, may synergistically contribute to slow the progression of AD, when intervention(s) begins at the early stages of the disease processes [296]. Other major focuses are multi-targeted drug development and drug repositioning in AD [43].

Conclusions

AD is a complex and multifactorial disease for which the mechanisms remain to be fully elucidated. The lack of success in the Aβ-centric single target approach is compelling evidence that the paradigm of AD drug design needs to be shifted. As new insights into AD pathogenesis and progression are gained, developing or repurposing drugs with the capacity to target different aspects of the disease pathogenesis at once become promising in AD therapies. In addition, the development of novel biomarkers and imaging tools in AD has advanced dramatically in the past decade. However, the application of these tools in clinical trial practice is yet to be fully optimized. Finally, we are entering the era of "big data". The concept of precision medicine has been introduced into AD field with the goal to utilize patient-centered approaches focusing on early screening for risks and detection of pathophysiology. Using customized multi-targeted and biomarker-guided strategies, we can achieve both effective and safe preventive therapies, based on the disease characteristics of each individual patient.

Abbreviations

3C Study: The three city study; 7,8-DHF: Flavone 7,8-dihydroxyflavone; A4 Trial: Anti-amyloid treatment in asymptomatic alzheimer's disease trial; ACCORD-MIND: Action to control cardiovascular risk in diabetes trial with memory in diabetes; ACHEI: Cholinesterase inhibitors; ACTIVE: Advanced cognitive training for independent and vital elderly; AD: Alzheimer's disease; ADAD: API autosomal-dominant AD; ADCOMS: Alzheimer's disease composite score; ADCS-ADL: Alzheimer's disease cooperative study – activities of daily living; APECS: Amyloid-b production and effects on cognition study; APH-1: Anterior pharynx defective 1; ApoE: Apolipoprotein E; APP: Amyloid Precursor Protein (APP); ARIA: Amyloid-related imaging abnormalities; ARIA-E: Amyloid-related imaging abnormalities edema; Aβ: Amyloid-beta; BACE-1: b-site APP cleaving enzyme 1; BBB: Blood brain barrier; CAP: Collaboration for Alzheimer's prevention; CBS: Corticobasal syndrome; CDK5: Cyclin dependent kinase 5; CDR-SB: Clinical dementia rating sum of boxes; CNS: Central nervous system; CSF: Cerebrospinal fluid; DIAN-TU: DIAN trials unit; FABS: Fitness for the aging brain study; FAD: Familial Alzheimer's disease; FDG-PET: Flurodeoxyglucose positron emission tomography; FINGER: Finnish geriatric intervention study to prevent cognitive impairment and disability; GEM: Ginkgo evaluation of memory; GI: Gastrointestinal; HPS: Heart protection study; LTD: Long term depression; LTP: Long term potentiation; MAO: Monoamine Oxidase; MAPT: Multidomain alzheimer preventive trial; MCI: Mild cognitive impairment; MIDAS: Memory Improvement with Docasahexaenoic Acid Study; MIND Diet: Mediterranean-DASH intervention for neurodegenerative delay diet; MIND-ADMINI: Multimodal preventative trial for AD; MMSE: Mini mental state examination; MT: Microtubule; NCT: Nicastrin; NFT: Neurofibrillary tangles; NGF: Nerve growth factor; NIC5--15: Pinitol; NMDA: N-methyl-D-aspartate; NSAIDs: Non-steroidal anti-inflammatory drugs; NT: Neurotrophins; PEN-2: Presenilin enhancer 2; PHF: Paired helical filaments; PK: Protein kinase; PP: Protein phosphatase; PPARγ: Proliferator-activated receptor gamma; PreDIVA: Prevention of dementia by intensive vascular care study; PROSPER: Prospective study of pravastatin in the elderly at risk; PS: Presenilin; PSP: Progressive supranuclear palsy; RXR: Retinoid X receptor; SNIFF: Study of nasal insulin to fight forgetfulness; Syst-Eur Trial: Systolic hypertension in europe trial; Tg: Transgenic; Trk: Tropomyosin receptor kinase

Acknowledgements

We thank Margaret Zhong, Larry Zhang, Hannah Escow and Caroline Wang for critical reading of the manuscript.

Funding

DC is supported by NIH R01 (1R01AG048923) and RF1 (1RF1AG054014), by Department of Veteran Affairs BLR&D (1I01BX003380) and RR&D (1I01RX002290), as well as by New York State SCI Foundation. JC is supported by NNSFC (81771162) and RF1 (1RF1AG054014 for DC). PJ is supported by NNSFC (81771162).

Authors' contributions

DC constructed the idea, participated in literature search and interpretation, as well as in manuscript writing. JC participated in literature search and manuscript writing. PJ participated in manuscript writing. All authors read and approved the final manuscript.

Competing interests

The authors declare that they have no competing interests.

Author details

[1]James J Peters VA Medical Center, Research & Development, Bronx, NY 10468, USA. [2]Department of Neurology, Alzheimer Disease Research Center, Icahn School of Medicine at Mount Sinai, New York, NY 10029, USA. [3]The Central Hospital of The Hua Zhong University of Science and Technology, Wuhan, China.

References

1. Alzheimer's Association. 2012 Alzheimer's disease facts and figures. Alzheimers Dement. 2012;8:131–68.
2. Minino AM, Murphy SL, Xu J, Kochanek KD. Deaths: final data for 2008. Natl Vital Stat Rep. 2011;59:1–126.
3. Thies W, Bleiler L. Alzheimer's disease facts and figures. Alzheimers Dement. 2013;2013(9):208–45.
4. Freudenberg-Hua Y, Li W, Davies P. The role of genetics in advancing precision medicine for Alzheimer's disease-a narrative review. Front Med. 2018;5:108.
5. Van Cauwenberghe C, Van Broeckhoven C, Sleegers K. The genetic landscape of Alzheimer disease: clinical implications and perspectives. Genet Med. 2016;18:421–30.
6. Verheijen J, Sleegers K. Understanding Alzheimer disease at the Interface between genetics and transcriptomics. Trends Genet. 2018;34:434–47.
7. Sorbi S. Molecular genetics of Alzheimer's disease. Aging (Milano). 1993;5: 417–25.
8. Scheltens P, Blennow K, Breteler MM, de Strooper B, Frisoni GB, Salloway S, Van der Flier WM. Alzheimer's disease. Lancet. 2016;388:505–17.
9. Bradley WG. Alzheimer's disease: theories of causation. Adv Exp Med Biol. 1990;282:31–8.
10. Armstrong RA. What causes alzheimer's disease? Folia Neuropathol. 2013;51: 169–88.
11. Morris JC. Early-stage and preclinical Alzheimer disease. Alzheimer Dis Assoc Disord. 2005;19:163–5.
12. Kennedy ME, Stamford AW, Chen X, Cox K, Cumming JN, Dockendorf MF, Egan M, Ereshefsky L, Hodgson RA, Hyde LA, et al. The BACE1 inhibitor

verubecestat (MK-8931) reduces CNS beta-amyloid in animal models and in Alzheimer's disease patients. Sci Transl Med. 2016;8:363ra150.
13. May PC, Willis BA, Lowe SL, Dean RA, Monk SA, Cocke PJ, Audia JE, Boggs LN, Borders AR, Brier RA, et al. The potent BACE1 inhibitor LY2886721 elicits robust central Abeta pharmacodynamic responses in mice, dogs, and humans. J Neurosci. 2015;35:1199–210.
14. May PC, Dean RA, Lowe SL, Martenyi F, Sheehan SM, Boggs LN, Monk SA, Mathes BM, Mergott DJ, Watson BM, et al. Robust central reduction of amyloid-beta in humans with an orally available, non-peptidic beta-secretase inhibitor. J Neurosci. 2011;31:16507–16.
15. Hung SY, Fu WM. Drug candidates in clinical trials for Alzheimer's disease. J Biomed Sci. 2017;24:47.
16. Moussa CE. Beta-secretase inhibitors in phase I and phase II clinical trials for Alzheimer's disease. Expert Opin Investig Drugs. 2017;26:1131–6.
17. Hu X, Das B, Hou H, He W, Yan R. BACE1 deletion in the adult mouse reverses preformed amyloid deposition and improves cognitive functions. J Exp Med. 2018;215(3):927–40.
18. De Strooper B, Iwatsubo T, Wolfe MS. Presenilins and gamma-secretase: structure, function, and role in Alzheimer disease. Cold Spring Harb Perspect Med. 2012;2:a006304.
19. Zhang X, Li Y, Xu H, Zhang YW. The gamma-secretase complex: from structure to function. Front Cell Neurosci. 2014;8:427.
20. Barton AJ, Crook BW, Karran EH, Brown F, Dewar D, Mann DM, Pearson RC, Graham DI, Hardy J, Hutton M, et al. Alteration in brain presenilin 1 mRNA expression in early onset familial Alzheimer's disease. Neurodegeneration. 1996;5:213–8.
21. Borchelt DR, Thinakaran G, Eckman CB, Lee MK, Davenport F, Ratovitsky T, Prada CM, Kim G, Seekins S, Yager D, et al. Familial Alzheimer's disease-linked presenilin 1 variants elevate Abeta1-42/1-40 ratio in vitro and in vivo. Neuron. 1996;17:1005–13.
22. De Strooper B, Saftig P, Craessaerts K, Vanderstichele H, Guhde G, Annaert W, Von Figura K, Van Leuven F. Deficiency of presenilin-1 inhibits the normal cleavage of amyloid precursor protein. Nature. 1998;391:387–90.
23. Herreman A, Serneels L, Annaert W, Collen D, Schoonjans L, De Strooper B. Total inactivation of gamma-secretase activity in presenilin-deficient embryonic stem cells. Nat Cell Biol. 2000;2:461–2.
24. Li YM, Lai MT, Xu M, Huang Q, DiMuzio-Mower J, Sardana MK, Shi XP, Yin KC, Shafer JA, Gardell SJ. Presenilin 1 is linked with gamma-secretase activity in the detergent solubilized state. Proc Natl Acad Sci U S A. 2000;97:6138–43.
25. Li YM, Xu M, Lai MT, Huang Q, Castro JL, DiMuzio-Mower J, Harrison T, Lellis C, Nadin A, Neduvelil JG, et al. Photoactivated gamma-secretase inhibitors directed to the active site covalently label presenilin 1. Nature. 2000;405: 689–94.
26. Naruse S, Thinakaran G, Luo JJ, Kusiak JW, Tomita T, Iwatsubo T, Qian X, Ginty DD, Price DL, Borchelt DR, et al. Effects of PS1 deficiency on membrane protein trafficking in neurons. Neuron. 1998;21:1213–21.
27. Scheuner D, Eckman C, Jensen M, Song X, Citron M, Suzuki N, Bird TD, Hardy J, Hutton M, Kukull W, et al. Secreted amyloid beta-protein similar to that in the senile plaques of Alzheimer's disease is increased in vivo by the presenilin 1 and 2 and APP mutations linked to familial Alzheimer's disease. Nat Med. 1996;2:864–70.
28. Zhang Z, Nadeau P, Song W, Donoviel D, Yuan M, Bernstein A, Yankner BA. Presenilins are required for gamma-secretase cleavage of beta-APP and transmembrane cleavage of Notch-1. Nat Cell Biol. 2000;2:463–5.
29. Haapasalo A, Kovacs DM. The many substrates of presenilin/gamma-secretase. J Alzheimers Dis. 2011;25:3–28.
30. Dovey HF, John V, Anderson JP, Chen LZ, de Saint AP, Fang LY, Freedman SB, Folmer B, Goldbach E, Holsztynska EJ, et al. Functional gamma-secretase inhibitors reduce beta-amyloid peptide levels in brain. J Neurochem. 2001; 76:173–81.
31. Lanz TA, Wood KM, Richter KE, Nolan CE, Becker SL, Pozdnyakov N, Martin BA, Du P, Oborski CE, Wood DE, et al. Pharmacodynamics and pharmacokinetics of the gamma-secretase inhibitor PF-3084014. J Pharmacol Exp Ther. 2010;334:269–77.
32. Searfoss GH, Jordan WH, Calligaro DO, Galbreath EJ, Schirtzinger LM, Berridge BR, Gao H, Higgins MA, May PC, Ryan TP. Adipsin, a biomarker of gastrointestinal toxicity mediated by a functional gamma-secretase inhibitor. J Biol Chem. 2003;278:46107–16.
33. Wong GT, Manfra D, Poulet FM, Zhang Q, Josien H, Bara T, Engstrom L, Pinzon-Ortiz M, Fine JS, Lee HJ, et al. Chronic treatment with the gamma-secretase inhibitor LY-411,575 inhibits beta-amyloid peptide production and alters lymphopoiesis and intestinal cell differentiation. J Biol Chem. 2004; 279:12876–82.
34. Albright CF, Dockens RC, Meredith JE Jr, Olson RE, Slemmon R, Lentz KA, Wang JS, Denton RR, Pilcher G, Rhyne PW, et al. Pharmacodynamics of selective inhibition of gamma-secretase by avagacestat. J Pharmacol Exp Ther. 2013;344:686–95.
35. Coric V, van Dyck CH, Salloway S, Andreasen N, Brody M, Richter RW, Soininen H, Thein S, Shiovitz T, Pilcher G, et al. Safety and tolerability of the gamma-secretase inhibitor avagacestat in a phase 2 study of mild to moderate Alzheimer disease. Arch Neurol. 2012;69:1430–40.
36. Doody RS, Aisen PS, Iwatsubo T. Semagacestat for treatment of Alzheimer's disease. N Engl J Med. 2013;369:1661.
37. Doody RS, Raman R, Farlow M, Iwatsubo T, Vellas B, Joffe S, Kieburtz K, He F, Sun X, Thomas RG, et al. A phase 3 trial of semagacestat for treatment of Alzheimer's disease. N Engl J Med. 2013;369:341–50.
38. Netzer WJ, Dou F, Cai D, Veach D, Jean S, Li Y, Bornmann WG, Clarkson B, Xu H, Greengard P. Gleevec inhibits beta-amyloid production but not notch cleavage. Proc Natl Acad Sci U S A. 2003;100:12444–9.
39. Gillman KW, Starrett JE Jr, Parker MF, Xie K, Bronson JJ, Marcin LR, McElhone KE, Bergstrom CP, Mate RA, Williams R, et al. Discovery and evaluation of BMS-708163, a potent, selective and orally bioavailable gamma-secretase inhibitor. ACS Med Chem Lett. 2010;1:120–4.
40. Folch J, Petrov D, Ettcheto M, Abad S, Sanchez-Lopez E, Garcia ML, Olloquequi J, Beas-Zarate C, Auladell C, Camins A. Current research therapeutic strategies for Alzheimer's disease treatment. Neural Plast. 2016; 2016:8501693.
41. Weggen S, Eriksen JL, Das P, Sagi SA, Wang R, Pietrzik CU, Findlay KA, Smith TE, Murphy MP, Bulter T, et al. A subset of NSAIDs lower amyloidogenic Abeta42 independently of cyclooxygenase activity. Nature. 2001;414:212–6.
42. Green RC, Schneider LS, Amato DA, Beelen AP, Wilcock G, Swabb EA, Zavitz KH, Tarenflurbil Phase 3 Study G. Effect of tarenflurbil on cognitive decline and activities of daily living in patients with mild Alzheimer disease: a randomized controlled trial. JAMA. 2009;302:2557–64.
43. Bachurin SO, Bovina EV, Ustyugov AA. Drugs in clinical trials for Alzheimer's disease: the major trends. Med Res Rev. 2017;37:1186–225.
44. Lemere CA. Developing novel immunogens for a safe and effective Alzheimer's disease vaccine. Prog Brain Res. 2009;175:83–93.
45. Pasquier F, Sadowsky C, Holstein A, Leterme Gle P, Peng Y, Jackson N, Fox NC, Ketter N, Liu E, Ryan JM, Team ACCS. Two phase 2 multiple ascending-dose studies of Vanutide Cridificar (ACC-001) and QS-21 adjuvant in mild-to-moderate Alzheimer's disease. J Alzheimers Dis. 2016;51:1131–43.
46. Winblad B, Graf A, Riviere ME, Andreasen N, Ryan JM. Active immunotherapy options for Alzheimer's disease. Alzheimers Res Ther. 2014;6:7.
47. Davtyan H, Bacon A, Petrushina I, Zagorski K, Cribbs DH, Ghochikyan A, Agadjanyan MG. Immunogenicity of DNA- and recombinant protein-based Alzheimer disease epitope vaccines. Hum Vaccin Immunother. 2014;10: 1248–55.
48. Abushouk AI, Elmaraezy A, Aglan A, Salama R, Fouda S, Fouda R, AlSafadi AM. Bapineuzumab for mild to moderate Alzheimer's disease: a meta-analysis of randomized controlled trials. BMC Neurol. 2017;17:66.
49. Laske C. Phase 3 trials of solanezumab and bapineuzumab for Alzheimer's disease. N Engl J Med. 2014;370:1459.
50. Tucker S, Moller C, Tegerstedt K, Lord A, Laudon H, Sjodahl J, Soderberg L, Spens E, Sahlin C, Waara ER, et al. The murine version of BAN2401 (mAb158) selectively reduces amyloid-beta protofibrils in brain and cerebrospinal fluid of tg-ArcSwe mice. J Alzheimers Dis. 2015;43:575–88.
51. Sevigny J, Chiao P, Bussiere T, Weinreb PH, Williams L, Maier M, Dunstan R, Salloway S, Chen T, Ling Y, et al. The antibody aducanumab reduces Abeta plaques in Alzheimer's disease. Nature. 2016;537:50–6.
52. Maccecchini ML, Chang MY, Pan C, John V, Zetterberg H, Greig NH. Posiphen as a candidate drug to lower CSF amyloid precursor protein, amyloid-beta peptide and tau levels: target engagement, tolerability and pharmacokinetics in humans. J Neurol Neurosurg Psychiatry. 2012;83:894–902.
53. Sinha S, Du Z, Maiti P, Klarner FG, Schrader T, Wang C, Bitan G. Comparison of three amyloid assembly inhibitors: the sugar scyllo-inositol, the polyphenol epigallocatechin gallate, and the molecular tweezer CLR01. ACS Chem Neurosci. 2012;3:451–8.
54. Buee L, Bussiere T, Buee-Scherrer V, Delacourte A, Hof PR. Tau protein isoforms, phosphorylation and role in neurodegenerative disorders. Brain Res Brain Res Rev. 2000;33:95–130.

55. Drechsel DN, Hyman AA, Cobb MH, Kirschner MW. Modulation of the dynamic instability of tubulin assembly by the microtubule-associated protein tau. Mol Biol Cell. 1992;3:1141–54.
56. Nelson PT, Alafuzoff I, Bigio EH, Bouras C, Braak H, Cairns NJ, Castellani RJ, Crain BJ, Davies P, Del Tredici K, et al. Correlation of Alzheimer disease neuropathologic changes with cognitive status: a review of the literature. J Neuropathol Exp Neurol. 2012;71:362–81.
57. Fath T, Eidenmuller J, Brandt R. Tau-mediated cytotoxicity in a pseudohyperphosphorylation model of Alzheimer's disease. J Neurosci. 2002;22:9733–41.
58. Leschik J, Welzel A, Weissmann C, Eckert A, Brandt R. Inverse and distinct modulation of tau-dependent neurodegeneration by presenilin 1 and amyloid-beta in cultured cortical neurons: evidence that tau phosphorylation is the limiting factor in amyloid-beta-induced cell death. J Neurochem. 2007;101:1303–15.
59. Shahani N, Subramaniam S, Wolf T, Tackenberg C, Brandt R. Tau aggregation and progressive neuronal degeneration in the absence of changes in spine density and morphology after targeted expression of Alzheimer's disease-relevant tau constructs in organotypic hippocampal slices. J Neurosci. 2006;26:6103–14.
60. Tackenberg C, Brandt R. Divergent pathways mediate spine alterations and cell death induced by amyloid-beta, wild-type tau, and R406W tau. J Neurosci. 2009;29:14439–50.
61. Panza F, Solfrizzi V, Seripa D, Imbimbo BP, Lozupone M, Santamato A, Zecca C, Barulli MR, Bellomo A, Pilotto A, et al. Tau-centric targets and drugs in clinical development for the treatment of Alzheimer's disease. Biomed Res Int. 2016;2016:3245935.
62. Baddeley TC, McCaffrey J, Storey JM, Cheung JK, Melis V, Horsley D, Harrington CR, Wischik CM. Complex disposition of methylthioninium redox forms determines efficacy in tau aggregation inhibitor therapy for Alzheimer's disease. J Pharmacol Exp Ther. 2015;352:110–8.
63. Wischik CM, Staff RT, Wischik DJ, Bentham P, Murray AD, Storey JM, Kook KA, Harrington CR. Tau aggregation inhibitor therapy: an exploratory phase 2 study in mild or moderate Alzheimer's disease. J Alzheimers Dis. 2015;44:705–20.
64. Bakota L, Brandt R. Tau biology and tau-directed therapies for Alzheimer's disease. Drugs. 2016;76:301–13.
65. Pei JJ, Bjorkdahl C, Zhang H, Zhou X, Winblad B. p70 S6 kinase and tau in Alzheimer's disease. J Alzheimers Dis. 2008;14:385–92.
66. Jia Q, Deng Y, Qing H. Potential therapeutic strategies for Alzheimer's disease targeting or beyond beta-amyloid: insights from clinical trials. Biomed Res Int. 2014;2014:837157.
67. Hampel H, Ewers M, Burger K, Annas P, Mortberg A, Bogstedt A, Frolich L, Schroder J, Schonknecht P, Riepe MW, et al. Lithium trial in Alzheimer's disease: a randomized, single-blind, placebo-controlled, multicenter 10-week study. J Clin Psychiatry. 2009;70:922–31.
68. Tariot PN, Aisen PS. Can lithium or valproate untie tangles in Alzheimer's disease? J Clin Psychiatry. 2009;70:919–21.
69. del Ser T, Steinwachs KC, Gertz HJ, Andres MV, Gomez-Carrillo B, Medina M, Vericat JA, Redondo P, Fleet D, Leon T. Treatment of Alzheimer's disease with the GSK-3 inhibitor tideglusib: a pilot study. J Alzheimers Dis. 2013;33: 205–15.
70. Martinez A. Preclinical efficacy on GSK-3 inhibitors: towards a future generation of powerful drugs. Med Res Rev. 2008;28:773–96.
71. Sereno L, Coma M, Rodriguez M, Sanchez-Ferrer P, Sanchez MB, Gich I, Agullo JM, Perez M, Avila J, Guardia-Laguarta C, et al. A novel GSK-3beta inhibitor reduces Alzheimer's pathology and rescues neuronal loss in vivo. Neurobiol Dis. 2009;35:359–67.
72. Natarajan P, Priyadarshini V, Pradhan D, Manne M, Swargam S, Kanipakam H, Bhuma V, Amineni U. E-pharmacophore-based virtual screening to identify GSK-3beta inhibitors. J Recept Signal Transduct Res. 2016;36:445–58.
73. Tell V, Hilgeroth A. Recent developments of protein kinase inhibitors as potential AD therapeutics. Front Cell Neurosci. 2013;7:189.
74. Mushtaq G, Greig NH, Anwar F, Al-Abbasi FA, Zamzami MA, Al-Talhi HA, Kamal MA. Neuroprotective mechanisms mediated by CDK5 inhibition. Curr Pharm Des. 2016;22:527–34.
75. Wen Y, Yu WH, Maloney B, Bailey J, Ma J, Marie I, Maurin T, Wang L, Figueroa H, Herman M, et al. Transcriptional regulation of beta-secretase by p25/cdk5 leads to enhanced amyloidogenic processing. Neuron. 2008;57:680–90.
76. Min SW, Chen X, Tracy TE, Li Y, Zhou Y, Wang C, Shirakawa K, Minami SS, Defensor E, Mok SA, et al. Critical role of acetylation in tau-mediated neurodegeneration and cognitive deficits. Nat Med. 2015;21:1154–62.
77. Sohn PD, Tracy TE, Son HI, Zhou Y, Leite RE, Miller BL, Seeley WW, Grinberg LT, Gan L. Acetylated tau destabilizes the cytoskeleton in the axon initial segment and is mislocalized to the somatodendritic compartment. Mol Neurodegener. 2016;11:47.
78. Tracy TE, Sohn PD, Minami SS, Wang C, Min SW, Li Y, Zhou Y, Le D, Lo I, Ponnusamy R, et al. Acetylated tau obstructs KIBRA-mediated signaling in synaptic plasticity and promotes Tauopathy-related memory loss. Neuron. 2016;90:245–60.
79. Trzeciakiewicz H, Tseng JH, Wander CM, Madden V, Tripathy A, Yuan CX, Cohen TJ. A dual pathogenic mechanism links tau acetylation to sporadic Tauopathy. Sci Rep. 2017;7:44102.
80. Min SW, Sohn PD, Li Y, Devidze N, Johnson JR, Krogan NJ, Masliah E, Mok SA, Gestwicki JE, Gan L. SIRT1 deacetylates tau and reduces pathogenic tau spread in a mouse model of Tauopathy. J Neurosci. 2018;38:3680–8.
81. Albayram O, Kondo A, Mannix R, Smith C, Tsai CY, Li C, Herbert MK, Qiu J, Monuteaux M, Driver J, et al. Cis P-tau is induced in clinical and preclinical brain injury and contributes to post-injury sequelae. Nat Commun. 2017;8:1000.
82. Kondo A, Shahpasand K, Mannix R, Qiu J, Moncaster J, Chen CH, Yao Y, Lin YM, Driver JA, Sun Y, et al. Antibody against early driver of neurodegeneration cis P-tau blocks brain injury and tauopathy. Nature. 2015;523:431–6.
83. Lu KP, Kondo A, Albayram O, Herbert MK, Liu H, Zhou XZ. Potential of the antibody against cis-phosphorylated tau in the early diagnosis, treatment, and prevention of Alzheimer disease and brain injury. JAMA Neurol. 2016; 73:1356–62.
84. Hart GW, Slawson C, Ramirez-Correa G, Lagerlof O. Cross talk between O-GlcNAcylation and phosphorylation: roles in signaling, transcription, and chronic disease. Annu Rev Biochem. 2011;80:825–58.
85. Liu F, Shi J, Tanimukai H, Gu J, Gu J, Grundke-Iqbal I, Iqbal K, Gong CX. Reduced O-GlcNAcylation links lower brain glucose metabolism and tau pathology in Alzheimer's disease. Brain. 2009;132:1820–32.
86. Flight MH. Neurodegenerative disease: tau immunotherapy targets transcellular propagation. Nat Rev Drug Discov. 2013;12:904.
87. Goedert M, Eisenberg DS, Crowther RA. Propagation of tau aggregates and neurodegeneration. Annu Rev Neurosci. 2017;40:189–210.
88. Goedert M, Spillantini MG. Propagation of tau aggregates. Mol Brain. 2017; 10:18.
89. Kfoury N, Holmes BB, Jiang H, Holtzman DM, Diamond MI. Trans-cellular propagation of tau aggregation by fibrillar species. J Biol Chem. 2012;287: 19440–51.
90. Yanamandra K, Kfoury N, Jiang H, Mahan TE, Ma S, Maloney SE, Wozniak DF, Diamond MI, Holtzman DM. Anti-tau antibodies that block tau aggregate seeding in vitro markedly decrease pathology and improve cognition in vivo. Neuron. 2013;80:402–14.
91. Yanamandra K, Jiang H, Mahan TE, Maloney SE, Wozniak DF, Diamond MI, Holtzman DM. Anti-tau antibody reduces insoluble tau and decreases brain atrophy. Ann Clin Transl Neurol. 2015;2:278–88.
92. Chukwu JE, Pedersen JT, Pedersen LO, Volbracht C, Sigurdsson EM, Kong XP. Tau antibody structure reveals a molecular switch defining a pathological conformation of the tau protein. Sci Rep. 2018;8:6209.
93. Rajamohamedsait H, Rasool S, Rajamohamedsait W, Lin Y, Sigurdsson EM. Prophylactic active tau immunization leads to sustained reduction in both tau and amyloid-beta pathologies in 3xTg mice. Sci Rep. 2017;7:17034.
94. Gruninger F. Invited review: drug development for tauopathies. Neuropathol Appl Neurobiol. 2015;41:81–96.
95. Dai CL, Chen X, Kazim SF, Liu F, Gong CX, Grundke-Iqbal I, Iqbal K. Passive immunization targeting the N-terminal projection domain of tau decreases tau pathology and improves cognition in a transgenic mouse model of Alzheimer disease and tauopathies. J Neural Transm. 2015;122:607–17.
96. Dai CL, Hu W, Tung YC, Liu F, Gong CX, Iqbal K. Tau passive immunization blocks seeding and spread of Alzheimer hyperphosphorylated tau-induced pathology in 3 × Tg-AD mice. Alzheimers Res Ther. 2018;10:13.
97. Dai CL, Tung YC, Liu F, Gong CX, Iqbal K. Tau passive immunization inhibits not only tau but also Abeta pathology. Alzheimers Res Ther. 2017;9:1.
98. Malia TJ, Teplyakov A, Ernst R, Wu SJ, Lacy ER, Liu X, Vandermeeren M, Mercken M, Luo J, Sweet RW, Gilliland GL. Epitope mapping and structural basis for the recognition of phosphorylated tau by the anti-tau antibody AT8. Proteins. 2016;84:427–34.
99. Mayeux R. Epidemiology of neurodegeneration. Annu Rev Neurosci. 2003; 26:81–104.

100. Castellano JM, Kim J, Stewart FR, Jiang H, DeMattos RB, Patterson BW, Fagan AM, Morris JC, Mawuenyega KG, Cruchaga C, et al. Human apoE isoforms differentially regulate brain amyloid-beta peptide clearance. Sci Transl Med. 2011;3:89ra57.
101. Cataldo AM, Peterhoff CM, Troncoso JC, Gomez-Isla T, Hyman BT, Nixon RA. Endocytic pathway abnormalities precede amyloid beta deposition in sporadic Alzheimer's disease and Down syndrome: differential effects of APOE genotype and presenilin mutations. Am J Pathol. 2000;157:277–86.
102. Li J, Kanekiyo T, Shinohara M, Zhang Y, LaDu MJ, Xu H, Bu G. Differential regulation of amyloid-beta endocytic trafficking and lysosomal degradation by apolipoprotein E isoforms. J Biol Chem. 2012;287:44593–601.
103. Holtzman DM, Herz J, Bu G. Apolipoprotein E and apolipoprotein E receptors: normal biology and roles in Alzheimer disease. Cold Spring Harb Perspect Med. 2012;2:a006312.
104. Liu CC, Kanekiyo T, Xu H, Bu G. Apolipoprotein E and Alzheimer disease: risk, mechanisms and therapy. Nat Rev Neurol. 2013;9:106–18.
105. Kuszczyk MA, Sanchez S, Pankiewicz J, Kim J, Duszczyk M, Guridi M, Asuni AA, Sullivan PM, Holtzman DM, Sadowski MJ. Blocking the interaction between apolipoprotein E and Abeta reduces intraneuronal accumulation of Abeta and inhibits synaptic degeneration. Am J Pathol. 2013;182:1750–68.
106. Liu Q, Wu WH, Fang CL, Li RW, Liu P, Lei P, Hu J, Sun X, Zheng YZ, Zhao YF, Li YM. Mapping ApoE/Abeta binding regions to guide inhibitor discovery. Mol BioSyst. 2011;7:1693–700.
107. Sadowski MJ, Pankiewicz J, Scholtzova H, Mehta PD, Prelli F, Quartermain D, Wisniewski T. Blocking the apolipoprotein E/amyloid-beta interaction as a potential therapeutic approach for Alzheimer's disease. Proc Natl Acad Sci U S A. 2006;103:18787–92.
108. Yang J, Ji Y, Mehta P, Bates KA, Sun Y, Wisniewski T. Blocking the apolipoprotein E/amyloid-beta interaction reduces fibrillar vascular amyloid deposition and cerebral microhemorrhages in TgSwDI mice. J Alzheimers Dis. 2011;24:269–85.
109. Cramer PE, Cirrito JR, Wesson DW, Lee CY, Karlo JC, Zinn AE, Casali BT, Restivo JL, Goebel WD, James MJ, et al. ApoE-directed therapeutics rapidly clear beta-amyloid and reverse deficits in AD mouse models. Science. 2012; 335:1503–6.
110. Kim J, Castellano JM, Jiang H, Basak JM, Parsadanian M, Pham V, Mason SM, Paul SM, Holtzman DM. Overexpression of low-density lipoprotein receptor in the brain markedly inhibits amyloid deposition and increases extracellular a beta clearance. Neuron. 2009;64:632–44.
111. Dodart JC, Marr RA, Koistinaho M, Gregersen BM, Malkani S, Verma IM, Paul SM. Gene delivery of human apolipoprotein E alters brain Abeta burden in a mouse model of Alzheimer's disease. Proc Natl Acad Sci U S A. 2005;102: 1211–6.
112. Hudry E, Dashkoff J, Roe AD, Takeda S, Koffie RM, Hashimoto T, Scheel M, Spires-Jones T, Arbel-Ornath M, Betensky R, et al. Gene transfer of human Apoe isoforms results in differential modulation of amyloid deposition and neurotoxicity in mouse brain. Sci Transl Med. 2013;5:212ra161.
113. Kim J, Eltorai AE, Jiang H, Liao F, Verghese PB, Kim J, Stewart FR, Basak JM, Holtzman DM. Anti-apoE immunotherapy inhibits amyloid accumulation in a transgenic mouse model of Abeta amyloidosis. J Exp Med. 2012;209:2149–56.
114. Liao F, Hori Y, Hudry E, Bauer AQ, Jiang H, Mahan TE, Lefton KB, Zhang TJ, Dearborn JT, Kim J, et al. Anti-ApoE antibody given after plaque onset decreases Abeta accumulation and improves brain function in a mouse model of Abeta amyloidosis. J Neurosci. 2014;34:7281–92.
115. Brodbeck J, McGuire J, Liu Z, Meyer-Franke A, Balestra ME, Jeong DE, Pleiss M, McComas C, Hess F, Witter D, et al. Structure-dependent impairment of intracellular apolipoprotein E4 trafficking and its detrimental effects are rescued by small-molecule structure correctors. J Biol Chem. 2011;286: 17217–26.
116. Chen HK, Liu Z, Meyer-Franke A, Brodbeck J, Miranda RD, McGuire JG, Pleiss MA, Ji ZS, Balestra ME, Walker DW, et al. Small molecule structure correctors abolish detrimental effects of apolipoprotein E4 in cultured neurons. J Biol Chem. 2012;287:5253–66.
117. Wang C, Najm R, Xu Q, Jeong DE, Walker D, Balestra ME, Yoon SY, Yuan H, Li G, Miller ZA, et al. Gain of toxic apolipoprotein E4 effects in human iPSC-derived neurons is ameliorated by a small-molecule structure corrector. Nat Med. 2018;24:647–57.
118. Donkin JJ, Stukas S, Hirsch-Reinshagen V, Namjoshi D, Wilkinson A, May S, Chan J, Fan J, Collins J, Wellington CL. ATP-binding cassette transporter A1 mediates the beneficial effects of the liver X receptor agonist GW3965 on object recognition memory and amyloid burden in amyloid precursor protein/presenilin 1 mice. J Biol Chem. 2010;285:34144–54.
119. Fitz NF, Cronican A, Pham T, Fogg A, Fauq AH, Chapman R, Lefterov I, Koldamova R. Liver X receptor agonist treatment ameliorates amyloid pathology and memory deficits caused by high-fat diet in APP23 mice. J Neurosci. 2010;30:6862–72.
120. Koldamova RP, Lefterov IM, Staufenbiel M, Wolfe D, Huang S, Glorioso JC, Walter M, Roth MG, Lazo JS. The liver X receptor ligand T0901317 decreases amyloid beta production in vitro and in a mouse model of Alzheimer's disease. J Biol Chem. 2005;280:4079–88.
121. Riddell DR, Zhou H, Comery TA, Kouranova E, Lo CF, Warwick HK, Ring RH, Kirksey Y, Aschmies S, Xu J, et al. The LXR agonist TO901317 selectively lowers hippocampal Abeta42 and improves memory in the Tg2576 mouse model of Alzheimer's disease. Mol Cell Neurosci. 2007;34:621–8.
122. Laskowitz DT, Lei B, Dawson HN, Wang H, Bellows ST, Christensen DJ, Vitek MP, James ML. The apoE-mimetic peptide, COG1410, improves functional recovery in a murine model of intracerebral hemorrhage. Neurocrit Care. 2012;16:316–26.
123. Laskowitz DT, McKenna SE, Song P, Wang H, Durham L, Yeung N, Christensen D, Vitek MP. COG1410, a novel apolipoprotein E-based peptide, improves functional recovery in a murine model of traumatic brain injury. J Neurotrauma. 2007;24:1093–107.
124. Vitek MP, Christensen DJ, Wilcock D, Davis J, Van Nostrand WE, Li FQ, Colton CA. APOE-mimetic peptides reduce behavioral deficits, plaques and tangles in Alzheimer's disease transgenics. Neurodegener Dis. 2012;10:122–6.
125. Wang H, Durham L, Dawson H, Song P, Warner DS, Sullivan PM, Vitek MP, Laskowitz DT. An apolipoprotein E-based therapeutic improves outcome and reduces Alzheimer's disease pathology following closed head injury: evidence of pharmacogenomic interaction. Neuroscience. 2007;144:1324–33.
126. Liu S, Breitbart A, Sun Y, Mehta PD, Boutajangout A, Scholtzova H, Wisniewski T. Blocking the apolipoprotein E/amyloid beta interaction in triple transgenic mice ameliorates Alzheimer's disease related amyloid beta and tau pathology. J Neurochem. 2014;128:577–91.
127. Mak AC, Pullinger CR, Tang LF, Wong JS, Deo RC, Schwarz JM, Gugliucci A, Movsesyan I, Ishida BY, Chu C, et al. Effects of the absence of apolipoprotein e on lipoproteins, neurocognitive function, and retinal function. JAMA Neurol. 2014;71:1228–36.
128. Heywood WE, Galimberti D, Bliss E, Sirka E, Paterson RW, Magdalinou NK, Carecchio M, Reid E, Heslegrave A, Fenoglio C, et al. Identification of novel CSF biomarkers for neurodegeneration and their validation by a high-throughput multiplexed targeted proteomic assay. Mol Neurodegener. 2015;10:64.
129. Martinez-Morillo E, Hansson O, Atagi Y, Bu G, Minthon L, Diamandis EP, Nielsen HM. Total apolipoprotein E levels and specific isoform composition in cerebrospinal fluid and plasma from Alzheimer's disease patients and controls. Acta Neuropathol. 2014;127:633–43.
130. Simon R, Girod M, Fonbonne C, Salvador A, Clement Y, Lanteri P, Amouyel P, Lambert JC, Lemoine J. Total ApoE and ApoE4 isoform assays in an Alzheimer's disease case-control study by targeted mass spectrometry (n= 669): a pilot assay for methionine-containing proteotypic peptides. Mol Cell Proteomics. 2012;11:1389–403.
131. Talwar P, Sinha J, Grover S, Agarwal R, Kushwaha S, Srivastava MV, Kukreti R. Meta-analysis of apolipoprotein E levels in the cerebrospinal fluid of patients with Alzheimer's disease. J Neurol Sci. 2016;360:179–87.
132. Boehm-Cagan A, Michaelson DM. Reversal of apoE4-driven brain pathology and behavioral deficits by bexarotene. J Neurosci. 2014;34:7293–301.
133. Burns MP, Vardanian L, Pajoohesh-Ganji A, Wang L, Cooper M, Harris DC, Duff K, Rebeck GW. The effects of ABCA1 on cholesterol efflux and Abeta levels in vitro and in vivo. J Neurochem. 2006;98:792–800.
134. Casali BT, Corona AW, Mariani MM, Karlo JC, Ghosal K, Landreth GE. Omega-3 fatty acids augment the actions of nuclear receptor agonists in a mouse model of Alzheimer's disease. J Neurosci. 2015;35:9173–81.
135. Escribano L, Simon AM, Gimeno E, Cuadrado-Tejedor M, Lopez de Maturana R, Garcia-Osta A, Ricobaraza A, Perez-Mediavilla A, Del Rio J, Frechilla D. Rosiglitazone rescues memory impairment in Alzheimer's transgenic mice: mechanisms involving a reduced amyloid and tau pathology. Neuropsychopharmacology. 2010;35:1593–604.
136. Jiang Q, Lee CY, Mandrekar S, Wilkinson B, Cramer P, Zelcer N, Mann K, Lamb B, Willson TM, Collins JL, et al. ApoE promotes the proteolytic degradation of Abeta. Neuron. 2008;58:681–93.
137. LaClair KD, Manaye KF, Lee DL, Allard JS, Savonenko AV, Troncoso JC, Wong PC. Treatment with bexarotene, a compound that increases apolipoprotein-

E, provides no cognitive benefit in mutant APP/PS1 mice. Mol Neurodegener. 2013;8:18.
138. Skerrett R, Pellegrino MP, Casali BT, Taraboanta L, Landreth GE. Combined liver X receptor/peroxisome proliferator-activated receptor gamma agonist treatment reduces amyloid beta levels and improves behavior in amyloid precursor protein/Presenilin 1 mice. J Biol Chem. 2015;290:21591–602.
139. Tachibana M, Shinohara M, Yamazaki Y, Liu CC, Rogers J, Bu G, Kanekiyo T. Rescuing effects of RXR agonist bexarotene on aging-related synapse loss depend on neuronal LRP1. Exp Neurol. 2016;277:1–9.
140. Tai LM, Koster KP, Luo J, Lee SH, Wang YT, Collins NC, Ben Aissa M, Thatcher GR, LaDu MJ. Amyloid-beta pathology and APOE genotype modulate retinoid X receptor agonist activity in vivo. J Biol Chem. 2014;289:30538–55.
141. Vanmierlo T, Rutten K, Dederen J, Bloks VW, van Vark-van der Zee LC, Kuipers F, Kiliaan A, Blokland A, Sijbrands EJ, Steinbusch H, et al. Liver X receptor activation restores memory in aged AD mice without reducing amyloid. Neurobiol Aging. 2011;32:1262–72.
142. Cummings JL, Zhong K, Kinney JW, Heaney C, Moll-Tudla J, Joshi A, Pontecorvo M, Devous M, Tang A, Bena J. Double-blind, placebo-controlled, proof-of-concept trial of bexarotene Xin moderate Alzheimer's disease. Alzheimers Res Ther. 2016;8:4.
143. Hu J, Liu CC, Chen XF, Zhang YW, Xu H, Bu G. Opposing effects of viral mediated brain expression of apolipoprotein E2 (apoE2) and apoE4 on apoE lipidation and Abeta metabolism in apoE4-targeted replacement mice. Mol Neurodegener. 2015;10:6.
144. Yamazaki Y, Painter MM, Bu G, Kanekiyo T. Apolipoprotein E as a therapeutic target in Alzheimer's disease: a review of basic research and clinical evidence. CNS Drugs. 2016;30:773–89.
145. Zhong N, Scearce-Levie K, Ramaswamy G, Weisgraber KH. Apolipoprotein E4 domain interaction: synaptic and cognitive deficits in mice. Alzheimers Dement. 2008;4:179–92.
146. Zhong N, Weisgraber KH. Understanding the association of apolipoprotein E4 with Alzheimer disease: clues from its structure. J Biol Chem. 2009;284: 6027–31.
147. Kanekiyo T, Xu H, Bu G. ApoE and Abeta in Alzheimer's disease: accidental encounters or partners? Neuron. 2014;81:740–54.
148. Hanson AJ, Bayer-Carter JL, Green PS, Montine TJ, Wilkinson CW, Baker LD, Watson GS, Bonner LM, Callaghan M, Leverenz JB, et al. Effect of apolipoprotein E genotype and diet on apolipoprotein E lipidation and amyloid peptides: randomized clinical trial. JAMA Neurol. 2013;70:972–80.
149. Tai LM, Bilousova T, Jungbauer L, Roeske SK, Youmans KL, Yu C, Poon WW, Cornwell LB, Miller CA, Vinters HV, et al. Levels of soluble apolipoprotein E/ amyloid-beta (Abeta) complex are reduced and oligomeric Abeta increased with APOE4 and Alzheimer disease in a transgenic mouse model and human samples. J Biol Chem. 2013;288:5914–26.
150. Youmans KL, Tai LM, Nwabuisi-Heath E, Jungbauer L, Kanekiyo T, Gan M, Kim J, Eimer WA, Estus S, Rebeck GW, et al. APOE4-specific changes in Abeta accumulation in a new transgenic mouse model of Alzheimer disease. J Biol Chem. 2012;287:41774–86.
151. Tai LM, Mehra S, Shete V, Estus S, Rebeck GW, Bu G, LaDu MJ. Soluble apoE/ Abeta complex: mechanism and therapeutic target for APOE4-induced AD risk. Mol Neurodegener. 2014;9:2.
152. Vance JE, Hayashi H. Formation and function of apolipoprotein E-containing lipoproteins in the nervous system. Biochim Biophys Acta. 1801;2010:806–18.
153. Zhu L, Zhong M, Elder GA, Sano M, Holtzman DM, Gandy S, Cardozo C, Haroutunian V, Robakis NK, Cai D. Phospholipid dysregulation contributes to ApoE4-associated cognitive deficits in Alzheimer's disease pathogenesis. Proc Natl Acad Sci U S A. 2015;112:11965–70.
154. Hanson AJ, Craft S, Banks WA. The APOE genotype: modification of therapeutic responses in Alzheimer's disease. Curr Pharm Des. 2015;21: 114–20.
155. Salloway S, Sperling R, Fox NC, Blennow K, Klunk W, Raskind M, Sabbagh M, Honig LS, Porsteinsson AP, Ferris S, et al. Two phase 3 trials of bapineuzumab in mild-to-moderate Alzheimer's disease. N Engl J Med. 2014;370:322–33.
156. Szekely CA, Breitner JC, Fitzpatrick AL, Rea TD, Psaty BM, Kuller LH, Zandi PP. NSAID use and dementia risk in the cardiovascular health study: role of APOE and NSAID type. Neurology. 2008;70:17–24.
157. Altmann A, Tian L, Henderson VW, Greicius MD, Alzheimer's Disease Neuroimaging Initiative I. Sex modifies the APOE-related risk of developing Alzheimer disease. Ann Neurol. 2014;75:563–73.
158. Farrer LA, Cupples LA, Haines JL, Hyman B, Kukull WA, Mayeux R, Myers RH, Pericak-Vance MA, Risch N, van Duijn CM. Effects of age, sex, and ethnicity on the association between apolipoprotein E genotype and Alzheimer disease. A meta-analysis. APOE and Alzheimer disease Meta analysis consortium. JAMA. 1997;278:1349–56.
159. Nyarko JNK, Quartey MO, Pennington PR, Heistad RM, Dea D, Poirier J, Baker GB, Mousseau DD. Profiles of beta-amyloid peptides and key secretases in brain autopsy samples differ with sex and APOE epsilon4 status: impact for risk and progression of Alzheimer disease. Neuroscience. 2018;373:20–36.
160. Abram M, Wegmann M, Fokuhl V, Sonar S, Luger EO, Kerzel S, Radbruch A, Renz H, Zemlin M. Nerve growth factor and neurotrophin-3 mediate survival of pulmonary plasma cells during the allergic airway inflammation. J Immunol. 2009;182:4705–12.
161. Bergmann I, Reiter R, Toyka KV, Koltzenburg M. Nerve growth factor evokes hyperalgesia in mice lacking the low-affinity neurotrophin receptor p75. Neurosci Lett. 1998;255:87–90.
162. Dyck PJ, Peroutka S, Rask C, Burton E, Baker MK, Lehman KA, Gillen DA, Hokanson JL, O'Brien PC. Intradermal recombinant human nerve growth factor induces pressure allodynia and lowered heat-pain threshold in humans. Neurology. 1997;48:501–5.
163. Malcangio M, Lessmann V. A common thread for pain and memory synapses? Brain-derived neurotrophic factor and trkB receptors. Trends Pharmacol Sci. 2003;24:116–21.
164. Pezet S, Malcangio M, McMahon SB. BDNF: a neuromodulator in nociceptive pathways? Brain Res Brain Res Rev. 2002;40:240–9.
165. Sah DW, Ossipo MH, Porreca F. Neurotrophic factors as novel therapeutics for neuropathic pain. Nat Rev Drug Discov. 2003;2:460–72.
166. Shu XQ, Mendell LM. Neurotrophins and hyperalgesia. Proc Natl Acad Sci U S A. 1999;96:7693–6.
167. Pardridge WM. Neurotrophins, neuroprotection and the blood-brain barrier. Curr Opin Investig Drugs. 2002;3:1753–7.
168. Poduslo JF, Curran GL. Permeability at the blood-brain and blood-nerve barriers of the neurotrophic factors: NGF, CNTF, NT-3, BDNF. Brain Res Mol Brain Res. 1996;36:280–6.
169. Saltzman WM, Mak MW, Mahoney MJ, Duenas ET, Cleland JL. Intracranial delivery of recombinant nerve growth factor: release kinetics and protein distribution for three delivery systems. Pharm Res. 1999;16:232–40.
170. Tuszynski MH, Thal L, Pay M, Salmon DP, U HS, Bakay R, Patel P, Blesch A, Vahlsing HL, Ho G, et al. A phase 1 clinical trial of nerve growth factor gene therapy for Alzheimer disease. Nat Med. 2005;11:551–5.
171. Rafii MS, Baumann TL, Bakay RA, Ostrove JM, Siffert J, Fleisher AS, Herzog CD, Barba D, Pay M, Salmon DP, et al. A phase1 study of stereotactic gene delivery of AAV2-NGF for Alzheimer's disease. Alzheimers Dement. 2014;10:571–81.
172. Tuszynski MH, Yang JH, Barba D, U HS, Bakay RA, Pay MM, Masliah E, Conner JM, Kobalka P, Roy S, Nagahara AH. Nerve growth factor gene therapy: activation of neuronal responses in Alzheimer disease. JAMA Neurol. 2015; 72:1139–47.
173. Rafii MS, Tuszynski MH, Thomas RG, Barba D, Brewer JB, Rissman RA, Siffert J, Aisen PS, Team ANS. Adeno-associated viral vector (serotype 2)-nerve growth factor for patients with Alzheimer disease: a randomized clinical trial. JAMA Neurol. 2018;75(7):834–41.
174. Longo FM, Massa SM. Small-molecule modulation of neurotrophin receptors: a strategy for the treatment of neurological disease. Nat Rev Drug Discov. 2013;12:507–25.
175. Massa SM, Xie Y, Yang T, Harrington AW, Kim ML, Yoon SO, Kraemer R, Moore LA, Hempstead BL, Longo FM. Small, nonpeptide p75NTR ligands induce survival signaling and inhibit proNGF-induced death. J Neurosci. 2006;26:5288–300.
176. Tep C, Lim TH, Ko PO, Getahun S, Ryu JC, Goettl VM, Massa SM, Basso M, Longo FM, Yoon SO. Oral administration of a small molecule targeted to block proNGF binding to p75 promotes myelin sparing and functional recovery after spinal cord injury. J Neurosci. 2013;33:397–410.
177. Knowles JK, Simmons DA, Nguyen TV, Vander Griend L, Xie Y, Zhang H, Yang T, Pollak J, Chang T, Arancio O, et al. Small molecule p75NTR ligand prevents cognitive deficits and neurite degeneration in an Alzheimer's mouse model. Neurobiol Aging. 2013;34:2052–63.
178. Nguyen TV, Shen L, Vander Griend L, Quach LN, Belichenko NP, Saw N, Yang T, Shamloo M, Wyss-Coray T, Massa SM, Longo FM. Small molecule p75NTR ligands reduce pathological phosphorylation and misfolding of tau, inflammatory changes, cholinergic degeneration, and cognitive deficits in AbetaPP(L/S) transgenic mice. J Alzheimers Dis. 2014;42:459–83.

179. Simmons DA, Knowles JK, Belichenko NP, Banerjee G, Finkle C, Massa SM, Longo FM. A small molecule p75NTR ligand, LM11A-31, reverses cholinergic neurite dystrophy in Alzheimer's disease mouse models with mid- to late-stage disease progression. PLoS One. 2014;9:e102136.
180. Aboulkassim T, Tong XK, Tse YC, Wong TP, Woo SB, Neet KE, Brahimi F, Hamel E, Saragovi HU. Ligand-dependent TrkA activity in brain differentially affects spatial learning and long-term memory. Mol Pharmacol. 2011;80: 498–508.
181. Scarpi D, Cirelli D, Matrone C, Castronovo G, Rosini P, Occhiato EG, Romano F, Bartali L, Clemente AM, Bottegoni G, et al. Low molecular weight, non-peptidic agonists of TrkA receptor with NGF-mimetic activity. Cell Death Dis. 2012;3:e389.
182. Wang J, Hancock MK, Dudek JM, Bi K. Cellular assays for high-throughput screening for modulators of Trk receptor tyrosine kinases. Curr Chem Genomics. 2008;1:27–33.
183. Zhang Q, Descamps O, Hart MJ, Poksay KS, Spilman P, Kane DJ, Gorostiza O, John V, Bredesen DE. Paradoxical effect of TrkA inhibition in Alzheimer's disease models. J Alzheimers Dis. 2014;40:605–17.
184. Schmid DA, Yang T, Ogier M, Adams I, Mirakhur Y, Wang Q, Massa SM, Longo FM, Katz DM. A TrkB small molecule partial agonist rescues TrkB phosphorylation deficits and improves respiratory function in a mouse model of Rett syndrome. J Neurosci. 2012;32:1803–10.
185. Simmons DA, Belichenko NP, Yang T, Condon C, Monbureau M, Shamloo M, Jing D, Massa SM, Longo FM. A small molecule TrkB ligand reduces motor impairment and neuropathology in R6/2 and BACHD mouse models of Huntington's disease. J Neurosci. 2013;33:18712–27.
186. Devi L, Ohno M. 7,8-dihydroxyflavone, a small-molecule TrkB agonist, reverses memory deficits and BACE1 elevation in a mouse model of Alzheimer's disease. Neuropsychopharmacology. 2012;37:434–44.
187. Jang SW, Liu X, Yepes M, Shepherd KR, Miller GW, Liu Y, Wilson WD, Xiao G, Blanchi B, Sun YE, Ye K. A selective TrkB agonist with potent neurotrophic activities by 7,8-dihydroxyflavone. Proc Natl Acad Sci U S A. 2010;107:2687–92.
188. Zhang Z, Liu X, Schroeder JP, Chan CB, Song M, Yu SP, Weinshenker D, Ye K. 7,8-dihydroxyflavone prevents synaptic loss and memory deficits in a mouse model of Alzheimer's disease. Neuropsychopharmacology. 2014;39: 638–50.
189. Zhou W, Li X, Huang D, Zhou W, Li T, Song W. No significant effect of 7,8-dihydroxyflavone on APP processing and Alzheimer-associated phenotypes. Curr Alzheimer Res. 2015;12:47–52.
190. Volinsky N, Kholodenko BN. Complexity of receptor tyrosine kinase signal processing. Cold Spring Harb Perspect Biol. 2013;5:a009043.
191. Heneka MT, Kummer MP, Latz E. Innate immune activation in neurodegenerative disease. Nat Rev Immunol. 2014;14:463–77.
192. Perry VH, Holmes C. Microglial priming in neurodegenerative disease. Nat Rev Neurol. 2014;10:217–24.
193. Prokop S, Miller KR, Heppner FL. Microglia actions in Alzheimer's disease. Acta Neuropathol. 2013;126:461–77.
194. Zhang B, Gaiteri C, Bodea LG, Wang Z, McElwee J, Podtelezhnikov AA, Zhang C, Xie T, Tran L, Dobrin R, et al. Integrated systems approach identifies genetic nodes and networks in late-onset Alzheimer's disease. Cell. 2013;153:707–20.
195. Mathur R, Ince PG, Minett T, Garwood CJ, Shaw PJ, Matthews FE, Brayne C, Simpson JE, Wharton SB, Function MRCC, Ageing Neuropathology Study G. A reduced astrocyte response to beta-amyloid plaques in the ageing brain associates with cognitive impairment. PLoS One. 2015;10:e0118463.
196. Mrak RE, Griffinbc WS. The role of activated astrocytes and of the neurotrophic cytokine S100B in the pathogenesis of Alzheimer's disease. Neurobiol Aging. 2001;22:915–22.
197. Paradisi S, Sacchetti B, Balduzzi M, Gaudi S, Malchiodi-Albedi F. Astrocyte modulation of in vitro beta-amyloid neurotoxicity. Glia. 2004;46:252–60.
198. Thal DR. The role of astrocytes in amyloid beta-protein toxicity and clearance. Exp Neurol. 2012;236:1–5.
199. Tuppo EE, Arias HR. The role of inflammation in Alzheimer's disease. Int J Biochem Cell Biol. 2005;37:289–305.
200. Holmes C, Cunningham C, Zotova E, Woolford J, Dean C, Kerr S, Culliford D, Perry VH. Systemic inflammation and disease progression in Alzheimer disease. Neurology. 2009;73:768–74.
201. Sudduth TL, Schmitt FA, Nelson PT, Wilcock DM. Neuroinflammatory phenotype in early Alzheimer's disease. Neurobiol Aging. 2013;34:1051–9.
202. von Bernhardi R, Cornejo F, Parada GE, Eugenin J. Role of TGFbeta signaling in the pathogenesis of Alzheimer's disease. Front Cell Neurosci. 2015;9:426.
203. Garwood CJ, Cooper JD, Hanger DP, Noble W. Anti-inflammatory impact of minocycline in a mouse model of tauopathy. Front Psychiatry. 2010;1:136.
204. Parachikova A, Vasilevko V, Cribbs DH, LaFerla FM, Green KN. Reductions in amyloid-beta-derived neuroinflammation, with minocycline, restore cognition but do not significantly affect tau hyperphosphorylation. J Alzheimers Dis. 2010;21:527–42.
205. Green HF, Nolan YM. GSK-3 mediates the release of IL-1beta, TNF-alpha and IL-10 from cortical glia. Neurochem Int. 2012;61:666–71.
206. Hu J, Ferreira A, Van Eldik LJ. S100beta induces neuronal cell death through nitric oxide release from astrocytes. J Neurochem. 1997;69:2294–301.
207. Liu B, Hong JS. Role of microglia in inflammation-mediated neurodegenerative diseases: mechanisms and strategies for therapeutic intervention. J Pharmacol Exp Ther. 2003;304:1–7.
208. Malinski T. Nitric oxide and nitroxidative stress in Alzheimer's disease. J Alzheimers Dis. 2007;11:207–18.
209. Swerdlow RH, Burns JM, Khan SM. The Alzheimer's disease mitochondrial cascade hypothesis: progress and perspectives. Biochim Biophys Acta. 1842; 2014:1219–31.
210. Bharadwaj PR, Bates KA, Porter T, Teimouri E, Perry G, Steele JW, Gandy S, Groth D, Martins RN, Verdile G. Latrepirdine: molecular mechanisms underlying potential therapeutic roles in Alzheimer's and other neurodegenerative diseases. Transl Psychiatry. 2013;3:e332.
211. Shevtsova EF, Vinogradova DV, Kireeva EG, Reddy VP, Aliev G, Bachurin SO. Dimebon attenuates the Abeta-induced mitochondrial permeabilization. Curr Alzheimer Res. 2014;11:422–9.
212. Condello C, Yuan P, Schain A, Grutzendler J. Microglia constitute a barrier that prevents neurotoxic protofibrillar Abeta42 hotspots around plaques. Nat Commun. 2015;6:6176.
213. Wang A, Das P, Switzer RC 3rd, Golde TE, Jankowsky JL. Robust amyloid clearance in a mouse model of Alzheimer's disease provides novel insights into the mechanism of amyloid-beta immunotherapy. J Neurosci. 2011;31: 4124–36.
214. Lee S, Varvel NH, Konerth ME, Xu G, Cardona AE, Ransohoff RM, Lamb BT. CX3CR1 deficiency alters microglial activation and reduces beta-amyloid deposition in two Alzheimer's disease mouse models. Am J Pathol. 2010; 177:2549–62.
215. Liu Z, Condello C, Schain A, Harb R, Grutzendler J. CX3CR1 in microglia regulates brain amyloid deposition through selective protofibrillar amyloid-beta phagocytosis. J Neurosci. 2010;30:17091–101.
216. Cederblad L, Rosengren B, Ryberg E, Hermansson NO. AZD8797 is an allosteric non-competitive modulator of the human CX3CR1 receptor. Biochem J. 2016;473:641–9.
217. Bhaskar K, Konerth M, Kokiko-Cochran ON, Cardona A, Ransohoff RM, Lamb BT. Regulation of tau pathology by the microglial fractalkine receptor. Neuron. 2010;68:19–31.
218. Lopez-Lopez A, Gelpi E, Lopategui DM, Vidal-Taboada JM. Association of the CX3CR1-V249I variant with neurofibrillary pathology progression in late-onset Alzheimer's disease. Mol Neurobiol. 2018;55:2340–9.
219. Niess JH, Brand S, Gu X, Landsman L, Jung S, McCormick BA, Vyas JM, Boes M, Ploegh HL, Fox JG, et al. CX3CR1-mediated dendritic cell access to the intestinal lumen and bacterial clearance. Science. 2005;307:254–8.
220. Condello C, Yuan P, Grutzendler J. Microglia-Mediated Neuroprotection, TREM2, and Alzheimer's Disease: Evidence From Optical Imaging. Biol Psychiatry. 2018;83:377–87.
221. Singer AC, Martorell AJ, Douglas JM, Abdurrob F, Attokaren MK, Tipton J, Mathys H, Adaikkan C, Tsai LH. Noninvasive 40-Hz light flicker to recruit microglia and reduce amyloid beta load. Nat Protoc. 2018;13:1850–68.
222. Iaccarino HF, Singer AC, Martorell AJ, Rudenko A, Gao F, Gillingham TZ, Mathys H, Seo J, Kritskiy O, Abdurrob F, et al. Gamma frequency entrainment attenuates amyloid load and modifies microglia. Nature. 2016; 540:230–5.
223. Iaccarino HF, Singer AC, Martorell AJ, Rudenko A, Gao F, Gillingham TZ, Mathys H, Seo J, Kritskiy O, Abdurrob F, et al. Author correction: gamma frequency entrainment attenuates amyloid load and modifies microglia. Nature. 2018;562:E1.
224. Eimer WA, Vijaya Kumar DK, Navalpur Shanmugam NK, Rodriguez AS, Mitchell T, Washicosky KJ, Gyorgy B, Breakefield XO, Tanzi RE, Moir RD. Alzheimer's disease-associated beta-amyloid is rapidly seeded by Herpesviridae to protect against brain infection. Neuron. 2018;99:56–63 e53.
225. Kumar DK, Choi SH, Washicosky KJ, Eimer WA, Tucker S, Ghofrani J, Lefkowitz A, McColl G, Goldstein LE, Tanzi RE, Moir RD. Amyloid-beta

peptide protects against microbial infection in mouse and worm models of Alzheimer's disease. Sci Transl Med. 2016;8:340ra372.
226. Readhead B, Haure-Mirande JV, Funk CC, Richards MA, Shannon P, Haroutunian V, Sano M, Liang WS, Beckmann ND, Price ND, et al. Multiscale analysis of independent Alzheimer's cohorts finds disruption of molecular, genetic, and clinical networks by human herpesvirus. Neuron. 2018;99:64–82 e67.
227. Buckley JS, Salpeter SR. A risk-benefit assessment of dementia medications: systematic review of the evidence. Drugs Aging. 2015;32:453–67.
228. Johnson JW, Kotermanski SE. Mechanism of action of memantine. Curr Opin Pharmacol. 2006;6:61–7.
229. Olivares D, Deshpande VK, Shi Y, Lahiri DK, Greig NH, Rogers JT, Huang X. N-methyl D-aspartate (NMDA) receptor antagonists and memantine treatment for Alzheimer's disease, vascular dementia and Parkinson's disease. Curr Alzheimer Res. 2012;9:746–58.
230. Patel L, Grossberg GT. Combination therapy for Alzheimer's disease. Drugs Aging. 2011;28:539–46.
231. Deardorff WJ, Shobassy A, Grossberg GT. Safety and clinical effects of EVP-6124 in subjects with Alzheimer's disease currently or previously receiving an acetylcholinesterase inhibitor medication. Expert Rev Neurother. 2015;15:7–17.
232. Thomsen MS, Hansen HH, Timmerman DB, Mikkelsen JD. Cognitive improvement by activation of alpha7 nicotinic acetylcholine receptors: from animal models to human pathophysiology. Curr Pharm Des. 2010;16:323–43.
233. Wilkinson D, Windfeld K, Colding-Jorgensen E. Safety and efficacy of idalopirdine, a 5-HT6 receptor antagonist, in patients with moderate Alzheimer's disease (LADDER): a randomised, double-blind, placebo-controlled phase 2 trial. Lancet Neurol. 2014;13:1092–9.
234. Atri A, Frolich L, Ballard C, Tariot PN, Molinuevo JL, Boneva N, Windfeld K, Raket LL, Cummings JL. Effect of Idalopirdine as adjunct to cholinesterase inhibitors on change in cognition in patients with Alzheimer disease: three randomized clinical trials. JAMA. 2018;319:130–42.
235. Grove RA, Harrington CM, Mahler A, Beresford I, Maruff P, Lowy MT, Nicholls AP, Boardley RL, Berges AC, Nathan PJ, Horrigan JP. A randomized, double-blind, placebo-controlled, 16-week study of the H3 receptor antagonist, GSK239512 as a monotherapy in subjects with mild-to-moderate Alzheimer's disease. Curr Alzheimer Res. 2014;11:47–58.
236. Haig GM, Pritchett Y, Meier A, Othman AA, Hall C, Gault LM, Lenz RA. A randomized study of H3 antagonist ABT-288 in mild-to-moderate Alzheimer's dementia. J Alzheimers Dis. 2014;42:959–71.
237. Youdim MB. The path from anti Parkinson drug selegiline and rasagiline to multifunctional neuroprotective anti Alzheimer drugs ladostigil and m30. Curr Alzheimer Res. 2006;3:541–50.
238. Bansal Y, Silakari O. Multifunctional compounds: smart molecules for multifactorial diseases. Eur J Med Chem. 2014;76:31–42.
239. Weinreb O, Amit T, Bar-Am O, Yogev-Falach M, Youdim MB. The neuroprotective mechanism of action of the multimodal drug ladostigil. Front Biosci. 2008;13:5131–7.
240. Weinreb O, Amit T, Bar-Am O, Youdim MB. Ladostigil: a novel multimodal neuroprotective drug with cholinesterase and brain-selective monoamine oxidase inhibitory activities for Alzheimer's disease treatment. Curr Drug Targets. 2012;13:483–94.
241. Youdim MB. Multi target neuroprotective and neurorestorative anti-Parkinson and anti-Alzheimer drugs ladostigil and m30 derived from rasagiline. Exp Neurobiol. 2013;22:1–10.
242. Hongpaisan J, Sun MK, Alkon DL. PKC epsilon activation prevents synaptic loss, Abeta elevation, and cognitive deficits in Alzheimer's disease transgenic mice. J Neurosci. 2011;31:630–43.
243. Grant SG, O'Dell TJ, Karl KA, Stein PL, Soriano P, Kandel ER. Impaired long-term potentiation, spatial learning, and hippocampal development in fyn mutant mice. Science. 1992;258:1903–10.
244. Kojima N, Ishibashi H, Obata K, Kandel ER. Higher seizure susceptibility and enhanced tyrosine phosphorylation of N-methyl-D-aspartate receptor subunit 2B in fyn transgenic mice. Learn Mem. 1998;5:429–45.
245. Nakazawa T, Komai S, Tezuka T, Hisatsune C, Umemori H, Semba K, Mishina M, Manabe T, Yamamoto T. Characterization of Fyn-mediated tyrosine phosphorylation sites on GluR epsilon 2 (NR2B) subunit of the N-methyl-D-aspartate receptor. J Biol Chem. 2001;276:693–9.
246. Prybylowski K, Chang K, Sans N, Kan L, Vicini S, Wenthold RJ. The synaptic localization of NR2B-containing NMDA receptors is controlled by interactions with PDZ proteins and AP-2. Neuron. 2005;47:845–57.
247. Isosaka T, Hattori K, Kida S, Kohno T, Nakazawa T, Yamamoto T, Yagi T, Yuasa S. Activation of Fyn tyrosine kinase in the mouse dorsal hippocampus is essential for contextual fear conditioning. Eur J Neurosci. 2008;28:973–81.
248. Kaufman AC, Salazar SV, Haas LT, Yang J, Kostylev MA, Jeng AT, Robinson SA, Gunther EC, van Dyck CH, Nygaard HB, Strittmatter SM. Fyn inhibition rescues established memory and synapse loss in Alzheimer mice. Ann Neurol. 2015;77:953–71.
249. Nygaard HB, van Dyck CH, Strittmatter SM. Fyn kinase inhibition as a novel therapy for Alzheimer's disease. Alzheimers Res Ther. 2014;6:8.
250. Um JW, Strittmatter SM. Amyloid-beta induced signaling by cellular prion protein and Fyn kinase in Alzheimer disease. Prion. 2013;7:37–41.
251. Ittner LM, Ke YD, Delerue F, Bi M, Gladbach A, van Eersel J, Wolfing H, Chieng BC, Christie MJ, Napier IA, et al. Dendritic function of tau mediates amyloid-beta toxicity in Alzheimer's disease mouse models. Cell. 2010;142:387–97.
252. Nygaard HB, Wagner AF, Bowen GS, Good SP, MacAvoy MG, Strittmatter KA, Kaufman AC, Rosenberg BJ, Sekine-Konno T, Varma P, et al. A phase Ib multiple ascending dose study of the safety, tolerability, and central nervous system availability of AZD0530 (saracatinib) in Alzheimer's disease. Alzheimers Res Ther. 2015;7:35.
253. Prickaerts J, Heckman PRA, Blokland A. Investigational phosphodiesterase inhibitors in phase I and phase II clinical trials for Alzheimer's disease. Expert Opin Investig Drugs. 2017;26:1033–48.
254. Garcia-Osta A, Cuadrado-Tejedor M, Garcia-Barroso C, Oyarzabal J, Franco R. Phosphodiesterases as therapeutic targets for Alzheimer's disease. ACS Chem Neurosci. 2012;3:832–44.
255. Arai H, Takahashi T. A combination therapy of donepezil and cilostazol for patients with moderate Alzheimer disease: pilot follow-up study. Am J Geriatr Psychiatry. 2009;17:353–4.
256. Ihara M, Nishino M, Taguchi A, Yamamoto Y, Hattori Y, Saito S, Takahashi Y, Tsuji M, Kasahara Y, Takata Y, Okada M. Cilostazol add-on therapy in patients with mild dementia receiving donepezil: a retrospective study. PLoS One. 2014;9:e89516.
257. Taguchi A, Takata Y, Ihara M, Kasahara Y, Tsuji M, Nishino M, Stern D, Okada M. Cilostazol improves cognitive function in patients with mild cognitive impairment: a retrospective analysis. Psychogeriatrics. 2013;13:164–9.
258. Sperling RA, Jack CR Jr, Aisen PS. Testing the right target and right drug at the right stage. Sci Transl Med. 2011;3:111cm133.
259. Norton S, Matthews FE, Barnes DE, Yaffe K, Brayne C. Potential for primary prevention of Alzheimer's disease: an analysis of population-based data. Lancet Neurol. 2014;13:788–94.
260. Hsu D, Marshall GA. Primary and secondary prevention trials in Alzheimer disease: looking Back, Moving Forward. Curr Alzheimer Res. 2017;14:426–40.
261. Sperling RA, Jack CR Jr, Black SE, Frosch MP, Greenberg SM, Hyman BT, Scheltens P, Carrillo MC, Thies W, Bednar MM, et al. Amyloid-related imaging abnormalities in amyloid-modifying therapeutic trials: recommendations from the Alzheimer's Association research roundtable workgroup. Alzheimers Dement. 2011;7:367–85.
262. Kozauer N, Katz R. Regulatory innovation and drug development for early-stage Alzheimer's disease. N Engl J Med. 2013;368:1169–71.
263. Forette F, Seux ML, Staessen JA, Thijs L, Birkenhager WH, Babarskiene MR, Babeanu S, Bossini A, Gil-Extremera B, Girerd X, et al. Prevention of dementia in randomised double-blind placebo-controlled systolic hypertension in Europe (Syst-Eur) trial. Lancet. 1998;352:1347–51.
264. Satizabal C, Beiser AS, Seshadri S. Incidence of dementia over three decades in the Framingham heart study. N Engl J Med. 2016;375:93–4.
265. McGuinness B, Craig D, Bullock R, Passmore P. Statins for the prevention of dementia. Cochrane Database Syst Rev. 2009;(2):CD003160. https://doi.org/10.1002/14651858.CD003160.pub2.
266. Heart Protection Study Collaborative G. MRC/BHF heart protection study of cholesterol lowering with simvastatin in 20,536 high-risk individuals: a randomised placebo-controlled trial. Lancet. 2002;360:7–22.
267. Shepherd J, Blauw GJ, Murphy MB, Bollen EL, Buckley BM, Cobbe SM, Ford I, Gaw A, Hyland M, Jukema JW, et al. Pravastatin in elderly individuals at risk of vascular disease (PROSPER): a randomised controlled trial. Lancet. 2002; 360:1623–30.
268. Launer LJ, Miller ME, Williamson JD, Lazar RM, Gerstein HC, Murray AM, Sullivan M, Horowitz KR, Ding J, Marcovina S, et al. Effects of intensive glucose lowering on brain structure and function in people with type 2 diabetes (ACCORD MIND): a randomised open-label substudy. Lancet Neurol. 2011;10:969–77.

269. Dineley KT, Jahrling JB, Denner L. Insulin resistance in Alzheimer's disease. Neurobiol Dis. 2014;72(Pt A):92–103.
270. Freiherr J, Hallschmid M, Frey WH 2nd, Brunner YF, Chapman CD, Holscher C, Craft S, De Felice FG, Benedict C. Intranasal insulin as a treatment for Alzheimer's disease: a review of basic research and clinical evidence. CNS Drugs. 2013;27:505–14.
271. Craft S, Baker LD, Montine TJ, Minoshima S, Watson GS, Claxton A, Arbuckle M, Callaghan M, Tsai E, Plymate SR, et al. Intranasal insulin therapy for Alzheimer disease and amnestic mild cognitive impairment: a pilot clinical trial. Arch Neurol. 2012;69:29–38.
272. Reger MA, Watson GS, Green PS, Baker LD, Cholerton B, Fishel MA, Plymate SR, Cherrier MM, Schellenberg GD, Frey WH 2nd, Craft S. Intranasal insulin administration dose-dependently modulates verbal memory and plasma amyloid-beta in memory-impaired older adults. J Alzheimers Dis. 2008;13: 323–31.
273. Reger MA, Watson GS, Green PS, Wilkinson CW, Baker LD, Cholerton B, Fishel MA, Plymate SR, Breitner JC, DeGroodt W, et al. Intranasal insulin improves cognition and modulates beta-amyloid in early AD. Neurology. 2008;70:440–8.
274. Yarchoan M, Arnold SE. Repurposing diabetes drugs for brain insulin resistance in Alzheimer disease. Diabetes. 2014;63:2253–61.
275. Perez MJ, Quintanilla RA. Therapeutic actions of the Thiazolidinediones in Alzheimer's disease. PPAR Res. 2015;2015:957248.
276. Feart C, Samieri C, Rondeau V, Amieva H, Portet F, Dartigues JF, Scarmeas N, Barberger-Gateau P. Adherence to a Mediterranean diet, cognitive decline, and risk of dementia. JAMA. 2009;302:638–48.
277. Morris MC, Tangney CC, Wang Y, Sacks FM, Barnes LL, Bennett DA, Aggarwal NT. MIND diet slows cognitive decline with aging. Alzheimers Dement. 2015;11:1015–22.
278. Morris MC, Tangney CC, Wang Y, Sacks FM, Bennett DA, Aggarwal NT. MIND diet associated with reduced incidence of Alzheimer's disease. Alzheimers Dement. 2015;11:1007–14.
279. Stephen R, Hongisto K, Solomon A, Lonnroos E. Physical activity and Alzheimer's disease: a systematic review. J Gerontol A Biol Sci Med Sci. 2017; 72:733–9.
280. Lautenschlager NT, Cox KL, Flicker L, Foster JK, van Bockxmeer FM, Xiao J, Greenop KR, Almeida OP. Effect of physical activity on cognitive function in older adults at risk for Alzheimer disease: a randomized trial. JAMA. 2008; 300:1027–37.
281. Scarmeas N, Luchsinger JA, Schupf N, Brickman AM, Cosentino S, Tang MX, Stern Y. Physical activity, diet, and risk of Alzheimer disease. JAMA. 2009;302: 627–37.
282. Rebok GW, Ball K, Guey LT, Jones RN, Kim HY, King JW, Marsiske M, Morris JN, Tennstedt SL, Unverzagt FW, et al. Ten-year effects of the advanced cognitive training for independent and vital elderly cognitive training trial on cognition and everyday functioning in older adults. J Am Geriatr Soc. 2014;62:16–24.
283. Farina N, Llewellyn D, Isaac MG, Tabet N. Vitamin E for Alzheimer's dementia and mild cognitive impairment. Cochrane Database Syst Rev. 2017;1: CD002854.
284. Dysken MW, Guarino PD, Vertrees JE, Asthana S, Sano M, Llorente M, Pallaki M, Love S, Schellenberg GD, McCarten JR, et al. Vitamin E and memantine in Alzheimer's disease: clinical trial methods and baseline data. Alzheimers Dement. 2014;10:36–44.
285. Dysken MW, Sano M, Asthana S, Vertrees JE, Pallaki M, Llorente M, Love S, Schellenberg GD, McCarten JR, Malphurs J, et al. Effect of vitamin E and memantine on functional decline in Alzheimer disease: the TEAM-AD VA cooperative randomized trial. JAMA. 2014;311:33–44.
286. DeKosky ST, Williamson JD, Fitzpatrick AL, Kronmal RA, Ives DG, Saxton JA, Lopez OL, Burke G, Carlson MC, Fried LP, et al. Ginkgo biloba for prevention of dementia: a randomized controlled trial. JAMA. 2008;300:2253–62.
287. Williamson JD, Vellas B, Furberg C, Nahin R, Dekosky ST. Comparison of the design differences between the Ginkgo evaluation of memory study and the GuidAge study. J Nutr Health Aging. 2008;12:73S–9S.
288. Vellas B, Coley N, Ousset PJ, Berrut G, Dartigues JF, Dubois B, Grandjean H, Pasquier F, Piette F, Robert P, et al. Long-term use of standardised Ginkgo biloba extract for the prevention of Alzheimer's disease (GuidAge): a randomised placebo-controlled trial. Lancet Neurol. 2012;11:851–9.
289. Fotuhi M, Mohassel P, Yaffe K. Fish consumption, long-chain omega-3 fatty acids and risk of cognitive decline or Alzheimer disease: a complex association. Nat Clin Pract Neurol. 2009;5:140–52.
290. Yurko-Mauro K, McCarthy D, Rom D, Nelson EB, Ryan AS, Blackwell A, Salem N Jr, Stedman M, Investigators M. Beneficial effects of docosahexaenoic acid on cognition in age-related cognitive decline. Alzheimers Dement. 2010;6: 456–64.
291. Ngandu T, Lehtisalo J, Solomon A, Levalahti E, Ahtiluoto S, Antikainen R, Backman L, Hanninen T, Jula A, Laatikainen T, et al. A 2 year multidomain intervention of diet, exercise, cognitive training, and vascular risk monitoring versus control to prevent cognitive decline in at-risk elderly people (FINGER): a randomised controlled trial. Lancet. 2015;385:2255–63.
292. Bateman RJ, Xiong C, Benzinger TL, Fagan AM, Goate A, Fox NC, Marcus DS, Cairns NJ, Xie X, Blazey TM, et al. Clinical and biomarker changes in dominantly inherited Alzheimer's disease. N Engl J Med. 2012;367:795–804.
293. Albert MS, DeKosky ST, Dickson D, Dubois B, Feldman HH, Fox NC, Gamst A, Holtzman DM, Jagust WJ, Petersen RC, et al. The diagnosis of mild cognitive impairment due to Alzheimer's disease: recommendations from the National Institute on Aging-Alzheimer's Association workgroups on diagnostic guidelines for Alzheimer's disease. Alzheimers Dement. 2011;7: 270–9.
294. McKhann GM, Knopman DS, Chertkow H, Hyman BT, Jack CR Jr, Kawas CH, Klunk WE, Koroshetz WJ, Manly JJ, Mayeux R, et al. The diagnosis of dementia due to Alzheimer's disease: recommendations from the National Institute on Aging-Alzheimer's Association workgroups on diagnostic guidelines for Alzheimer's disease. Alzheimers Dement. 2011;7:263–9.
295. Panza F, Solfrizzi V, Imbimbo BP, Logroscino G. Amyloid-directed monoclonal antibodies for the treatment of Alzheimer's disease: the point of no return? Expert Opin Biol Ther. 2014;14:1465–76.
296. Hane FT, Robinson M, Lee BY, Bai O, Leonenko Z, Albert MS. Recent Progress in Alzheimer's disease research, part 3: diagnosis and treatment. J Alzheimers Dis. 2017;57:645–65.

6

Gene-environment interaction between lead and Apolipoprotein E4 causes cognitive behavior deficits in mice

Anna K. Engstrom[1], Jessica M. Snyder[2], Nobuyo Maeda[3] and Zhengui Xia[1*]

Abstract

Background: Alzheimer's disease (AD) is characterized by progressive cognitive decline and memory loss. Environmental factors and gene-environment interactions (GXE) may increase AD risk, accelerate cognitive decline, and impair learning and memory. However, there is currently little direct evidence supporting this hypothesis.

Methods: In this study, we assessed for a GXE between lead and ApoE4 on cognitive behavior using transgenic knock-in (KI) mice that express the human Apolipoprotein E4 allele (ApoE4-KI) or Apolipoprotein E3 allele (ApoE3-KI). We exposed 8-week-old male and female ApoE3-KI and ApoE4-KI mice to 0.2% lead acetate via drinking water for 12 weeks and assessed for cognitive behavior deficits during and after the lead exposure. In addition, we exposed a second (cellular) cohort of animals to lead and assessed for changes in adult hippocampal neurogenesis as a potential underlying mechanism for lead-induced learning and memory deficits.

Results: In the behavior cohort, we found that lead reduced contextual fear memory in all animals; however, this decrease was greatest and statistically significant only in lead-treated ApoE4-KI females. Similarly, only lead-treated ApoE4-KI females exhibited a significant decrease in spontaneous alternation in the T-maze. Furthermore, all lead-treated animals developed persistent spatial working memory deficits in the novel object location test, and this deficit manifested earlier in ApoE4-KI mice, with female ApoE4-KI mice exhibiting the earliest deficit onset. In the cellular cohort, we observed that the maturation, differentiation, and dendritic development of adult-born neurons in the hippocampus was selectively impaired in lead-treated female ApoE4-KI mice.

Conclusions: These data suggest that GXE between ApoE4 and lead exposure may contribute to cognitive impairment and that impaired adult hippocampal neurogenesis may contribute to these deficits in cognitive behavior. Together, these data suggest a role for GXE and sex differences in AD risk.

Keywords: Lead, Apolipoprotein E, Cognitive behavior, Adult hippocampal neurogenesis, Learning and memory

* Correspondence: zxia@u.washington.edu
[1]Toxicology Program, Department of Environmental and Occupational Health Sciences, University of Washington, Box 357234, Seattle, WA 98195, USA
Full list of author information is available at the end of the article

Background

Alzheimer's disease (AD) is the most common age-related neurodegenerative disorder [1]. Autosomal dominant mutations account for less than 5% of all Alzheimer's cases [2], thus, most AD cases are likely due to a combination of environmental and genetic risk factors [3–5]. A gene-environment interaction (GXE) between genetic risk factors and environmental exposures may perturb hippocampus-dependent learning and memory, accelerate cognitive decline, and contribute to neurodegenerative diseases, including AD. However, there is a paucity of information supporting this GXE hypothesis.

Apolipoprotein E4 allele (ApoE4) is the strongest genetic risk factor for late-onset AD [6]; it increases the frequency and decreases the age at onset of AD in a gene dose-dependent manner [6]. ApoE4 carriers also have a worse prognosis following traumatic brain injury, a higher prevalence of mild cognitive impairment, and accelerated cognitive decline [7–11].

ApoE4 impairs hippocampus-dependent learning and memory in an age- and sex-dependent manner in transgenic knock-in (KI) mouse models [12–14]. In contrast to aging ApoE3-KI mice or male ApoE4-KI mice, female transgenic ApoE4-KI mice exhibit spatial learning and memory deficits starting at 16 months of age [12, 14]. Interestingly, female human ApoE4 carriers have an increased risk of AD compared to males, and female ApoE4 carriers with mild cognitive impairment experience greater hippocampal volume loss and reduced memory performance [15, 16]. Due to the negative effects of ApoE4 on cognition, ApoE4 carriers, particularly female carriers, may be more susceptible to toxicant-induced cognitive impairment compared to ApoE4 non-carriers.

Lead is a ubiquitous environmental contaminant and a significant public health concern in the U.S. and globally [17–19]. This is exemplified by the recent water crisis in Flint, Michigan, where the water supply was contaminated with lead due to lead leaching from old water pipes. The fact that many U.S. cities still have lead service pipes for water distribution underscores the continuing risk of lead exposure in the U.S. [20].

Both animal and epidemiological studies have reported an association between lead exposure and accelerated cognitive decline and/or AD-associated neuropathology in adults [21–25]. Interestingly, among workers occupationally exposed to lead, those with at least one ApoE4 allele experienced accelerated cognitive decline relative to ApoE4 non-carriers [26]. This epidemiological finding suggests that an interaction between lead and ApoE4 may accelerate cognitive decline. However, an experimental model is necessary in order to directly assess for a GXE between ApoE4 and lead regarding cognitive impairment. In this study, we used homozygous male and female ApoE3-KI and ApoE4-KI mice as an experimental model in order to assess the effect of lead exposure and ApoE4 on cognitive behavior and to examine any potential sex differences in susceptibility. We used deficits in hippocampus-dependent learning and memory as a measure of cognitive decline and AD-related memory impairment because the hippocampus is one of the earliest brain regions affected in AD patients and deficits in hippocampus-dependent spatial learning and memory may develop prior to the onset of a clinical diagnosis [27–29].

Interestingly, perturbation of adult hippocampal neurogenesis may cause cognitive behavior deficits, accelerate cognitive decline, and increase AD risk [30]. During adult hippocampal neurogenesis, adult neural precursor cells in the dentate gyrus (DG) of the hippocampus continuously generate adult-born neurons [31] which contribute to hippocampus-dependent learning and memory [32–37]. Various factors have been shown to modulate adult neurogenesis [31, 33, 34, 37, 38], however, little is known about whether toxicants or GXE may impair adult hippocampal neurogenesis. ApoE is expressed in adult neural precursor cells in the DG [6, 31, 39], and in vivo studies using ApoE4-KI mice found that ApoE4 alters adult-born neuron survival and maturation in an age- and sex-dependent fashion [12–14, 40]. Furthermore, we previously reported that lead can impair the proliferation, survival, and differentiation of adult neural precursor cells from the DG of the hippocampus in vitro [41]. No study to date has assessed the effect of adult-only lead exposure on adult hippocampal neurogenesis and cognitive behavior. Thus, we also investigated whether impaired adult hippocampal neurogenesis may contribute to this GXE between ApoE4 and lead exposure regarding cognitive impairment.

Methods

Mice

Humanized Apolipoprotein E3 and E4 knock-in (ApoE3-KI and ApoE4-KI) mice were generated as previously described [42] and provided by Dr. Nobuyo Maeda at the University of North Carolina, Chapel Hill. The human E3 or E4 allele in the ApoE3-KI or ApoE4-KI mice is expressed at physiological levels under control of the endogenous mouse ApoE promoter [13]. ApoE3-KI and ApoE4-KI animals were maintained as homozygous lines and all animals were housed in standard conditions (12 h light/dark cycle) with food and water provided ad libitum.

Reagents

Animal drinking water with 0.2% lead (II) acetate (Cat. 316512, Sigma-Aldrich, St. Louis, MO) was prepared from a stock lead acetate solution and replaced weekly. The preparation, use, and disposal of hazardous agents was carried out according to the Environmental Health and Safety Office at the University of Washington.

Lead exposure

Male and female ApoE3-KI and ApoE4-KI animals were weaned at 28 days and littermates of the same sex were randomly mixed into groups of 3–5 animals per cage. At 8 weeks of age, the mice were either switched to drinking water with 0.2% lead acetate (lead-treated) or kept on normal animal drinking water (control). Body weight was recorded every 1–2 weeks throughout the exposure. Water consumption was monitored for the first week of the exposure period. Lead-treated animals were exposed to lead drinking water for 12 weeks, at which point all the animals were switched to normal drinking water for the remaining duration of the study for the behavior cohort. We used separate cohorts of animals, one for behavior and one for cellular studies, to assess cognitive behavior and adult hippocampal neurogenesis, respectively. The behavior cohorts had $n = 8–13$ animals per genotype/treatment/sex and the cellular cohorts had $n = 6–10$ animals per genotype/treatment/sex.

Open field test

The open field test was conducted before and after the lead exposure to assess for the development of any lead-induced locomotor deficits or anxiety. Briefly, each animal was placed into a TruScan Photo Beam Tracking arena (Colbourn Instruments, Whitehall, PA) with Plexiglas walls (10″ X 10″ X 16″) and their movement was monitored with two sets of infrared breams. The animal was allowed to freely explore the arena for 20 min and the data was collected by TruScan 2.0 software (Colbourn Instruments).

Elevated plus maze

We conducted the elevated plus maze test in order to assess the effect of lead exposure on anxiety. The maze (26″ x 26″ x 15.25″; San Diego Instruments, San Diego, CA) consisted of four plastic arms with 7″ walls (two enclosed and two open), and it was placed in the center of the behavior room. Each animal was placed into the center of the maze facing an open arm and allowed to freely explore the maze for 5 min. The open and closed arm ends were defined as the distal 1/3 of the arms. ANYmaze software (San Diego Instruments) was used to collect data on the animal's movement during the test.

Novel object location test

In order to assess hippocampus-dependent, short-term spatial working memory, we used the 1 h novel object location (NOL) test. This test was performed as previously described with a few modifications [34]. Briefly, each animal was placed into an open field arena (Colbourn Instruments) with two identical objects in two different locations. During training, the animal was allowed to freely explore the two objects for 5 min and then returned to its home cage. After 1 h, the animal was returned to the arena with the same two objects; one object remained in its original location and one object had been moved to a novel location. The time the animal spent actively investigating each object during the training and testing was quantified. Each training and testing session was recorded and scored offline by an experimenter blinded to the animal's genotype and treatment. We calculated the discrimination index by dividing the difference in exploration time between the novel (C) and familiar (A) locations by the total exploration time.

Cued-contextual fear-conditioning

Contextual fear conditioning is another form of hippocampus-dependent learning and memory [33, 37, 43]. We tested 5–6-month-old animals and used a weak foot shock conditioning paradigm (3 x 0.3 mA, 2 s shocks with 2 min inter-trial intervals) as previously described [33]. For conditioning, the mouse was placed into the foot shock context (10″ x 10″ x 16″ arena with grid shock floor (Colbourn Instruments) and star-shaped wallpaper) and allowed to freely explore the arena for 2 min before the presentation of a 90 dB, 30 s tone (conditioned stimulus, CS). During the last 2 s of the tone presentation, a 0.3 mA foot shock (unconditioned stimulus, US) was delivered via the grid shock floor. This cycle was repeated two more times for a total of three cycles before the animal was returned to its home cage. The CS and US were automated and delivered by TruScan software (Colbourn Instruments). The contextual fear memory test was conducted 24 h after conditioning. The mouse was placed back into the foot shock context for 2 min in the absence of any foot shock. For the cued test (performed 2 h after context test), the animal was placed into a different context (new room; hexagonal Plexiglas arena; cartoon wallpaper) and allowed to freely explore for 2 min followed by the presentation of the CS for 2 min. For the novel context test (performed 2 h after the cued test), the mouse was placed into a novel context (new room; rat cage; striped wallpaper) and allowed to freely explore without any CS or US presentation. In all three tests, persistent freezing behavior (four paws on the ground, no head or body movement besides breathing) was recorded manually every 5 s during the 2 min scoring periods by an experimenter blinded to animal genotype and treatment.

T-maze continuous alternation task

We assessed spontaneous alternation in 12–13- month-old animals using a continuous alternation T-maze protocol with slight modifications [44]. Briefly, the black, plastic T-maze had two goal arms and a start arm (12.2″ x 4.5″ x 8.26″), and was placed on a platform (22.5″) in the center of a room. The test consisted of a first-forced trial followed by 14 free-choice trials. For the first-forced trial, one of the goal arms was (randomly) blocked with a plastic guillotine door. The animal was sequestered in the distal one-third of the start arm for 5 s before the guillotine door was raised and the animal was allowed to enter the unblocked goal arm. Once the animal returned to the start arm, it was sequestered in the start arm for 5 s before the start of the 14 free-choice trials. For each free-choice trial, the mouse was allowed to enter either of the unblocked goal arms; once it entered a goal arm, the other goal arm was blocked with a guillotine door. The animal eventually returned to the start arm and was sequestered for 5 s while all of the goal arms were unblocked. This was repeated for a total of 14 free-choice trials. The alternation percentage was calculated by dividing the number of times the animal entered alternating arms by 14 (free-choice trials). We defined arm entry as the animal's tail tip entering the arm and defined repetitive arm entries as an animal re-entering the same arm three times in a row (e.g., 5 sequential entries into the same arm is 3 repetitive entries). An experimenter blinded to animal genotype and treatment scored each test.

Brain and blood lead analysis

We collected blood and brain tissue for lead analysis at sacrifice after the cessation of the lead exposure from a subset of the mice in the cellular cohort (20 weeks old; n = 3–5 per genotype/sex/treatment). The Environmental Health Laboratory at the University of Washington measured blood lead levels using inductively coupled plasma mass spectrometry (ICP-MS; Agilent 7500ce, Agilent Technologies, Santa Clara, CA). The spatial distribution and semi-quantitative measurement of lead and zinc levels (ppm) in 30 µm brain hemisphere sections from 20-week-old ApoE4-KI control or lead-treated females was determined by laser ablation ICP-MS (LA-ICP-MS) using an NWR213 laser ablation system (ESI, Portland, OR) connected to an Agilent 7500ce ICP-MS (Agilent Technologies, Santa Clara, CA). Quantification was achieved using spiked protein matrix as external standards.

TUNEL staining

TUNEL staining was performed using the Trevigen TACS 2 TdT-fluor In situ Apoptosis Detection Kit (Cat. 4812-30-K, Sigma-Aldrich, St. Louis, MO) on 30 µm fresh frozen coronal brain sections according to the manufacturer's instructions. The cells were permeabilized using Trevigen's Cytonin™ permeabilization buffer and an experimental positive control was included (treated with TACS-Nuclease™).

Quantification of dentate gyrus volume

The volume of the dentate gyrus was quantified using coronal images (20X magnification) from 15-month-old female ApoE3-KI and ApoE4-KI mice from the behavior cohorts as previously described [45].

BrdU administration

5-bromo-2′-deoxyuridine (BrdU) was from Sigma (Cat. B9285, Sigma-Aldrich, St. Louis, MO) and stored as a 20 mg/ml stock in saline with 0.007% NaOH at -20 °C. After 9 weeks of lead exposure, the mice in one of the cellular cohorts were dosed with 100 mg/kg BrdU by intraperitoneal injection 5 times in 1 day (every 2 h) and sacrificed 3 weeks later (at the end of the 12 week lead exposure) in order to assess the maturation of BrdU-labeled adult-born cells. A second cellular cohort was dosed with BrdU 1 X 100 mg/kg 2 h prior to sacrifice (at the end of the 12 week lead exposure period) in order to assess for proliferative BrdU-labeled cells.

Immunohistochemistry

The primary antibodies and dilutions used in immunohistochemistry were: rat monoclonal anti-BrdU (1:500, Bio-Rad Laboratories AbD Serotec, Raleigh, NC), mouse monoclonal anti-NeuN (1:1000, Millipore, Billerica, MA), mouse monoclonal anti-GAD67 (1:2000, Millipore, Billerica, MA), and donkey polyclonal anti-DCX (1:200, Santa Cruz Biotechnology, Dallas, TX), Goat anti-rat, goat anti-mouse, and donkey anti-rat Alexa Fluor-conjugated secondary antibodies as well as Hoechst 33342 (2.5 µg/ml) were from Invitrogen (Carlsbad, CA). All of the primary and secondary antibodies were diluted into the appropriate blocking buffer (10% donkey or goat serum and 1% BSA).

Mice were anesthetized with ketamine/xylazine and then euthanized by decapitation. One brain hemisphere was freshly frozen for brain lead analysis or other biochemical analysis, while the other hemisphere was post-fixed in 10% neutral-buffered formalin for 3–4 days followed by 30% (w/v) sucrose in phosphate-buffered saline (PBS, pH 7.4) at 4 °C for 3–4 days until saturated. Each post-fixed hemisphere was then stored in cryoprotectant media (30% glycerol; 30% ethylene glycol; 40% PBS) at -80 °C until sectioning. Coronal brain sections (30 µm thick) were used for immunohistochemistry (IHC) using the free-floating antibody staining method as previously described [38].

Quantification and imaging of immunostained cells

Immunostained cells were quantified as previously described [34, 38]. Every eighth serial section (30 µm) was immunostained for each IHC marker (or combination of markers). An experimenter blinded to treatment and genotype quantified marker$^+$ cells in the subgranular zone and granule cell layer of the DG. This number was multiplied by 8 in order to estimate the total number of marker$^+$ cells per DG. Marker colocalization (double-positive cell) was defined as overlapping fluorescent signals in a single cell using a Z-series stack. All the marker$^+$ cells from at least 9 coronal sections per mouse ($n = 3–5$ mice per genotype/sex/treatment) were quantified for each immuno marker or marker combination. All images were captured with an Olympus Fluoview-1000 laser scanning confocal microscope with the following lenses: numerical aperture (NA) 0.75 10X, NA 0.75 20X, NA1.3 40X (oil), or NA 1.35 60X (oil). Optical Z-sections (1 μm thick) were collected and processed using ImageJ software (NIH, Bethesda, MD). Images were uniformly adjusted for color, brightness, and contrast with Adobe Photoshop CS4 (Adobe Systems Inc., San Jose, CA).

Quantification of dendritic morphology

The dendritic morphology of DCX$^+$ cells in control and lead-treated ApoE3-KI and ApoE4-KI mice (at least 13 individual neurons per genotype/sex/treatment) was assessed by Sholl analysis as previously described [34].

Histology

Kidney and liver sections from control and lead-treated ApoE3-KI and ApoE4-KI males and females ($n = 3–4$ per genotype/treatment) were fixed in 10% neutral buffered formalin, paraffin embedded, cut into 4- to 5-μm sections, routinely stained with hematoxylin and eosin (H&E), and evaluated by a board-certified veterinary pathologist. Slides were coded to remove information regarding genotype and treatment. Kidneys were scored semi-quantitatively using a 0–4 scale, in which "0" was normal; "1" indicated minimal expansion of the glomerular mesangial matrix and minimal multifocal tubular protein; "2" indicated mild changes of the glomerulus with mild interstitial fibrosis, interstitial nephritis, and tubular protein; "3" indicated moderate multifocal to coalescing changes characterized by more pronounced glomerular, tubular and interstitial changes; and "4" indicated end stage disease with obsolescent glomeruli and severe multifocal to coalescing interstitial nephritis and fibrosis with or without dilation of the renal pelvis (hydronephrosis). Intranuclear inclusion bodies within the proximal renal tubules were noted when present. Livers were assessed using modified criteria from a previous study [46] and scored semi-quantitatively for changes including necrotic foci, cytoplasmic vacuolation, and mononuclear cell infiltration on a 0–4 system in which "0" was normal; "1" indicated minimal changes; "2" indicated mild changes; "3" indicated moderate changes; and "4" indicated severe changes. Images of representative lesions were acquired using NIS-Elements BR 3.2 64-bit and plated in Adobe Photoshop Elements. Image brightness and contrast was adjusted using Auto Smart Fix and Auto White Balance manipulations applied to the entire image.

Statistical analysis

Statistical analyses were conducted using GraphPad Prism software (version 6.0 h for Mac, GraphPad Software Inc., San Diego, CA, USA) and Stata (version 12.0 for Mac, StataCorp LP, College Station, TX, USA). Two-way analysis of variance (ANOVA) with the Holm-Sidak *post-test* ($\alpha = 0.05$) was used to analyze the open field, elevated plus maze, contextual fear, and T-maze data in order to account for the main effect of genotype (ApoE3-KI vs. ApoE4-KI), treatment (control vs. lead), or time. Two-tailed *t*-test ($\alpha = 0.05$) was used for within-genotype comparisons for the NOL data. Multilevel mixed-effects linear regression ($\alpha = 0.05$) was used for longitudinal analysis of within-genotype NOL discrimination index data. Two-way analysis of variance (ANOVA) with Fisher's LSD *post-test* ($\alpha = 0.05$) was used to analyze all of the cellular data. All data represent mean ± SEM, n.s. not significant; * $p < 0.05$; ** $p < 0.01$; *** $p < 0.001$.

Results

ApoE3-KI and ApoE4-KI mice do not exhibit weight loss, locomotor deficits, or anxiety following lead exposure

We exposed 8-week-old male and female ApoE3-KI and ApoE4-KI mice to 0.2% lead acetate (lead-treated) or normal drinking water (control) for 12 weeks to model sub-chronic environmental and occupational exposure through ingestion (Fig. 1). We used 0.2% lead acetate in our study because this concentration has been used extensively in the literature to study lead neurotoxicity in mice [47–52]. We recorded body weight every 1–2 weeks during the lead exposure period and did not observe any weight loss in any of the lead-exposed animals at any time during lead exposure (Fig. 1b). Lead-treated ApoE3-KI mice were slightly heavier than their controls at several time points, but this weight gain was not associated with any locomotor deficits. There was no significant difference in body weight between control and lead-treated ApoE4-KI mice.

We conducted the open field test for all of the animals in the behavior cohort before and after the 12-week lead exposure in order to assess locomotor activity and anxiety. The pre-exposure test was performed to exclude any intrinsic differences between the control and lead-treated cohorts that could complicate data interpretation. Although there were some small differences in locomotor activity between the two genotypes, with ApoE4-KI mice exhibiting slightly higher baseline activity than ApoE3-KI mice, there were no significant differences in open field activity between control and lead-treated cohorts prior to the lead exposure of either genotype (data not shown).

After lead exposure, the lead-treated females, both ApoE3-KI and ApoE4-KI, traveled further, spent more time moving, and moved slightly faster than their respective controls (Fig. 2). There was no significant effect of lead on locomotor activity in male mice. It is

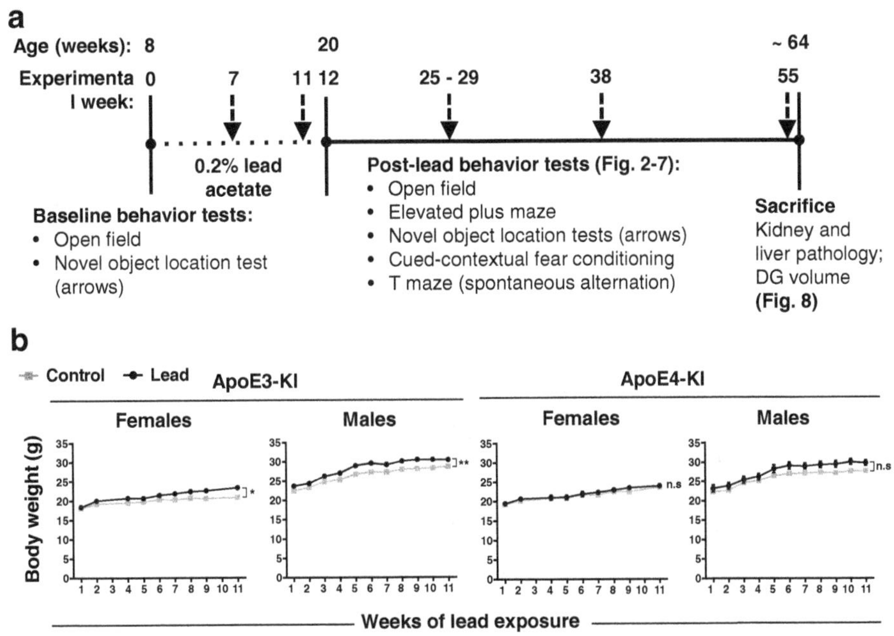

Fig. 1 Adult male and female ApoE3-KI and ApoE4-KI mice do not exhibit weight loss upon exposure to 0.2% lead acetate for 12 weeks. **a** Experimental design and timeline for the behavior cohort. **b** Body weight was measured every 1–2 weeks during the lead exposure window. The lead-treated mice did not exhibit any weight loss relative to controls of the same sex and genotype. ApoE3-KI mice exposed to lead weighed slightly but significantly more at several time points than control mice during the lead exposure. Data are mean ± SEM with $n = 8$–13 per genotype/sex/treatment. Two-way ANOVA, significant main effect of treatment: n.s., not significant; * $p < 0.05$; ** $p < 0.01$

important to note that there were no significant differences in locomotor activity between lead-treated ApoE3-KI and ApoE4-KI mice of either sex.

We also used the open field test to determine if lead treatment caused anxiety, measured as more time or distance in the margin, less time or distance in the center, or reduced center entries. Lead treatment did not change these parameters in males (Fig. 3a-f). Lead-treated ApoE3-KI females traveled a greater distance in the center of the open field and made more center entries compared to ApoE3-KI control females (Fig. 3d-f). Notably, there were no significant differences in center distance traveled and center entry between lead-treated ApoE3-KI and ApoE4-KI females.

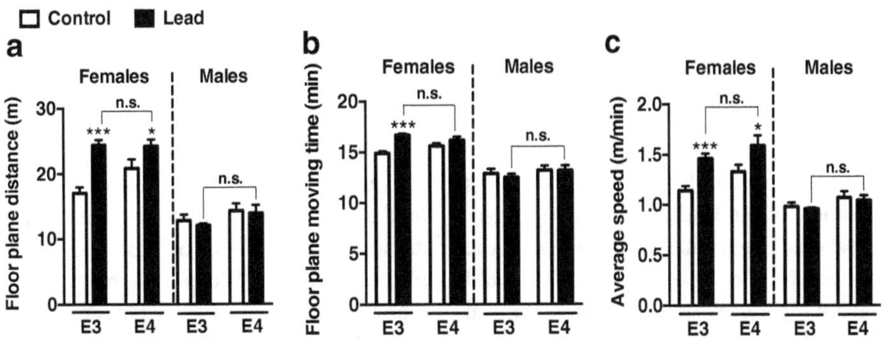

Fig. 2 Lead-treated ApoE3-KI and ApoE4-KI male and female mice do not exhibit locomotor deficits in the open field test compared to controls. Mice were exposed to lead as previously described and the open field test was conducted after the cessation of the lead exposure. There was a significant main effect of lead treatment in female animals on floor plane distance, moving time, and average speed (Two-way ANOVA: floor plane distance, $F(1,31) = 22.85$, $p < 0.0001$; moving time, $F(1,31) = 20.47$, $p < 0.0001$; average speed, $F(1,31) = 20.49$, $p < 0.0001$). *Post-hoc* analyses found that lead-treated ApoE3-KI and/or ApoE4-KI females traveled a (**a**) greater distance, (**b**) spent the same or more time moving, and (**c**) traveled slightly faster than controls. There were no significant differences between lead and control ApoE3-KI and ApoE4-KI males or between lead-treated ApoE3-KI and ApoE4-KI mice (males or females) in any of the locomotor endpoints. Data are mean ± SEM with $n = 8$–13 per genotype/sex/treatment. Two-way ANOVA with Holm-Sidak *post-hoc* tests: n.s., not significant; * $p < 0.05$; *** $p < 0.001$

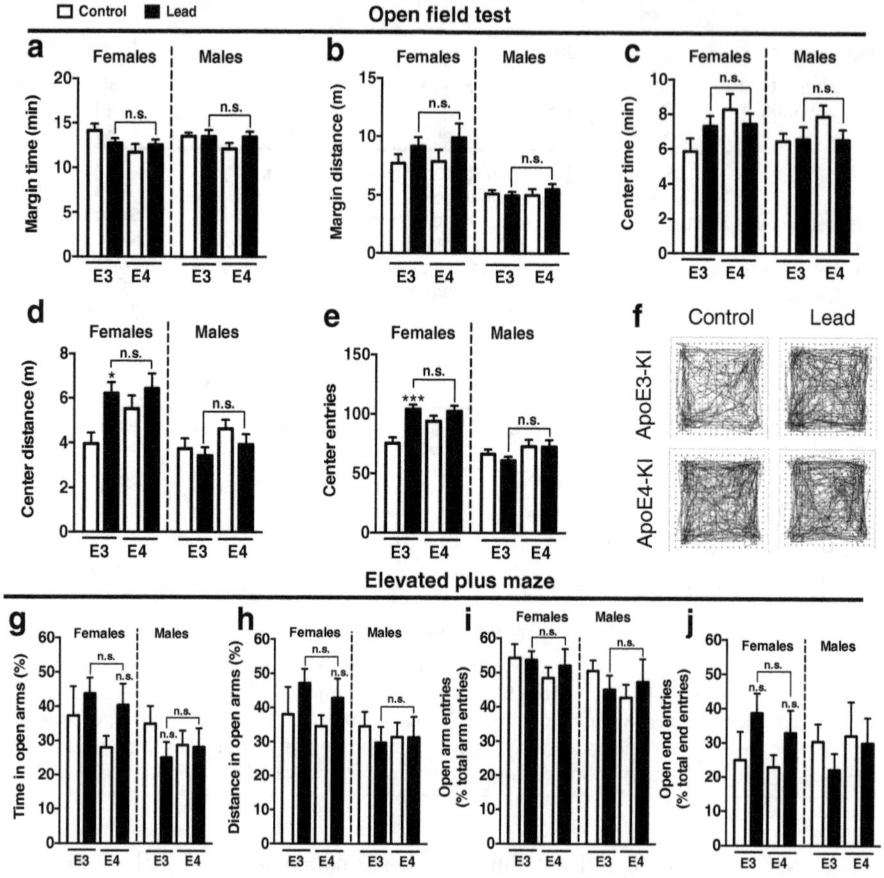

Fig. 3 Male and female ApoE3-KI and ApoE4-KI mice exposed to lead do not exhibit overt anxiety in the open field test or elevated plus maze. The open field test was used to determine if lead treatment causes anxiety, measured as more time or distance in the margin, less time or distance in the center, or reduced center entries. There was a significant main effect of lead treatment in female mice on center distance and center entries (Two-way ANOVA: center distance, $F_{(1,31)} = 5.936$, $p = 0.0208$; center entries, $F_{(1,31)} = 14.76$, $p = 0.0006$). *Post-hoc* analyses found that there were no significant differences between lead-treated ApoE3-KI and ApoE4-KI mice (males and females) on the (**a**) time or (**b**) distance traveled in the margins, the (**c**) time or (**d**) distance traveled in the center, or the (**e**) number of center entries in the open field test. *D*, ApoE3-KI females treated with lead traveled a slightly greater distance in the center and *E*, made more center entries than controls. There were no significant differences between control and lead-treated ApoE4-KI females, ApoE3-KI males, or ApoE4-KI males in the open field test. **f** Representative open field track plots from female control and lead-treated ApoE3-KI and ApoE4-KI mice. In the elevated plus maze, both male and female ApoE3-KI and ApoE4-KI mice exposed to lead spent a (**g**) similar or greater amount of time and traveled a (**h**) similar or greater distance in the open arms of the maze compared to controls. Lead-treated males and females did not exhibit reduced (**i**) open arm or (**j**) open arm end entries compared to control animals. Data are mean ± SEM with $n = 8–13$ per genotype/treatment. Two-way ANOVA with Holm-Sidak *post-hoc* tests: n.s., not significant; * $p < 0.05$; *** $p < 0.001$

We also conducted the elevated plus maze test to assess anxiety after the cessation of the lead exposure (Fig. 3g-j). The elevated plus maze is commonly used to assess the anxiogenic and anxiolytic effects of toxicological and pharmacological agents. It relies on a mouse's natural avoidance of heights and open spaces and it's preference for dark, sheltered spaces [53]. There was no significant effect of genotype or lead exposure on the percent of total time males or females spent or the total distance they traveled in the open arms by two-way ANOVA (Fig. 3g, h). In addition, there was no significant effect of genotype or treatment on the number of open arm entries or open arm end entries among males or females (Fig. 3i, j).

Thus, subchronic exposure of 8-week-old mice to 0.2% lead acetate did not decrease locomotor activity or cause anxiety in ApoE3-KI or ApoE4-KI mice. Although lead exposure may result in a slight hyperactive phenotype in ApoE3-KI and ApoE4-KI females and a slight anxiolytic phenotype in ApoE3-KI females, there were no significant differences between lead-treated ApoE3-KI and ApoE4-KI mice of either sex.

ApoE4-KI females exposed to lead exhibit impaired contextual fear memory

We also conducted a contextual fear-conditioning test (age of mice: 5–6 months old) to characterize the effect of lead

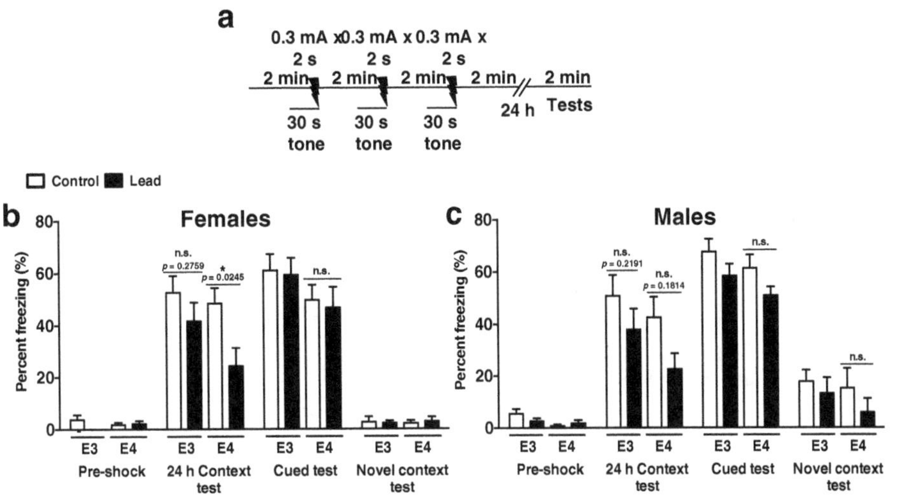

Fig. 4 Lead impairs contextual fear memory in lead-treated ApoE4-KI females at 22–24 weeks of age. **a** Schematic of cued and contextual fear conditioning test performed post-lead exposure. **b, c** Female and male mice had low baseline freezing behavior (Pre-shock). In the 24 h Context test, there was a significant main effect of lead treatment on freezing behavior in both males and females (Two-way ANOVA: females, $F_{(1,33)} = 6.803$, $p = 0.0136$; males, $F_{(1,42)} = 4.435$, $p = 0.0412$). Although lead treatment reduced contextual memory in all animals (manifested as reduced freezing 24 h after fear conditioning) *post-hoc* tests revealed that this was only statistically significant between control and lead-treated ApoE4-KI females (Holm-Sidak *post-hoc* test: $F_{(1,33)} = 2.648$, $p = 0.0245$). Auditory-cued (hippocampus-independent) fear memory was not affected (Cued test) in any lead-exposed animals. All animals did not freeze when placed into a novel, non-shock context (Novel context test). Data are mean ± SEM with $n = 8$–13 per sex/genotype/treatment. Two-way ANOVA with Holm-Sidak *post-hoc* test. n.s. not significant; * $p < 0.05$

and ApoE4 on hippocampus-dependent learning and memory (Fig. 4a). We used a 0.3 mA x 3 foot shock paradigm because we previously reported that this paradigm is sensitive to changes in contextual fear memory and adult neurogenesis [33]. All mice showed minimal freezing behavior at baseline before foot shock (Fig. 4b, c). We performed the context test 24 h after fear-conditioning in order to assess contextual fear memory. Interestingly, lead-treated ApoE4-KI females had significantly reduced contextual fear memory compared to ApoE4-KI controls (Fig. 4b). Male ApoE4-KI mice and both male and female ApoE3-KI mice exposed to lead exhibited a statistically non-significant reduction in freezing behavior upon lead treatment (Fig. 4b, c). Lead treatment did not cause any statistically significant changes in any animals in auditory-cued fear memory–a form of amygdala-dependent, but hippocampus-independent memory–or in general freezing in a novel context. Furthermore, lead treatment did not affect animals' shock sensitivity (data not shown). Thus, lead exposure impairs the formation and/or retrieval of contextual fear memory in ApoE4-KI female mice.

ApoE4-KI females exhibit decreased spontaneous alternation and increased repetitive arm entry in a T-maze

We assessed spontaneous alternation using the T-maze in 12–13-month-old animals. Rodents spontaneously alternate the arms they enter in the T-maze, and this is likely due to a combination of novelty-elicited exploratory behavior as well as spatial working memory [44, 54]. Interestingly, lead-treated ApoE4-KI females exhibited a significant reduction in spontaneous alternation (Fig. 5a) and had a significant increase in repetitive arm entries compared to control ApoE4-KI females (Fig. 5b). These behavior changes were specific to females and were not observed in males. There were no significant differences between control and lead-treated animals on the ratio of left/right arm entries or mean session duration in either females or males (Fig. 5c, d). These data suggest that there may be a GXE interaction between lead and ApoE4 on spontaneous alternation and repetitive entries. Furthermore, lead-treated female ApoE4-KI mice are more sensitive than males. These differences are not due to a bias in arm entries or significant differences in task completion time.

ApoE3-KI and ApoE4-KI mice exposed to lead exhibit a GXE interaction and sex differences in the onset of short-term spatial memory deficits in the novel objection location test (NOL)

We conducted a 1 h NOL test to assess hippocampus-dependent spatial working memory before, during, and after the lead exposure. Importantly, at each NOL time point (baseline through 10 months post-lead), none of the mice exhibited a preference for either object or location during the training session, and there was no difference in

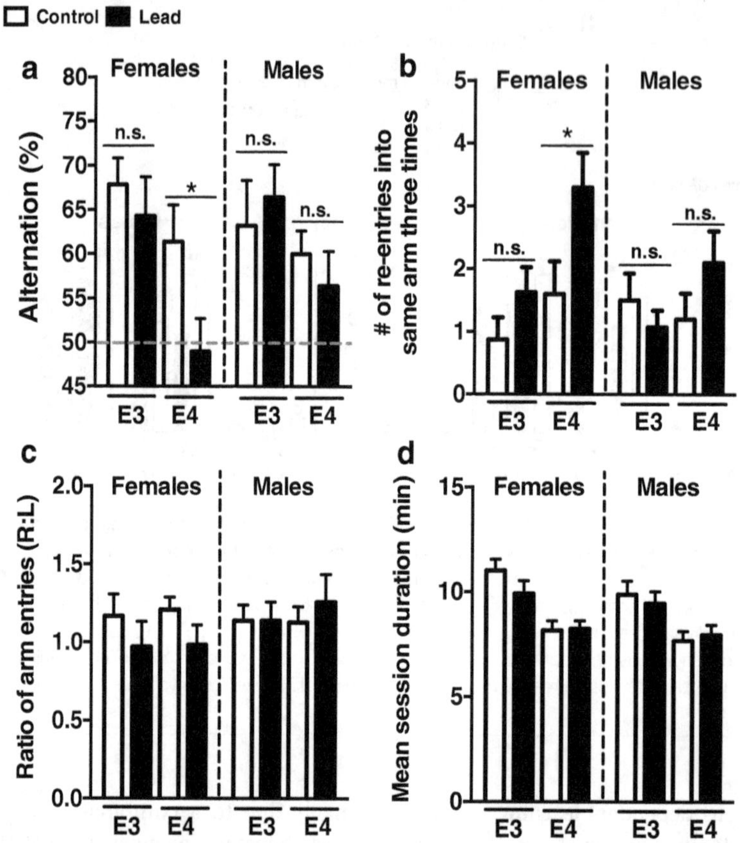

Fig. 5 Lead impairs spontaneous alternation and increases repetitive arm entry in lead-treated ApoE4-KI females. Spontaneous alternation was assessed using the T-maze at 12–13 months of age. **a** There was a significant main effect of genotype on spontaneous alternation in females (Two-way ANOVA: genotype, $F_{(1,32)} = 7.666$, $p = 0.0093$). Lead-treated ApoE4-KI female mice exhibited reduced spontaneous alternation compared to female ApoE4-KI control mice (Holm-Sidak *post-test*: $F_{(1,32)} = 2.356$, $p = 0.0490$). **b** There was a significant main effect of both genotype and treatment on repetitive arm entries in females (Two-way ANOVA: genotype, $F_{(1,32)} = 5.915$, $p = 0.0208$; treatment, $F_{(1,32)} = 6.164$, $p = 0.0185$). ApoE4-KI females exposed to lead exhibited significantly increased repetitive arm entries compared to control ApoE4-KI female mice (Holm-Sidak *post-test:* $F_{(1,32)} = 2.584$, p 0.0289). There was no significant difference in spontaneous alternation or arm re-entries in lead-treated ApoE3-KI and ApoE4-KI male mice. **c** Female and male mice did not exhibit any arm preference. **d** There was a significant main effect of genotype on mean session duration in both the females and males, with ApoE4-KI mice completing the alternation task slightly faster than ApoE3-KI mice of the same sex (Two-way ANOVA: females, $F_{(1,30)} = 19.50$, $p = 0.0001$; males $F_{(1,41)} = 9.803$, $p = 0.0032$). There was no significant difference in mean session duration between control and lead-treated animals of the same genotype and sex. Data are mean ± SEM with n = 8–13 per sex/genotype/treatment. n.s. not significant; * $p < 0.05$

the total exploration time between lead-treated and control mice (data not shown).

Before lead exposure, all of the ApoE3-KI and ApoE4-KI females and males spent significantly more time exploring the object in the novel vs. familiar (C vs. A) location during the test period, indicating that they remembered the original object location (Fig. 6A). Seven weeks into the lead exposure, all of the mice spent significantly more time exploring the novel location except for lead-treated ApoE4-KI females, which did not discriminate between the old vs. new object locations (Fig. 6B). After 11 weeks of lead exposure, both the lead-treated ApoE4-KI females and males no longer discriminated between the familiar and novel object locations while the lead-treated ApoE3-KI mice continued to spend significantly more time exploring the novel object location (Fig. 6C). Both the lead-treated ApoE4-KI females and males continued to exhibit a deficit in spatial working memory at 3, 6, and 10 months post-lead exposure (Fig. 6D and data not shown). Lead-treated ApoE3-KI mice still spent significantly more time exploring the novel object location at 3, 6, and 10 months post-lead exposure (Fig. 6D and data not shown). However, the differences in exploration time between the new vs. old object locations became smaller over time among the ApoE3-KI mice exposed to lead indicating poorer spatial memory.

We calculated the discrimination index for each NOL test, and the discrimination indices at each time point are summarized by genotype and sex in Fig. 7. There was an effect of lead exposure on the discrimination index in all lead-exposed animals (Multiple mixed-effects linear

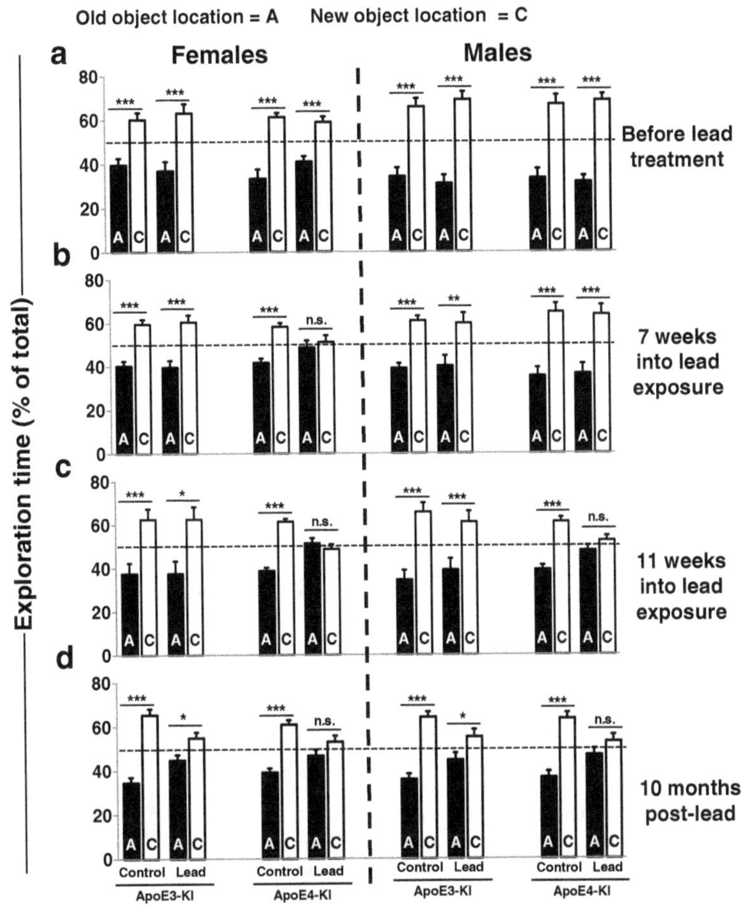

Fig. 6 The effect of lead on short-term spatial memory in the NOL test. The NOL test was performed before, during, and after the lead exposure to assess for spatial working memory deficits. The time animals spent investigating the object in the old (location A) vs. new (location C) locations was quantified. More time spent exploring the object in the novel vs. old location indicates memory for the old location. ***(A)*** All the animals had intact spatial memory prior to the lead exposure. ***(B)*** At 7 weeks into the lead exposure, only the lead-treated ApoE4-KI females did not discriminate between the old vs. new object locations (Two-tailed *t*-test (A vs. C): $p = 1.000$). ***(C)*** At 11 weeks, both the lead-treated ApoE4-KI females and males no longer discriminated between the object locations (females, $p = 0.4042$; males, $p = 0.1959$) while the ApoE3-KI females and males spent significantly more time exploring the novel object location (females, $p = 0.0107$; males, $p = 0.0098$). ***(D)*** Lead-treated ApoE4-KI females and males continued to exhibit a deficit in spatial working memory at 10 months post-lead exposure (females, $p = 0.0961$; males, $p = 0.1855$). Lead-treated ApoE3-KI mice still spent statistically significantly more time exploring the novel object location at 10 months post-lead exposure (females, $p = 0.0186$; males, $p = 0.0320$). Data are mean ± SEM with $n = 8$–13 per genotype/treatment. Two-tailed *t*–test: n.s. not significant, * $p < 0.05$; ** $p < 0.01$; *** $p < 0.001$

regression: ApoE3-KI females, $p = 0.001$; ApoE4-KI females, $p < 0.0001$; ApoE3-KI males, $p = 0.019$; ApoE4-KI males, $p < 0.0001$). During the lead exposure period, there was no difference in the discrimination index between control and lead-treated ApoE3-KI females (Fig. 7a). However, lead-treated ApoE3-KI females had a significantly lower discrimination index at 3 and 10 months post-lead exposure compared to controls.

Interestingly, the lead-treated ApoE4-KI females had a significantly lower discrimination index than control ApoE4-KI females starting at 7 weeks into the lead exposure, and this decrease persisted through 10 months post-lead (Fig. 7b). Thus, lead-treated ApoE3-KI and ApoE4-KI females exhibited persistent deficits in short-term spatial memory, with ApoE4-KI females exhibiting a significant decrease in the discrimination index starting at 7 weeks into the lead exposure, much earlier than lead-treated ApoE3-KI females at 3 months post-lead exposure.

Lead-treated ApoE3-KI males had a significantly lower discrimination index at 6 and 10 months post-lead compared to controls (Fig. 7c), suggesting that spatial memory deficits can develop long after lead exposure. In contrast, lead-treated ApoE4-KI males had a significantly lower discrimination index than controls starting at 11 weeks into the lead exposure and this effect persisted through 10 months post-lead exposure (Fig. 7d). Thus, both ApoE3-KI and ApoE4-KI males exposed to lead exhibited persistent deficits in short-term spatial memory, but the lead-treated ApoE4-KI males showed these

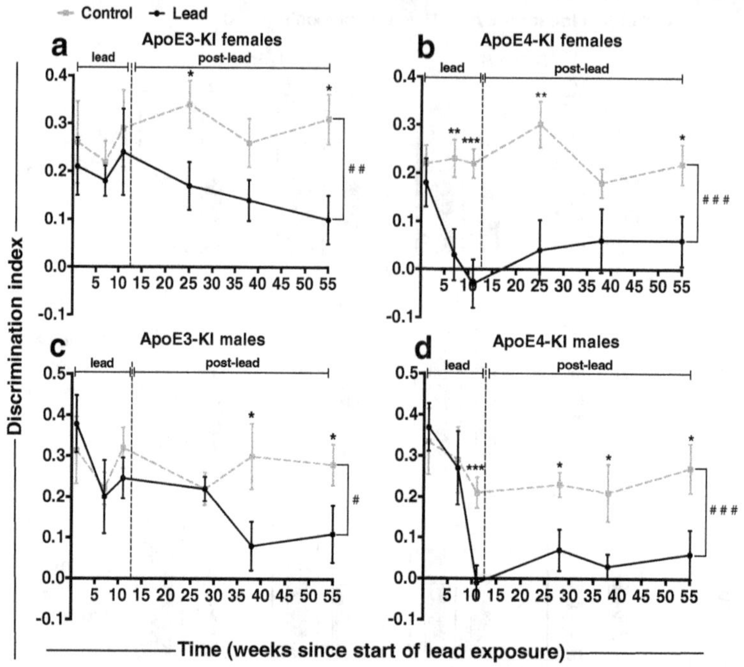

Fig. 7 Genotype and sex differences in lead-induced reduction of discrimination index over time. The discrimination index in the NOL test was calculated by dividing the difference in exploration time between the novel (**c**) and familiar (**a**) locations by the total exploration time, and used to compare changes of spatial memory over time. There was a main effect of lead exposure on the discrimination index in all lead-exposed animals (Multiple mixed-effects linear regression: ApoE3-KI females, $p = 0.001$; ApoE4-KI females, $p < 0.0001$; ApoE3-KI males, $p = 0.019$; ApoE4-KI males, $p < 0.0001$). **a** There was no difference in the discrimination index between control and lead-treated ApoE3-KI females during the lead exposure (Two-tailed *t*-test: 7 week, $p = 0.3046$; 11 week, $p = 0.9977$). Lead-treated ApoE3-KI females had a significantly lower discrimination index at 3 and 10 months post-lead exposure (3 months, $p = 0.0268$; 10 months, $p = 0.0156$) and a non-significant decrease 6 months post-lead ($p = 0.0901$) compared to controls. **b** Lead-treated ApoE4-KI females had a significantly lower discrimination index than ApoE4-KI control mice starting at 7 weeks into the lead exposure and this persisted through 10 months post-lead (7 weeks, $p = 0.0016$; 11 weeks, $p = 0.0002$; 3 months, $p = 0.0030$; 10 months, $p = 0.0269$). The lead-treated ApoE4-KI discrimination index was lower than controls at 6 months post-lead but not statistically significant ($p = 0.0713$). **c** Lead-treated ApoE3-KI males had a significantly lower discrimination index at 6 and 10 months post-lead compared to controls (6 months, $p = 0.0356$; 10 months, $p = 0.0418$). **d** In contrast, lead-treated ApoE4-KI males had a significantly lower discrimination index than controls starting at 11 weeks into the lead exposure and this effect persisted through 10 months post-lead exposure (11 weeks, $p = 0.0064$; 4 months, $p = 0.0433$; 6 months, $p = 0.0382$; 10 months, $p = 0.0275$). Data are mean ± SEM with n = 8–13 per sex/genotype/treatment. Multi-level mixed-effects linear regression; significant effect of treatment: # $p < 0.05$; ## $p < 0.01$; ### $p < 0.001$. Two-tailed *t*-test; significant difference between control and lead: n.s., not significant; * $p < 0.05$; ** $p < 0.01$; *** $p < 0.001$

deficits much earlier (starting at 11 weeks into the lead exposure vs. 6 months post-lead).

Together, data in Figs. 6 and 7 demonstrate that ApoE4-KI mice exposed to lead developed impaired spatial working memory much earlier than lead-treated ApoE3-KI mice, in both males and females. When we compare males and females of the same genotype, lead-induced spatial memory deficits manifested earlier in females than in males for both the ApoE3-KI and ApoE4-KI mice. These data suggest a GXE between lead exposure and ApoE4 on cognitive impairment as well as sex differences in the onset of cognitive deficits.

Lead-treated ApoE3-KI and ApoE4-KI mice do not exhibit significant pathology in the DG and other tissues

In order to determine if lead exposure causes systemic toxicity, we assessed for pathological changes in the liver and kidney of 64-week-old (~15-month-old) male and female ApoE3-KI and ApoE4-KI mice after various behavioral testing. There were no significant differences in kidney or liver pathology scores between control and lead-treated mice of either sex or genotype (Fig. 8a-d and data not shown). Furthermore, there were no changes in the volume of the DG of the hippocampus in ApoE3-KI or ApoE4-KI females upon lead exposure (Fig. 8e). In addition, we did not observe an increase in $TUNEL^+$ cells in the hippocampus or cortex of lead-treated animals (Fig. 9). Thus, the lead exposure regimen used in this study did not result in gross pathological changes in the DG, kidney, or liver.

Adult lead exposure results in elevated blood lead levels and lead deposition in the brain

We collected blood and brain tissue for lead analysis from the cellular cohort at sacrifice after the 12-week lead exposure. Lead exposure significantly raised blood lead levels in

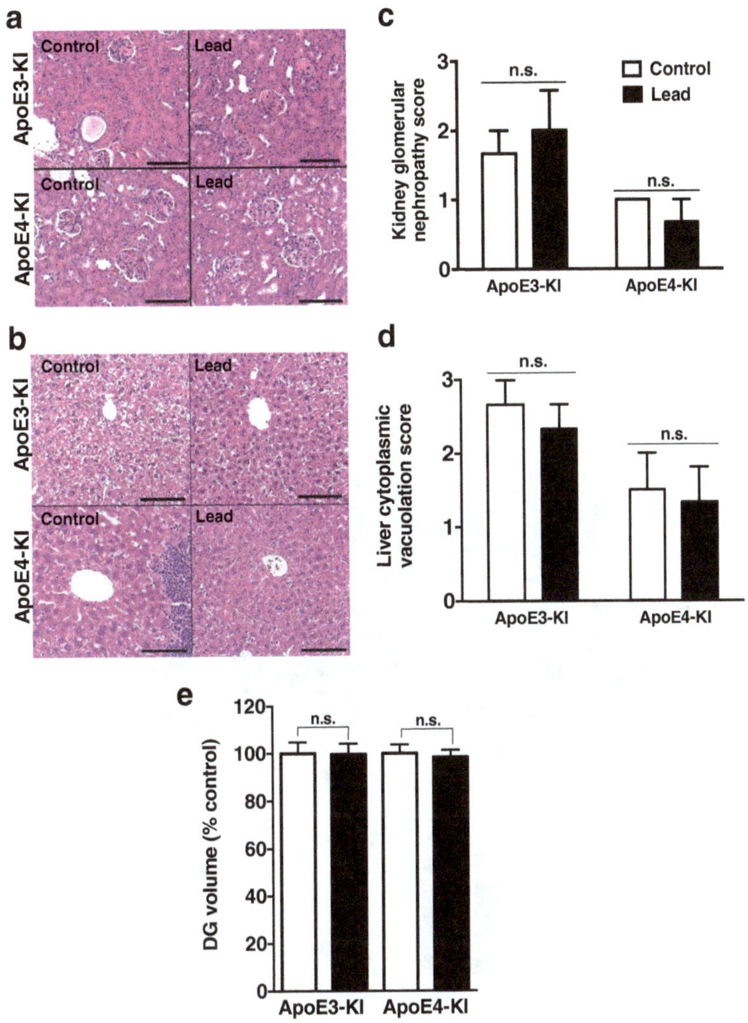

Fig. 8 Adult lead does not cause significant liver or kidney toxicity or DG volume loss in aged ApoE3-KI and ApoE4-KI mice. 8-week-old female ApoE3-KI and ApoE4-KI mice were exposed to 0.2% lead acetate for 12 weeks, then switched to normal drinking water and sacrificed 43–45 weeks post-lead exposure (14.5–15 months old). H&E staining of **a** kidney and **b** liver sections and quantification of **c** kidney glomerular nephropathy and **d** liver cytoplasmic vacuolation in female ApoE3-KI and ApoE4-KI mice. **e** DG volume was measured in female ApoE3-KI and ApoE4-KI mice using ImageJ analysis of confocal images of coronal sections from one brain hemisphere. Data are mean ± SEM. $n = 3$–5 per genotype/treatment. Two-way ANOVA with Fisher's LSD *post-test*: n.s., not significant. Scale bars, 100 μm

all animals relative to controls at the end of the 12 week exposure, and lead levels were higher in exposed females than males of the same genotype (Fig. 10a). Lead-exposed animals also had significantly higher brain lead levels relative to their controls at the end of the 12-week exposure, with the highest levels in ApoE4-KI female brains (Fig. 10b). Low-resolution LA-ICP-MS of sections from a control and a lead-treated female ApoE4-KI mouse illustrate that adult-only lead exposure is sufficient to cause increased lead deposition throughout the brain (Fig. 10c-f), while levels of the essential metal zinc (an internal control for the imaging and exposure) were not significantly different between control and lead-treated mice (data not shown).

Lead decreases proliferation of adult-born cells in the hippocampus in all lead-exposed mice

Adult hippocampal neurogenesis is the process whereby adult neural stem cells in the DG of the hippocampus generate adult-born neurons [31]. These adult-born neurons can influence hippocampus-dependent learning and memory [33, 34, 37, 55]. Interestingly, ApoE4 alters adult-born neuron differentiation and maturation in the DG of female ApoE4-KI mice [40]. Thus, we examined whether adult lead exposure inhibits adult neurogenesis in the hippocampus and whether there is a GXE between lead exposure and ApoE4 on this process using a second cohort (the cellular cohort) of mice.

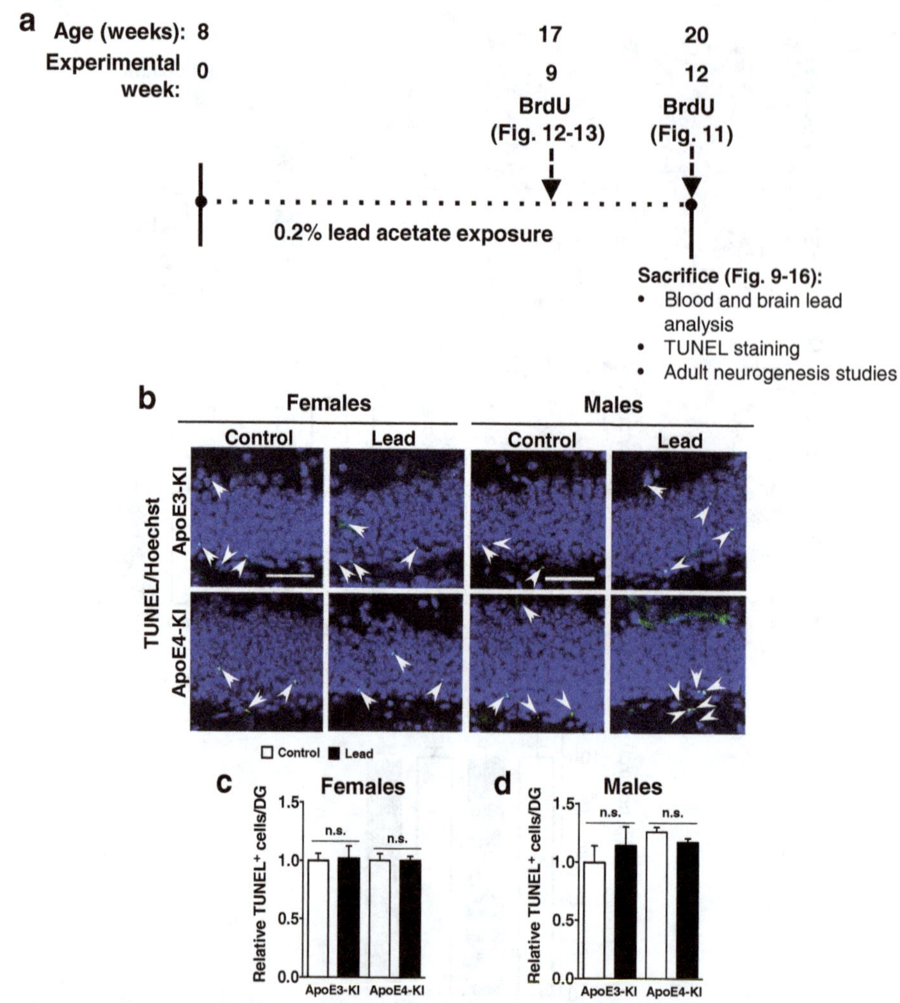

Fig. 9 Adult-only lead exposure does not increase the number of TUNEL$^+$ apoptotic cells in the DG of the hippocampus. **a** Experimental design and timeline for cellular studies (BrdU dosing) for Figs. 9, 10, 11, 12, 13, 14, 15 and 16. **b** Representative images of TUNEL$^+$ (green) cells in the DG of control and lead-treated ApoE3-KI and ApoE4-KI males and females. Quantification of TUNEL$^+$ cells per DG in ApoE3-KI and ApoE4-KI **c** females and **d** males. Data are mean ± SEM with $n = 3$–4 per genotype/sex/treatment. Two-way ANOVA with Fisher's LSD *post-test*: n.s., not significant. Scale bar, 50 μm

To determine if adult-only lead exposure is sufficient to impair cell proliferation during adult neurogenesis, we treated half of the cellular cohort of mice with BrdU 2 h prior to sacrifice at the end of the 12-week lead exposure in order to label actively proliferating cells in S-phase of the cell cycle (Fig. 11). We found that lead significantly reduced the total number of BrdU$^+$ cells in all lead-treated animals compared to their respective controls of the same genotype and sex (Fig. 11a-d). The percent change in BrdU$^+$ cells in lead-treated mice compared to control mice was not statistically significantly different between ApoE3-KI and ApoE4-KI mice, in either sex (Fig. 11e-f). These data suggest that adult-only lead exposure for 12 weeks is sufficient to significantly decrease adult-born cell proliferation in the DG of the hippocampus of all mice. Although this cellular mechanism does not explain the behavior differences observed between ApoE3-KI vs. ApoE4-KI mice, or between males and females, it may contribute to the eventual memory loss in all lead-exposed mice, such as that observed in the novel object location test.

Lead impairs adult-born neuron differentiation and decreases the dendritic complexity of immature neurons in the DG of female ApoE4-KI mice

We examined the effect of lead on neuronal differentiation of adult-born cells in the DG, using immunostaining for DCX and NeuN as markers of immature and mature neurons, respectively (Figs. 12a and 13a). BrdU was administered to the remaining half of the cellular cohort of mice at 9 weeks into the lead exposure (3 weeks prior to sacrifice) in order to label 3-week-old

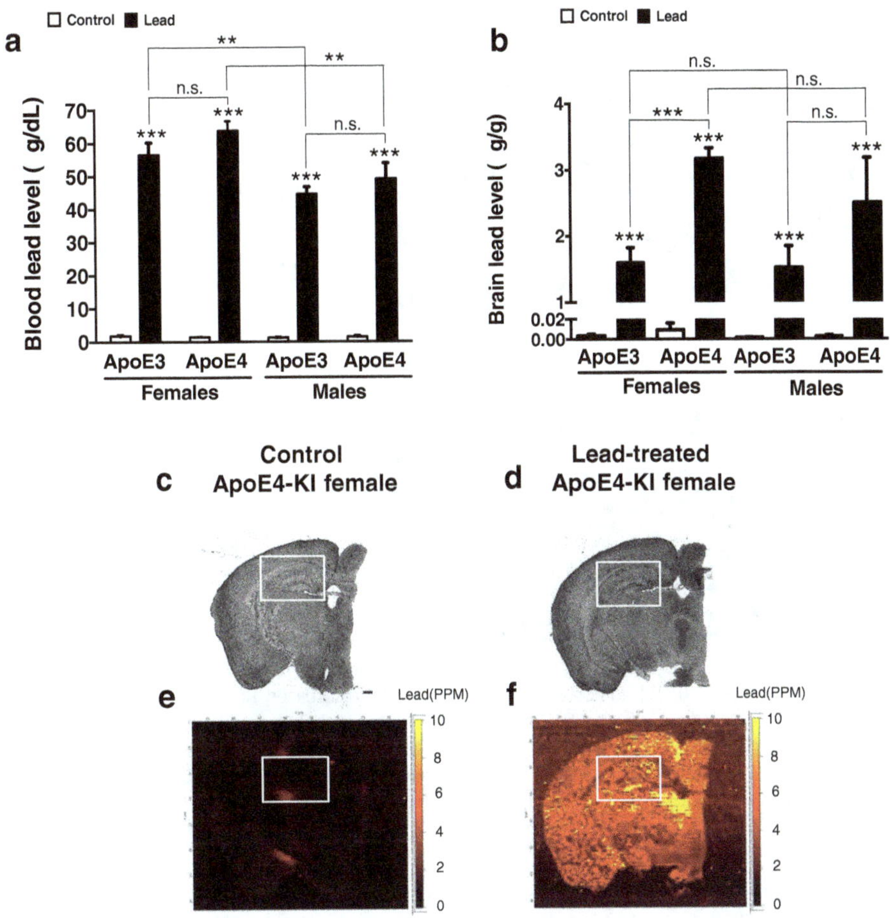

Fig. 10 Adult-only lead exposure results in elevated blood lead levels and lead deposition in the brain. 8-week-old ApoE3-KI and ApoE4-KI male and female mice were exposed to 0.2% lead acetate for 12 weeks and then sacrificed. Blood and one brain hemisphere were collected at sacrifice and (**a**) blood lead and (**b**) brain lead levels were measured using ICP-MS. Brightfield images of one brain hemisphere from a female (**c**) control and (**d**) lead-treated ApoE4-KI mouse after the 12 week lead exposure. Semi-quantitative measurement of lead in the brain of a (**e**) control and (**f**) lead-treated ApoE4-KI mouse using LA-ICP-MS. Two-way ANOVA with Fisher's LSD *post-test*: n.s., not significant; ** $p < 0.01$; *** $p < 0.001$. Scale bars, 100 μm

adult-born cells. Lead treatment significantly reduced the proportion of adult-born cells that express DCX ($BrdU^+DCX^+$/total $BrdU^+$) or NeuN ($BrdU^+NeuN^+$/total $BrdU^+$) in female ApoE4-KI mice, but not in other lead-treated mice (Fig. 12b-c, and Fig. 13b-c), suggesting that lead inhibits neuronal differentiation of adult-born neurons in the hippocampus and that female ApoE4-KI mice are more sensitive. There was also a statistically significant decrease in the number of total adult-born mature neurons ($BrdU^+NeuN^+$) in both male and female ApoE4-KI mice, although the effect was smaller in males than in females (Fig. 13d-e).

We also assessed the dendritic morphology, a measure of neuronal maturation, of adult-born neurons in this same cohort of mice. Because the acid treatment necessary for BrdU staining damages neuronal processes, we used DCX immunostaining alone to visualize neuronal processes of newly generated neurons (Fig. 14a-b, 15a-b). Neurite tracing and Sholl analysis showed that lead treatment significantly decreased the total dendritic length (Fig. 14c) and the number of dendritic crossings (Fig. 14e) in female ApoE4-KI mice. This effect was not seen in female ApoE3-KI mice (Fig. 14d) or any of the male mice (Fig. 15). These data suggest that ApoE4-KI females are more sensitive to the effects of lead on neuronal differentiation and maturation.

Lead reduces the number of GABAergic interneurons in the DG of ApoE4-KI female mice

GABAergic interneurons play an important role in adult hippocampal neurogenesis [56]. Previous studies report that ApoE4-KI female mice exhibit an age-dependent decrease in the number of GABAergic interneurons in the DG of the hippocampus, starting at 6 months of age [12, 14, 40]. Thus, we examined the effect of lead on the number of GABAergic neurons at the end of the 12-

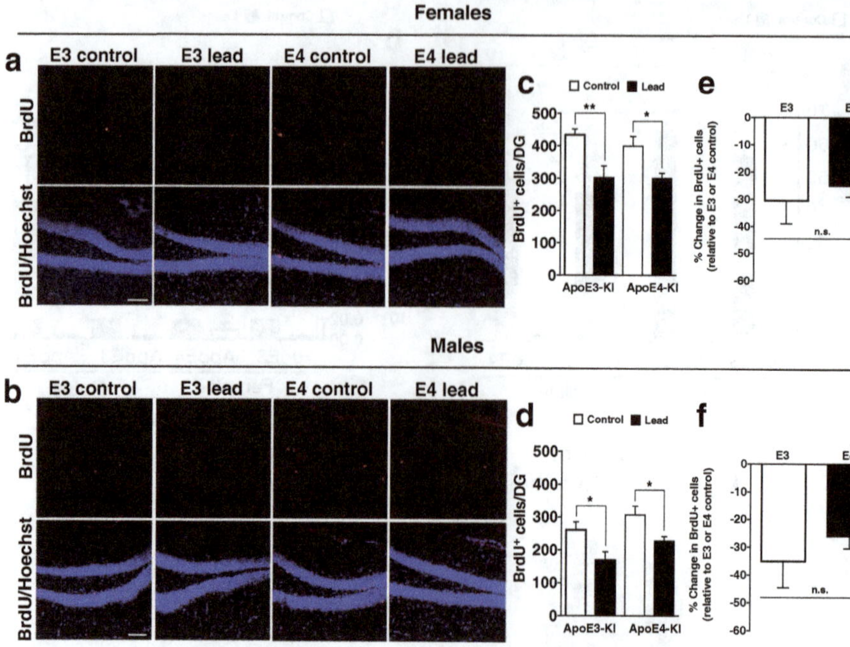

Fig. 11 Adult lead exposure decreases adult-born cell proliferation in the DG of the hippocampus of all mice. 8-week-old male and female ApoE3- and ApoE4-KI mice were exposed to 0.2% lead acetate for 12 weeks and then sacrificed. BrdU was administered 2 h prior to sacrifice (1 x 100 mg/kg). Representative images of BrdU (red) immunostaining in the DG of 20-week-old (**a**) female and (**b**) male ApoE3-KI and ApoE4-KI control and lead-treated mice. Quantification of the total BrdU+ cells per DG in (**c**) females and (**d**) males. Quantification of the percent change in total BrdU+ cells in lead-treated mice relative to ApoE3-KI or ApoE4-KI control (**e**) females and (**f**) males. Data are mean ± SEM with $n = 3$–5 per genotype/sex/treatment. Two-way ANOVA with Fisher's LSD *post-test*: n.s., not significant; * $p < 0.05$; ** $p < 0.01$. Scale bars, 100 μm

week lead exposure (20-weeks old) using GAD67 staining as a marker (Fig. 16a). There was no significant difference in the total number of GABAergic neurons between control ApoE3-KI and ApoE4-KI mice in either sex (Fig. 16b). However, lead treatment significantly decreased the number of $GAD67^{+}$ cells in the DG of ApoE4-KI females but not in other mice.

Discussion

AD currently affects nearly 35 million people and is projected to affect 117 million people worldwide by 2050 [57]. AD and cognitive decline are associated with significant societal, financial, and health care costs. Yet, there is a paucity of research on the role of environmental exposures and GXE on neurodegenerative disease risk and AD pathogenesis. Thus, additional investigation into how environmental factors and GXE may influence AD risk or accelerate cognitive decline is of immense public health importance.

Functional impairment in cognition is often used as a proxy to estimate the presence and degree of AD-associated neuropathology [58, 59]. Here, we used humanized transgenic knock-in mice as an animal model of human ApoE4 carriers to assess whether there is a GXE between lead and ApoE4 on cognitive behavior, and potentially on AD risk. ApoE3-KI and ApoE4-KI female mice develop spontaneous learning and memory deficits starting at 15–18 months [12–14]. Consequently, we assessed learning and memory prior to 15 months of age to determine if lead can accelerate the onset of cognitive behavior deficits. We defined a GXE as a different effect of lead exposure on cognitive behavior in mice expressing the human ApoE4 allele from those expressing the human ApoE3 allele. Based on this definition, we concluded that lead interacts with ApoE4 because we observed statistically significant deficits in contextual fear memory and spontaneous alternation in lead-treated ApoE4-KI female mice but not in other animals. In addition, lead causes an earlier onset of spatial working memory deficits in the NOL test in lead-treated ApoE4-KI mice compared to ApoE3-KI mice, for both males and females. Together, these data suggest that the effect of lead exposure on cognitive behavior is different depending on ApoE genotype. More specifically, a GXE between lead and ApoE4 may accelerate cognitive decline, contribute to a more rapid progression from cognitive aging to mild cognitive impairment, and potentially contribute to AD. Furthermore, females may be more susceptible to this GXE.

We found that lead exposure decreased spontaneous alternation in the T-maze in female ApoE4-KI animals. While alternation is not strictly hippocampus-dependent,

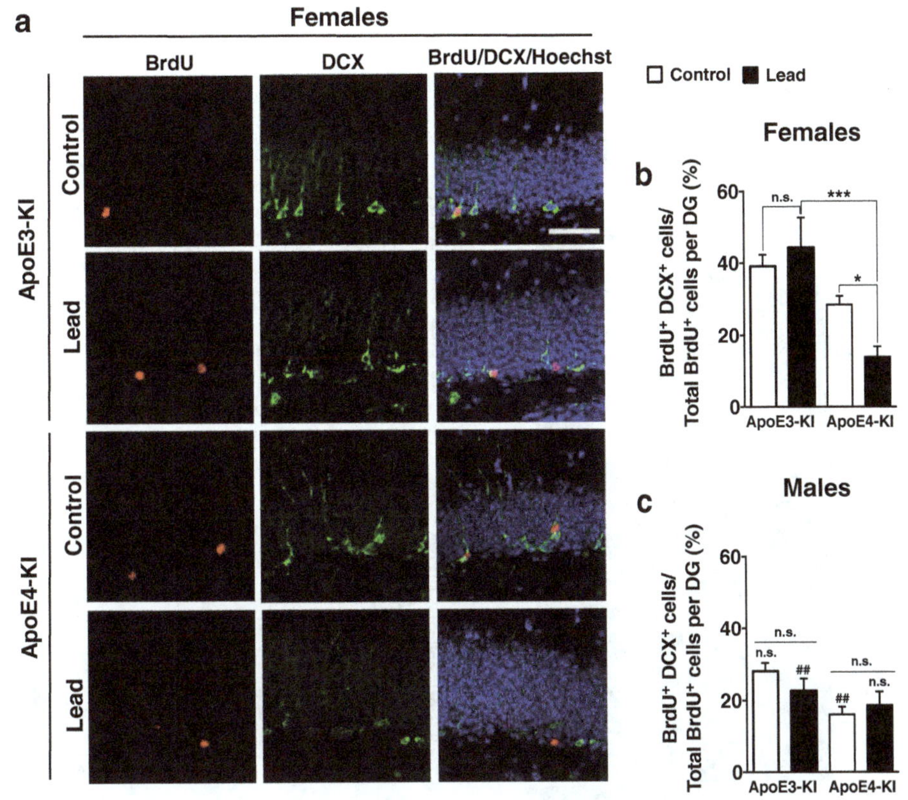

Fig. 12 Lead decreases adult-born immature neuron maturation in the DG of ApoE4-KI female mice. 8-week-old male and female ApoE3- and ApoE4-KI mice were exposed to 0.2% lead acetate for 12 weeks and then sacrificed. 100 mg/kg BrdU was administered 5 times in 1 day (every 2 h) 3 weeks prior to sacrifice (i.e., at 9 weeks into lead exposure). **a** Representative images of BrdU (red) and DCX (green) immunostaining in the DG of control and lead-treated female ApoE3-KI and ApoE4-KI animals. Quantification of the percent of total $BrdU^+$ cells that are $BrdU^+DCX^+$ per DG in females (**b**) and males (**c**) respectively. Data are mean ± SEM with $n = 4–5$ per genotype/sex/treatment. Two-way ANOVA with Fisher's LSD *post-test*: Comparison between control and lead-treated: n.s., not significant; * $p < 0.05$; *** $p < 0.001$. Comparison between males and females of the same genotype and treatment: n.s., not significant; ##, $p < 0.01$. Scale bar, 50 μm

alternation performance is very sensitive to hippocampal lesions [44, 54, 60]. More importantly, impaired alternation and/or repetitive arm entry has been reported in several different AD-mouse models, including models with presenilin and amyloid precursor protein mutations [61–64].

Lead exposure also impaired hippocampus-dependent spatial memory in the NOL test in all lead-treated animals. Interestingly, lead-exposed ApoE3-KI male mice developed memory loss in the NOL test at 6 months post-lead exposure. Moreover, the memory loss in all lead-exposed animals was persistent through 10 months post-lead. These data suggest that sub-chronic adult lead exposure alone is sufficient to cause long lasting or irreversible memory impairment, and that this behavior phenotype can occur long after exposure has ended. These findings are pertinent to human health because irreversible loss of memory formation is characteristic of AD, senile dementia, and up to 50% of Parkinson's disease cases [65]. Importantly, the aging population in the U.S. experienced high lead exposure in early life [66]. Thus, it is possible that lead exposure may lead to cognitive impairment later in life and contribute to cognitive decline associated with aging and neurodegeneration, such as late-onset AD.

Epidemiological reports suggest an increased risk of late-onset AD and increased cognitive decline with mild cognitive impairment in women [15, 16]. We observed that lead impaired contextual fear memory and working memory in the T-maze in female but not male ApoE4-KI mice. Furthermore, lead-induced spatial memory impairment in the NOL test manifested earlier in females than males for both ApoE3-KI and ApoE4-KI mice. These data provide strong evidence for sex differences in susceptibility to lead-induced cognitive decline in an animal model and suggest that women may be more susceptible to cognitive impairment and/or AD following exposure to toxicants such as lead.

We report average peak blood lead levels of 44.4–63.4 μg/dL, similar to previous animal studies and comparable to some occupational exposure settings in the 20th century [49, 67–69]. Elevated blood lead levels (≥10 μg/dL for adults) can still be encountered among U.S. workers,

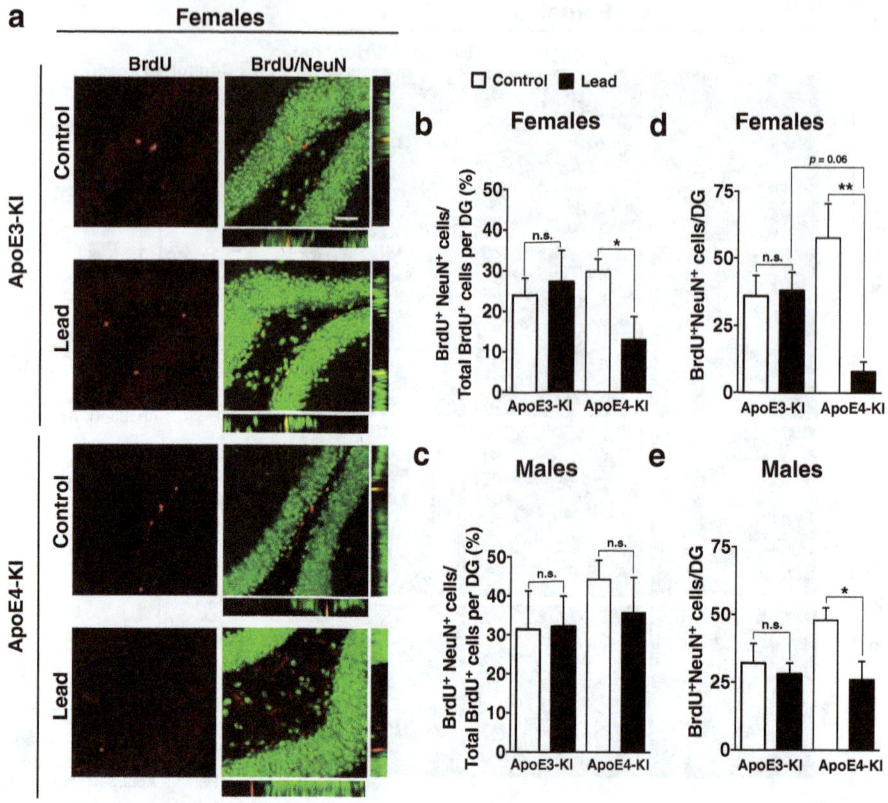

Fig. 13 Lead decreases adult-born neuron differentiation in the DG of ApoE4-KI female mice. 8-week-old male and female ApoE3-KI and ApoE4-KI mice were exposed to 0.2% lead acetate for 12 weeks and then sacrificed. 100 mg/kg BrdU was administered 5 times in 1 day (every 2 h) 3 weeks prior to sacrifice (i.e., at 9 weeks into lead exposure). **a** Representative images of BrdU (red) and NeuN (green) immunostaining in the DG of control and lead-treated female ApoE3-KI and ApoE4-KI animals. Quantification of the percent of total BrdU+ cells that are BrdU + NeuN+ per DG in **b** females and **c** males, respectively. Quantification of the total number of BrdU + NeuN+ cells in **d** females and **e** males, respectively. Data are mean ± SEM with $n = 4$–5 per genotype/sex/treatment. Two-way ANOVA with Fisher's LSD *post-test*: n.s., not significant; * $p < 0.05$; ** $p < 0.01$. Scale bar, 50 μm

and Occupational Safety & Health Administration regulations do not require U.S. workers to be removed from their job sites until they have a blood lead level ≥ 50 μg/dL. [70]. Importantly, high levels of lead exposure from environmental sources and in occupational settings are still a major concern in developing countries [18, 71]. Therefore, 0.2% lead acetate serves as an experimental model for occupational exposures globally, for environmental exposure in developing countries, and for the US population who were exposed to high levels of environmental lead prior to the ban of leaded gasoline and paint.

Brain and blood lead levels were highest in female ApoE4-KI mice. There were no differences in water consumption during the first week but water consumption thereafter was not monitored. Although we cannot formally exclude the possibility that ApoE4-KI females drank more water than other animals after the first week of lead exposure, there was no statistically significant difference between blood lead levels of female ApoE3-KI and ApoE4-KI mice. Thus, it seems unlikely that higher water consumption alone led to more lead deposition in the brain of female ApoE4-KI.

It is possible that the ApoE4-KI enhances lead deposition in the brain and differences in brain lead disposition may contribute to the GXE between ApoE4 and lead. Interestingly, ApoE4-KI mice exhibit decreased basement membrane thickness, reduced collagen and tight junction protein expression, as well as increased matrix metalloproteinase 9 activity in the blood-brain barrier, suggesting that more lead may accumulate in the brain of ApoE4-KI mice due to reduced blood-brain barrier integrity [72–74]. Furthermore, human ApoE4 carriers with AD also exhibit a thinner basement membrane, increased fibrin extravasion, and pericyte loss in the blood-brain barrier compared to ApoE3-KI carriers with AD or non-AD controls [75, 76]. Thus, effects of E4 on the blood-brain barrier may increase the accumulation of lead in the brain in ApoE4-KI mice or maybe even in humans, and contribute to more severe or earlier onset of learning and memory impairments.

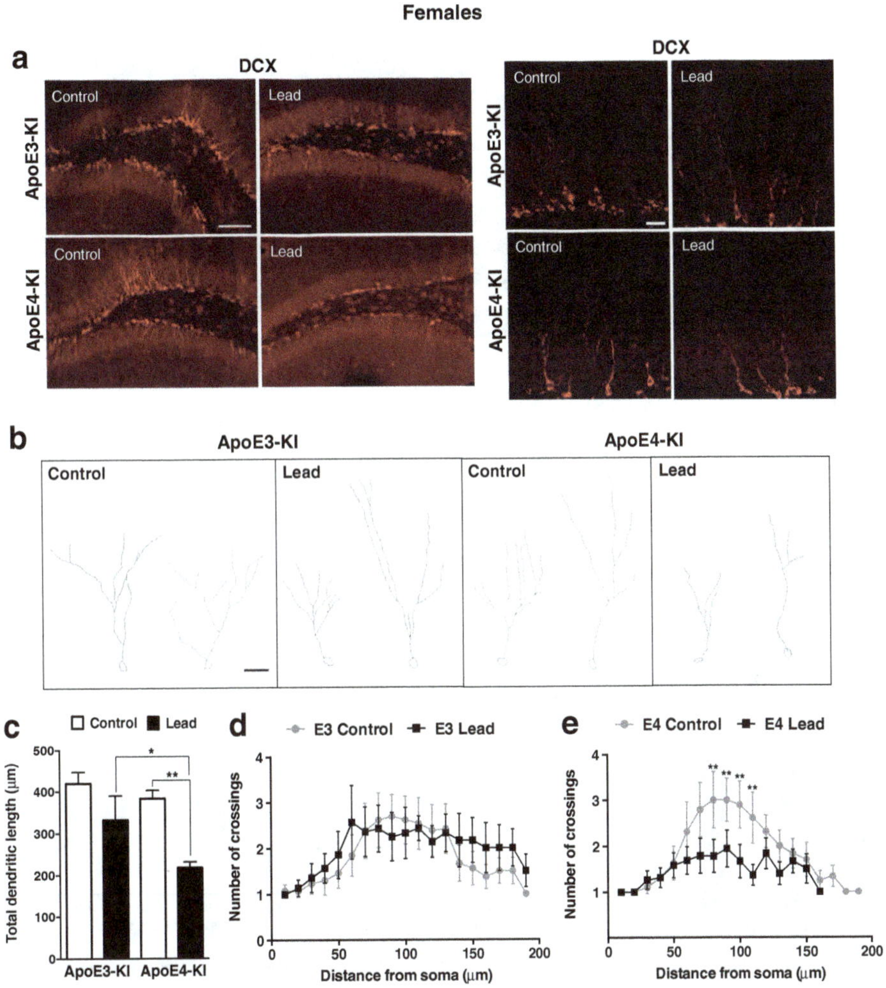

Fig. 14 Lead decreases the dendritic complexity of immature neurons in the DG of ApoE4-KI female mice. **a**, Representative confocal images of DCX (red) immunostaining in the DG of 20-week-old female ApoE3-KI and ApoE4-KI control and lead-treated mice (left scale bar, 100 μm; right scale bar, 25 μm). **b**, Representative examples of DCX+ neurons from female ApoE3-KI and ApoE4-KI control and lead-treated mice traced using the ImageJ Simple Neurite Tracer plug-in (scale bar, 25 μm). **c**, Quantification of the total dendritic length of DCX+ neurons in the DG. Sholl analysis of DCX+ neurons from (**d**) ApoE3-KI and (**e**) ApoE4-KI female mice. Data are mean ± SEM with $n = 4–5$ per genotype/treatment. Two-way ANOVA with Fisher's LSD *post-test* for analysis of total dendritic length; two-tailed *t-test* for within genotype comparisons of the number of crossings in control vs. lead-treated mice: * $p < 0.05$; ** $p < 0.01$

We previously found that lead can impair the survival, proliferation, and differentiation of adult neural precursor cells in vitro [41]. Thus, we sought to determine whether lead can interact with ApoE4 to impair adult hippocampal neurogenesis in vivo and whether this could be an underlying mechanism for the observed cognitive deficits. We exposed mice to lead starting at 8 weeks of age in order to avoid the cumulative effects of lead on both the developing and adult brain [77]. Unlike previous reports using the ApoE3-KI and ApoE4-KI models, we did not see a significant effect of ApoE4 alone on adult-born cell proliferation and maturation. This may be due to the fact that the effects of ApoE4 are age-dependent and we analyzed adult neurogenesis 1.5–2.5 months earlier (in 4.6-month-old vs. 6–7-month-old mice) than previous studies [12, 14, 40]. Data presented here demonstrate that adult lead exposure impairs adult-born cell proliferation in all lead-treated animals; this mechanism may contribute to lead impairment of spatial memory in the novel object location test that eventually develop in all lead-treated mice. Furthermore, lead exposure significantly impaired adult-born neuron differentiation and decreased dendritic complexity specifically in ApoE4-KI females. These cellular changes correlate with the fact that lead impairment of cognition is most pronounced in ApoE4-KI females. There was also a statistically significant reduction in the number of adult-born mature neurons ($BrdU^+NeuN^+$ cells) in male ApoE4-KI mice, although the reduction is smaller than that in females. This cellular change occurs at the end of the 12-week lead exposure and

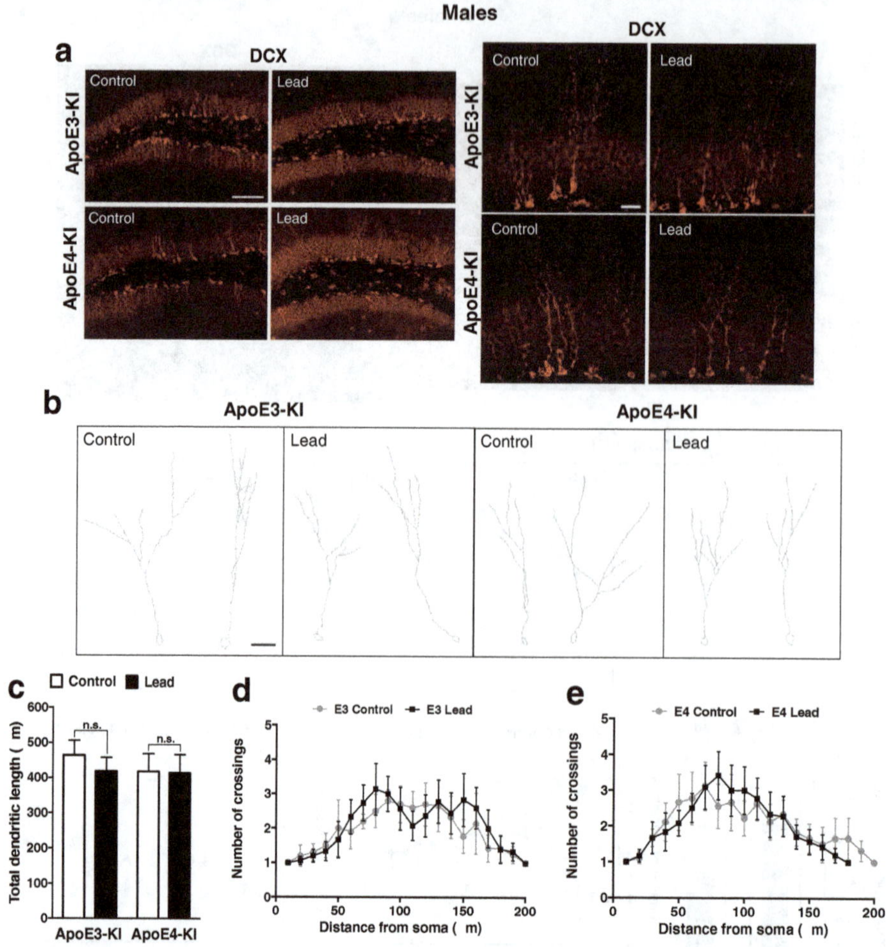

Fig. 15 Lead does not impair the dendritic complexity of immature neurons in the DG of male mice. **a**, Representative confocal images of DCX (red) immunostaining in the DG of 20-week-old male ApoE3-KI and ApoE4-KI control and lead-treated mice (left scale bar, 100 μm; right scale bar, 25 μm). **b**, Representative examples of DCX+ neurons from male ApoE3-KI and ApoE4-KI control and lead-treated mice traced using the ImageJ Simple Neurite Tracer plug-in (scale bar, 25 μm). **c**, Quantification of the total dendritic length of DCX+ neurons in the DG. Sholl analysis of DCX+ neurons from **d** ApoE3-KI and **e** ApoE4-KI male mice. Data are mean ± SEM with $n = 4$–5 per genotype/treatment. Two-way ANOVA with Fisher's LSD *post-test*: n.s., not significant

correlates with the onset of NOL deficits in the lead-treated ApoE4-KI males in the behavior cohort. Together, these data suggest that lead and ApoE4 may interact to perturb neuronal differentiation and maturation during adult hippocampal neurogenesis, and that this mechanism may contribute to the lead and ApoE4 interaction on accelerated cognitive impairment in ApoE4 mice and the heightened sensitivity of ApoE4 females.

The survival and integration of adult-born neurons is activity-dependent and occurs at approximately three weeks after neuronal birth [78, 79]. Several different cell types and inputs facilitate the survival and maturation of adult-born cells during this window, including GABAergic interneurons that may exert trophic effects on adult-born immature neuron survival and maturation [56, 80, 81]. Previous studies found that there are basal sex differences in the number of GAD67$^+$ interneurons in ApoE3-KI and ApoE4-KI mice, with female mice having significantly more GAD67$^+$ interneurons, and that female ApoE4-KI mice have significantly fewer GAD67$^+$ cells than ApoE3-KI mice starting at 6–7 months of age [40]. We found that lead significantly decreased the total number of GAD67$^+$ cells in 20-week-old, lead-treated ApoE4-KI females. This cellular effect correlates closely with our observation of significantly reduced adult-born neuron maturation and dendritic complexity in ApoE4-KI females, suggesting that an interaction between lead and ApoE4 may contribute to earlier impairment of GABAergic input and contribute to the observed impairment in immature neuron maturation in ApoE4-KI females.

Adult-born, immature neurons play a critical role in synaptic plasticity within the DG [79, 82, 83]. Notably, the increased responsiveness and excitability of newborn

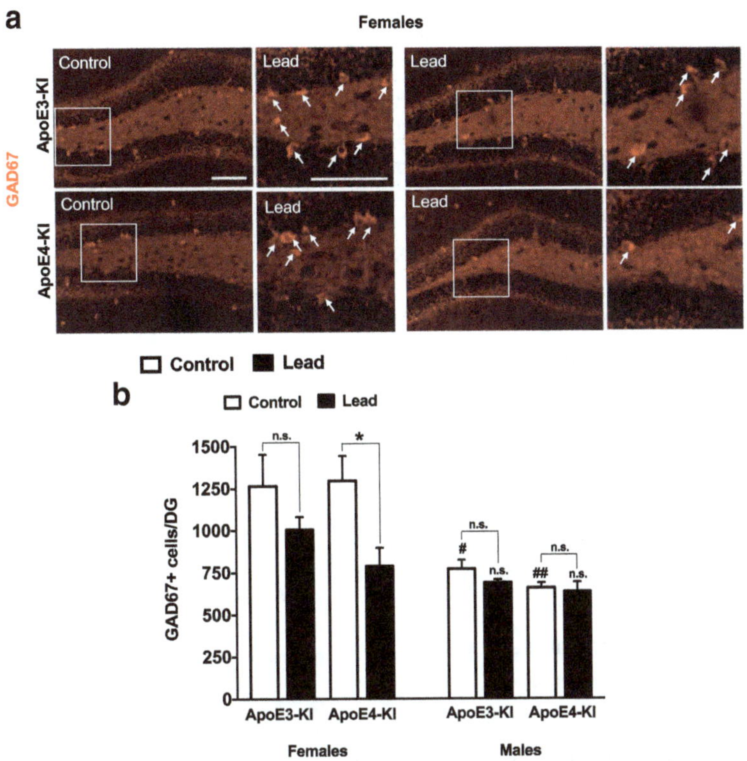

Fig. 16 Lead decreases the total number of GAD67+ GABAergic interneurons in 20-week-old female ApoE4-KI mice. 8-week-old male and female ApoE3-KI and ApoE4-KI mice were exposed to 0.2% lead acetate for 12 weeks and sacrificed. **a** Representative images of GAD67 (red) immunostaining in the DG of 20-week-old female ApoE3-KI and ApoE4-KI control and lead-treated mice. **b** Quantification of the total number of GAD67+ cells in the DG of 20-week-old ApoE3-KI and ApoE4-KI females and males. Data are mean ± SEM with $n = 3–5$ per genotype/treatment. Two-way ANOVA with Fisher's LSD *post-test*. Comparison between control and lead-treated: n.s., not significant; * $p < 0.05$. Comparison between males and females of the same genotype and treatment: n.s., not significant; #, $p < 0.05$; ##, $p < 0.01$. Scale bars, 100 μm

granule cells may give these adult-born cells a specific and significant role in learning and memory [55, 84]. In rats, a greater proportion of young, adult-born neurons are activated during spatial exploration compared to existing granule cells [85, 86]. Similarly, the selective loss of immature neurons impairs long-term spatial memory retention and contextual fear extinction [36]. Thus, the disruption of adult-born immature neuron maturation in lead-treated ApoE4-KI females may be associated with the impaired hippocampus-dependent learning and memory in these mice.

Although lead was deposited in the mouse brain broadly including the hippocampus and no regional specific deposition was found, we did not observe overt motor impairment. In humans, high levels of lead exposure can cause fine and gross motor impairments. However, lead exposure during development, which interferes with the proper development of the nervous system, likely plays a significant role in these cases. In the present study, mice were exposed to lead beginning at 8 weeks of age, eliminating the effect of lead on the developing nervous system. We only measured gross motor function (open field test), so we cannot rule out if lead exposure caused fine motor dysfunction. We did not observe a significant increase in TUNEL^{+} cells in the hippocampus or cortex of lead-treated animals. However, lead impaired adult neurogenesis in the hippocampus, with the greatest effect seen in female ApoE4-KI mice. Thus, newborn cells and neurons in the hippocampus, especially those in mice expressing human ApoE4 allele, may be more vulnerable than neurons in other regions of the brain to lead toxicity in the adult mice.

Similar to other studies that have reported basal sex differences in adult neurogenesis in these mice [14], we report baseline differences in the total number of adult-born cells (total BrdU^{+} cells), and the total number of GAD67^{+} cells in the DG between control males and females. However, we do not think these differences alter the conclusions of this study. For example, we found that all control mice performed equally well in tests for contextual fear memory, spontaneous alternation in the T-maze, and memory for novel object location (NOL). In addition, while ApoE3-KI and ApoE4-KI male mice had a lower number of BrdU^{+} and GAD67^{+} cells, they did not show statistically significant memory deficits after lead exposure when tested for contextual fear memory or spontaneous alternation in the T-maze. They also exhibited a later onset of deficits in the NOL test than their respective females of the same genotype. These data suggest that the lower basal adult neurogenesis in males does not affect their basal shot-term spatial and contextual memory, nor lead to higher sensitivity to lead impairment of cognition.

Conclusions

Although it has been hypothesized that exposure to environmental factors and a GXE interaction may increase AD risk, there is little direct evidence supporting this hypothesis. In this study, we found that adult lead exposure is sufficient to impair hippocampus-dependent learning and memory and that these deficits are more severe or occur earlier in female ApoE4-KI mice. These findings provide some of the first direct evidence for a GXE interaction between lead and ApoE4 on cognitive impairment. Furthermore, impaired adult hippocampal neurogenesis may be a potential mechanism underlying this GXE interaction. These results also provide new insight into how environmental toxicants and genetic risk factors may interact to contribute to cognitive decline and neurodegeneration in non-AD patients.

Abbreviations

AD: Alzheimer's disease; ApoE3-KI and ApoE4-KI: Apolipoprotein E3 or E4 knock-in mouse model; BrdU: 5-bromo-2'-deoxyuridine; DG: Dentate gyrus; GXE: Gene-environment interaction; H&E: Hematoxylin and eosin; iCP-MS: Inductively coupled mass spectrometry; NOL: Novel Object Location

Acknowledgements

We thank Mike Paulsen, Dr. Christopher Simpson, and the Environmental Health Laboratory at the University of Washington for providing LA-ICP-MS services. We thank Dr. Daniel Storm and members of the Xia laboratory for critically reading the manuscript and scientific discussions.

Funding

This work was supported by the National Institutes of Health (R01 MH95840 and ES026591 to Z.X., T32ES015459 to A.E.).

Authors' contributions

A.E. and Z.X. designed the research; A.E. performed the behavior and cellular experiments; J.S. performed histology and pathology experiments; N.M. contributed unpublished reagents/analytic tools; A.E. and Z.X. analyzed data; A.E., J.S., and Z.X. wrote the paper. All authors read and approved the final manuscript.

Competing interests

The authors declare that they have no competing interests.

Author details

[1]Toxicology Program, Department of Environmental and Occupational Health Sciences, University of Washington, Box 357234, Seattle, WA 98195, USA. [2]Department of Comparative Medicine, School of Medicine, University of Washington, Seattle, WA 98195, USA. [3]Department of Pathology and Laboratory Medicine, University of North Carolina, Chapel Hill, NC 27599, USA.

References

1. Ott A, Breteler MM, van Harskamp F, Claus JJ, van der Cammen TJ, Grobbee DE, Hofman A. Prevalence of Alzheimer's disease and vascular dementia: association with education. The Rotterdam study. BMJ. 1995;310(6985):970–3.
2. Wu JF, Basha R, Zawia NH. The environment, epigenetics and amyloidogenesis. Journal of Molecular Neuroscience. 2008;34(1):1–7.
3. Gatz M, Fratiglioni L, Johansson B, Berg S, Mortimer JA, Reynolds CA, Fiske A, Pedersen NL. Complete ascertainment of dementia in the Swedish Twin Registry: the HARMONY study. Neurobiol Aging. 2005;26(4):439–47.
4. Raiha I, Kaprio J, Koskenvuo M, Rajala T, Sourander L. Alzheimer's disease in twins. Biomed Pharmacother. 1997;51(3):101–4.
5. Ketelaar ME, Hofstra EM, Hayden MR. What monozygotic twins discordant for phenotype illustrate about mechanisms influencing genetic forms of neurodegeneration. Clin Genet. 2012;81(4):325–33.
6. Liu CC, Kanekiyo T, Xu HX, Bu GJ. Apolipoprotein E and Alzheimer disease: risk, mechanisms and therapy. Nature Reviews Neurology. 2013;9(2):106–18.
7. Mortensen EL, Hogh P. A gender difference in the association between APOE genotype and age-related cognitive decline. Neurology. 2001;57(1):89–95.
8. Cosentino S, Scarmeas N, Helzner E, Glymour MM, Brandt J, Albert M, Blacker D, Stern Y. APOE epsilon 4 allele predicts faster cognitive decline in mild Alzheimer disease. Neurology. 2008;70(19 Pt 2):1842–9.
9. Whitehair DC, Sherzai A, Emond J, Raman R, Aisen PS, Petersen RC, Fleisher AS, Alzheimer's Disease Cooperative S. Influence of apolipoprotein E varepsilon4 on rates of cognitive and functional decline in mild cognitive impairment. Alzheimers Dement. 2010;6(5):412–9.
10. Beydoun MA, Boueiz A, Abougergi MS, Kitner-Triolo MH, Beydoun HA, Resnick SM, O'Brien R, Zonderman AB. Sex differences in the association of the apolipoprotein E epsilon 4 allele with incidence of dementia, cognitive impairment, and decline. Neurobiol Aging. 2012;33(4):720–31. e724.
11. Blair CK, Folsom AR, Knopman DS, Bray MS, Mosley TH, Boerwinkle E, Atherosclerosis Risk in Communities Study I. APOE genotype and cognitive decline in a middle-aged cohort. Neurology. 2005;64(2):268–76.
12. Andrews-Zwilling Y, Bien-Ly N, Xu Q, Li G, Bernardo A, Yoon SY, Zwilling D, Yan TX, Chen LG, Huang YD. Apolipoprotein E4 Causes Age- and Tau-Dependent Impairment of GABAergic Interneurons, Leading to Learning and Memory Deficits in Mice. Journal Of Neuroscience. 2010;30(41):13707–17.
13. Bour A, Grootendorst J, Vogel E, Kelche C, Dodart JC, Bales K, Moreau PH, Sullivan PM, Mathis C. Middle-aged human apoE4 targeted-replacement mice show retention deficits on a wide range of spatial memory tasks. Behav Brain Res. 2008;193(2):174–82.
14. Leung L, Andrews-Zwilling Y, Yoon SY, Jain S, Ring K, Dai J, Wang MM, Tong L, Walker D, Huang YD. Apolipoprotein E4 Causes Age- and Sex-Dependent Impairments of Hilar GABAergic Interneurons and Learning and Memory Deficits in Mice. Plos One. 2012;7(12):18.
15. Fleisher A, Grundman M, Jack Jr CR, Petersen RC, Taylor C, Kim HT, Schiller DH, Bagwell V, Sencakova D, Weiner MF, et al. Sex, apolipoprotein E epsilon 4 status, and hippocampal volume in mild cognitive impairment. Arch Neurol. 2005;62(6):953–7.
16. Bretsky PM, Buckwalter JG, Seeman TE, Miller CA, Poirier J, Schellenberg GD, Finch CE, Henderson VW. Evidence for an interaction between apolipoprotein E genotype, gender, and Alzheimer disease. Alzheimer Dis Assoc Disord. 1999;13(4):216–21.
17. Cox DD, Gary; O; Haver, Robert; Salatino, Brendon: American Healthy Homes Survey: Lead and Arsenic Findings. In.: U.S. Department of Housing and Urban Development, Office of Healthy Homes and Lead Hazard Control; 2011.
18. Brosche S, Denney V, Weinberg J, Calonzo M, Withanage H, Clark S. Asia Regional Paint Report. In: IPEN. 2014. p. 3–34.
19. Willmsen C, Kamb Lewis, Mayo J. Loaded with lead. In: Seattle Times. Seattle, WA: Seattle Times; 2014.

20. Rabin R. The lead industry and lead water pipes "A Modest Campaign". Am J Public Health. 2008;98(9):1584–92.
21. Basha MR, Wei W, Bakheet SA, Benitez N, Siddiqi HK, Ge YW, Lahiri DK, Zawia NH. The fetal basis of amyloidogenesis: exposure to lead and latent overexpression of amyloid precursor protein and beta-amyloid in the aging brain. J Neurosci. 2005;25(4):823–9.
22. Stewart WF, Schwartz BS, Davatzikos C, Shen D, Liu D, Wu X, Todd AC, Shi W, Bassett S, Youssem D. Past adult lead exposure is linked to neurodegeneration measured by brain MRI. Neurology. 2006;66(10):1476–84.
23. Weisskopf MG, Wright RO, Schwartz J, Spiro 3rd A, Sparrow D, Aro A, Hu H. Cumulative lead exposure and prospective change in cognition among elderly men: the VA Normative Aging Study. Am J Epidemiol. 2004;160(12):1184–93.
24. Wu J, Basha MR, Brock B, Cox DP, Cardozo-Pelaez F, McPherson CA, Harry J, Rice DC, Maloney B, Chen D, et al. Alzheimer's disease (AD)-like pathology in aged monkeys after infantile exposure to environmental metal lead (Pb): evidence for a developmental origin and environmental link for AD. J Neurosci. 2008;28(1):3–9.
25. Bihaqi SW, Zawia NH. Enhanced taupathy and AD-like pathology in aged primate brains decades after infantile exposure to lead (Pb). Neurotoxicology. 2013;39:95–101.
26. Stewart WF, Schwartz BS, Simon D, Kelsey K, Todd AC. ApoE genotype, past adult lead exposure, and neurobehavioral function. Environ Health Perspect. 2002;110(5):501–5.
27. Buccione I, Perri R, Carlesimo GA, Fadda L, Serra L, Scalmana S, Caltagirone C. Cognitive and behavioural predictors of progression rates in Alzheimer's disease. Eur J Neurol. 2007;14(4):440–6.
28. Johnson DK, Storandt M, Morris JC, Galvin JE. Longitudinal study of the transition from healthy aging to Alzheimer disease. Arch Neurol. 2009;66(10):1254–9.
29. Weintraub S, Wicklund AH, Salmon DP. The neuropsychological profile of Alzheimer disease. Cold Spring Harb Perspect Med. 2012;2(4):a006171.
30. Lazarov O, Marr RA. Neurogenesis and Alzheimer's disease: at the crossroads. Exp Neurol. 2010;223(2):267–81.
31. Ming GL, Song H. Adult neurogenesis in the mammalian brain: significant answers and significant questions. Neuron. 2011;70:687–702.
32. Garthe A, Behr J, Kempermann G. Adult-generated hippocampal neurons allow the flexible use of spatially precise learning strategies. PLoS One. 2009;4:e5464.
33. Pan YW, Chan GCK, Kuo CT, Storm DR, Xia Z. Inhibition of Adult Neurogenesis by Inducible and Targeted Deletion of ERK5 Mitogen-Activated Protein Kinase Specifically in Adult Neurogenic Regions Impairs Contextual Fear Extinction and Remote Fear Memory. J Neurosci. 2012;32:6444–55.
34. Wang W, Pan YW, Zou J, Li T, Abel GM, Palmiter RD, Storm DR, Xia Z. Genetic Activation of ERK5 MAP Kinase Enhances Adult Neurogenesis and Extends Hippocampus-Dependent Long-Term Memory. J Neurosci. 2014; 34(6):2130–47.
35. Clelland CD, Choi M, Romberg C, Clemenson Jr GD, Fragniere A, Tyers P, Jessberger S, Saksida LM, Barker RA, Gage FH, et al. A functional role for adult hippocampal neurogenesis in spatial pattern separation. Science. 2009;325(5937):210–3.
36. Deng W, Saxe MD, Gallina IS, Gage FH. Adult-born hippocampal dentate granule cells undergoing maturation modulate learning and memory in the brain. J Neurosci. 2009;29:13532–42.
37. Pan YW, Storm DR, Xia Z. The maintenance of established remote contextual fear memory requires ERK5 MAP kinase and ongoing adult neurogenesis in the hippocampus. PLoS One. 2012;7(11):e50455.
38. Pan YW, Zou J, Wang W, Sakagami H, Garelick MG, Abel G, Kuo CT, Storm DR, Xia Z: Inducible and conditional deletion of extracellular signal-regulated kinase 5 disrupts adult hippocampal neurogenesis. *J Biol Chem* 2012, (in press).
39. Yang CP, Gilley JA, Zhang G, Kernie SG. ApoE is required for maintenance of the dentate gyrus neural progenitor pool. Development. 2011;138(20):4351–62.
40. Li G, Bien-Ly N, Andrews-Zwilling Y, Xu Q, Bernardo A, Ring K, Halabisky B, Deng CH, Mahley RW, Huang YD. GABAergic Interneuron Dysfunction Impairs Hippocampal Neurogenesis in Adult Apolipoprotein E4 Knockin Mice. Cell Stem Cell. 2009;5(6):634–45.
41. Engstrom A, Wang H, Xia Z. Lead decreases cell survival, proliferation, and neuronal differentiation of primary cultured adult neural precursor cells through activation of the JNK and p38 MAP kinases. Toxicol In Vitro. 2015;29(5):1146–55.
42. Xu PT, Schmechel D, Rothrock-Christian T, Burkhart DS, Qiu HL, Popko B, Sullivan P, Maeda N, Saunders AM, Roses AD, et al. Human apolipoprotein E2, E3, and E4 isoform-specific transgenic mice: human-like pattern of glial and neuronal immunoreactivity in central nervous system not observed in wild-type mice. Neurobiol Dis. 1996;3(3):229–45.
43. Shan Q, Chan GC, Storm DR. Type 1 adenylyl cyclase is essential for maintenance of remote contextual fear memory. J Neurosci. 2008;28(48):12864–7.
44. Spowart-Manning L, van der Staay FJ. The T-maze continuous alternation task for assessing the effects of putative cognition enhancers in the mouse. Behav Brain Res. 2004;151(1–2):37–46.
45. Sahay A, Scobie KN, Hill AS, O'Carroll CM, Kheirbek MA, Burghardt NS, Fenton AA, Dranovsky A, Hen R. Increasing adult hippocampal neurogenesis is sufficient to improve pattern separation. Nature. 2011;472:466–70.
46. Mabrouk A, Bel Hadj Salah I, Chaieb W, Ben Cheikh H. Protective effect of thymoquinone against lead-induced hepatic toxicity in rats. Environmental science and pollution research international. 2016;23(12):12206–15.
47. Bihaqi SW, Bahmani A, Subaiea GM, Zawia NH. Infantile exposure to lead and late-age cognitive decline: relevance to AD. Alzheimers Dement. 2014;10(2):187–95.
48. Masoud AM, Bihaqi SW, Machan JT, Zawia NH, Renehan WE. Early-Life Exposure to Lead (Pb) Alters the Expression of microRNA that Target Proteins Associated with Alzheimer's Disease. J Alzheimers Dis. 2016;51(4):1257–64.
49. Dosunmu R, Alashwal H, Zawia NH. Genome-wide expression and methylation profiling in the aged rodent brain due to early-life Pb exposure and its relevance to aging. Mechanisms of ageing and development. 2012;133(6):435–43.
50. Patkova J, Vojtisek M, Tuma J, Vozeh F, Knotkova J, Santorova P, Wilhelm J. Evaluation of lipofuscin-like pigments as an index of lead-induced oxidative damage in the brain. Exp Toxicol Pathol. 2012;64(1–2):51–6.
51. Yu H, Li T, Cui Y, Liao Y, Wang G, Gao L, Zhao F, Jin Y. Effects of lead exposure on D-serine metabolism in the hippocampus of mice at the early developmental stages. Toxicology. 2014;325:189–99.
52. Liu F, Xue Z, Li N, Huang H, Ying Y, Li J, Wang L, Li W. Effects of lead exposure on the expression of amyloid beta and phosphorylated tau proteins in the C57BL/6 mouse hippocampus at different life stages. Journal of trace elements in medicine and biology : organ of the Society for Minerals and Trace Elements. 2014;28(2):227–32.
53. Walf AA, Frye CA. The use of the elevated plus maze as an assay of anxiety-related behavior in rodents. Nat Protoc. 2007;2(2):322–8.
54. Gerlai R. A new continuous alternation task in T-maze detects hippocampal dysfunction in mice. A strain comparison and lesion study. Behav Brain Res. 1998;95(1):91–101.
55. Deng W, Aimone JB, Gage FH. New neurons and new memories: how does adult hippocampal neurogenesis affect learning and memory? Nat Rev Neurosci. 2010;11:339–50.
56. Tozuka Y, Fukuda S, Namba T, Seki T, Hisatsune T. GABAergic excitation promotes neuronal differentiation in adult hippocampal progenitor cells. Neuron. 2005;47:803–15.
57. Qiu C, Kivipelto M, von Strauss E. Epidemiology of Alzheimer's disease: occurrence, determinants, and strategies toward intervention. Dialogues Clin Neurosci. 2009;11(2):111–28.
58. Jones RN, Manly J, Glymour MM, Rentz DM, Jefferson AL, Stern Y. Conceptual and measurement challenges in research on cognitive reserve. J Int Neuropsychol Soc. 2011;17(4):593–601.
59. Yassa MA, Lacy JW, Stark SM, Albert MS, Gallagher M, Stark CE. Pattern separation deficits associated with increased hippocampal CA3 and dentate gyrus activity in nondemented older adults. Hippocampus. 2011;21(9):968–79.
60. Dudchenko PA. An overview of the tasks used to test working memory in rodents. Neurosci Biobehav Rev. 2004;28(7):699–709.
61. Holcomb L, Gordon MN, McGowan E, Yu X, Benkovic S, Jantzen P, Wright K, Saad I, Mueller R, Morgan D, et al. Accelerated Alzheimer-type phenotype in transgenic mice carrying both mutant amyloid precursor protein and presenilin 1 transgenes. Nat Med. 1998;4(1):97–100.
62. Arendash GW, King DL, Gordon MN, Morgan D, Hatcher JM, Hope CE, Diamond DM. Progressive, age-related behavioral impairments in transgenic mice carrying both mutant amyloid precursor protein and presenilin-1 transgenes. Brain Res. 2001;891(1–2):42–53.
63. Laursen B, Mork A, Plath N, Kristiansen U, Bastlund JF. Impaired hippocampal acetylcholine release parallels spatial memory deficits in Tg2576 mice subjected to basal forebrain cholinergic degeneration. Brain Res. 2014;1543:253–62.
64. Holcomb LA, Gordon MN, Jantzen P, Hsiao K, Duff K, Morgan D. Behavioral changes in transgenic mice expressing both amyloid precursor protein and presenilin-1 mutations: lack of association with amyloid deposits. Behav Genet. 1999;29(3):177–85.

65. Arnaldi D, Campus C, Ferrara M, Fama F, Picco A, De Carli F, Accardo J, Brugnolo A, Sambuceti G, Morbelli S, et al. What predicts cognitive decline in de novo Parkinson's disease? Neurobiol Aging. 2012;33(6):1127. e1111-1120.
66. ATSDR. Toxicological profile for lead. Atlanta, GA, US: U.S. Department of Health and Human Services, Public Health Serivce, Agency for Toxic Substances and Disease Registry; 2007.
67. Mantere P, Hanninen H, Hernberg S. Subclinical neurotoxic lead effects: two-year follow-up studies with psychological test methods. Neurobehav Toxicol Teratol. 1982;4(6):725–7.
68. Williamson AM, Teo RK. Neurobehavioural effects of occupational exposure to lead. British journal of industrial medicine. 1986;43(6):374–80.
69. Lucchini R, Albini E, Cortesi I, Placidi D, Bergamaschi E, Traversa F, Alessio L. Assessment of neurobehavioral performance as a function of current and cumulative occupational lead exposure. Neurotoxicology. 2000;21(5):805–11.
70. OSHA: 2005d. Toxic and Hazardous Substances. Occupational safety and health standards. Washington, DC: Occupational Safety and Health Administration. Code of Federal Regulations. 29 CFR 1910.1025. In.; March 25, 2005.
71. Ilyas F. City air heavily polluted with lead, cadmium, and CO. In: DAWNcom. 2014.
72. Tai LM, Thomas R, Marottoli FM, Koster KP, Kanekiyo T, Morris AW, Bu G. The role of APOE in cerebrovascular dysfunction. Acta Neuropathol. 2016;131(5): 709–23.
73. Alata W, Ye Y, St-Amour I, Vandal M, Calon F. Human apolipoprotein E varepsilon4 expression impairs cerebral vascularization and blood-brain barrier function in mice. J Cereb Blood Flow Metab. 2015;35(1):86–94.
74. Bell RD, Winkler EA, Singh I, Sagare AP, Deane R, Wu Z, Holtzman DM, Betsholtz C, Armulik A, Sallstrom J, et al. Apolipoprotein E controls cerebrovascular integrity via cyclophilin A. Nature. 2012;485(7399):512–6.
75. Salloway S, Gur T, Berzin T, Tavares R, Zipser B, Correia S, Hovanesian V, Fallon J, Kuo-Leblanc V, Glass D, et al. Effect of APOE genotype on microvascular basement membrane in Alzheimer's disease. J Neurol Sci. 2002;203–204:183–7.
76. Halliday MR, Rege SV, Ma Q, Zhao Z, Miller CA, Winkler EA, Zlokovic BV. Accelerated pericyte degeneration and blood-brain barrier breakdown in apolipoprotein E4 carriers with Alzheimer's disease. Journal of Cerebral Blood Flow and Metabolism. 2016;36(1):216–27.
77. Bayer SA, Altman J, Russo RJ, Zhang X. Timetables of neurogenesis in the human brain based on experimentally determined patterns in the rat. Neurotoxicology. 1993;14(1):83–144.
78. Tashiro A, Sandler VM, Toni N, Zhao C, Gage FH. NMDA-receptor-mediated, cell-specific integration of new neurons in adult dentate gyrus. Nature. 2006;442:929–33.
79. Marin-Burgin A, Schinder AF. Requirement of adult-born neurons for hippocampus-dependent learning. Behav Brain Res. 2012;227(2):391–9.
80. Ge S, Goh EL, Sailor KA, Kitabatake Y, Ming GL, Song H. GABA regulates synaptic integration of newly generated neurons in the adult brain. Nature. 2006;439:589–93.
81. Kim WR, Christian K, Ming GL, Song H. Time-dependent involvement of adult-born dentate granule cells in behavior. Behav Brain Res. 2012; 227(2):470–9.
82. Snyder JS, Kee N, Wojtowicz JM. Effects of adult neurogenesis on synaptic plasticity in the rat dentate gyrus. J Neurophysiol. 2001;85:2423–31.
83. Esposito MS, Piatti VC, Laplagne DA, Morgenstern NA, Ferrari CC, Pitossi FJ, Schinder AF. Neuronal differentiation in the adult hippocampus recapitulates embryonic development. J Neurosci. 2005;25:10074–86.
84. Pan YW, Storm DR, Xia Z. Role of adult neurogenesis in hippocampus-dependent memory, contextual fear extinction and remote contextual memory: new insights from ERK5 MAP kinase. Neurobiol Learn Mem. 2013;105:81–92.
85. Ramirez-Amaya V, Marrone DF, Gage FH, Worley PF, Barnes CA. Integration of new neurons into functional neural networks. J Neurosci. 2006;26:12237–41.
86. Sandoval CJ, Martinez-Claros M, Bello-Medina PC, Perez O, Ramirez-Amaya V. When are new hippocampal neurons, born in the adult brain, integrated into the network that processes spatial information? PLoS One. 2011;6(3): e17689.

7

Predominant expression of Alzheimer's disease-associated BIN1 in mature oligodendrocytes and localization to white matter tracts

Pierre De Rossi[1†], Virginie Buggia-Prévot[1†], Benjamin L. L. Clayton[2], Jared B. Vasquez[3], Carson van Sanford[3], Robert J. Andrew[1], Ruben Lesnick[1], Alexandra Botté[1], Carole Deyts[1], Someya Salem[1], Eshaan Rao[1], Richard C. Rice[1], Angèle Parent[1], Satyabrata Kar[4], Brian Popko[2], Peter Pytel[5], Steven Estus[3] and Gopal Thinakaran[1,2,5*]

Abstract

Background: Genome-wide association studies have identified *BIN1* within the second most significant susceptibility locus in late-onset Alzheimer's disease (AD). *BIN1* undergoes complex alternative splicing to generate multiple isoforms with diverse functions in multiple cellular processes including endocytosis and membrane remodeling. An increase in *BIN1* expression in AD and an interaction between BIN1 and Tau have been reported. However, disparate descriptions of BIN1 expression and localization in the brain previously reported in the literature and the lack of clarity on brain BIN1 isoforms present formidable challenges to our understanding of how genetic variants in *BIN1* increase the risk for AD.

Methods: In this study, we analyzed BIN1 mRNA and protein levels in human brain samples from individuals with or without AD. In addition, we characterized the BIN1 expression and isoform diversity in human and rodent tissue by immunohistochemistry and immunoblotting using a panel of BIN1 antibodies.

Results: Here, we report on BIN1 isoform diversity in the human brain and document alterations in the levels of select BIN1 isoforms in individuals with AD. In addition, we report striking BIN1 localization to white matter tracts in rodent and the human brain, and document that the large majority of BIN1 is expressed in mature oligodendrocytes whereas neuronal BIN1 represents a minor fraction. This predominant non-neuronal BIN1 localization contrasts with the strict neuronal expression and presynaptic localization of the BIN1 paralog, Amphiphysin 1. We also observe upregulation of BIN1 at the onset of postnatal myelination in the brain and during differentiation of cultured oligodendrocytes. Finally, we document that the loss of BIN1 significantly correlates with the extent of demyelination in multiple sclerosis lesions.

Conclusion: Our study provides new insights into the brain distribution and cellular expression of an important risk factor associated with late-onset AD. We propose that efforts to define how genetic variants in *BIN1* elevate the risk for AD would behoove to consider BIN1 function in the context of its main expression in mature oligodendrocytes and the potential for a role of BIN1 in the membrane remodeling that accompanies the process of myelination.

Keywords: Alzheimer's disease, Oligodendrocyte, BIN1, Amphiphysin 1, Multiple sclerosis, Late-onset Alzheimer's disease, Isoform diversity, Alternative splicing, Myelination, Immunohistochemistry

* Correspondence: gopal@uchicago.edu
†Equal contributors
[1]Department of Neurobiology, The University of Chicago, JFK R212, 924 East 57th Street, Chicago, IL 60637, USA
[2]Department of Neurology, The University of Chicago, Chicago, IL 60637, USA
Full list of author information is available at the end of the article

Background

The *B*ridging *IN*tegrator-1 (BIN1; also referred to as amphiphysin II and SH3P9) is a member of the Bin/Amphiphysin/Rvs (BAR) family of adaptor proteins that regulates membrane dynamics in a variety of cellular functions [1]. BIN1 was first identified as a protein that interacted with the N-terminus of the MYC oncoprotein [2], and cloned based on sequence similarity to Amphiphysin 1, a protein predominantly expressed in the brain [3–8]. Based on sequence similarity to Amphiphysin 1, it has been proposed that BIN1 might function in synaptic vesicle endocytosis [9]. However, neuronal cultures prepared from *Bin1*$^{-/-}$ mice failed to reveal a deficiency in basal synaptic vesicle uptake [10], raising the possibility that BIN1 and Amphiphysin 1 may have divergent functions in the brain. Unlike its close paralog Amphiphysin 1, BIN1 is broadly expressed in several tissues, with the highest expression in skeletal muscle [2, 4, 6, 11]. Alternate splicing of the 20 exons in *BIN1* gene generates at least 10 transcripts encoding ubiquitous and tissue-specific isoforms, which differ not only in their tissue distribution but also in subcellular localization and cellular function [2, 4–6, 12, 13].

All isoforms of BIN1 contain an N-terminal BAR domain, which functions in sensing and generating membrane curvature and is critical for BIN1 function in membrane tubulation and budding/vesicle formation. A C-terminal SH3 domain, also found in all isoforms, mediates BIN1 interaction with proteins involved in endocytosis, such as dynamin, synaptojanin, and endophilin [1, 4–6, 14]. The CLathrin-Associated Protein binding region (CLAP domain), encoded by alternatively spliced exons present only in the neuronal BIN1 isoforms, is important for BIN1's function in clathrin-mediated endocytosis and synaptic vesicle recycling [1, 9]. Crystal structure and functional studies predicted that the BIN1 CLAP domain is critical to recruiting dynamin and regulate its self-assembly at the clathrin-coated pit [15]. Moreover, the residues encoded by the alternatively spliced exon 7 within the BAR domain promotes BIN1 interaction with dynamin 2 [16, 17]. In addition to proteins involved in endocytosis, the BIN1 SH3 domain can interact with a number of other proteins including the tyrosine kinase c-Abl, the actin nucleation-promoting factor N-WASP, actin, myosin, and Tau, suggesting the involvement of the cytoskeleton in BIN1 function [18–21].

Very little is known about BIN1 expression in the brain. The identification of polymorphisms upstream of *BIN1* that act as a major genetic risk factor for late-onset AD has stimulated an interest in understanding BIN1's role in the central nervous system [22–24]. It is notable that *BIN1* is ranked in the AlzGene database as the second most statistically significant AD susceptibility gene based on a meta-analysis [25]. In vitro assays and analysis of mutant flies lacking the expression of the *Drosophila* BIN1 ortholog *Amphiphysin* have suggested that BIN1 modifies AD risk through Tau pathology [26] or β-amyloid production [27] and studies have reported altered expression of BIN1 in Alzheimer Disease, albeit with discrepancies [26, 28–31]. Nevertheless, since functional BIN1 variants are yet to be identified, the precise link between *BIN1* and the susceptibility to AD remains elusive. A survey of the published literature reveals conflicting information on the cellular and subcellular localization of BIN1 in the brain. Previous studies have described the presence of BIN1 in apical dendrites, initial axon segments, along the axons, nerve terminals, or the nodes of Ranvier [4, 26, 30]. Although it has been generally assumed that BIN1 is mainly expressed in neurons, *Bin1* was found among the top 50 highly expressed genes in cultured oligodendrocytes by genomic analysis [32]. A precise description of its expression and localization in the nervous system is a prerequisite for understanding BIN1 function and dysfunction in the brain. Here, we report the prominent non-neuronal expression of BIN1 in mouse and the human brain, which contrasts with neuronal expression of Amphiphysin 1. We detail BIN1 expression in mature oligodendrocytes and its enrichment in the white matter and characterize BIN1 isoform diversity in the gray and white matter of individuals with and without AD. The upregulation of BIN1 during in vitro oligodendrocyte maturation and the period of myelination in vivo, and the loss of BIN1 within brain lesions of patients with multiple sclerosis are all consistent and point to a potential role for BIN1 in mature oligodendrocytes in the brain.

Methods

Human autopsy tissue

The RNA analyses were performed on human anterior cingulate brain tissue samples, which were supplied by the University of Kentucky AD Center Neuropathology Core. These samples have been previously described [33–35]. Evaluation of AD status was conducted by the AD Center Neuropathology and Clinical Cores using guidelines set forth by the National Institute on Aging Reagan Institute that included evaluation of neurofibrillary tangles and neuritic senile plaques [36–38]. Age at death for the cognitively intact, i.e. non-AD donors, was 82.3 ± 8.6 (mean ± SD, $n = 29$) while AD donors were 81.7 ± 6.3 (mean ± SD, $n = 28$). The post-mortem interval for non-AD and AD donors was 2.8 ± 0.9 and 3.4 ± 0.6 h, respectively. The samples used for immunoblotting and immunohistochemistry were obtained from the University of Chicago autopsy archives and NIH Neurobiobank (Table 1).

Primary cultures

Greater than 95% pure cultures of rat oligodendrocyte progenitor cells (OPCs) were isolated from cortices of

Table 1 List of human samples used for immunohistochemistry and immunoblot analysis[a]

Patient ID	Disease	Age	Gender	PMI (h)
10152	Control	68	F	19
121405	Control	76	M	22
61220	Control	70	F	18
91412	Control	76	M	8
41524	Control	79	F	14
41522	Control	44	M	40
15109	Control	68	F	13
51501	Control	59	F	23
4320	Control	87	F	9
4064	Control	75	F	15
4294	Control	80	M	19
4307	Control	84	M	12
4308	Control	70	M	12
121115	MS	66	F	24
90712	MS	69	M	22
120213	MS	53	F	25
10618	MS	38	F	24
40317	MS	75	F	23
71202	AD; Braak 5	88	F	40
101208	AD; Braak 5	93	F	41
4279	AD Braak 5	76	M	14
4313	AD Braak 5	66	F	16
4414	AD Braak 5	69	F	15
4454	AD Braak 2-3	82	M	9
4466	AD Braak 5	81	M	16

[a]AD ($n = 29$) and non-AD ($n = 28$) human samples used for qPCR analysis have been previously described (Cited Ref: [19, 32, 68])
PMI post mortem interval

6–7 day old pups as described by sequential immunopanning on dishes coated with antibodies against Ran-2, GalC, and O4 [39]. Ran-2$^-$, GalC$^-$, O4$^+$ OPCs were cultured in medium supplemented with the mitogen PDGFα (Peprotech). Mature oligodendrocytes were generated by differentiating OPCs in medium containing the hormone 3-3'-5-Triiodo-L-thyronine (Sigma). Primary rat hippocampal neurons and astrocytes were cultured as described [40].

Analysis of gene expression

The expression levels of *BIN1* isoforms that lack exon 7 (Delta-7-BIN1 (D7-BIN1) or include exon 7 (BIN1 + Ex7) were determined by quantitative polymerase chain reactions (qPCR). The primers for BIN1 + Ex7 were: exon 5 sense 5'-CCTGCTGTGGATGGATTACC-3' and exon 7 antisense 5'-GCTTTCTCAAGCAGCGAGAC-3'. D7-BIN1 reactions used the same exon 5 sense primer and a junctional antisense primer, 5'-GCTTTCTCAAGCAGC GAGAC-3', corresponding to the last 6 nucleotides of exon 6 and the first 11 nucleotides of exon 8. Each 20 μL reaction mixture contained 20 ng of cDNA, 1 μM of each primer, and 2X SYBR Green (Quanta Biosciences) and was subjected to a PCR profile of 40 cycles at 95 °C for 15 sec, 60 °C for 30 sec, and 72 °C for 20 sec. A melting curve was performed after each qPCR run to ensure specific amplification. The *BIN1* isoform copy number in samples was determined by using a standard curve generated in parallel. Copy numbers were normalized to the geometric mean of reference genes *EIF4H* and *RPL32*. Levels of cell type-specific genes were determined similarly. Primer sequences for microglial and endothelial cells were reported previously [41, 42]. Additional primer sequences were as follows: *SYP* (synaptophysin), 5'-AGG GAACACATGCAAGGAG-3' and 5'-CCTTAAACACGA ACCACAGG-3'; *MBP*, 5'-AAGGCCAGAGACCAGGAT TT-3', and 5'-TAGCCATGGGTGATCCAGA-3'; *GFAP* 5'-AAGAGATCCGCACGCAGTAT-3' and 5'-GTAGTCGT TGGCTTCGTGCT-3'. Assays were repeated at least two times. The extent that *BIN1* mRNA levels were associated with AD-status or cell type-specific gene expression was determined by using a general linear model (SPSS v.19).

BIN1 alternate splicing in RNA isolated from human anterior cingulate samples was determined by PCR. Assays included an exon 12 sense primer 5'-GAGT CAACCACGAGCCAGAG-3' and exon 18 antisense primer 5'-GAAGGTCTCCACCACGACAG-3'. Each 20 μL reaction mixture contained 20 ng of cDNA, 1 μM of each primer, and Platinum Taq (Life Technologies) and was subjected to a PCR profile of 30 cycles at 95 °C for 15 sec, 59 °C for 30 sec, and 72 °C for 20 sec. Assays were performed in triplicate and PCR amplicons were excised from gels and sequenced.

Immunofluorescence labeling of transfected cells

HEK293 cells cultured on glass coverslips were transiently transfected with an expression plasmid that encodes FLAG-tagged human BIN1 isoform 7 (lacking exons 7, 11, 13–15) [generously provided by Dr. Zhou, Merck Research Laboratories]. The following day, the cells were fixed, permeabilized, and stained with mAb against FLAG or BIN1 antibodies as described [43].

Human brain immunohistochemistry

5 μm-thick paraffin embedded brain sections from individuals with and without multiple sclerosis were rehydrated, treated with antigen retrieval buffer (DAKO) in a steamer for 20 min, followed by a 5 min incubation with 3% H_2O_2 and permeabilized with PBST (phosphate-buffered saline containing 0.025% Triton-X 100). Sections were blocked with 10% normal rabbit serum-PBST for 1 h and then incubated with the indicated primary

antibodies (Additional file 1: Table S1) for 1 h followed by species-specific secondary antibodies. The antigen-antibody reactions were detected by Envision + kit (Dako) or Vectastain Elite-kit (Vector laboratories). Nuclei were counterstained using hematoxylin. The slides were scanned using CRi Pannoramic Scan Whole Slide Scanner and analyzed by Pannoramic Viewer (3DHISTECH).

Immunofluorescence labeling and analysis

Wild-type C57/BL6 mice (between 1-month and 5-month-old) or adult rats were fixed by perfusion with 4% paraformaldehyde containing 4% sucrose. Immunofluorescence labeling was performed on 40 µm-thick sections. Floating brain sections were subjected to epitope retrieval by incubation in 10 mM trisodium citrate pH 6 and 0.05% Tween20 for 30 min at 90°C prior to blocking. The sections were sequentially incubated with the indicated primary antibodies (Additional file 1: Table S1) and Alexa Fluor-conjugated secondary antibodies (Molecular Probes) diluted in Tris-buffered saline containing 1% BSA and 0.25% Triton-X 100, for 48 h and 2 h, respectively. Nuclei were labeled using Hoechst stain (Molecular Probes) before mounting the sections on slides. Confocal images were acquired on a Leica SP5 II STED-CW Superresolution Laser Scanning Confocal microscope and analyzed by ImageJ [44].

Immunoblot analysis

Frontal cortex and deep frontal white matter regions were weighed and homogenized (20% weight/volume) in ice-cold lysis buffer [150 mM NaCl, 50 mM Tris–HCl pH 7.4, 0.5% NP-40, 0.5% sodium deoxycholate, 5 mM EDTA, 0.25 mM PMSF and protease inhibitor cocktail (Sigma)]. An equal volume of lysis buffer containing 2% SDS was then added to each sample and briefly sonicated. Cultured cells were lysed in 150 mM NaCl, 50 mM Tris pH 7.5, 1 mM EDTA, 1% Triton-X 100, 0.5% sodium deoxycholate, 0.1% SDS. Aliquots of lysates were fractionated by 10% or 4-20% polyacrylamide gel electrophoresis. Primary antibodies used for Western blot analysis are listed in Additional file 1: Table S1. After incubation with infrared dye-conjugated secondary antibodies, signals were recorded by the Odyssey infrared imaging system (LI-COR Biosciences) and quantified using ImageJ [44].

Results

Differential expression of BIN1 isoforms in the gray and white matter

We performed qPCR assays to quantify *BIN1* expression in non-AD and AD anterior cingulate brain tissue samples. Since the inclusion of exon 7 is suggested to vary by cell type [45], we used primers specific for *BIN1* isoforms that contained exon 7 (BIN1 + Ex7) and lacked exon 7 [Delta-7-BIN1 (D7-BIN1)]. Sample results were compared to standard curves for each isoform that were analyzed in parallel to determine absolute *BIN1* copy numbers. We found that *BIN1* was expressed at moderate abundance with 2,000-30,000 copies per ~20 ng cDNA. These values were normalized relative to the geometric mean of two housekeeping genes, ribosomal protein L32 (*RPL32*) and eukaryotic initiation factor 4H (*EIF4H*). The percentage of *BIN1* expressed as the D7-BIN1 isoform was 62 ± 15% (mean ± SD, range 23-93%, $n = 57$). We observed that the expression of BIN1 + Ex7 and D7-BIN1 was not correlated (Fig. 1a). We interpret this result as suggesting that the isoforms are either not expressed coordinately or that they are expressed in different cell types with the proportion of these cell types varying among samples.

To investigate this question, the expression of BIN1 + Ex7 and D7-BIN1 was compared to that of genes with cell-type specific expression. Inspection of the results suggested that BIN1 + Ex7 expression was associated positively with synaptophysin expression (neuronal marker) but not with the markers of oligodendrocytes, astrocytes, microglia, or endothelial cells (Fig. 1c and d, Additional file 2: Figure S1A-C). This association was confirmed statistically by evaluating with a general linear model that included BIN1 + Ex7 as the dependent variable and synaptophysin and AD as independent variables. This produced a moderately significant model (adjusted $R^2 = 0.264$). BIN1 + Ex7 was significantly associated with synaptophysin ($p = 1.07X10^{-4}$) and modestly with AD ($p = 0.046$, note the limited power of 0.517) (Fig. 1c and Additional file 3: Table S2). If the model was expanded to include the AD-associated *BIN1* single-nucleotide polymorphism rs7561528 [46], the BIN1 + Ex7 association with synaptophysin was unchanged. However, rs7561528 was not associated with BIN1 + Ex7 expression ($p = 0.3$) and including the single-nucleotide polymorphism in the model pushed AD from significance ($p = 0.068$) (data not shown). The increase in BIN1 + Ex7 expression in AD appears to be a fairly modest 18% (Additional file 4: Table S3). These results are in accordance with the findings reported by Chapuis et al. where the data were normalized to either actin or an apparent microglia gene, *GUSB* [26].

In contrast to BIN1 + Ex7, inspection of the graphs of the D7-BIN1 isoform relative to cell-specific mRNAs suggested that the D7-BIN1 isoform was associated positively with myelin basic protein (MBP), a marker for mature oligodendrocytes and the white matter (Fig. 1e and f) but not with other cell types (Additional 2: Figure S1D–F). We confirmed this notion by qPCR analysis of RNA isolated from gray matter and white matter and found that ~90% of *BIN1* in the white matter corresponds to D7-BIN1 isoforms (Fig. 1b). Using a linear model that included MBP and AD status, we found a

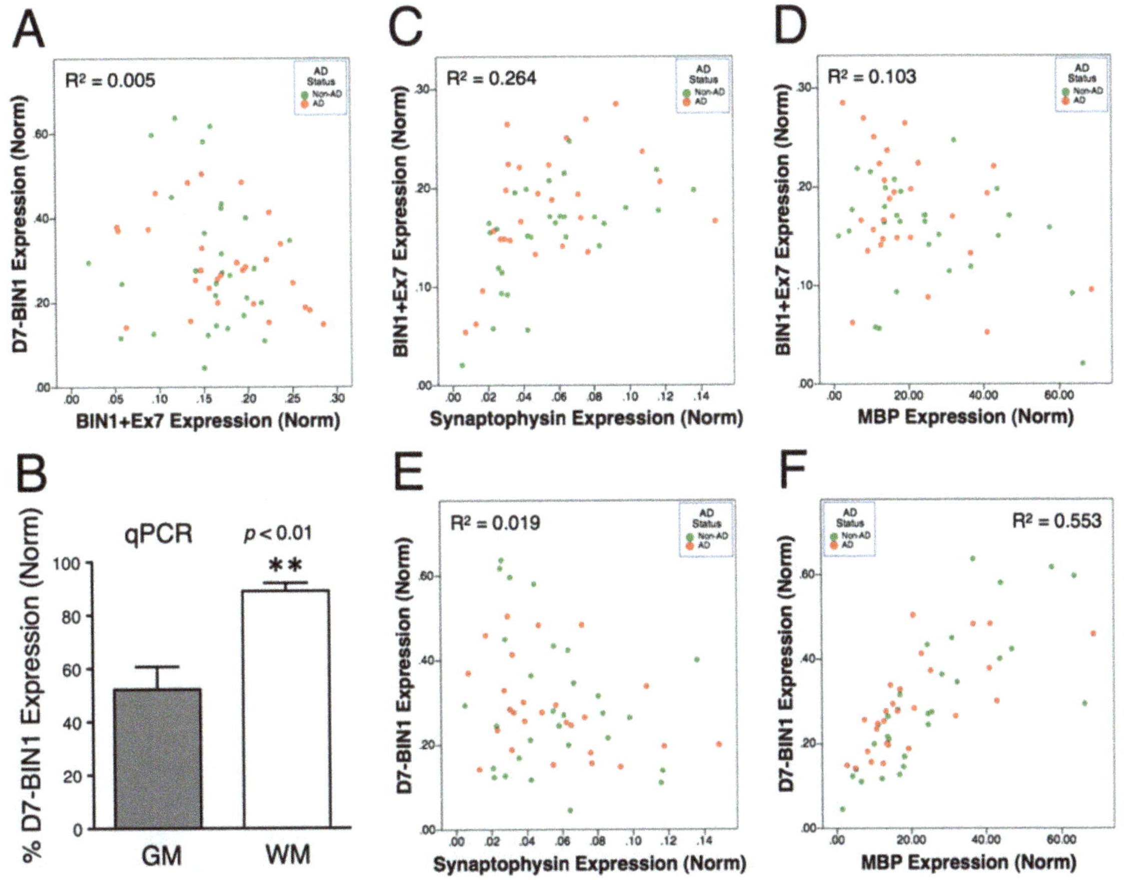

Fig. 1 Quantification of *BIN1* transcript levels in brains with and without AD. **a** Scatter plot of the normalized levels of *BIN1* isoforms generated by alternative splicing of exon 7 in each sample (quantified by qPCR analysis) reveals a lack of correlation between D7 + Ex7 and D7-BIN1 expression. **b** qPCR analysis of *BIN1* exon 7 alternative splicing in the human brain shows a significantly higher proportion of *BIN1* transcripts lacking exon 7 in white matter (WM) as compared with gray matter (GM). **c–f** Scatter plots of BIN1 + Ex7 and D7-*BIN1* expression compared to *SYP* (synaptophysin) and *MBP* expression. AD = AD; Norm = normalized expression. The indicated R^2 values (A, C-F) are adjusted R^2 values, reflecting the presence of two independent variables in the analysis, i.e., AD status and *BIN1*, *SYP* or *MBP* expression

significant model ($R^2 = 0.553$) wherein D7-BIN1 was significantly associated with MBP ($p = 2.97\text{X}10^{-11}$). However, we observed no significant association between AD and D7-BIN1 expression ($p = 0.4$) (Additional file 5: Table S4). Additional analyses did not find a significant association between D7-BIN1 and the AD-associated single-nucleotide polymorphism ($p = 0.6$). These results reveal that the association between *BIN1* expression and AD status is more complicated than previously understood due to the expression of alternatively spliced *BIN1* transcripts, and raise the possibility that *BIN1* expression may not be limited to neurons.

BIN1 is enriched in the human brain white matter

To confirm the above results, we performed immunoblots of homogenates prepared from human brain white matter and gray matter tissue using antibodies raised against non-overlapping epitopes of BIN1: rabbit polyclonal antibody (pAb) BSH3 raised against epitopes encoded by exons 17–20 (reacts with all BIN1 isoforms; Additional file 6: Figure S2); monoclonal antibody (mAb) 2 F11, raised against a junctional epitope generated by the juxtaposition of residues encoded by exons 6 and 8 (thus specific for D7-BIN1 isoforms) [13]; and mAb 99D, raised against an epitope encoded by exon 17 within the Myc-binding domain [47] (Fig. 2a). The specificities of the two BIN1 mAbs have been well established [10, 13, 47] and confirmed by transfection studies in HEK293 cells using BIN1 isoform 7 [which lacks the exon 7-encoded sequences] (Additional file 6: Figure 2SC). Cell-specific marker proteins expected to be enriched in the gray matter (post-synaptic density protein 95 [PSD95] and synaptophysin) and the white matter (MBP and aspartoacylase [ASPA]) were used to assess the purity of the samples (Fig. 2b). Immunoblot analysis revealed two primary BIN isoforms in the gray matter, migrating at ~90 and ~65 kDa (Fig. 2c). The longest BIN1 isoform was detected at low levels by pAb BSH3 (which can detect all

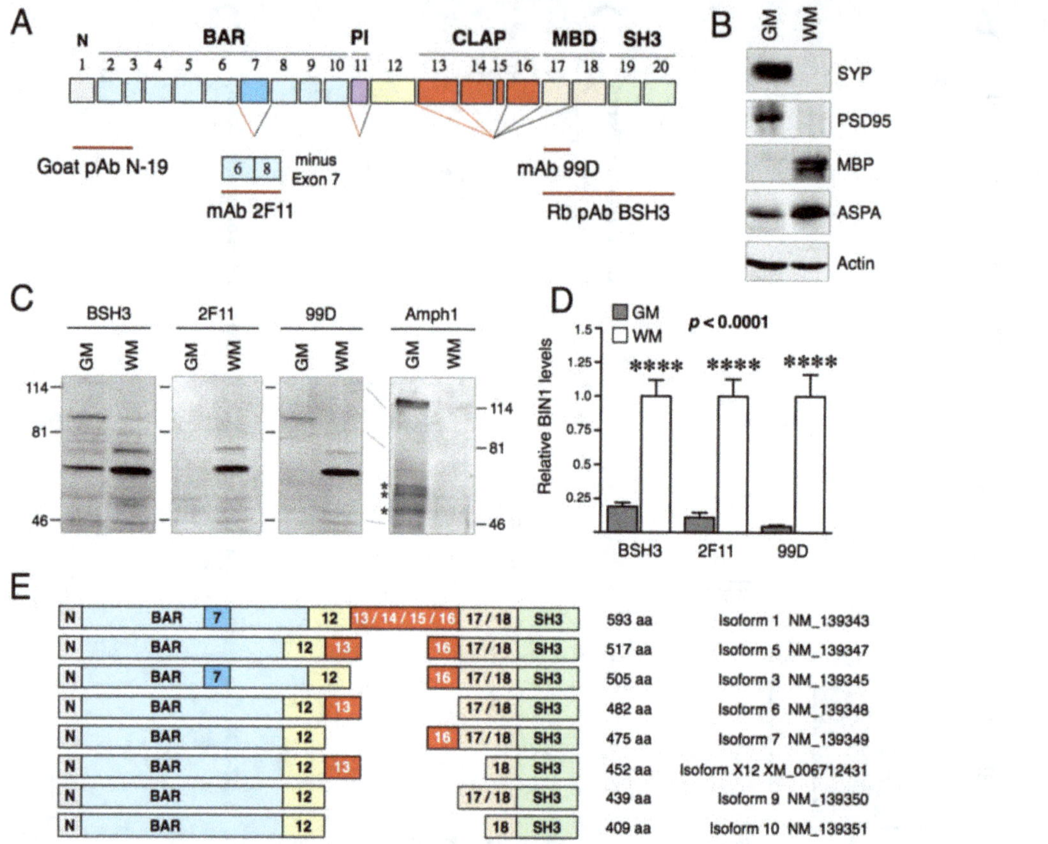

Fig. 2 Immunoblot and RT-PCR analysis of BIN1 isoform diversity in the human brain. **a** The schematic structure of BIN1 indicating the epitopes of the antibodies used in this study. **b** Immunoblot analysis of neuronal and oligodendrocyte marker protein levels in extracts prepared from the human brain gray matter and white matter. **c** Immunoblot analysis of BIN1 and Amphiphysin 1 levels. The pAb BSH3 reacts with all BIN1 isoforms whereas mAb 2 F11 and 99D react with D7-BIN1 and + exon 17 BIN1 isoforms, respectively. The asterisks indicate non-specific signals. **d** The signal intensities of BIN1 were quantified using the Li-COR system, normalized to actin and plotted as mean ± SEM ($n = 8$). Statistical significance was assessed by ANOVA. **e** Schematic illustration of the alternatively spliced human brain BIN1 isoforms identified in this study. Five independent human brain samples were subjected to RT-PCR analysis by using primers corresponding to sequences within exons 12 and 18 and the resulting amplicons were fractionated by electrophoresis. The bands were excised and individually sequenced to identify the major isoforms generated by alternate splicing of exons 13–17. The exclusion of BIN1 exon 11 in brain and inclusion of exon 7 in isoforms 1 and 3 were inferred from the published literature and the RT-PCR and immunoblot results of our study

isoforms) only in the gray matter. Based on its detection by 99D (detects isoforms containing exon 17) but not by 2 F11 (detects isoforms that lack exon 7) the ~90 kDa band corresponds to BIN1 isoform 1, often referred to as the "neuronal BIN1 isoform" (henceforth referred as BIN1:H). The ~65 kDa BIN1 gray matter isoforms failed to react with both mAb 2 F11 and 99D, which indicates that they contain exon 7-encoded residues and lack exon 17-encoded residues.

All three BIN1 antibodies revealed significantly higher BIN1 levels in the white matter (Fig. 2c and d). Quantification revealed that in comparison to the gray matter, the white matter overall contains ~3-fold higher levels of BIN1 (normalized to actin) (p <0.0001 by ANOVA) (Fig. 2d). The predominant white matter BIN1 isoforms migrated at ~65-75 kDa and were uniformly detectible by all three antibodies. This observation suggested that the white matter BIN1 isoforms, for the most part, lacked exon 7-encoded residues and contained exon 17-encoded residues. In contrast to its selective expression in the gray matter, BIN1:H isoform was conspicuously absent in the white matter. Our detection of lower molecular weight ~65-75 kDa BIN1 isoforms (henceforth referred as BIN1:L) in the brain are consistent with the size of the non-neuronal and ubiquitous BIN1 isoforms lacking the intact CLAP domain (encoded by exons 13–16). To confirm this notion, we performed RT-PCR analysis of mRNA isolated from human brain using forward and reverse primers within the exons 12 and 18, respectively. By sequence analysis of the PCR products, we identified multiple BIN1 isoforms generated by variable alternate splicing of BIN1 exons 13–16 (Additional file 7: Figure S3 and Fig. 2e). Finally, for comparison with BIN1 expression, we also assessed the levels of Amphiphysin 1, the brain-specific BIN1 homolog [3, 5, 48]. We found that Amphiphysin 1 is enriched in the gray matter, consistent with previous studies describing Amphiphysin 1 as the neuron-specific homolog of BIN1 (Fig. 2c). This finding supports the idea that Amphiphysin 1 and BIN1:H isoform differed in their cell type expression when compared to the BIN1:L isoforms.

Alteration in the levels of BIN1 isoforms in AD

The diversity of the brain BIN1 isoforms and differential expression of BIN1 isoforms in the gray and white matter raised the question as to the significance of these findings to AD. To address this issue, we examined BIN1 levels in tissue samples from individuals with AD and age-matched controls. In the gray matter samples from AD cases, we observed a marked decrease in the levels of BIN1:H isoform, while there was an increase in the levels of BIN1:L isoforms (Fig. 3a and b). The relative levels of BIN1:L isoform were significantly higher in the gray matter of AD cases as compared with the controls (Fig. 3c). These findings are in agreement with an AD-associated decrease in the larger BIN1 isoform and an increase of the smaller BIN1 isoforms in various regions of the cortex and the hippocampus reported in a previous study [30]. Unlike the case of increased BIN:L levels in the gray matter, comparable levels of BIN1:L levels were found in the white matter samples (Fig. 3a).

We considered the possibility that the apparent AD-associated decrease in BIN1:H isoform could be the result of an overall neuronal loss in the gray matter. Therefore, we simultaneously quantified the levels of Amphiphysin 1 in the samples and normalized the data to the levels of actin. The results show significant differences in Amphiphysin 1 levels between controls and AD samples (Fig. 3a and b). Similar to BIN1:H isoform, the levels of Amphiphysin1 were markedly lower in the gray matter AD samples in comparison with the controls, with a high degree of correlation (Pearson r 0.934; $p = 0.02$). To extend this observation, we performed a series of immunoblots to quantify the levels of markers of neurons

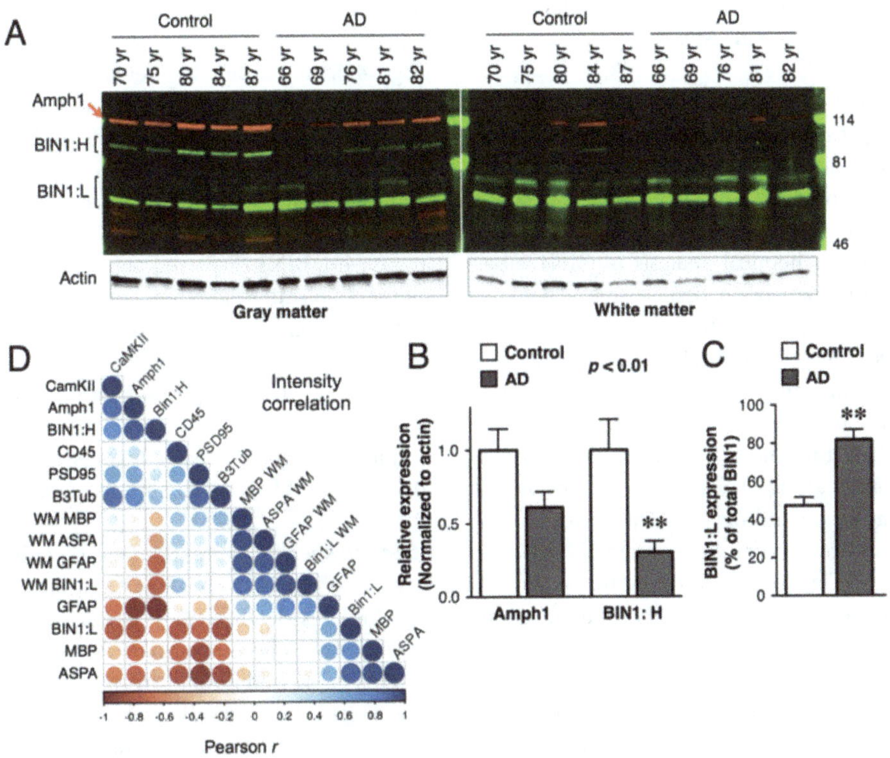

Fig. 3 AD-associated changes in the levels of BIN1 isoforms. **a** Immunoblot analysis of BIN1 and Amphiphysin 1 levels in the brain samples from controls and AD cases. The age of each individual is listed. The blots were simultaneously probed with BIN1 and Amphiphysin 1 antibodies. The levels of actin were used as the control for loading. Note that the gray and white matter blots were scanned using different conditions to achieve equivalent signals. **b** The levels of Amphiphysin 1 and BIN1 isoforms in the gray matter were quantified using the Li-COR system and normalized to the levels of actin. The relative expression levels of Amphiphysin 1 and BIN1: H (~90 kDa) were plotted as mean ± SEM ($n = 5$). The statistical significance was analyzed by ANOVA. **c** The plot shows the percentage of BIN1:L (~65-75 kDa) isoform relative to all BIN1 isoforms in the gray matter of each tissue sample. **d** Pearson r correlation matrix analysis. The levels of multiple cellular markers were quantified as described above and the relative expression level differences in AD samples relative to the controls were used to generate the correlation matrix. Larger blue-colored circles represent a higher degree of correlation, and larger red-colored circles represent an inverse correlation. Smaller neutral-colored circles represent a lack of correlation. A color scale is drawn at the bottom. GM = gray matter; WM = white matter; Amph 1 = Amphiphysin 1

(CamKII, PSD-95, and Class III β-tubulin), oligodendrocytes (MBP, ASPA), astrocytes (glial fibrillary acidic protein [GFAP]), and microglia/macrophages (CD45). We calculated the relative difference in the levels of each marker protein in AD versus control samples, and then performed a Pearson correlation matrix analysis to assess the degree of relationship between the levels of BIN1 isoforms with the cell-type markers (Fig. 3d). The results show a significant correlation between BIN1:H and Amphiphysin 1 with neuronal markers in their relative expression level differences between controls and AD cases. In contrast, BIN1:L isoforms showed an inverse correlation with neuronal markers. Moreover, AD-associated changes in the levels of BIN1:L isoforms in the gray matter showed a high degree of correlation with the oligodendrocyte marker ASPA (Pearson r 0.897; $p < 0.05$). Significant correlation was also observed between the levels of BIN1:L isoforms and GFAP in the white matter (Pearson r 0.936; $p < 0.02$). Taken together, the results of qPCR and quantitative immunoblot analyses suggest neuronal and non-neuronal expression of BIN1, and reveal that the expression of BIN1 isoforms is differentially affected in brains of patients with AD.

Predominant white matter localization and oligodendrocyte expression of BIN1 in the human brain

Whereas BIN1 expression in brain has been previously reported, the cellular profile of BIN1 expression in human has not been characterized in detail [4, 5, 12, 26, 30]. We performed immunohistochemical analysis of BIN1 labeling in post-mortem human brain tissue using a panel of four BIN1 antibodies (Fig. 2a). In hippocampus and parahippocampal gyrus of the human brain, all four antibodies revealed similar strong immunolabeling of the white matter and weaker immunolabeling of the gray matter (Figs. 4a–c and 5a). Within the white matter, BIN1 immunolabeling was found along densely-packed myelinated fiber tracts and in oligodendrocytes, which display the "fried egg" appearance commonly observed in non-perfused brain tissue (Fig. 4b and d). In the hippocampus, intense BIN1 immunolabeling was observed along axons of the perforant path and the alveus (Fig. 4a and 5a). More importantly, we observed little BIN1 immunostaining in neuronal soma within the cortex or the hippocampus. Instead, in the outer layers of the cortex, strong BIN1 labeling was found in smaller cells with radial morphology and highly ramified processes and in numerous patchy/punctate processes (Fig. 4c).

Oligodendrocytes are responsible for axon myelination in the brain. Based on the intense white matter immunolabeling, we predicted that BIN1 is predominantly expressed in oligodendrocytes. In order to formally determine the identity of BIN1-positive cells in the human brain, we performed labeling of adjacent sections with multiple BIN1 antibodies and specific markers for mature oligodendrocytes, astrocytes, and microglia. Immunolabeling with an antibody against tubulin polymerisation-promoting protein p25 (TPPP), a marker for mature oligodendrocytes, revealed a cellular pattern of immunolabeling very similar to that of BIN1 antibodies in all brain regions studied. For example, TPPP stained nearly all the cells in the cerebral peduncle, which contains a large number of myelinating oligodendrocytes whose processes ensheath the axons that project to the cerebellum and the spinal cord (Fig. 4d). Adjacent sections stained with three BIN1 antibodies revealed intense labeling of the fiber tracts and labeling of the oligodendrocyte cell bodies within the cerebral peduncle. In contrast, BIN1 immunolabeling of oligodendrocytes and their fine processes in the CA1 region, as well as the intense immunolabeling of fiber tracks in the alveus, were strikingly distinct from the evenly dispersed Ionized calcium-binding adapter molecule 1 (Iba1) and GFAP immunolabeling of microglia and astrocytes, respectively (Fig. 4e). The predominant oligodendrocyte cell-type immunolabeling of BIN1 is also discernable based on a comparison of the structure of the stained population of cells, each with their distinctive cellular morphology (Fig. 4f). In order to determine more precisely the localization of BIN1 in myelinated axons, we performed two-color immunostaining with antibodies against BIN1 and Caspr (Contactin-associated protein), an axonal membrane protein. In comparison to Caspr, which becomes concentrated in the paranodal junctions of myelinated axons [49], BIN1 displayed patchy distribution along short segments of interdigitating processes without an apparent concentration in the nodes or the paranodal area (Fig. 4g). Moreover, we also observed annular immunolabeling of BIN1, which likely represent cross-sections of traversing myelinated axons. Together, these results show predominant oligodendrocyte expression and white matter localization of BIN1 in the human brain.

Cell-type specific expression and complementary localization of BIN1 and Amphiphysin 1

The findings detailed above were surprising because it is generally assumed, and in a few papers described, that BIN1 is expressed in neurons [4, 26, 30]. In order to carefully assess the distribution of BIN1 in the human brain, we performed immunohistochemical analysis of BIN1 and compared it to the distribution of Amphiphysin 1. Strikingly, adjacent sections stained with antibodies against Amphiphysin 1 and BIN1 revealed a near complementary pattern of expression in the cortex, hippocampal CA fields, hilus, subiculum, fimbria, caudate nucleus, lateral geniculate nucleus, and cerebral peduncle (Fig. 5a). Amphiphysin 1 was widely expressed in neurons throughout the cortex and hippocampus. Notably, Amphiphysin 1 immunolabeling was apparent in neuronal soma and was

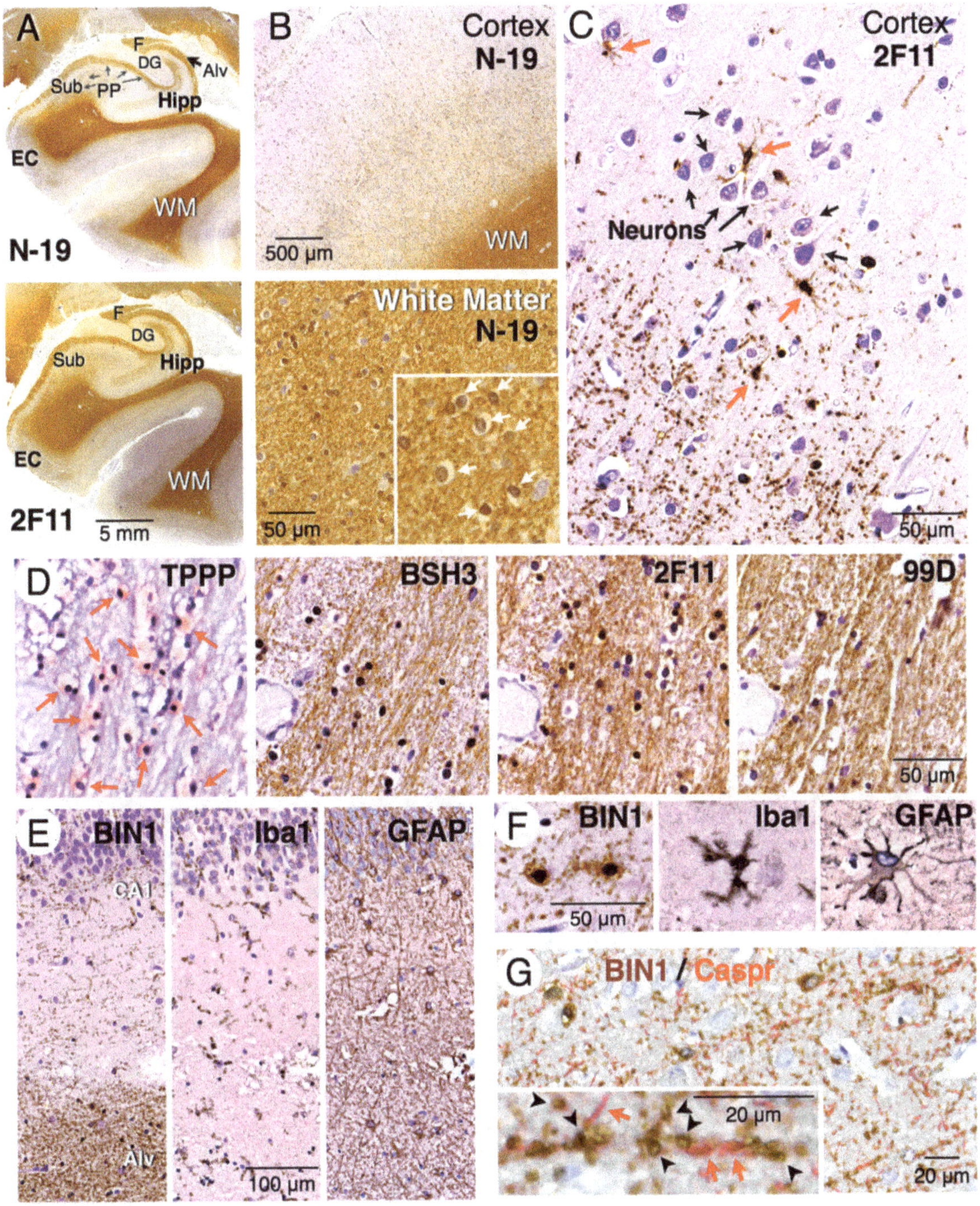

Fig. 4 White matter localization and oligodendrocyte expression of BIN1 in the human brain. **a** Immunohistochemical staining of the hippocampus and parahippocampal gyrus using goat pAb N-19 (top) and mAb 2 F11 (bottom) reveal prominent white matter labeling. In the hippocampus, the perforant path axons and the alveus are labeled. **b** Higher magnification images of N-19 shows relatively weaker labeling in the cortex and intense labeling in the white matter. Note the labeling of mature oligodendrocytes (*white arrows*) in the enlarged area. **c** Higher magnification of mAb 2 F11 labeling reveals intense BIN1 labeling of smaller cells with a radial morphology and ramified processes (*red arrows*), and only a weak labeling of larger neuronal cell bodies (*black arrows*). In addition punctate and discontinuous staining along fine linear processes is also visible. **d** TPPP immunolabeling identifies mature oligodendrocytes in cerebral peduncle (*red arrows*). Analysis of adjacent serial sections reveal BIN1 labeling of mature oligodendrocytes and traversing myelinated fibers. **e, f** Immunohistochemical analysis of adjacent sections of hippocampal CA1 region reveals that the BIN1 cellular labeling pattern is distinct from that of microglia (Iba1) and astrocytes (GFAP). **g** Two-color immunostaining of BIN1 and Caspr. The inset shows a magnified area where the localization of BIN1 (brown) and Caspr (red) along adjacent segments of the axon tracts can be seen. BIN1 immunolabeling of annular structures likely represents cross sections of myelinated axons that lie perpendicular to the plane of the section. WM = white matter; Alv = alveus; Hipp = hippocampus; EC = entorhinal cortex; F = fimbria; DG = dentate gyrus; Sub = subiculum; PP = perforant path; CA1 = *Cornu Ammonis* area 1

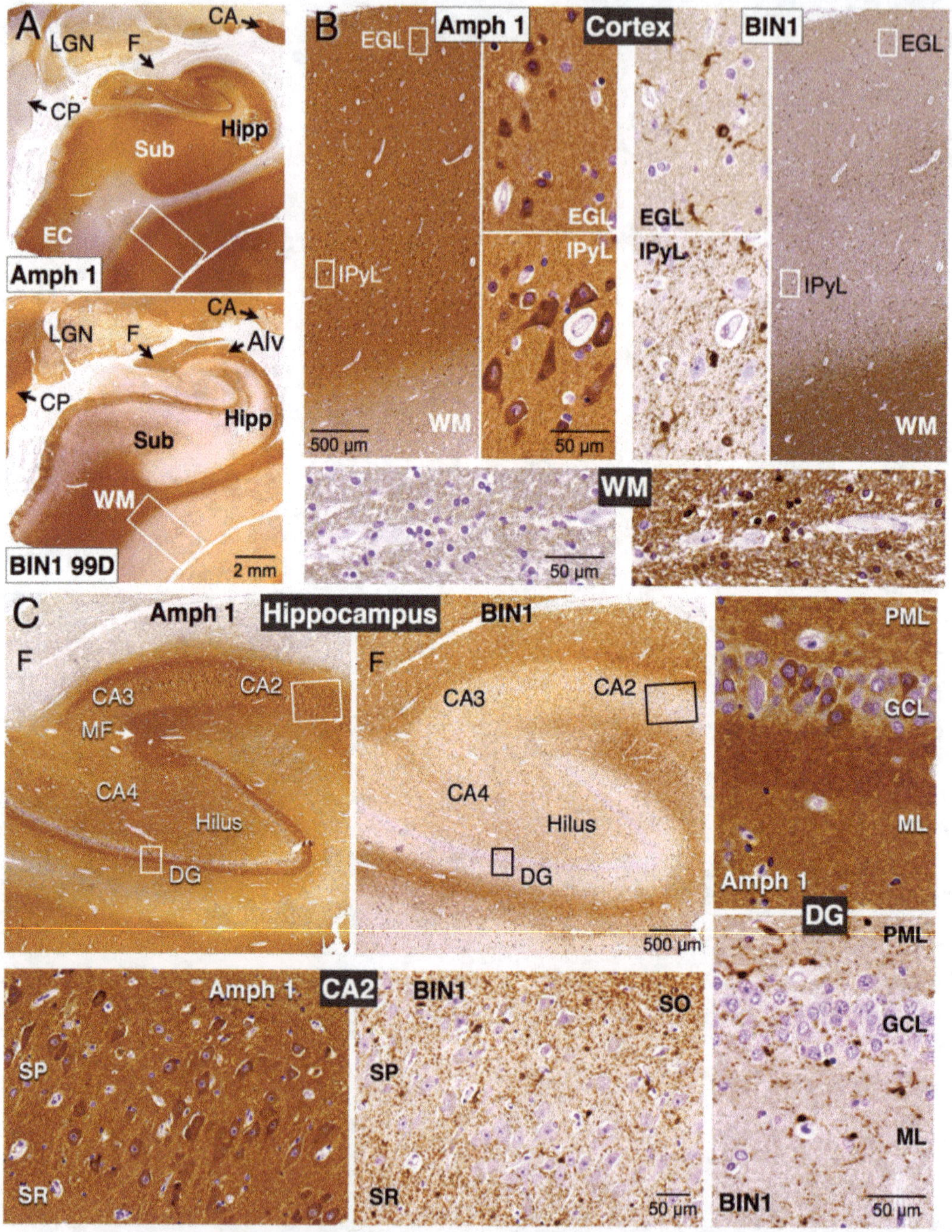

Fig. 5 Distinct cellular localization of BIN1 and Amphiphysin 1 in the human brain. **a** Immunohistochemical labeling of adjacent sections of the hippocampus and parahippocampal gyrus using mAb against Amphiphysin 1 or BIN1 (99D) reveals near complementary pattern of labeling. Amphiphysin 1 antibody does not stain the white matter whereas intense BIN1 labeling is observed in the white matter. **b** Amphiphysin 1 and BIN1 immunolabeling of the cortex (the boxed area in panel A) and a section of the white matter are shown at a higher magnification. Boxed regions in the external granule layer and internal pyramidal layer are also shown at further magnification to visualize the cells that are immunoreactive. Amphiphysin 1 and BIN1 labeling of morphologically distinct neurons and oligodendrocytes, respectively, are quite obvious. **c** Amphiphysin 1 and BIN1 labeling of the hippocampal area. A higher magnification of the boxed area of CA2 and dentate gyrus is shown at the bottom and on the right, respectively. In all areas, Amphiphysin 1 mAb stains the neuronal soma and the neuropil whereas BIN1 mAb stains smaller cells and profuse branched processes. Very little BIN1 signal is found in neurons. Amphiphysin 1 but not BIN1 localizes to the terminal fields of hippocampal mossy fibers, which are non-myelinated. Amph 1 = Amphiphysin 1; WM = white matter; Alv = alveus; Hipp = hippocampus; Sub = subiculum; EC = entorhinal cortex; CA = caudate nucleus; CP = cerebral peduncle; F = fimbria; LGN = lateral geniculate nucleus; EGL = external granular layer; IPyL = internal pyramidal layer; DG = dentate gyrus; CA2-CA4 = *Cornu Ammonis* areas 2–4; MF = mossy fibers; PML = polymorphic layer; GCL = granule cell layer; ML = molecular layer; SO = *stratum oriens*; SP = *stratum pyramidale*; SR = *stratum raidatum*

also intense in the neuropil (Fig. 5b and c). In comparison, we observed little, if any, neuronal or neuropil BIN1 immunolabeling in the cortex or hippocampus (Fig. 5b and c). On the contrary, BIN1 immunolabeling showed a strong signal in the white matter. Interestingly, whereas Amphiphysin 1 antibody labeled the mossy fiber terminal field in the hippocampus, these unmyelinated axons of the dentate gyrus granule cells are not labeled by the BIN1 antibody (Fig. 5c). Similarly, the Amphiphysin 1 antibody labeled the terminal zones of the associational and commissural pathways, as well as the perforant pathway in the molecular layer of the dentate gyrus, whereas BIN1 immunolabeling in this area was restricted to a few ramified cells and their processes (Fig. 5c). Thus, immunohistochemical staining and immunoblot analysis with independent antibodies support the assertion that BIN1 is enriched in the human brain white matter and shows little overlap with the expression and neuronal localization of its close homolog Amphiphysin 1.

BIN1 expression in mature oligodendrocytes and localization in the white matter tracts in rodent brain

In order to ascertain the cellular distribution of BIN1, we performed immunofluorescence labeling of mouse and rat brain tissue. Labeling with three BIN1 antibodies revealed striking localization of BIN1 in the corpus callosum (Fig. 6a and b, and Additional file 8: Figure S4). In the cortex, BIN1 immunolabeling was observed in the soma of numerous cells dispersed in all cortical layers (Fig. 6c). Within the corpus callosum, the BIN1 antibodies stained linear arrays of cells characteristic of interfascicular oligodendrocytes (Fig. 6b and Additional file 8: Figure S4C and D). In addition to the arciform BIN1 immunolabeling of the soma, punctate BIN1 immunolabeling was apparent in the cortex along the processes with short barbed branches and in the white matter along parallel oriented tracks, as visualized by high-resolution confocal microscopy (Fig. 6b). Double-immunofluorescence labeling analysis revealed that BIN1 immunolabeling essentially overlapped with MBP localization in the corpus callosum (Fig. 6a), in corticostriatal projections (Fig. 6d) and in the cerebellar white matter (Fig. 6e). In contrast to the intense NeuN labeling of the hippocampal neurons, BIN1 labeling was not readily discernable (Fig. 6a and f). Instead, BIN1 immunolabeling was observed in a few smaller cells and fine processes in the hippocampus. Similarly, easily distinguishable large neurons in striatum stained positive for Amphiphysin 1, whereas BIN1 localized to smaller cells and intersecting myelinated fiber bundles consistent with prominent non-neuronal BIN1 expression (Fig. 6g).

Examination of BIN1 and Amphiphysin 1 distribution in the cerebellum revealed the most intense BIN1 labeling in the white matter, whereas Amphiphysin labeling was present in the molecular layer along with synaptophysin (Fig. 7a and b). Within the granule cell layer, BIN1 immunolabeling was mainly found in processes, which were in close proximity to synaptophysin-positive glomeruli (multisynaptic agglomerations of mossy fiber terminals), but essentially with little overlap as revealed by line scan analysis (Fig. 7c). A comparison of the distribution of BIN1 with the paranodal marker Caspr in the cortex and the hippocampus revealed that BIN1 localized to discontinuous segments along slender processes adjacent to Caspr, with little or no overlap (Fig. 7d), suggesting its localization to the internode sections. The results described above provide compelling evidence for the paucity of BIN1 in neurons and its enrichment in the white matter tracts in rodent brain mirroring our observations in the human brain.

Finally, BIN1-positive cells in the cortex and corpus callosum were positive for ASPA, TPPP, and CC1 epitope, markers for mature oligodendrocytes (Fig. 7e and f, and data not shown). Immunolabeling using an antibody against neural/glial antigen 2 (NG2) showed little or no expression of BIN1 in oligodendrocyte progenitor cells (Fig. 7g and h). Similarly, BIN1 was not expressed in microglia or astrocytes (Fig. 7i and j). BIN1 was not detected at appreciable levels in dendrites (identified by microtubule-associated protein 2 [MAP2] labeling) or presynaptic sites (synapsin 1 labeling) in the cortex (data not shown). As expected from BIN1 localization in myelinating oligodendrocytes, BIN1 immunolabeling showed overlap with the axonal marker phospho-neurofilament (data not shown). Together, the results described above are consistent with high-level BIN1 expression in mature oligodendrocytes and their processes in the brain.

Upregulation of BIN1 during developmental myelination and oligodendrocyte maturation

Myelin formation in the rodent brain begins in the first postnatal week and peak myelination occurs 2–3 weeks after birth. In order to characterize BIN1 expression during this period, we analyzed BIN1 expression in post-natal rat brain at 7 days, 15 days and 21 days. Multiple alternatively spliced BIN1 isoforms in the range of ~ 55–115 kDa were detectible using pAb BSH3 (Fig. 8a). Quantitative immunoblot analysis revealed a significant increase in all BIN1 isoforms during the post-natal period of oligodendrocyte generation and intense myelination ($p < 0.01$). Furthermore, following the initial increase, high-level BIN1 expression was maintained in the adult rodent brain (Fig. 8c). Moreover, like in the human brain BIN1:L isoforms were relatively more abundant than the BIN1:H isoform, which is presumably expressed in neurons. To confirm these results, we assessed BIN1 expression during in vitro differentiation of cultured rat oligodendrocyte progenitor cells isolated from rat brain. Immunoblot

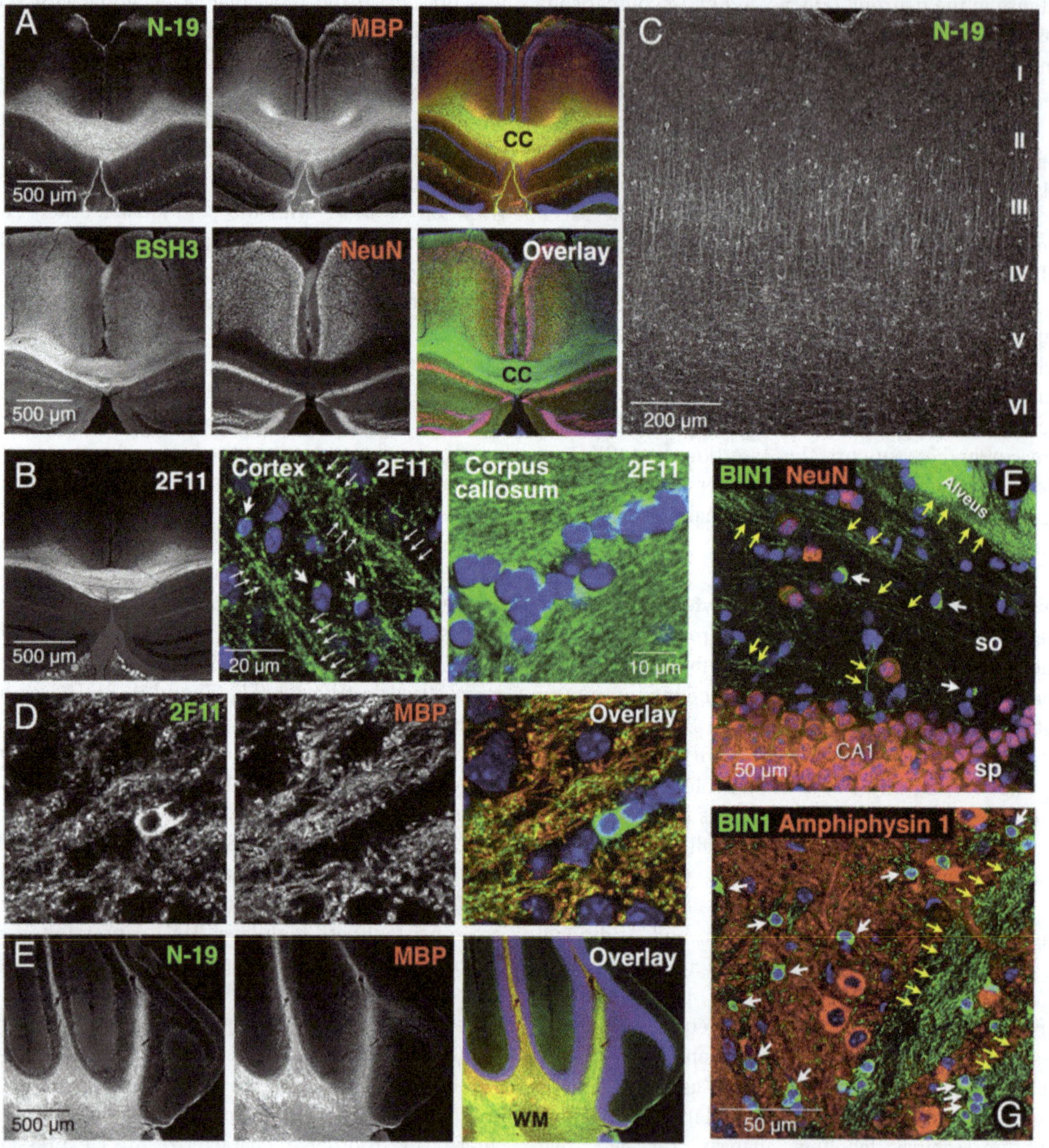

Fig. 6 The distribution of BIN1 in mouse brain. BIN1 immunolabeling is in green and the marker labeling is in red. Nuclear staining with Hoechst is in blue. **a** Immunofluorescence labeling of coronal sections with antibodies against BIN1 (N-19 or BSH3) shows overlap with MBP but not with NeuN labeling. **b**–**g** Confocal microscopy analysis of BIN1 immunolabeling. **b** A low magnification image of BIN1 labeling with mAb 2 F11. A higher magnification of the cortex and corpus callosum is shown in the middle and right panels. *Thick* and *thin arrows* point to BIN1 labeling of the cell body and barbarized processes in the cortex. **c** N-19 labeling reveals BIN1-positive cells dispersed throughout the cortical layers. **d** and **e** BIN1 and MBP labeling overlap along corticostriatal projections and in the cerebellar white matter. **f** BIN1 and NeuN labeling are largely distinct in the hippocampus and striatum. BIN1-positive cell bodies (*white arrows*) and processes in *stratum oriens* or fiber bundles in alveus (*yellow arrows*) are indicated. **g** BIN1 immunolabeling of cell bodies (*white arrows*) and fiber bundles (*yellow arrows*) in the striatum does not overlap with neuronal and neuropil labeling of Amphiphysin 1. CC = corpus callosum; CA1 = *Cornu Ammonis* area 1; SO = *stratum oriens*; SP = *stratum pyramidale*

analysis revealed a significant upregulation of BIN1 levels, specifically BIN1:L isoforms, during oligodendrocyte maturation (Fig. 8b). In parallel, we assessed BIN1 expression in cultured neurons following in vitro differentiation for 21 days and found that BIN1 expression was only weakly detectable in mature neurons. In contrast, Amphiphysin 1 was expressed at high levels in mature neurons but not in cultured oligodendrocytes (Fig. 8b). These findings corroborated previous studies that reported high levels of *Bin1* transcripts in mature oligodendrocytes [32, 45] and are entirely in agreement with our in vivo localization of BIN1 and Amphiphysin 1 in mature oligodendrocytes and

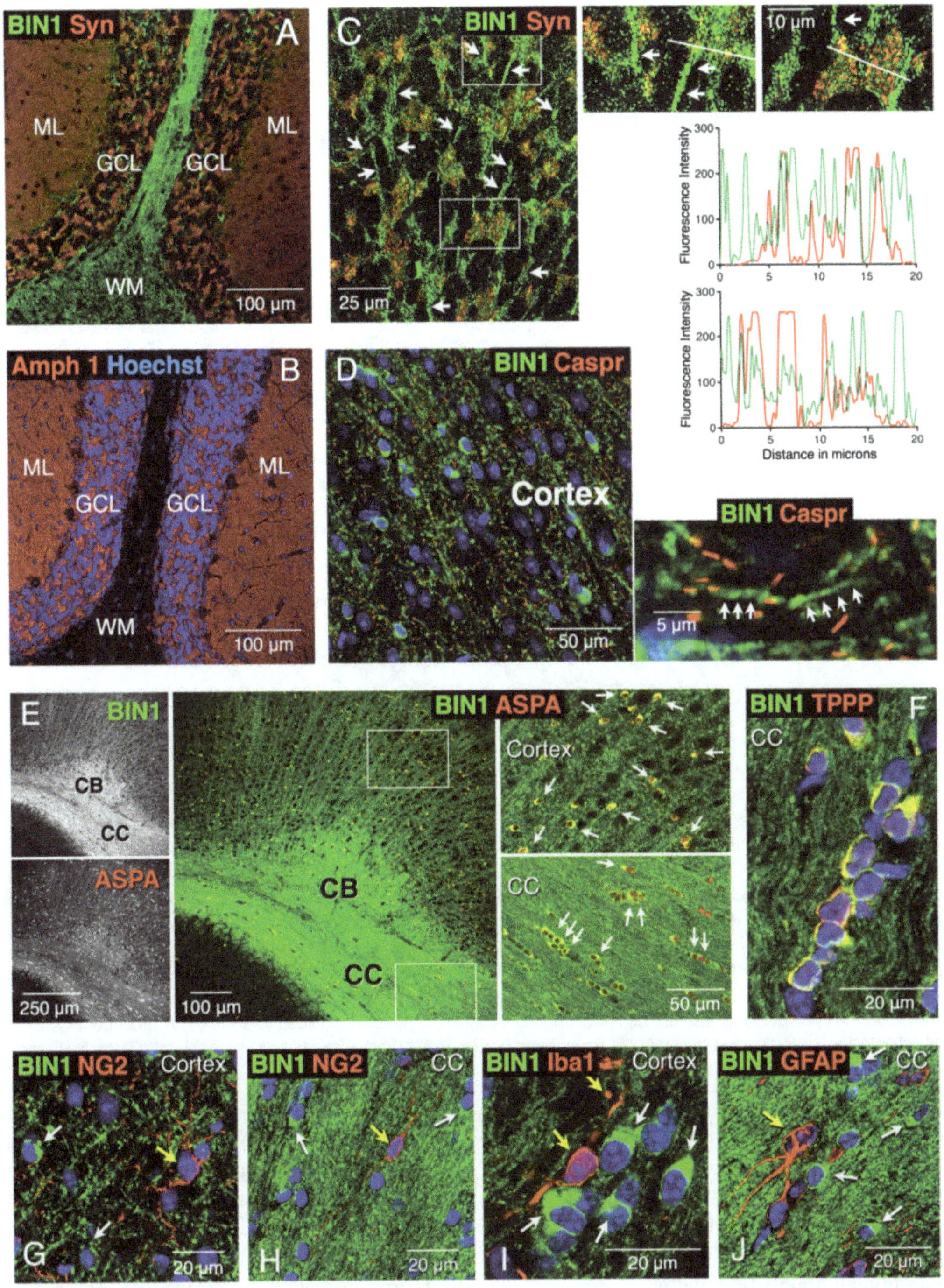

Fig. 7 Expression of BIN1 in mature oligodendrocytes. BIN1 immunolabeling is in green and the marker labeling is in red. Nuclear staining with Hoechst is in blue. **a-c** Sagittal sections of the cerebellum were labeled with the indicated antibodies. BIN1 labeling is prominent in the white matter whereas no labeling for Amphiphysin was observed in the white matter. Synaptophysin and Amphiphysin 1 labeling are prominent in the molecular layer synaptic terminals and in the granule cell layer mossy fibers. Higher magnification of the granule cell layer reveals BIN1-positive processes (*arrows*) around synaptophysin-positive mossy fibers **c**. The areas indicated by the rectangles are enlarged on the right. Line-scan analysis of BIN1 and synaptophysin fluorescence intensities plotted as graphs shows that the proteins localize to distinct structures. **d** BIN1 labeling in the cortex is found along the internodal segments of processes (*arrows*) adjacent to the paranodal localization of Caspr. **e** and **f** All BIN1-positive cells (*arrows*) are also positive for ASPA and TPPP, which are markers of mature oligodendrocytes. A higher magnification of the boxed areas is shown. **g**–**j** BIN labeling in cortex and corpus callosum (*white arrows*) does not overlap with NG2-labeled OPCs, Iba1-labeled microglia or GFAP-labeled astrocytes (*yellow arrows*). Syn = synaptophysin; Amph 1 = Amphiphysin 1; WM = white matter; ML = molecular layer; GCL = granule cell layer; CC = corpus callosum; CB = cingulum bundle

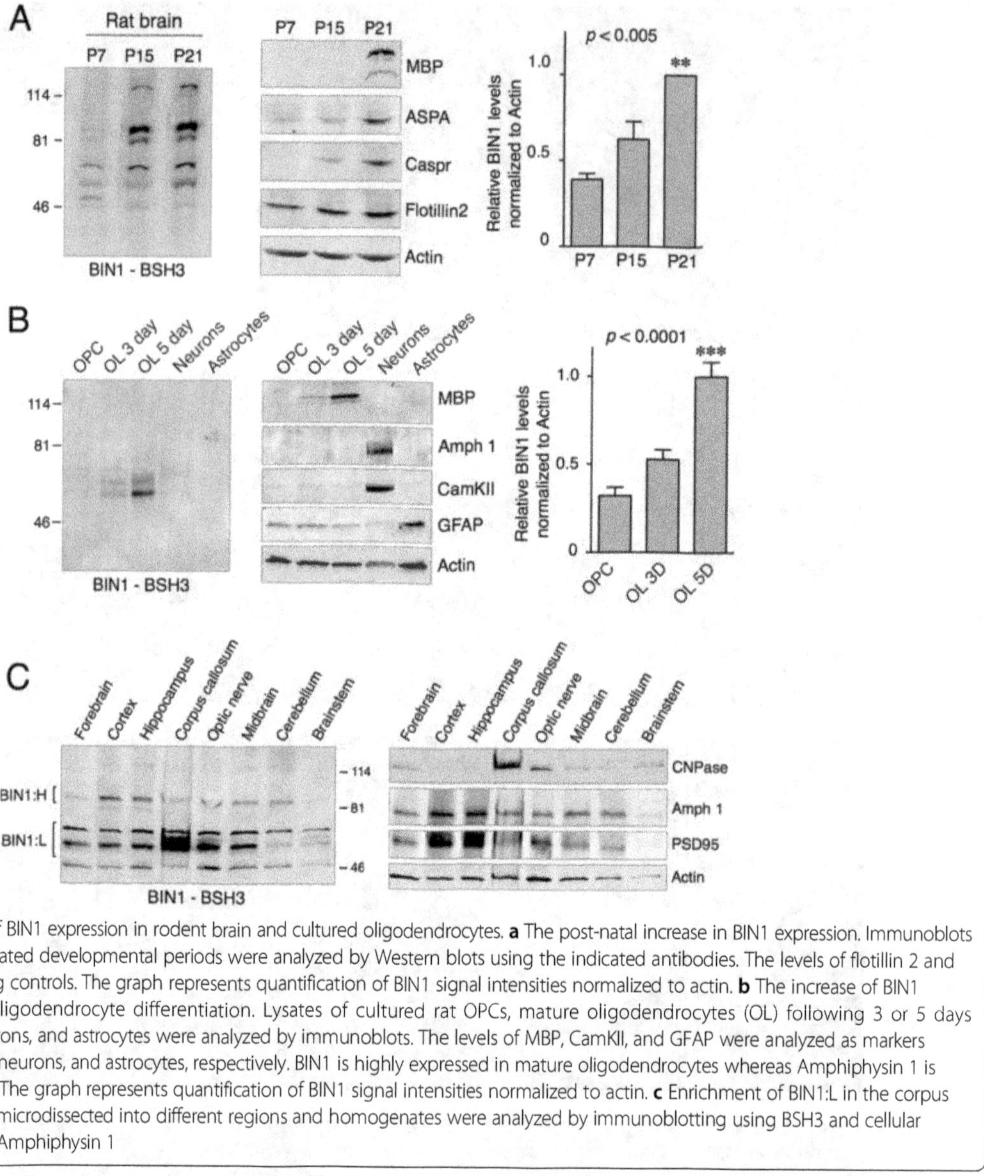

Fig. 8 Immunoblot analysis of BIN1 expression in rodent brain and cultured oligodendrocytes. **a** The post-natal increase in BIN1 expression. Immunoblots of brain lysates from the indicated developmental periods were analyzed by Western blots using the indicated antibodies. The levels of flotillin 2 and actin were assessed as loading controls. The graph represents quantification of BIN1 signal intensities normalized to actin. **b** The increase of BIN1 expression during in vitro oligodendrocyte differentiation. Lysates of cultured rat OPCs, mature oligodendrocytes (OL) following 3 or 5 days of differentiation, mature neurons, and astrocytes were analyzed by immunoblots. The levels of MBP, CamKII, and GFAP were analyzed as markers for mature oligodendrocytes, neurons, and astrocytes, respectively. BIN1 is highly expressed in mature oligodendrocytes whereas Amphiphysin 1 is abundant in mature neurons. The graph represents quantification of BIN1 signal intensities normalized to actin. **c** Enrichment of BIN1:L in the corpus callosum. Adult rat brain was microdissected into different regions and homogenates were analyzed by immunoblotting using BSH3 and cellular marker antibodies. Amph 1 = Amphiphysin 1

neurons, respectively, by immunohistochemical staining. Finally, we analyzed BIN1 isoform expression by dissecting different regions of adult rat brain. From this analysis, it became clear that BIN1:L isoforms were uniquely enriched in the corpus callosum (Fig. 8c), consistent with the results from human brain white matter.

Loss of BIN1 immunolabeling in demyelinated plaques of patients with multiple sclerosis

The results outlined above showing expression of BIN1 in the myelin tracts prompted us to examine BIN1 immunolabeling in the brains of individuals with multiple sclerosis, as a disease model for demyelination. In a pilot study, we performed BIN1 labeling of autopsy brain samples from a set of confirmed cases of multiple sclerosis and compared the results to the staining of Luxol fast blue, a commonly used myelin stain. Fig. 9a shows Luxol fast blue staining of an inactive/chronic multiple sclerosis plaque, revealing a well-demarcated area of hypocellularity with myelin pallor. An adjacent serial section stained with BIN1 antibody reveals the loss of BIN1 immunolabeling within the lesion relative to an intense periplaque normal white matter labeling (Fig. 9a). We also analyzed the similarities in Luxol fast blue and BIN1 staining intensities in active multiple sclerosis plaques with demyelination and activated macrophages, and in shadow plaques where the axons maintain uniformly thin myelin sheaths. The results from three BIN1 antibodies reveal the high degree of similarity between BIN1 labeling intensity and the extent of myelin loss in multiple sclerosis lesions (Fig. 9b and Additional file 9: Figure S5). BIN1 immunolabeling in shadow plaques

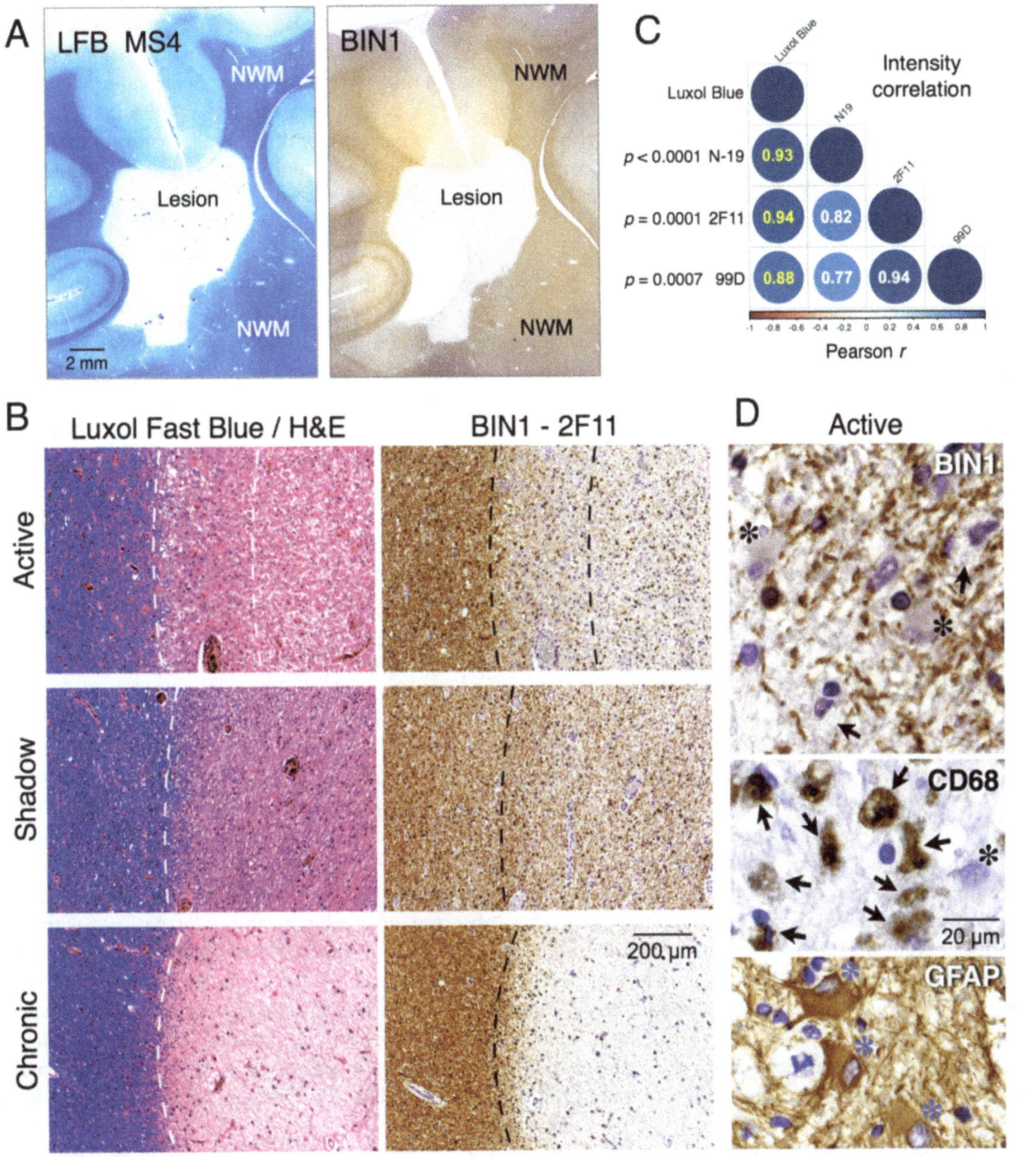

Fig. 9 Loss of BIN1 parallels myelin loss in multiple sclerosis brain lesions. **a** Staining of adjacent serial autopsy brain sections with Luxol fast blue (left) and BIN1 antibody (right) shows myelin loss that parallels striking loss of BIN1 labeling intensity within a chronic/inactive multiple sclerosis plaque. **b** Adjacent sections of samples from multiple sclerosis patients were analyzed by histology or immunohistochemistry. Images correspond to an active lesion (top), shadow plaque (middle) and chronic plaque (bottom). Dashed lines mark the lesion border. **c** Luxol fast blue (not shown) and BIN1 antibody staining intensities were quantified from digitized images. The percentage difference in the staining intensities within lesions in comparison to adjacent normal white matter was calculated. Correlation matrix analysis reveals a significant correlation between myelin loss and reduction in BIN1 immunolabeling intensities. **d** Higher magnification of the border of an active lesion depicting myelin fragmentation and loss of BIN1 immunoreactivity. CD68 staining of foamy macrophages (arrows) and GFAP staining of hypertrophic astrocytes (asterisks) are also shown in the bottom panels. NWM = normal white matter

was more intense in comparison to chronic plaques, consistent with remyelination in these lesions. In all cases, BIN1 immunolabeling appeared to be restricted to cells with oligodendrocyte morphology. Notably, BIN1 immunolabeling was not detectable in CD45-positive perivascular cells (Additional file 10: Figure S6B), or in CD68-positive foamy macrophages and GFAP-positive reactive astrocytes located in the periphery of the active lesions (Fig. 9d). Correlation matrix analysis, comparing the intensity difference of Luxol blue staining or BIN1 antibody labeling within the lesion relative to the peri-plaque region, revealed a significant correlation between the loss of myelin and the decrease of BIN1 immunolabeling (Fig. 9c). The diminution of BIN1 within chronic lesions and its reemergence during remyelination within the multiple sclerosis lesions are consistent with BIN1 expression in myelinating oligodendrocytes.

Discussion

In this paper, we document prominent BIN1 expression in mature oligodendrocytes and its localization within the white matter in the brain, which strikingly contrasts with neuronal and presynaptic localization of the BIN1 paralog, Amphiphysin 1. Our study reveals the upregulation of BIN1 expression during in vivo myelination as well as oligodendrocyte maturation in vitro. Moreover, we reveal the diversity of brain BIN1 isoforms and report on the alteration of select BIN1 isoform expression in patients with AD. Finally, we show that the loss of BIN1 immunoreactivity closely parallels myelin loss within brain lesions of individuals with multiple sclerosis in a pilot study. Altogether, our findings bring clarity to the issue of BIN1 expression and isoform diversity in the brain and provide novel insights on a possible non-neuronal role for BIN1, which has been genetically characterized as the second most significant risk factor for late-onset AD.

Predominant oligodendrocyte expression of BIN1

Previous studies have reported conflicting descriptions of BIN1 expression and localization in the brain. An earlier study characterized BIN1 by fractionation and immunolocalization and reported that BIN1 was enriched in nerve terminals in a manner similar to Amphiphysin 1 [5]. Concurrently, another study reported distinct localization of BIN1 in initial axon segments and nodes of Ranvier, with no overlap with the punctate nerve terminal immunolabeling of Amphiphysin 1 [4]. These differences likely resulted from the utilization of isoform-specific BIN1 antibodies. Using a large panel of antibodies, our results from immunohistochemical analyses of adjacent human brain sections for BIN1 and Amphiphysin 1 provides compelling evidence that these homologs are expressed in distinct cell types (Fig. 5). These findings were confirmed with detailed confocal microscopy analysis of BIN1 expression in rodent brain (Table 2). Overall, the results reveal that BIN1 is predominantly expressed in mature oligodendrocytes and highly enriched in the white matter in rodent and the human brain. Immunoblot analysis of human and rat brain tissue reveals that the neuronal BIN1:H isoform is expressed at lower levels only in the gray matter as compared with the more abundant BIN1:L isoforms, which are expressed in both the gray matter and white matter. Entirely consistent with our findings, BIN1 was one of the 308 proteins identified in both human and mouse brain myelin preparations by mass spectrometry [50].

Previous studies using the same antibodies employed in our analysis identified similar immunolabeling in the human brain as reported here, but attributed the labeling to neuronal soma or nucleus without comparing BIN1 immunolabeling with markers for neurons or oligodendrocytes [13, 26, 30]. Our results clearly show that, unlike Amphiphysin 1, the large majority of BIN1 immunoreactivity is not associated with neurons in the human brain (Fig. 5). In addition, it is clear that very little overlap exists between the cellular immunolabeling of NeuN and BIN1 throughout the rodent brain. Mature oligodendrocyte expression of BIN1 was established in our experiments using three commonly used cellular markers of oligodendrocytes. While our results are in agreement with a previous study reporting presynaptic localization of Amphiphysin 1 resembling that of synaptophysin in the cerebellum [3], they reveal that BIN1 localization markedly differs from that of synaptophysin. Specifically, BIN1 is highly enriched in white matter tracts in the cerebellum where it overlaps with MBP; in contrast synaptophysin and Amphiphysin 1 do not localize to the white matter (Figs. 5 and 6).

Although *BIN1* mRNA expression in microglia acutely-isolated from mouse brain was observed in RNA-seq experiments [45], our results show little evidence in support of microglial localization of BIN1 at the protein level in the human or mouse brain. Similar to our findings, no overlap in the cellular expression of BIN1 and Iba1 was observed in the hippocampus of patients with AD [26]. Furthermore, our study reveals BIN1 immunolabeling of morphologically distinct cell types from those stained by Iba1, CD45, and CD68, arguing against detectable levels of BIN1 expression in mouse or human brain microglia or macrophages in situ (Figs. 3, 6, 8, and Additional file 10: Figure S6). These findings are summarized in Table 2.

The significance of BIN1 expression in oligodendrocytes

High-level BIN1 protein expression in mature oligodendrocytes and the white matter in our studies are in agreement with the Barres lab's identification of *Bin1* among the top 50 highly expressed genes in cultured oligodendrocytes in a microarray study [32], and proteomic identification of BIN1 in human and mouse brain myelin preparations [50]. Our results show an increase of BIN1 levels both during oligodendrocyte maturation in vitro and critical period of myelination in vivo. Upregulation of BIN1 during synchronous differentiation of cultured oligodendrocytes is consistent with earlier microarray and recent RNAseq datasets [32, 45]. Similarly, a significant decrease in *BIN1* expression was observed in

Table 2 Summary of BIN1 expression in the brain analysed using cellular markers

Markers Brain tissue	Neurons	Mature	Immature	Microglia	Astrocytes	Macrophages
		Oligodendrocytes				
	NeuN, Amph 1, Calbindin, Parvalbumin	ASPA, TPP25, CNPase, CC1	NG2	Iba1, CD45	GFAP	CD68
Mouse/rat	–	++++	–	–	–	–
Human	–	++++	ND	–	–	–

The cellular markers employed to determine BIN1 expression in different cell types are indicated. ++++ = strong expression; – = no expression; +/– weak or occasional expression; *ND* not determined

microarray analysis of multiple sclerosis brain lesions in comparison with control brain samples (GEO DataSet GDS4218) [51]. In agreement, our analysis of brain tissue from patients with multiple sclerosis shows a close correlation between BIN1 levels and the intensity of myelin labeling across the different types of lesions. Notably, BIN1 labeling within the shadow plaques indicates possible reemergence of BIN1 expression during remyelination. Thus, BIN1 upregulation during oligodendrocyte maturation and its localization to myelinating oligodendrocytes have potential implications not only for normal physiology in the healthy brain but also for myelin repair under pathological conditions. OPCs remain abundant in the adult brain as lineage-restricted cells, which retain their capacity to proliferate and mature into myelinating oligodendrocytes as needed in response to demyelination resulting from injury or disease conditions. The lack of BIN1 expression in NG2-positive OPCs and the coordinate upregulation of BIN1 along with myelin-specific proteins suggest a possible role for BIN1 in membrane remodeling that accompanies the transition from the progenitors into myelinating oligodendrocytes with long arborized processes.

BIN1 isoform diversity in the brain

We report two important insights based on the results of our immunohistochemistry and immunoblot analyses. First, BIN1 levels are enriched in the human white matter in comparison to the gray matter. This finding is in agreement with the comparison of *BIN1* transcript levels between the human white matter and the gray matter reported from independent microarray analyses [50, 52, 53]. Second, the isoform distribution of BIN1 between the gray matter and white matter differs significantly, as revealed by different BIN1 antibodies. The ~90 kDa BIN1 isoform is expressed only in the gray matter at lower levels, whereas the ~65-75 kDa BIN1 isoforms are the predominant forms in the gray matter and white matter. Expression of seven brain-specific and two ubiquitous BIN1 isoforms have been reported previously [4, 6, 7]. Consistent with the previous characterization that the neuronal BIN1 isoform 1 contains the intact CLAP domain responsible for binding to clathrin, we clearly see an enrichment of the ~90 kDa BIN1 (the largest BIN1 isoform in the brain) in the gray matter. However, it is somewhat surprising that the BIN1 isoform 1 is not the predominant BIN1 species in the human brain. Our immunoblot analysis of controls and AD patients revealed that the majority of BIN1 isoforms expressed in the brain corresponded to ~65-75 kDa, the reported size of the ubiquitous BIN1 isoforms, raising the possibility that they may lack the CLAP domain.

By direct sequencing of the human brain RT-PCR products, we have confirmed variable alternate splicing of *BIN1* exons 13–16, which encodes the CLAP domain (Additional file 7: Figure S3). Thus, the results from immunoblot and RT-PCR analysis show that several human brain BIN1 isoforms lack the CLAP domain, entirely or at least partially. Our findings are similar to the previously reported RT-PCR analysis of BIN1 isoform composition in rat brain and peripheral tissue [7]. Since the CLAP domain is required for BIN1 interaction with clathrin, these observations raise the possibility that large proportion of BIN1 expressed in the brain may not participate in clathrin-mediated endocytosis [54]. Evidence from the analysis of *Drosophila* Amphiphysin, encoded by the unique *Amphiphysin* gene (and thought to be a BIN1 ortholog), show that absence of the CLAP domain results in no detectable defects in synaptic vesicle endocytosis in mutant flies [55–57]. Thus, the precise cellular functions of the major BIN1 isoforms in the brain remain to be established.

BIN1 expression in the brains of patients with AD

The functional connection between *BIN1* and the susceptibility to AD remains to be elucidated. Initial attempts to determine whether *BIN1* expression might be altered in AD have resulted in discordant findings. While two studies have reported significantly increased *BIN1* transcripts levels in brains of individuals with AD [26, 31], another found a positive correlation between *BIN1* expression levels and later age at onset of the disease [28]. Apparent disagreements were also reported by immunoblot analysis of BIN1 expression in individuals with AD. Whereas, a significant decrease in BIN1 levels was observed by immunoblot analysis in one study [29], an increase in BIN1 levels was reported in another study [30]. A comparison of the findings from these two reports with the results of our study offers some clarity to this apparent discrepancy. Uniformly, all three studies report a decrease of the ~90 kDa BIN1:H isoform and an increase of the ~65-75 kDa BIN1:L isoforms (Fig. 3). Further, we show that the decrease of the BIN1:H isoform correlated with a decrease in Amphiphysin 1 and neuronal markers, concurrent with the loss of neurons observed in AD. While BIN1:L expression highly correlated with oligodendrocyte markers, as expected from our immunostaining analysis, the correlation with GFAP or CD45 could also suggest an increase in BIN1:L expression in parallel with activation of astrocytes and microglia as well as infiltration of macrophages during pathogenesis. While this manuscript was under review, Adams and colleagues reported BIN1 expression in white matter and oligodendrocytes in the brain but not in neurons in healthy controls [58], consistent with our results. Interestingly, their study revealed weak BIN1 immunoreactivity in a subset of neurons in patients with AD. The findings described here complement the report by Adams et al. by identifying selective alterations of BIN1 isoforms in the gray matter of patients with AD.

A potential function for BIN1 in AD pathogenesis

There is substantial interest in understanding the functional connection between BIN1 and AD pathogenesis. In an earlier study, RNAi-mediated silencing of BIN1 expression in HeLa cells resulted in a 1.5- and 2-fold increase in Aβ40 and Aβ42 secretion, respectively [59]. It is tempting to speculate that this effect could have resulted from alterations in proteolytic processing of APP in endosomes in cells lacking BIN1 expression. However, the lack of a significant change in sAPPβ production argues against a simple model whereby the loss of BIN1 had an effect on endocytic trafficking of APP or BACE1, thus promoting amyloidogenic processing of APP. Moreover, the loss of BIN1 function neither impaired endocytic transferrin uptake in *Bin1−/−* fibroblasts nor phagocytic internalization of zymosan [10]. Thus, it is unlikely that RNAi knockdown of BIN1 introduced endocytic defects that altered Aβ generation. Interestingly, partial or total loss of *Amphiphysin* expression attenuated the rough eye phenotype induced by the overexpression of human Tau but not Aβ42 in *Drosophila* eye. A previous study showed an interaction between fly Amphiphysin and human Tau in a fly model of AD Tau pathology [26]. Whether this functional interaction between BIN1 and Tau enhances AD risk in mammalian brain awaits experimental confirmation. In this regard, it is worth noting that Tau is expressed in mature oligodendrocytes and Tau recruitment to the sites of process outgrowth is a critical step in the initiation of myelination [60, 61]. Whether a functional interaction between BIN1 and Tau in oligodendrocytes has physiological and/or pathological implications in myelination is a topic worth investigating in the future.

AD pathology in the white matter includes the loss of myelin and a decrease in oligodendrocyte proteins [62–68]. The exposure of oligodendrocytes to Aβ induces apoptotic cell death [69] and studies in AD transgenic mouse models show defects in myelin integrity [70, 71]. Moreover, analysis of human post-mortem brain tissue suggests an age-related reduction in myelin repair capacity associated with AD pathogenesis [71]. Therefore, insights into BIN1's function in oligodendrocytes will advance our understanding of its involvement as an AD risk factor.

Conclusions

BIN1 is the most significant late-onset AD susceptibility locus identified via the genome-wide association studies. Multiple BIN1 isoforms are expressed in the human brain and there are significant changes in the levels of select BIN1 isoforms in the brains of individuals with late-onset AD. BIN1 is predominantly expressed by the myelinating cells in the brain and its expression is upregulated during myelin formation in vitro and in vivo. BIN is enriched in the white matter in the human and rodent brain and its diminution correlates with the extent of demyelination within subcortical plaques of patients with Multiple Sclerosis. Our results suggest a potential role for BIN1 in mature oligodendrocytes in the brain.

Additional files

Additional file 1: Table S1. List of antibodies used in this study.

Additional file 2: Figure S1. Quantification of *BIN1* transcript levels in the brains of patients with and without Alzheimer's disease. (A-C) Scatter plots of BIN1+Ex7 expression in comparison with cellular marker expression. (D-F) Scatter plots of D7-Ex7 expression in comparison with cellular marker expression. AD = Alzheimer's disease; Norm = normalized expression. The results do not support an association between *BIN1* expression and the expression of cellular markers of astrocytes (*GFAP*), microglia [geometric mean of CD11b (*ITGAM*) and Iba1 (*AIF1*) expression (Malik et al., 2013)], and endothelial cells [geometric mean of von Willebrand Factor (*VWF*) and CD31 (*PECAM1*) expression (Parikh et al., 2014).

Additional file 3: Table S2. BIN1+ Ex7 expression is correlated with AD status and synaptophysin expression.

Additional file 4: Table S3. Quantification of BIN1+Ex7 expression relative to AD status.

Additional file 5: Table S4. D7-BIN1 expression is correlated with MBP expression but not AD status

Additional file 6: Figure S2. Characterization of polyclonal BIN1 antibody BSH3. (A) Schematic illustration of the exon structure of *BIN1* and possible alternate splicing. The protein structures of BIN1 isoforms 6-10 generated by alternate splicing of exons 13-17, which encode the CLAP and MBD are depicted. Note that exons 18-20 are invariable in all BIN1 isoforms. (B) Immunoblot analysis of C-terminally FLAG-tagged BIN1 isoforms 6-10 expressed in HEK293 cells [expression plasmids were generously provided by Dr. Zhou, Merck Research Laboratories]. Blots were probed with pAb BSH3 or anti-FLAG mAb. BSH3 was raised against residues encoded by exons 17-20. The results show that BSH3 is capable of reacting with isoform 10, which lacks exon 17 encoded residues. Thus, this antibody reacts with epitopes common to all BIN1 isoforms, encoded by exons 18-20. N = NH_2 terminus; BAR = Bin-amphiphysin-Rvs domain; PI = phosphoinositide binding domain; CLAP = clathrin/Adaptor protein 2 binding domain; MBD = MYC-binding domain; SH3 = SRC homology 3 domain. (C) Immunofluorescence analysis of antibody specificity. HEK293 cells transiently transfected with FLAG-tagged human BIN1 isoform 7 were stained with a combination of antibodies against the FLAG epitope tag or the indicated BIN1 antibodies. Wide-field images acquired on a Nikon TE2000 microscope using a 100X objective reveal that each BIN1 antibody strongly stains transfected cells.

Additional file 7: Figure S3. Identification of human brain *BIN1* isoforms. (A) Schematic illustration of the exon structure of *BIN1* and possible alternate splicing. (B) Analysis of human brain RT-PCR products. Human brain samples were subjected to RT-PCR analysis by using primers corresponding to sequences within exons 12 and 18 and the resulting amplicons were separated by polyacrylamide gel electrophoresis. Individual bands were excised from the gels and analyzed by sequencing to identify the major isoforms generated by alternate splicing of exons 13-17. The relative amounts of the isoforms within samples are semi-quantitative given that the smaller PCR amplicons could have been preferentially amplified as these samples underwent 30 cycles of PCR amplification.

Additional file 8: Figure S4. The distribution of BIN1 in rat brain. BIN1 staining is in green and nuclei stained with Hoechst are in blue. (A and B) Immunofluorescence staining of coronal sections with antibodies N-19 or 2F11 reveals BIN1 immunoreactivity in the cortex with intense straining of the corpus callosum (CC). (C and D) Higher magnification images of 2F11 staining of oligodendrocytes dispersed in the cortex and arranged as linear arrays in the corpus callosum.

Additional file 9: Figure S5. Loss of BIN1 staining in multiple sclerosis brain lesions. Staining of adjacent serial autopsy brain sections with Luxol fast blue (left) and BIN1 antibodies N19 and 99D shows that myelin loss parallels the loss of BIN1 staining intensity within multiple sclerosis plaques. Images correspond to an active lesion (top), shadow plaque (middle) and chronic plaque (bottom). Dashed lines mark the lesion border.

Additional file 10: Figure S6. BIN1 is not expressed in human brain microglial cells. (A) Immunohistochemical staining of adjacent sections of normal human brain cortex with antibodies against BIN1 or Iba1 reveals that BIN1 immunoreactive cells that are morphologically distinct from microglia. The boxed region is shown at a higher magnification on the right. (B) Single and two-color immunostaining of the human brain using antibodies against BIN1 and CD45 reveals that perivenular CD45-positive cells of the hematopoietic lineage do not express BIN1.

Abbreviations

ASPA, aspartoacylase; BAR, Bin/Amphiphysin/Rvs; BIN1, Bridging Integrator 1; Caspr, contactin-associated protein; CC1, crenarchaeal chromatin protein 1; cDNA, complementary DNA; CLAP, CLathrin-Associated Protein binding region; CNPase, 2',3'-Cyclic-Nucleotide 3'-Phosphodiesterase; GFAP, glial fibrillary acidic protein; Iba1, ionized calcium-binding adapter molecule 1; LOAD, late-onset alzheimer's disease; mAb, monoclonal antibody; MAP2, microtubule-associated protein 2; MBP, myelin basic protein; NG2, neural/glial antigen 2; OPC, oligodendrocyte progenitor cell; pAb, polyclonal antibody; PSD95, post-synaptic density protein 95; qPCR, quantitative polymerase chain reaction; RT, reverse transcription; TPPP/p25, tubulin polymerisation-promoting protein p25

Acknowledgements

We thank the University of Kentucky AD Center Neuropathology Core for providing the human brain specimens used for RNA analysis. Postmortem tissue specimens for biochemical analysis were provided by NIH Neurobiobank through the Human Brain and Spinal Fluid Resource Center, VA West Los Angeles Healthcare Center, which is sponsored by NINDS/NIMH, National Multiple Sclerosis Society, and the Department of Veterans Administration. We thank the Histology Core Facility at the University of Chicago Human Tissue Resource Center for immunostaining of human tissue. We thank Dr. Manuel F. Utset for helpful suggestions during the course of this study.

Funding

This study was supported by Cure Alzheimer's Fund (GT), National Multiple Sclerosis Society and Illinois Department of Public Health Multiple Sclerosis Research Fund Grant (GT), BrightFocus Foundation (SE), and National Institutes of Health grants AG019070 (GT), AG045775 (SE), and NS034939 (PB). P.D.R. was supported by an AD Research fellowship from the Illinois Department of Public Health and V.B.P was supported by a postdoctoral fellowship from BrightFocus Foundation. C.V.S. was supported by the National Center for Advancing Translational Sciences grant UL1TR000117. The authors acknowledge the University of Kentucky Alzheimer's Center (supported by P30-AG028383) for human tissue samples. Confocal imaging was performed at the Integrated Microscopy Core Facility at the University of Chicago (supported by S10OD010649). The use of University of Chicago's Core Facilities was supported by the National Center For Advancing Translational Sciences Award 5 UL1 TR 000430-09.

Authors' contributions

PDR, VBP, SE, and GT designed experiments and analyzed the data with the help of SK, BP, and PP. JBV, CVS, and SE performed human brain mRNA expression analysis. PDR, VBP, RL, AB, SS, RCR, and SK performed immunolabeling and PDR, VBP, SK, PP, and GT analyzed the data. PDR, RJA, ER, and CD performed immunoblotting and analyzed the data. BLLC, PDR, and BP characterized BIN1 expression in cultured oligodendrocytes and analyzed the data. PDR, VBP, and GT performed confocal imaging. PDR, VBP, SE, and GT wrote the manuscript. GT conceived of the study, coordinated data analysis, and prepared the final manuscript. All authors read and approved the final manuscript.

Competing interests

The authors declare that they have no competing interests.

Notes

Pierre De Rossi and Virginie Buggia-Prevot are co-first authors.
VBP's Present Address: The Neurodegeneration Consortium, The University of Texas MD Anderson Cancer Center, Houston, TX 77054, U.S.A.

Author details

[1]Department of Neurobiology, The University of Chicago, JFK R212, 924 East 57th Street, Chicago, IL 60637, USA. [2]Department of Neurology, The University of Chicago, Chicago, IL 60637, USA. [3]Sanders-Brown Center on Aging and Department of Physiology, University of Kentucky, Lexington, KY 40536, USA. [4]Centre for prions and protein folding diseases, University of Alberta, Edmonton, AB T6G 2B7, Canada. [5]Department of Pathology, The University of Chicago, Chicago, IL 60637, USA.

References

1. Prokic I, Cowling BS, Laporte J. Amphiphysin 2 (BIN1) in physiology and diseases. J Mol Med. 2014;92:453–63.
2. Sakamuro D, Elliott KJ, Wechsler-Reya R, Prendergast GC. BIN1 is a novel MYC-interacting protein with features of a tumour suppressor. Nat Genet. 1996;14:69–77.
3. Lichte B, Veh RW, Meyer HE, Kilimann MW. Amphiphysin, a novel protein associated with synaptic vesicles. EMBO J. 1992;11:2521–30.
4. Butler MH, David C, Ochoa GC, Freyberg Z, Daniell L, Grabs D, Cremona O, De Camilli P. Amphiphysin II (SH3P9; BIN1), a member of the amphiphysin/Rvs family, is concentrated in the cortical cytomatrix of axon initial segments and nodes of ranvier in brain and around T tubules in skeletal muscle. J Cell Biol. 1997;137:1355–67.
5. Ramjaun AR, Micheva KD, Bouchelet I, McPherson PS. Identification and characterization of a nerve terminal-enriched amphiphysin isoform. J Biol Chem. 1997;272:16700–6.
6. Leprince C, Romero F, Cussac D, Vayssiere B, Berger R, Tavitian A, Camonis JH. A new member of the amphiphysin family connecting endocytosis and signal transduction pathways. J Biol Chem. 1997;272:15101–5.
7. Tsutsui K, Maeda Y, Tsutsui K, Seki S, Tokunaga A. cDNA cloning of a novel amphiphysin isoform and tissue-specific expression of its multiple splice variants. Biochem Biophys Res Commun. 1997;236:178–83.
8. Wigge P, Kohler K, Vallis Y, Doyle CA, Owen D, Hunt SP, McMahon HT. Amphiphysin heterodimers: potential role in clathrin-mediated endocytosis. Mol Biol Cell. 1997;8:2003–15.
9. Wigge P, McMahon HT. The amphiphysin family of proteins and their role in endocytosis at the synapse. Trends Neurosci. 1998;21:339–44.

10. Muller AJ, Baker JF, DuHadaway JB, Ge K, Farmer G, Donover PS, et al. Targeted disruption of the murine Bin1/Amphiphysin II gene does not disable endocytosis but results in embryonic cardiomyopathy with aberrant myofibril formation. Mol Cell Biol. 2003;23:4295–306.
11. Prendergast GC, Muller AJ, Ramalingam A, Chang MY. BAR the door: cancer suppression by amphiphysin-like genes. Biochim Biophys Acta. 2009;1795:25–36.
12. Wechsler-Reya R, Sakamuro D, Zhang J, Duhadaway J, Prendergast GC. Structural analysis of the human BIN1 gene. Evidence for tissue-specific transcriptional regulation and alternate RNA splicing. J Biol Chem. 1997;272:31453–8.
13. DuHadaway JB, Lynch FJ, Brisbay S, Bueso-Ramos C, Troncoso P, McDonnell T, Prendergast GC. Immunohistochemical analysis of Bin1/Amphiphysin II in human tissues: diverse sites of nuclear expression and losses in prostate cancer. J Cell Biochem. 2003;88:635–42.
14. Micheva KD, Ramjaun AR, Kay BK, McPherson PS. SH3 domain-dependent interactions of endophilin with amphiphysin. FEBS Lett. 1997;414:308–12.
15. Owen DJ, Wigge P, Vallis Y, Moore JD, Evans PR, McMahon HT. Crystal structure of the amphiphysin-2 SH3 domain and its role in the prevention of dynamin ring formation. EMBO J. 1998;17:5273–85.
16. Nicot AS, Toussaint A, Tosch V, Kretz C, Wallgren-Pettersson C, Iwarsson E, et al. Mutations in amphiphysin 2 (BIN1) disrupt interaction with dynamin 2 and cause autosomal recessive centronuclear myopathy. Nat Genet. 2007;39:1134–9.
17. Ellis JD, Barrios-Rodiles M, Colak R, Irimia M, Kim T, Calarco JA, et al. Tissue-specific alternative splicing remodels protein-protein interaction networks. Mol Cell. 2012;46:884–92.
18. Kadlec L, Pendergast AM. The amphiphysin-like protein 1 (ALP1) interacts functionally with the cABL tyrosine kinase and may play a role in cytoskeletal regulation. Proc Natl Acad Sci U S A. 1997;94:12390–5.
19. Fernando P, Sandoz JS, Ding W, de Repentigny Y, Brunette S, Kelly JF, Kothary R, Megeney LA. Bin1 SRC homology 3 domain acts as a scaffold for myofiber sarcomere assembly. J Biol Chem. 2009;284:27674–86.
20. Falcone S, Roman W, Hnia K, Gache V, Didier N, Laine J, et al. N-WASP is required for Amphiphysin-2/BIN1-dependent nuclear positioning and triad organization in skeletal muscle and is involved in the pathophysiology of centronuclear myopathy. EMBO Mol Med. 2014;6:1455–75.
21. Sottejeau Y, Bretteville A, Cantrelle FX, Malmanche N, Demiaute F, Mendes T, et al. Tau phosphorylation regulates the interaction between BIN1's SH3 domain and Tau's proline-rich domain. Acta Neuropathol Commun. 2015;3:58.
22. Harold D, Abraham R, Hollingworth P, Sims R, Gerrish A, Hamshere ML, et al. Genome-wide association study identifies variants at CLU and PICALM associated with Alzheimer's disease. Nat Genet. 2009;41:1088–93.
23. Seshadri S, Fitzpatrick AL, Ikram MA, DeStefano AL, Gudnason V, Boada M, et al. Genome-wide analysis of genetic loci associated with Alzheimer disease. JAMA. 2010;303:1832–40.
24. Tan MS, Yu JT, Tan L. Bridging integrator 1 (BIN1): form, function, and Alzheimer's disease. Trends Mol Med. 2013;19:594–603.
25. Bertram L, McQueen MB, Mullin K, Blacker D, Tanzi RE. Systematic meta-analyses of Alzheimer disease genetic association studies: the AlzGene database. Nat Genet. 2007;39:17–23.
26. Chapuis J, Hansmannel F, Gistelinck M, Mounier A, Van Cauwenberghe C, Kolen KV, et al. Increased expression of BIN1 mediates Alzheimer genetic risk by modulating tau pathology. Mol Psychiatry. 2013;18:1225–34.
27. Miyagawa T, Ebinuma I, Morohashi Y, Hori Y, Chang MY, Hattori H, et al. BIN1 regulates BACE1 intracellular trafficking and amyloid-beta production. Hum Mol Genet. 2016
28. Karch CM, Jeng AT, Nowotny P, Cady J, Cruchaga C, Goate AM. Expression of novel Alzheimer's disease risk genes in control and Alzheimer's disease brains. PLoS One. 2012;7:e50976.
29. Glennon EB, Whitehouse IJ, Miners JS, Kehoe PG, Love S, Kellett KA, Hooper NM. BIN1 is decreased in sporadic but not familial Alzheimer's disease or in aging. PLoS One. 2013;8:e78806.
30. Holler CJ, Davis PR, Beckett TL, Platt TL, Webb RL, Head E, Murphy MP. Bridging integrator 1 (BIN1) protein expression increases in the Alzheimer's disease brain and correlates with neurofibrillary tangle pathology. J Alzheimers Dis. 2014;42:1221–7.
31. Martiskainen H, Viswanathan J, Nykanen NP, Kurki M, Helisalmi S, Natunen T, et al. Transcriptomics and mechanistic elucidation of Alzheimer's disease risk genes in the brain and in vitro models. Neurobiol Aging. 2015;36:1221. e1215-1228.
32. Dugas JC, Tai YC, Speed TP, Ngai J, Barres BA. Functional genomic analysis of oligodendrocyte differentiation. J Neurosci. 2006;26:10967–83.
33. Zou F, Gopalraj RK, Lok J, Zhu H, Ling IF, Simpson JF, et al. Sex-dependent association of a common low-density lipoprotein receptor polymorphism with RNA splicing efficiency in the brain and Alzheimer's disease. Hum Mol Genet. 2008;17:929–35.
34. Grear KE, Ling IF, Simpson JF, Furman JL, Simmons CR, Peterson SL, et al. Expression of SORL1 and a novel SORL1 splice variant in normal and Alzheimers disease brain. Mol Neurodegener. 2009;4:46.
35. Ling IF, Estus S. Role of SFRS13A in low-density lipoprotein receptor splicing. Hum Mutat. 2010;31:702–9.
36. Nelson PT, Abner EL, Scheff SW, Schmitt FA, Kryscio RJ, Jicha GA, Smith CD, Patel E, Markesbery WR. Alzheimer's-type neuropathology in the precuneus is not increased relative to other areas of neocortex across a range of cognitive impairment. Neurosci Lett. 2009;450:336–9.
37. Nelson PT, Braak H, Markesbery WR. Neuropathology and cognitive impairment in Alzheimer disease: a complex but coherent relationship. J Neuropathol Exp Neurol. 2009;68:1–14.
38. Nelson PT, Kukull WA, Frosch MP. Thinking outside the box: Alzheimer-type neuropathology that does not map directly onto current consensus recommendations. J Neuropathol Exp Neurol. 2010;69:449–54.
39. Way SW, Podojil JR, Clayton BL, Zaremba A, Collins TL, Kunjamma RB, et al. Pharmaceutical integrated stress response enhancement protects oligodendrocytes and provides a potential multiple sclerosis therapeutic. Nat Commun. 2015;6:6532.
40. Buggia-Prévot V, Fernandez CG, Udayar V, Vetrivel KS, Elie A, Roseman J, et al. A function for EHD family proteins in unidirectional retrograde dendritic transport of BACE1 and Alzheimer's disease Aβ production. Cell Rep. 2013;5:1552–63.
41. Parikh I, Fardo DW, Estus S. Genetics of PICALM expression and Alzheimer's disease. PLoS One. 2014;9:e91242.
42. Malik M, Simpson JF, Parikh I, Wilfred BR, Fardo DW, Nelson PT, Estus S. CD33 Alzheimer's risk-altering polymorphism, CD33 expression, and exon 2 splicing. J Neurosci. 2013;33:13320–5.
43. Buggia-Prevot V, Fernandez CG, Riordan S, Vetrivel KS, Roseman J, Waters J, Bindokas VP, Vassar R, Thinakaran G. Axonal BACE1 dynamics and targeting in hippocampal neurons: a role for Rab11 GTPase. Mol Neurodegener. 2014;9:1.
44. Rasband WS: ImageJ. Bethesda, Maryland, USA: U. S. National Institutes of Health; 1997–2016
45. Zhang Y, Chen K, Sloan SA, Bennett ML, Scholze AR, O'Keeffe S, et al. An RNA-sequencing transcriptome and splicing database of glia, neurons, and vascular cells of the cerebral cortex. J Neurosci. 2014;34:11929–47.
46. Naj AC, Jun G, Beecham GW, Wang LS, Vardarajan BN, Buros J, et al. Common variants at MS4A4/MS4A6E, CD2AP, CD33 and EPHA1 are associated with late-onset Alzheimer's disease. Nat Genet. 2011;43:436–41.
47. Wechsler-Reya R, Elliott K, Herlyn M, Prendergast GC. The putative tumor suppressor BIN1 is a short-lived nuclear phosphoprotein, the localization of which is altered in malignant cells. Cancer Res. 1997;57:3258–63.
48. David C, McPherson PS, Mundigl O, de Camilli P. A role of amphiphysin in synaptic vesicle endocytosis suggested by its binding to dynamin in nerve terminals. Proc Natl Acad Sci U S A. 1996;93:331–5.
49. Peles E, Nativ M, Lustig M, Grumet M, Schilling J, Martinez R, Plowman GD, Schlessinger J. Identification of a novel contactin-associated transmembrane receptor with multiple domains implicated in protein-protein interactions. EMBO J. 1997;16:978–88.
50. Ishii A, Dutta R, Wark GM, Hwang SI, Han DK, Trapp BD, Pfeiffer SE, Bansal R. Human myelin proteome and comparative analysis with mouse myelin. Proc Natl Acad Sci U S A. 2009;106:14605–10.
51. Han MH, Lundgren DH, Jaiswal S, Chao M, Graham KL, Garris CS, et al. Janus-like opposing roles of CD47 in autoimmune brain inflammation in humans and mice. J Exp Med. 2012;209:1325–34.
52. Su AI, Cooke MP, Ching KA, Hakak Y, Walker JR, Wiltshire T, et al. Large-scale analysis of the human and mouse transcriptomes. Proc Natl Acad Sci U S A. 2002;99:4465–70.
53. Holton P, Ryten M, Nalls M, Trabzuni D, Weale ME, Hernandez D, et al. Initial assessment of the pathogenic mechanisms of the recently identified Alzheimer risk Loci. Ann Hum Genet. 2013;77:85–105.
54. Elliott K, Ge K, Du W, Prendergast GC. The c-Myc-interacting adaptor protein Bin1 activates a caspase-independent cell death program. Oncogene. 2000;19:4669–84.
55. Leventis PA, Chow BM, Stewart BA, Iyengar B, Campos AR, Boulianne GL.

Drosophila Amphiphysin is a post-synaptic protein required for normal locomotion but not endocytosis. Traffic. 2001;2:839–50.
56. Razzaq A, Robinson IM, McMahon HT, Skepper JN, Su Y, Zelhof AC, Jackson AP, Gay NJ, O'Kane CJ. Amphiphysin is necessary for organization of the excitation-contraction coupling machinery of muscles, but not for synaptic vesicle endocytosis in Drosophila. Genes Dev. 2001;15:2967–79.
57. Zelhof AC, Bao H, Hardy RW, Razzaq A, Zhang B, Doe CQ. Drosophila Amphiphysin is implicated in protein localization and membrane morphogenesis but not in synaptic vesicle endocytosis. Development. 2001;128:5005–15.
58. Adams SL, Tilton K, Kozubek JA, Seshadri S, Delalle I. Subcellular Changes in Bridging Integrator 1 Protein Expression in the Cerebral Cortex During the Progression of Alzheimer Disease Pathology. J Neuropathol Exp Neurol. 2016
59. Bali J, Gheinani AH, Zurbriggen S, Rajendran L. Role of genes linked to sporadic Alzheimer's disease risk in the production of beta-amyloid peptides. Proc Natl Acad Sci U S A. 2012;109:15307–11.
60. LoPresti P, Szuchet S, Papasozomenos SC, Zinkowski RP, Binder LI. Functional implications for the microtubule-associated protein tau: localization in oligodendrocytes. Proc Natl Acad Sci U S A. 1995;92:10369–73.
61. Klein C, Kramer EM, Cardine AM, Schraven B, Brandt R, Trotter J. Process outgrowth of oligodendrocytes is promoted by interaction of fyn kinase with the cytoskeletal protein tau. J Neurosci. 2002;22:698–707.
62. Vlkolinský R, Cairns N, Fountoulakis M, Lubec G. Decreased brain levels of 2',3'-cyclic nucleotide-3'-phosphodiesterase in Down syndrome and Alzheimer's disease. Neurobiol Aging. 2001;22:547–53.
63. Roher AE, Weiss N, Kokjohn TA, Kuo Y-M, Kalback W, Anthony J, et al. Increased Aβ peptides and reduced cholesterol and myelin proteins characterize white matter degeneration in Alzheimer's disease. Biochemistry. 2002;41:11080–90.
64. Kamphuis W, Orre M, Kooijman L, Dahmen M, Hol EM. Differential cell proliferation in the cortex of the APPswePS1dE9 Alzheimer's disease mouse model. Glia. 2012;60:615–29.
65. Gagyi E, Kormos B, Castellanos KJ, Valyi-Nagy K, Korneff D, LoPresti P, Woltjer R, Valyi-Nagy T. Decreased oligodendrocyte nuclear diameter in Alzheimer's disease and Lewy body dementia. Brain pathology (Zurich, Switzerland). 2012;22:803–10.
66. Desai MK, Sudol KL, Janelsins MC, Mastrangelo MA, Frazer ME, Bowers WJ. Triple-transgenic Alzheimer's disease mice exhibit region-specific abnormalities in brain myelination patterns prior to appearance of amyloid and tau pathology. Glia. 2009;57:54–65.
67. Mitew S, Kirkcaldie MTK, Halliday GM, Shepherd CE, Vickers JC, Dickson TC. Focal demyelination in Alzheimer's disease and transgenic mouse models. Acta Neuropathol. 2010;119:567–77.
68. Gold BT, Johnson NF, Powell DK, Smith CD. White matter integrity and vulnerability to Alzheimer's disease: preliminary findings and future directions. Biochim Biophys Acta. 1822;2012:416–22.
69. Xu J, Chen S, Ahmed SH, Chen H, Ku G, Goldberg MP, Hsu CY. Amyloid-beta peptides are cytotoxic to oligodendrocytes. J Neurosci. 2001;21:RC118.
70. Desai MK, Mastrangelo MA, Ryan DA, Sudol KL, Narrow WC, Bowers WJ. Early oligodendrocyte/myelin pathology in Alzheimer's disease mice constitutes a novel therapeutic target. Am J Pathol. 2010;177:1422–35.
71. Behrendt G, Baer K, Buffo A, Curtis MA, Faull RL, Rees MI, Gotz M, Dimou L. Dynamic changes in myelin aberrations and oligodendrocyte generation in chronic amyloidosis in mice and men. Glia. 2013;61:273–86.

Chronic adiponectin deficiency leads to Alzheimer's disease-like cognitive impairments and pathologies through AMPK inactivation and cerebral insulin resistance in aged mice

Roy Chun-Laam Ng[1,4], On-Yin Cheng[1,4], Min Jian[1], Jason Shing-Cheong Kwan[1,4], Philip Wing-Lok Ho[1,2], Kenneth King-Yip Cheng[1,2], Patrick Ka Kit Yeung[5], Lena Lei Zhou[5], Ruby Lai-Chong Hoo[1,2], Sookja Kim Chung[2,3,5], Aimin Xu[1,2], Karen Siu-Ling. Lam[1,2,3,6*] and Koon Ho Chan[1,2,3,4,6*]

Abstract

Background: Insulin resistance is the major pathogenesis underlying type 2 diabetes mellitus (T2DM) and these patients have doubled risk of Alzheimer's disease (AD). Increasing evidence suggests that insulin resistance plays an important role in AD pathogenesis, possibly due to abnormal GSK3β activation, causing intra- and extracellular amyloid-beta (Aβ) accumulation. Adiponectin (APN) is an adipokine with insulin-sensitizing and anti-inflammatory effects. Reduced circulatory APN level is associated with insulin resistance and T2DM. The role of APN in AD has not been elucidated. In this study, we aim to examine if adiponectin deficiency would lead to cerebral insulin resistance, cognitive decline and Alzheimer's-like pathology in mice.

Methods: To study the role of adiponectin in cognitive functions, we employed adiponectin-knockout (APN-KO) mice and demonstrated chronic APN deficiency in their CNS. Behavioral tests were performed to study the cognitions of male APN-KO mice. Brains and tissue lysates were collected to study the pathophysiological and molecular changes in the brain of APN-KO mice. SH-SY5Y neuroblastoma cell line was used to study the molecular mechanism upon APN and insulin treatment.

Results: Aged APN-deficient mice displayed spatial memory and learning impairments, fear-conditioned memory deficit as well as anxiety. These mice also developed AD pathologies including increased cerebral $A\beta_{42}$ level, Aβ deposition, hyperphosphorylated Tau proteins, microgliosis and astrogliosis with increased cerebral IL-1β and TNFα levels that associated with increased neuronal apoptosis and reduced synaptic proteins levels, suggesting APN deficiency may lead to neuronal and synaptic loss in the brain. AD pathologies-associated APN-KO mice displayed attenuated AMPK phosphorylation and impaired insulin signaling including decreased Akt induction and increased GSK3β activation in the hippocampus and frontal cortex. Aged APN-KO mice developed hippocampal insulin resistance with reduced pAkt induction upon intracerebral insulin injection. Consistently, APN treatment in SH-SY5Y cells with insulin resistance and overexpressing Aβ induce higher pAkt levels through AdipoR1 upon insulin treatment whereas the induction was blocked by compound C, indicating APN can enhance neuronal insulin sensitivity through AMPK activation.
(Continued on next page)

* Correspondence: ksllam@hku.hk; koonho@hkucc.hku.hk
[1]Department of Medicine, LKS Faculty of Medicine, The University of Hong Kong, Hong Kong, Special Administrative Region, China
Full list of author information is available at the end of the article

(Continued from previous page)

Conclusion: Our results indicated that chronic APN deficiency inactivated AMPK causing insulin desensitization and elicited AD-like pathogenesis in aged mice which also developed significant cognitive impairments and psychiatric symptoms.

Keywords: Adiponectin, Alzheimer's disease, Insulin resistance, Aβ, AMPK, Cognitive impairments

Background

Alzheimer's disease (AD) is the most common cause of dementia in the elderlies. AD brain pathologies are characterized by deposition of extracellular amyloid-β (Aβ)-containing senile plaques, intracellular hyperphosphorylated Tau-containing neurofibrillary tangles (NFT), neuroinflammation, synaptic loss and neuronal death, leading to cognitive impairments. Aging and apolipoprotein E ε4 allele are known risk factors. Recently, type 2 diabetes mellitus (T2DM) is recognized as another risk factor of AD. Accumulating evidence demonstrated that T2DM and AD share similar pathophysiologies such as insulin resistance, disrupted glucose and lipid metabolism, inflammation and oxidative stress [1–5].

Cerebral insulin resistance is increasingly recognized as an important factor of AD pathogenesis. A series of studies has shown a strong association between insulin signaling and Aβ metabolism. Notably, Aβ oligomers, including dimers, trimers and dodecamers (Aβ*56), are the early neurotoxic species in AD. Cerebral insulin resistance results in glycogen synthase kinase 3β (GSK3β) activation, leading to increased Aβ production and Tau phosphorylation [6–8]. It was reported that insulin resistance increased extracellular Aβ deposition by enhancing γ-secretase activity, which is involved in Aβ production, thereby promoting Aβ secretion from neurons [9]. In contrast, insulin inhibits the GSK3β activity to prevent generation of Aβ and hyperphosphorylated Tau [8, 10]. Studies using transgenic AD mice models revealed that the transgenic mice exhibited hippocampal insulin resistance [11]. Leptin-deficient mice, a T2DM model, displayed impaired cerebral insulin signaling and cognitive impairments after treating with high-fat-diet [12, 13]. Postmortem study of AD brains indicated significant increase of insulin receptor substrate-1 (IRS-1) phosphorylation at serine residues, marker of insulin resistance. In addition, insulin resistance is associated with impaired synaptic plasticity [14]. Insulin administration reduced chronic neuroinflammation and microglia activation as well as enhanced synapse formation in AD mouse model [15, 16]. These studies established the associations between AD, cerebral insulin resistance and T2DM.

Adiponectin (APN) is an adipocyte-secreted circulating hormone, which exerts insulin sensitizing, anti-inflammatory and anti-oxidative effects to peripheral tissues. APN exists in three oligomeric forms in circulation, including trimers, hexamers and high molecular weight (HMW) oligomers [17]. T2DM patients and aged individuals have reduced circulating APN levels [18]. APN deficiency is associated with peripheral insulin resistance in mice and human, causing T2DM and DM-related syndromes [19, 20], whereas whether adiponectin is associated with cerebral insulin sensitivity has not been documented. Studies indicated APN can ameliorate insulin sensitivity by enhancing AMP-activated protein kinase (AMPK) phosphorylation, thereby, activating insulin receptor substrate (IRS) phosphorylation at Tyrosine residues. This promotes insulin signaling activities including insulin-mediated cell survival by inhibiting GSK3β and glucose uptake by enhancing translocation of GLUT4 transporter [21, 22].

The role of APN in the central nervous system (CNS) is not well characterized. Adiponectin receptors (AdipoR1 & AdipoR2) are abundantly expressed in the hippocampus, cortex and hypothalamus [23, 24]. Only trimeric and hexameric APN are detectable in human cerebrospinal fluid (CSF) suggesting that low molecular weight APN can cross the blood-brain barrier (BBB) and has a role in CNS [25]. APN has shown to be important in neurogenesis and proliferation of hippocampal neural stem cells [26, 27]. It has also been reported that APN-deficient mice exhibited depressive-like behavior [23]. Physical activities and environmental enrichment can increase cerebral APN levels that exerted anti-depressive effects and reduced neuroinflammation in mice [27]. Loss of APN in mice also exacerbated the severity of encephalomyelitis by activating lymphocytes in the mouse model of multiple sclerosis [28]. Clinical reports revealed association between decreased APN levels and ischemic stroke. APN treatment in mice with cerebral ischemia improved neurobehavioral performance and focal cerebral neurogenesis [29]. T2DM patients with lower serum APN levels have a lower mean hippocampal volume than T2DM patients with normal adiponectin levels [30]. Our previous findings demonstrated APN to be protective against Aβ neurotoxicity [31]. Although a recent publication showed an association between APN gene polymorphism and late onset AD [32], there are contradictory clinical reports on the difference of plasma APN level between non-demented control and AD or mild cognitive impairment patients [33–35]. The role of APN in AD remains uncertain. We, therefore, investigated if chronic APN deficiency would result in cerebral insulin resistance which is associated with AD-like pathologies, and cognitive impairments in aging mice.

In this study, we employed adiponectin knockout (APN-KO) mice to mimic the condition of chronic APN deficiency in T2DM patients and aged subjects, and demonstrated that there were cerebral insulin resistance and deregulated insulin signaling upon APN deficiency. The mice also exhibited memory decline and anxiety associated with AD pathologies including increased Aβ production, Tau phosphorylation, neuroinflammation and neurodegeneration. Our study provides novel evidence on the role of adiponectin in cerebral insulin sensitivity, development of AD-like pathologies and cognitive impairment.

Results

Chronic APN deficiency in CNS of APN-KO Mice

Trimeric APN could cross the BBB [27]. Recent studies showed that mRNA of adiponectin receptors were expressed in mouse brain. We performed immunofluorescent staining of AdipoR1 confirming that AdipoR1 protein is expressed in the cortex and hippocampus of mouse (Additional file 1). This indicated that the brain can respond to adiponectin present in the CNS. To verify if endogenous APN is present in WT mice and absent in APN-KO mice, the concentration of APN in CSF was determined by semi-quantitative dot-blot immunoassay. With reference to the standard curve (Additional file 1), concentrations of APN in CSF of 18-mth old WT mice were 428 ng/mL ± 156 ng/mL ($n = 4$, $p < 0.05$), whereas APN was undetectable in the CSF of aged APN-KO mice (Additional file 1). The APN-KO mice had chronic deficiency of APN, not only in peripheral tissues, but also in the CNS.

Aged APN-KO mice had anxiety, and impaired spatial learning and memory loss

To evaluate if psychiatric symptoms may be related to APN deficiency in aged individuals, we performed open field test to investigate the anxiety level in APN-KO mice. Both 9-mth-old & 18-mth-old APN-KO spent significantly longer time in the margin area and shorter time in the center area (14.05% ± 2.28% in 9-mth-old WT mice vs 7.34% ± 2.19% in 9-mth-old APN-KO mice, Fig. 1a; 15.99% ± 1.43% in 18-mth-old WT mice vs 10.32% ± 1.41% in 18-mth-old APN-KO mice, mean ± S.E.M, $p < 0.05$, Fig. 1b), indicating that chronic APN deficiency in mice was associated with increased anxiety level.

To assess the spatial learning and memory abilities of aging APN-KO mice, we employed a hidden platform version of the Morris-Water-Maze. Time required to locate the hidden platform during acquisition phase was analyzed. In the test, mice were trained with visible platform so that they could learn to locate the platform. The visible platform tests showed that both WT and APN-KO mice had a similar trend of escape latency in all 4 sessions ($p > 0.05$) by 9-mths-of-age and 18-mths-of-age, suggesting that aging did not significantly affect the locomotor activity and vision in WT and APN-KO mice. 9-mth old APN-KO adult mice showed no significant spatial learning and memory impairment ($p > 0.05$, Fig. 1c). However, we observed moderate prolongation in the latency of locating the hidden platform in 18-mth-old APN-KO mice. Although WT and APN-KO mice have had similar escape latency in the first two sessions, there were significant differences in the third and fourth sessions, suggesting that aged APN deficient mice had spatial memory and learning impairment ($p < 0.05$, Fig. 1d), which was not due to differences in swim speed, visual acuity or locomotor deficits as demonstrated by visible platform test and swim speed recording (Additional file 2). In addition, the probe tests indicated that 9-mth old APN-KO mice spent comparable time in the target quadrant (compared with WT, $p > 0.05$; Fig. 1e). In contrast, 18-mth-old APN-KO mice spent significantly less time in the target quadrant, suggesting there is a reference memory retention deficit in aged APN-KO mice ($p < 0.05$, Fig. 1f). These results revealed that chronic APN deficiency in aged mice was associated with spatial learning and memory impairments.

Hence, the APN-KO mice had increased anxiety level. To further confirm that aged APN-KO mice suffered from learning and memory deficits, we performed contextual and cue fear-conditioning test, a stress-associated memory task, governed by hippocampus, amygdala and is cortical-associated. 12-mth old WT mice displayed robust contextual fear conditioning 1 day later with freezing 68.58% ± 6.65%. In contrast, 12-mth old APN-KO mice froze significantly less (14.68% ± 3.08%; $p < 0.001$ versus WT mice; Additional file 3). When the mice were placed in a novel environment and experienced with the same cue without shock, APN-KO mice also froze less than the WT mice (51.71% ± 4.99% in WT mice vs 30.29% ± 3.93% in APN-KO mice; $p < 0.05$, Fig. 1g & Additional file 4). These results provided further support that chronic APN deficiency was associated with impaired hippocampus-dependent learning and memory upon aging.

Aged APN-KO mice had AD-like brain pathologies

To investigate if chronic APN deficiency could lead to increased Aβ production and Aβ oligomers, sections from 18-mth old wildtype and APN-KO mice were stained with antibody (clone 4G8) against Aβ. Faint Aβ-immunoreactive deposits were found in the cortex of APN-KO mice by 18 months but no plaque was present in the wildtype mice. ThioFlavin S staining also indicated the presence of Aβ deposits in APN-KO mice by

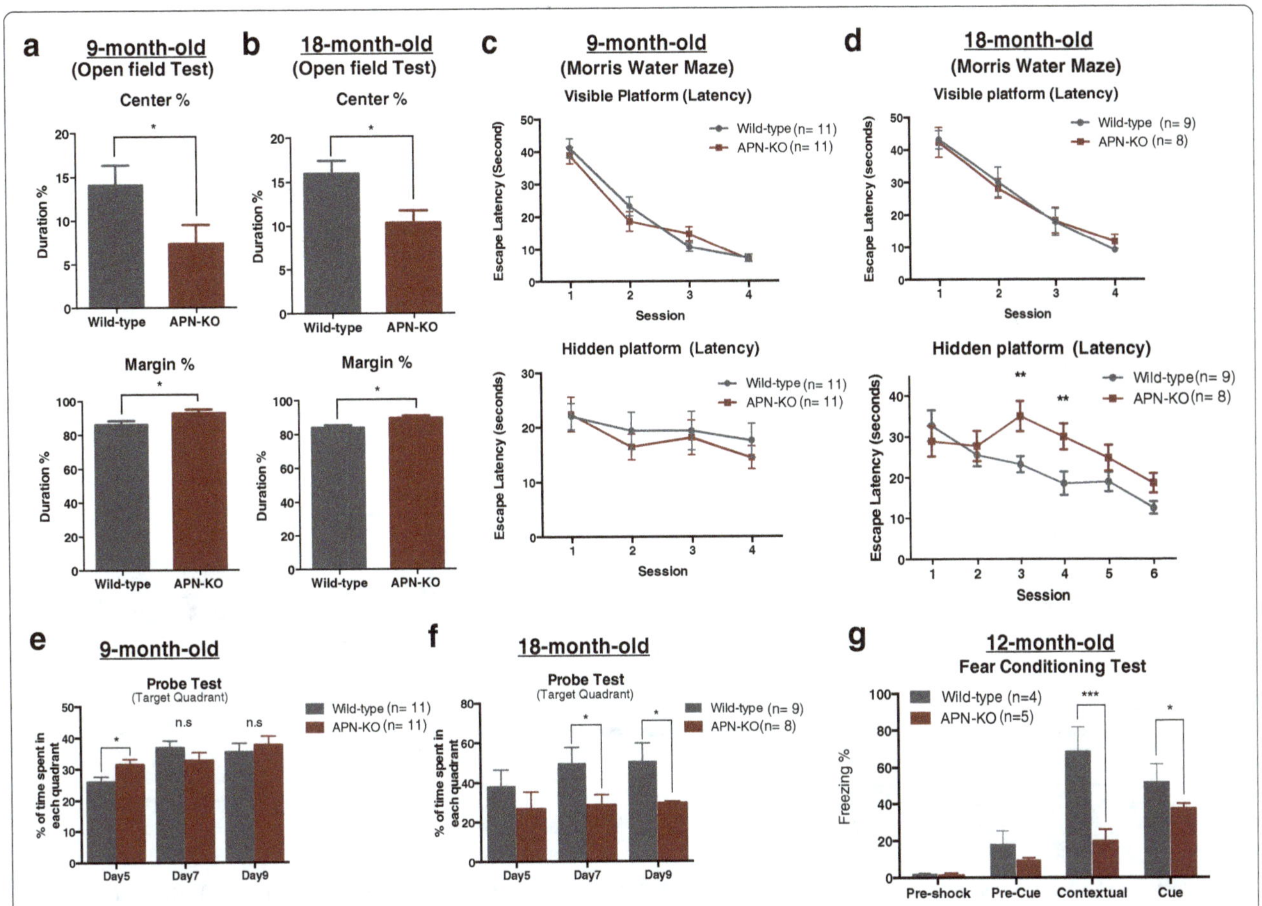

Fig. 1 Cognitive impairments of aged APN-KO mice in behavioral tests. In open-field test, time spent in marginal area and center area for both **(a)** 9-mth-old & **(b)** 18-mth-old wildtype and APN-KO mice were assessed. **c** 9-mth-old & **(d)** 18-mth-old APN-KO mice were trained with visible platform for 16 trials (4 trials/day) and hidden platform for 6 days (4 trials/day) to learn and search in the Morris-Water-Maze tests. Probe tests were performed for both **(e)** 9 mth & **(f)** 18-mth old mice, in which platform had been removed to investigate the time spent in platform quadrant. **(g)** Freezing times of the 12-mth-old mice were recorded in both contextual and cue test, indicating the APN-KO mice exhibited memory impairments. *$p < 0.05$, **$p < 0.01$, ***$p < 0.001$

18 months-of-age (Fig. 2a). Levels of Aβ1-42 in WT and APN-KO mice were also determined by Sandwich ELISA. Aβ1-42 levels in the hippocampus of 9-mth old APN-KO mice were comparable with that of WT mice (WT, 20.12 ± 2.16 pg/mg of protein vs APN-KO, 21.06 ± 8.96 pg/mg of protein; $p > 0.05$) (Fig. 2a). Moreover, soluble Aβ1-42 levels in the frontal cortex of 9-mth-old APN-KO mice were insignificantly higher than that of the WT mice (WT, 16.37 ± 2.29 pg/mg of protein vs APN-KO, 19.06 ± 2.08 pg/mg of protein; $p > 0.05$) (Fig. 2b). However, Aβ1-42 levels were significantly increased in both the hippocampus (WT, 13.45 ± 2.87 pg/mg of protein vs APN-KO, 46.77 ± 11.58 pg/mg of protein; $p < 0.05$) and frontal cortex (WT, 16.15 ± 3.52 pg/mg of protein vs APN-KO, 58.41 ± 16.67 pg/mg of protein; $p < 0.05$) of APN-KO mice relative to the wildtype mice by 18 month (Fig. 2b). In addition, we performed western blot by using 4G8 antibody to further verify the presence of Aβ oligomers in APN-KO mice. Interestingly, a distinct 56 kDa band was detected in the hippocampal and frontal cortical lysate of APN-KO mice by 18-month (Fig. 2c) but not by 9-month old. Aβ*56 is specific oligomeric species present in early AD mice and aged human subjects [36, 37]. These results suggested that chronic APN deficiency in aged mice led to increased cerebral Aβ accumulation.

To study whether Tau protein phosphorylation was increased in APN-KO mice, we evaluated the levels of $pTau^{S199/S202}$ & $pTau^{S396}$ in hippocampus and frontal cortex by western blot. Though Tau5 (total tau) expression varied between the WT and APN-KO mice, results revealed that 18-month old APN-KO mice had increased Tau phosphorylation at both $serine^{199/202}$ and $serine^{396}$ in hippocampus and frontal cortex relative to that of wildtype mice (Fig. 2d).

AD-like neuroinflammation, increased neuronal apoptosis and reduction of synaptic proteins in aged APN-KO mice

To determine if neuroinflammation was present in the brain of aged APN-KO mice, we initially examined

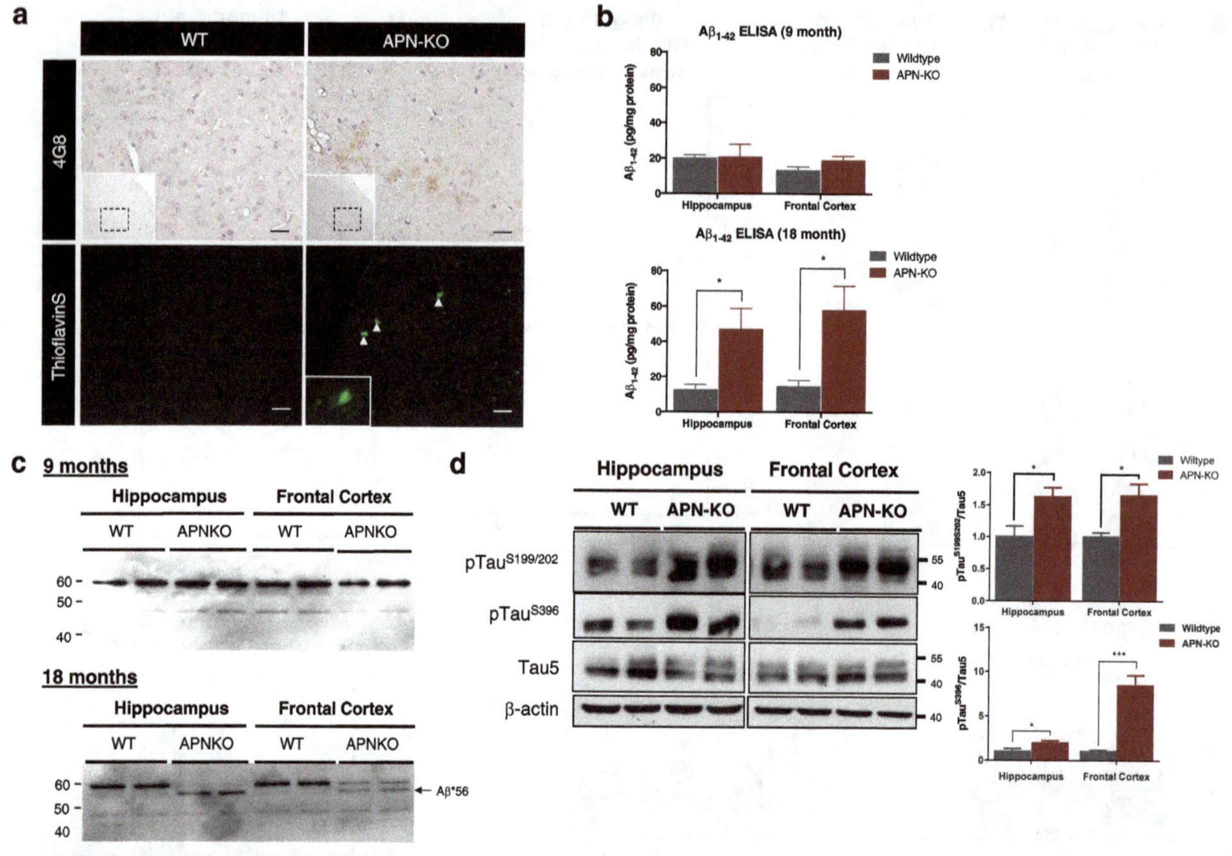

Fig. 2 Increase of Aβ production and Tau phosphorylation in aged APN-KO mice. **a** Immunohistochemistry analysis of anti-Aβ (4G8) showed accumulation of Aβ (*Brown*) in the cortex of 18-month APN-KO mice. **b** ELISA analysis of soluble $A\beta_{1-42}$ in the hippocampal and frontal cortical lysate of 9-month and 18-month old mice. **c** Immunoblotting of mouse Aβ by antibody 4G8 showing the presence of Aβ*56 in the hippocampus and frontal cortex of 18-mth old APN-KO mice. **d** Immunoblotting of pTau $serine^{199}$ & ^{202}, pTau $serine^{396}$ and Tau5 (total tau) in the hippocampus and frontal cortex of 18-mth old mice. Mean ± S.E.M.; *$p < 0.05$, **$p < 0.01$, *n.s. statistically not significant*; WT ($n = 4$) vs APN-KO ($n = 6$). Scale bar: 50 μm

changes of expression of Iba-1, a marker of microglia, in the cortex. Consistent with the robust inflammation reported in AD brains and AD mice model, higher number of Iba1-positive cells was observed in APN-KO by 18-mth (Fig. 3a). Astrogliosis is another pathological hallmark of AD, we then performed immunohistochemistry staining of GFAP in the brain sections of aged APN-KO mice. The number of GFAP-immunoreactive astrocytes in the CA1 regions of the hippocampus was significantly increased and astrocytes displayed hypertrophic changes. Quantitative analysis was also performed to confirm an increase in the number of Iba-1-positive cells in APN-KO mice, as compared with the wildtype mice. Furthermore, quantitative analysis revealed that the percentage of the area occupied by GFAP-positive cells was increased in the hippocampus of the APN-KO mice compared with the wildtype mice (Fig. 3b). We subsequently studied the expression of MHCII, a marker of proinflammatory activation (M1) of microglia, by western blot. The substantial increase of MHCII expression in both frontal cortex and hippocampus of 18-month old APN-KO mice indicated that the mice had reactivation of microglia and chronic cerebral inflammation (Fig. 3c). Reactivated microglia secrete proinflammatory cytokines (e.g., TNFα & IL-1β) that can cause synaptic loss [38, 39]. We then examined the cerebral levels of TNFα and IL-1β in APN-KO mice by ELISA assay. Both IL-1β and TNFα levels were increased in the aged APN-KO mice compared with wild-type mice of the same age (Fig. 3d). Together, these data suggested that APN deficiency led to neuroinflammation in aged mice.

To explore whether the cognitive impairments in aged APN-KO mice were associated with neurodegeneration, we evaluated neuronal apoptosis by double immunofluorescent staining of NeuN and TUNEL. Neuronal apoptotic cells in the hippocampus CA1 and cortex were markedly increased in aged APN-KO mice compared with wildtype mice (Fig. 4a). Quantitative analysis revealed that the estimated number of apoptotic cells in cortical defined regions in APN-KO was significantly higher than that of the wildtype mice (214.0 ± 26.2 vs

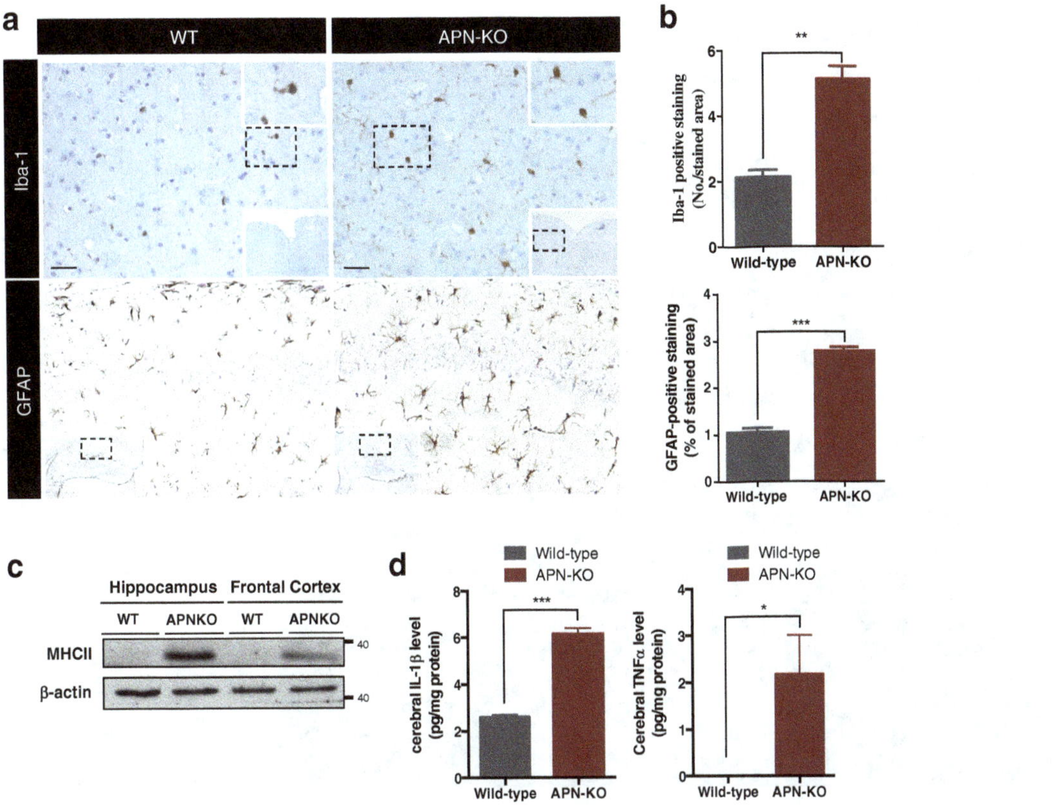

Fig. 3 Microglial reactivation and increased cerebral proinflammatory cytokines in APN-KO mice. **a** Representative image of immunohistochemistry staining of Iba-1 and GFAP represents the present of activated microglia (Brown, black arrows) and astrocytes respectively in the cortex of 18-mth old wildtype and APN-KO mice. **b** The percentage of Iba1 and GFAP positive stained area in the cortex of mice. **c** MHCII, M1 microglial activation marker, was detected in the frontal cortex and the hippocampus of APN-KO mice. **d** Cerebral IL-1β and TNFα levels detected by ELISA indicated significant increase in the 18-mth-old APN-KO mice. Mean ± S.E.M.; $^{*}p < 0.05$, $^{**}p < 0.01$, $^{***}p < 0.001$, *n.s. statistically not significant*; WT ($n = 3$) vs APN-KO ($n = 3$ or 4). Scale bar: 50 μm

46.3 ± 11.9; $p < 0.05$). In addition, the number of apoptotic cells in hippocampal CA1 region was also dramatically higher in APN-KO mice (44.0 ± 7.6 vs 11.3 ± 3.5; $p < 0.01$) than in wildtype mice, indicating that the number of apoptotic neurons was increased in APN-KO mice (Fig. 4b). To study whether the presence of Aβ oligomers and increased proinflammatory cytokines in the APN-KO mice were associated with synaptic loss, we examined the levels of spinophilin (post-synaptic protein) and synaptophysin (pre-synaptic protein) which are the common synaptic markers used to determine synaptic density. Western blot analysis showed that the level of synaptophysin was reduced significantly in the hippocampus and frontal cortex whereas spinophilin was reduced in the hippocampus of the aged APN-KO mice (Fig. 4c & d). Altogether these results suggested that chronic APN deficiency in CNS was associated with neuroinflammation and possibly led to neuronal apoptosis and synaptic loss. They provided an explanation for the cognitive impairments observed in the aged APN-KO mice.

Chronic APN deficiency led to attenuated AMPK activation causing deregulated insulin signaling pathways and cerebral insulin resistance

In peripheral tissues, APN signaling leads to AMPK activation, which reduces IRS-1 phosphorylation at serine residues to enhance insulin sensitivity [22, 40, 41]. To assess if there are changes of cerebral AMPK activities and insulin signaling between aged WT and APN-KO mice, we performed Western blot analysis to study the protein levels of main effectors in AMPK and insulin signaling. We found that there was drastic decrease of AMPK phosphorylation at threonine 172 (pAMPK^{T172}) in the frontal cortex and hippocampus of younger APN-KO mice (9-mth-old; Fig. 5a). Though AMPK phosphorylation was reduced insignificantly in the frontal cortex of APN-KO mice by 18-month-of-age, pAMPK^{T172} in the hippocampus was reduced significantly in APN-KO compared to aged WT mice (Fig. 5b). Concomitantly, pIRS-1^{S616} level was increased in the frontal cortex of aged APN-KO mice (18-mth-old; Fig. 5c), indicating that chronic APN deficiency might

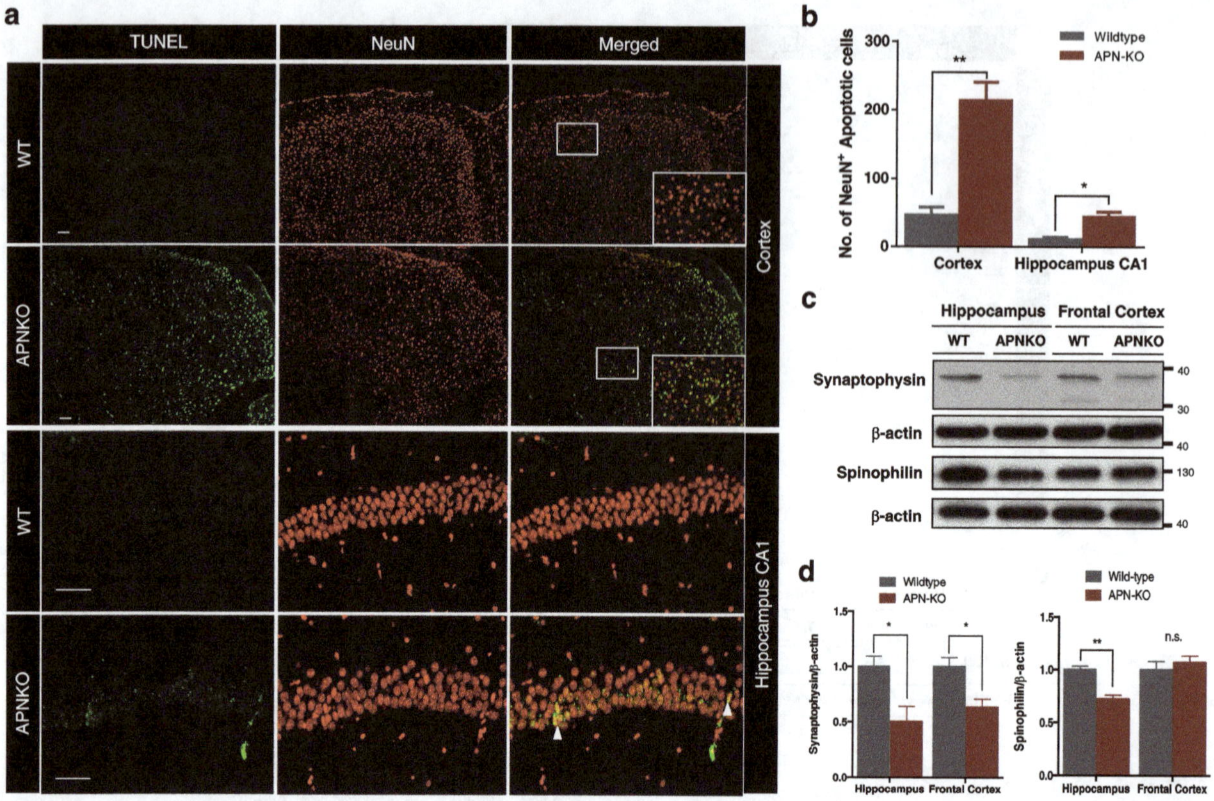

Fig. 4 Neuronal apoptosis and synaptic proteins reduction in 18-month old APN-KO mice. **a** Representative images show TUNEL-labeled (Red) apoptotic cells countered stained with DAPI (blue) in the cortex and hippocampus between 18-month old wildtype and APN-KO mice. **b** Graph demonstrates the differences of quantified numbers of TUNEL-labeled cells in the cortex and hippocampal CA1 region in wildtype and APN-KO mice. Two sampling regions (Blue square) in the cortex and one sampling region (red) in the hippocampal CA1 were defined. **c** Immunoblotting of synaptic proteins, synaptophysin and spinophilin in the hippocampus and frontal cortex of 18-mth old wildtype and APN-KO mice. **d** Densitometric analysis of synaptophysin and spinophilin demonstrating the differences of these synaptic proteins in the frontal cortex and hippocampus between wildtype and APN-KO mice. Mean ± S.E.M.; *$^*p < 0.05$, $^{**}p < 0.01$, $^{***}p < 0.001$, n.s. statistically not significant*; WT ($n = 4$) vs APN-KO ($n = 4$) Scale bar: 50 μm

lead to neuronal insulin resistance through inhibition of the AMPK-IRS1 signaling cascade.

pIRS-1^{S616} hinders the formation of activated form pIRS-1^{Tyr}, inactivating insulin signaling [6]. To examine whether chronic APN deficiency deregulated insulin signaling in neurons of aging mice, we performed western blotting to determine the level of phosphorylated Akt, GSK3α/β and Erk1/2. The levels of $pAkt^{S473}$, pGSK3α^{S21} (inhibitory form of GSK3α) and pGSK3β^{S9} (inhibitory form of GSK3β) were decreased while pGSK3β^{Y216} levels were drastically elevated in the frontal cortex and hippocampus of 9-mth-old APN-KO mice (Fig. 5d). We also found that level of pErk1/2 was reduced in both the frontal cortex and hippocampus of 9-mth old APN-KO mice, further indicating the disruption of insulin signaling (Additional file 5). In addition, there was no significant change in the level of insulin receptor (IR) suggesting that the reduced insulin signaling activities was not associated with reduced IR level (Additional file 6). Interestingly, the levels of IR, pAkt ^{S473}, pGSK3α^{S21}, pGSK3β^{S9} and pErk1/2 were increased significantly in the hippocampus of 18-mth-old APN-KO mice but reduced in the frontal cortex compared to WT mice. pGSK3α^{Y279}/β^{Y216} levels reduced insignificantly in the hippocampus between WT and APN-KO mice by 18-month old. However, the level of pGSK3β^{Y216} was higher in the frontal cortex of APN-KO mice (Fig. 5e, Additional file 5).

Since the endogenous plasma insulin level in APN-KO mice was comparable with the WT mice [42], the impaired insulin signaling activities may be due to changes in neuronal insulin sensitivity. To assess if there was changes in neuronal insulin sensitivity in aged APN-KO mice, we injected insulin (2 IU/kg body weight) to the right hippocampus of 12-mth-old APN-KO mice using a stereotaxic injection approach. We confirmed the position of injection by injecting a visible dye (Additional file 7). We found that induction of Akt activation after insulin injection to the right hippocampus was significantly reduced in the aged APN-KO mice compared to WT mice (Fig. 5f). The hippocampus of aged APN-KO mice was less sensitive to insulin compared to that of WT mice.

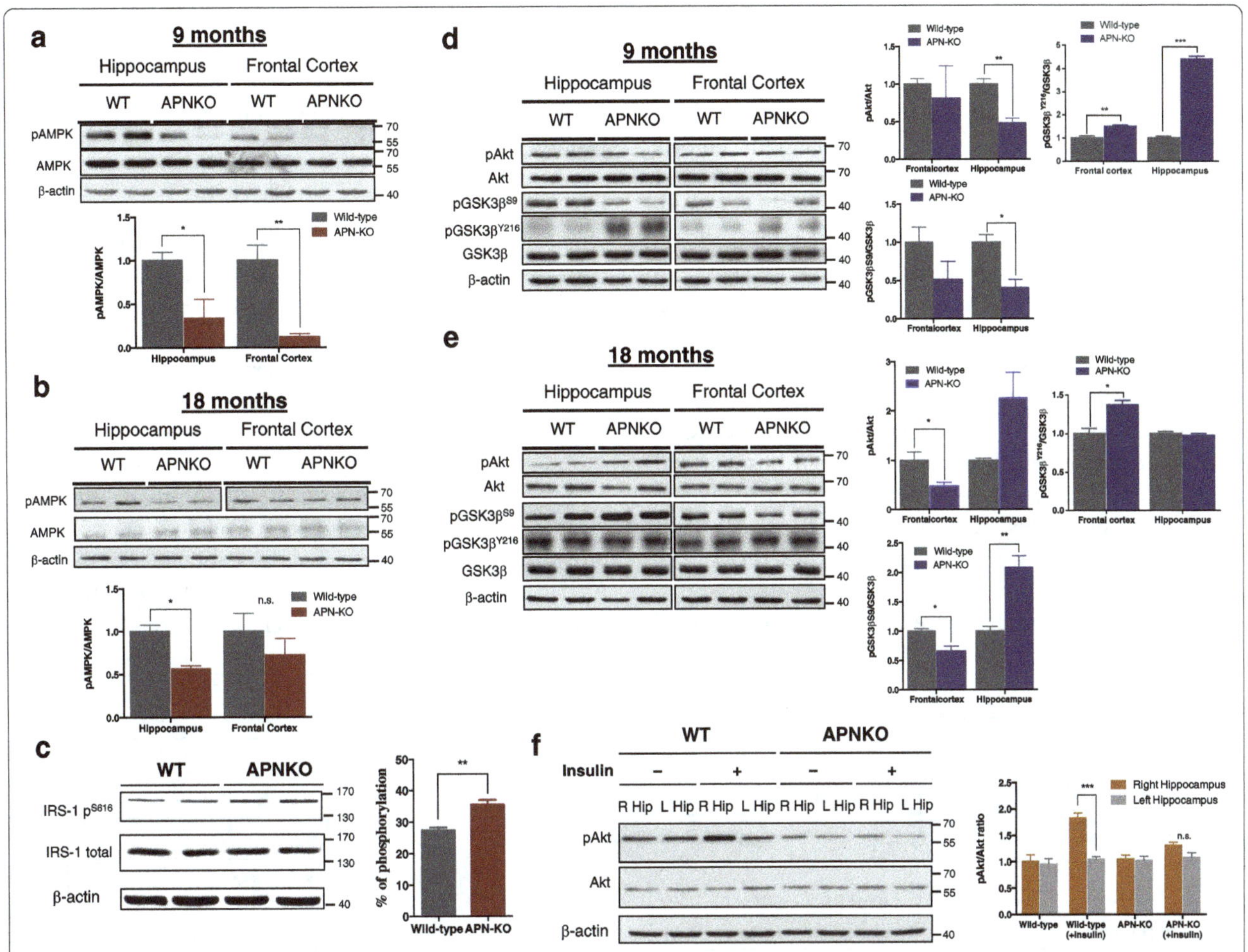

Fig. 5 APN deficiency attenuated AMPK phosphorylation causing insulin resistance and deregulated insulin signaling in APN-KO mice. Representative image of immunoblotting indicated reduction of pAMPK^{T172}/AMPK ratio in both the hippocampus and frontal cortex by **(a)** 9-mth-old and **(b)** 18-mth-old of APN-KO mice. **c** Increased level of IRS-1 phosphorylation at Serine ^{616} shown by immunoblotting in the frontal cortex of APN-KO mice. Representative immunoblotting analysis and densitometric analysis of the ratio of insulin signaling effectors (pAkt^{S473}/Akt, pGSK3β^{S9}/GSK3β, pGSK3β^{Y216}/GSK3β) in the hippocampus and frontal cortex of APN-KO mice or WT mice by **(d)** 9-mth-old & **(e)** 18-mth-old WT and APN-KO mice. **f** Representative image and densitometric analysis of pAkt level induction in the right hippocampus of WT mice and APN-KO mice in response to stereotaxic insulin injection. Mean ± S.E.M.; *$p < 0.05$, **$p < 0.01$, ***$p < 0.001$, *n.s. statistically not significant*; WT ($n = 3$) vs APN-KO ($n = 3$ or 4)

This indicated that chronic APN deficiency led to cerebral insulin resistance. Our results demonstrated that chronic APN deficiency was associated with cerebral insulin resistance and provided a possible molecular mechanism for the pathogenesis of AD in aged APN-KO mice.

APN ameliorates neuronal insulin sensitivity through AdipoR1-mediated AMPK activation

To study the insulin sensitization effect of APN in neuronal culture, human neuroblastoma SH-SY5Y cell line was induced with insulin resistance (SH-SY5Y$_{IR}$) by high concentration insulin. The pAkt level of SH-SY5Y$_{IR}$ cells did not increase after culturing with low concentration insulin (10 nmol/L) showing the presence of insulin resistance ($p > 0.05$). Mammalian trimeric APN restored the induction of pAkt and pGSK3β^{S9} levels in the SH-SY5Y$_{IR}$ cells with increased AMPK phosphorylation when cultured with 10 nmol/L insulin, demonstrating that APN could ameliorate neuronal insulin resistance. Furthermore, Compound C (2 μM), an AMPK inhibitor, blocked the insulin sensitizing effect of adiponectin as pAkt and pGSK3β^{S9} levels were reduced in the SH-SY5Y$_{IR}$ cells (Additional file 8). This indicated that APN enhanced neuronal insulin sensitivity to inhibit GSK3β activity by activating AMPK signaling.

We further examined which adiponectin receptor was involved in APN-enhanced insulin sensitivity in Aβ-producing neurons and whether APN can reduce Aβ production from neuronal cells. SH-SY5Y cells stably transfected with Swedish mutation of APP (SH-SY5Y$_{swAPP}$) produced Aβ oligomers, mimicking the AD neurons, as we reported previously [31]. SH-SY5Y$_{swAPP}$ transfected with a combination of siAdipoR1 and siAdipoR2 had reduced expression of AdipoR1 and AdipoR2 respectively (Fig. 6a). AMPK phosphorylation was blocked in both cells transfected with AdipoR1 and AdipoR2 RNAi duplex upon APN treatment (Fig. 6b). Addition of insulin induced pAkt and pGSK3β^{S9} levels while addition of mammalian trimeric APN (10 μg/mL) further enhanced higher levels of pAkt and pGSK3β^{S9} in SH-SY5Y$_{swAPP}$ cells when cultured with 10 nmol/L insulin. This implicated that APN could also enhance insulin sensitivity in Aβ-overproducing neuroblastoma cells. However, the pAkt and pGSK3β^{S9} levels were not increased in AdipoR1-RNAi-transfected SH-SY5Y$_{swAPP}$ when cultured with APN and insulin compared to the cells cultured with insulin only. In contrast, pAkt and pGSK3β^{S9} levels were further enhanced upon APN plus insulin treatment in SH-SY5Y$_{swAPP}$ cells transfected with AdipoR2 RNAi (Fig. 6c). APN reduced extracellular Aβ levels whereas the reduction was abrogated when SH-SY5Y$_{swAPP}$ cells were transfected with AdipoR1-RNAi. Interestingly, extracellular Aβ levels were also reduced though nonsignificant in AdipoR2-RNAi-transfected cells upon APN treatment (Fig. 6d). These data suggested APN was effective in neuronal insulin-sensitization through AdipoR1-AMPK activation and could be a possible therapeutic agent in AD.

Discussion

Our study demonstrated that aged mice with chronic APN deficiency in brain had spatial memory and fear-conditioned memory impairments as well as anxiety. Cognitive impairments in these aged mice were associated with AD-like pathologies including increased Aβ oligomers and hyperphosphorylated Tau. In addition, neuroinflammation was also found in aged APN-KO mice, as evidenced by substantial microglial reactivation together with elevated proinflammatory cytokines (TNFα and IL-1β levels. Increased apoptosis and reduction of hippocampal synaptic proteins suggested neuronal and synaptic loss in the aged APN-KO mice, which could be related to neurotoxic Aβ oligomers accumulation and elevated proinflammatory

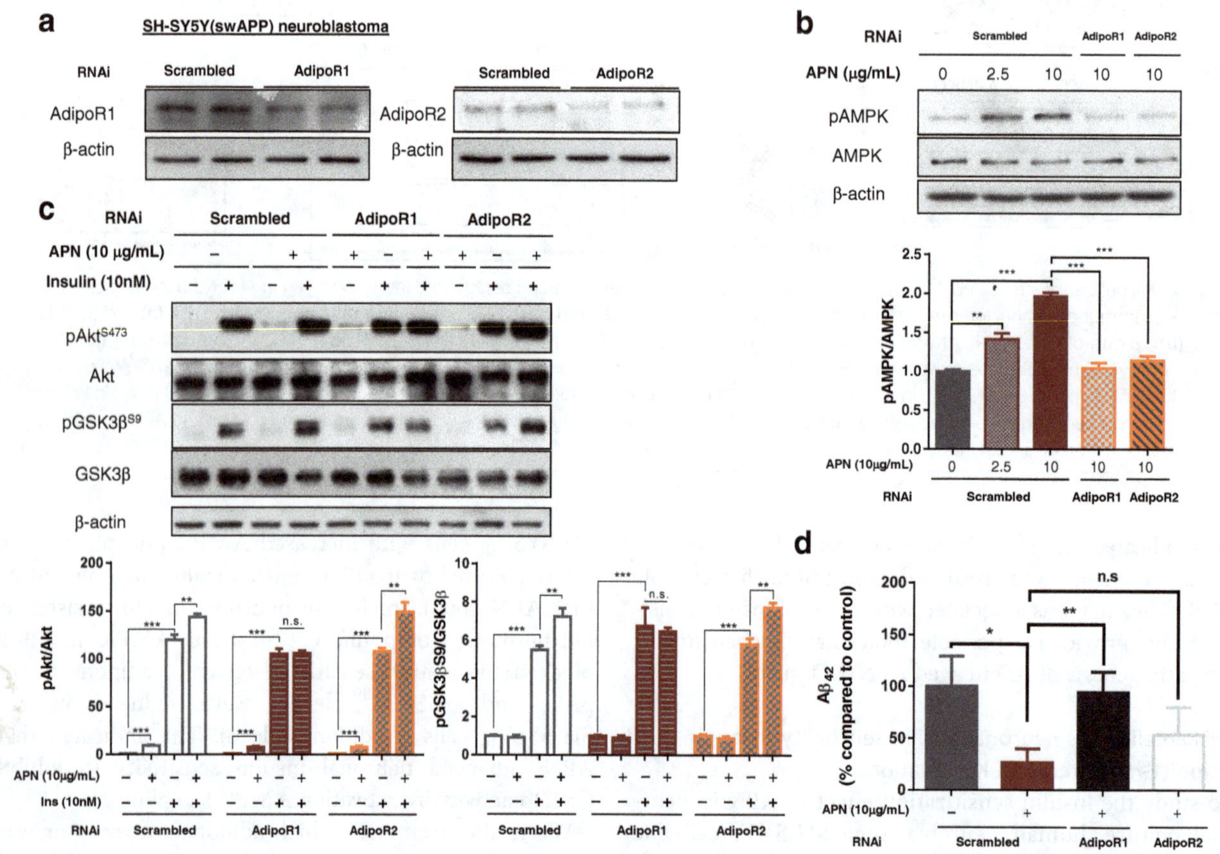

Fig. 6 APN enhanced neuronal insulin sensitivity *in vitro*. **a** AdipoR1 and AdipoR2 expressions in SH-SY5Y$_{swAPP}$ cells upon RNAi transfection. **b** Representative image of pAMPK levels upon APN treatment in SH-SY5Y$_{swAPP}$ cells transfected with scrambled, AdipoR1 or AdipoR2 RNAi duplex. **c** Representative images of western blot of pAkt, Akt, pGSK3β^{S9} and GSK3β in SH-SY5Y$_{swAPP}$ cells transfected with scrambled, AdipoR1 or AdipoR2 RNAi duplex that cultured with/without 10 nmol/L insulin, APN or with 10 μg/mL trimeric APN (APN^{Tri}) & 10 nmol/L insulin. **d** Levels of extracellular Aβ42 upon APN treatment in SH-SY5Y$_{swAPP}$ cells transfected with scrambled, AdipoR1 or AdipoR2 RNAi duplex. Mean ± S.E.M.; *$^{*}p < 0.05$, $^{**}p < 0.01$, $^{***}p < 0.001$, n.s. statistically not significant*

cytokines levels. Importantly, cerebral insulin resistance developed in the aged APN-KO mice with attenuated AMPK activation and impaired insulin signaling which was an underlying mechanism of AD pathogenesis. Concomitantly, our in vitro experiments showed that APN ameliorated neuronal insulin resistance. APN enhanced insulin sensitivity and reduced Aβ production through AdipoR1-mediated AMPK activation. The role of APN in molecular signal of AD pathogenesis was proposed based on findings of the present study (Fig. 7). All these supported the cognitive impairments in APN-deficient mice were associated with cerebral insulin resistance, AD-like brain pathologies and mimicked the phenotypes of AD patients and rodent models.

Accumulating evidence suggests that insulin resistance and inflammation are involved in the pathogenesis of both T2DM and AD [6, 39, 43]. Leptin, an adipokine has similar actions as APN in enhancing insulin sensitivity of peripheral tissues, has also been reported with neuroprotective effects. Leptin receptor-deficient mice, a T2DM model, had an age-dependent cognitive decline with reduced synaptic density and increased tau phosphorylation [13]. Despite that APN deficiency has a strong association with T2DM, the role of APN in AD is controversial. Considering the insulin sensitizing and anti-inflammatory effects of APN in peripheral tissues, APN may exert neuroprotective effects against AD pathogenesis. However, elevated plasma APN levels in AD patients were reported in some populations or specific gender [33, 44]. Meanwhile, another clinical study demonstrated that decreased serum APN level is associated with mild cognitive impairments and AD [34]. A recent publication reported that polymorphisms in the APN gene locus were associated with higher risk of AD [32]. Although it is believed that APN crosses the BBB from the systemic circulation to the CNS, the changes of circulatory APN level may not reflect the changes of APN level in the CNS. Most importantly, there was no significant difference of CSF adiponectin between normal subjects and AD patients, indicating AD onset might not be associated with increased level of CSF APN [35]. Moreover, the changes in plasma APN level in AD could be either the cause or consequence of AD onset. To assess the consequence of the changes in protein level, a knockout animal would be a better approach. Therefore, we employed APN-KO mice as the model. The aged mice were provided with chow diet, normal social interaction, minimized stress environment as well as prolonged APN deficiency to mimic the condition in T2DM patients and elderly. We confirmed the absence of APN in CSF by dot-blot immunoassay. The aged APN-KO mice had spatial memory impairments and anxiety. Remarkably, the mice also displayed AD-like pathologies including Aβ oligomers accumulation, Tau hyperphosphorylation, neuroinflammation and possibly synaptic loss. Our results suggested that chronic APN deficiency in CNS led to cognitive impairments. However, whether the elevated plasma APN levels reported in AD patients [44] was a compensatory mechanism for AD onset requires further investigation.

Aβ is believed to be one of the major neurotoxic species in AD pathogenesis. Our results have shown that soluble Aβ peptide production was increased along with the present of Aβ*56 (dodecamers) in APN-KO mice by 18-month. Unfortunately, low-molecular mass of mouse Aβ was hard to be detected by western blotting. We are the first group to show that Aβ*56 can be detected in mice without APP transgene. Aβ*56 is a specific oligomeric Aβ species present at higher levels in aging individuals with normal cognition and patients with mild cognitive impairments than patients with AD. This Aβ oligomeric species is positively correlated with Tau CP13 ($pTau^{S202}$) level and negatively correlated with synaptic proteins in AD patients [36]. Injection of Aβ*56 into healthy rat induced memory impairments suggesting this specific Aβ oligomer species might initiate age-associated memory impairments, and possibly the action was independent of neuronal loss but related to changes in synaptic functions [37]. It is observed that adiponectin level decreases in aging, hence delineating the molecular linkage between adiponectin and Aβ*56 formation may elucidate the mechanism of aged-related memory decline and even the onset of AD.

Our results clearly suggest that APN has an important role in cognitive functions of mammals. The mechanisms underlying APN activity in the CNS are poorly understood. It has been shown that APN receptors are abundantly expressed in the mammalian brain and APN can enhance hippocampal neural stem cells by inducing p38MAPK and inhibiting GSK3β activities [26]. These two molecules are important intracellular mediators of insulin signaling. Substantial evidence demonstrated that GSK3α/β activation led to AD pathologies including Aβ oligomerization, Tau hyperphosphorylation and synaptic loss [8, 10, 45]. It is well characterized that APN stimulates the activation of AMPK in peripheral tissues to enhance phosphorylation of IRS-1 at tyrosine residues that increase $pAkt^{S473}$ levels. $pAkt^{S473}$ can promote insulin-mediated inhibition of GSK3β. Postmortem studies revealed the increase of $pIRS\text{-}1^{S616}$ and activated GSK3β in AD brains [1]. Here, we propose that APN-AdipoR1-AMPK-induced insulin signaling activities may be important to protect aging brain from AD pathogenesis through GSK3β inhibition. These imply that APN is essential in enhancing cerebral insulin signaling to maintain normal cognitive functions. Future studies may be required to investigate if APN can regulate cerebral

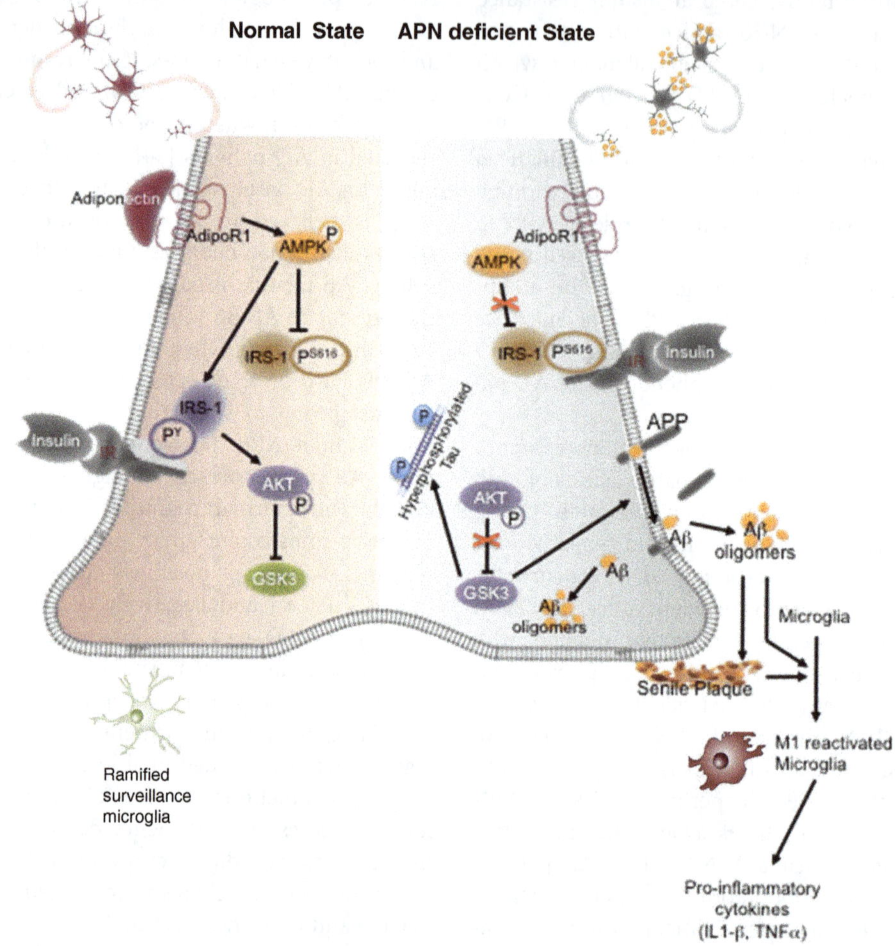

Fig. 7 Schematic presentation shows the Adiponectin signaling pathway in neuron under normal (*left*) and disease (*right*) conditions. We proposed that APN deficiency leads to decreased AMPK activation in neurons and increased IRS-1 phosphorylation at serine^{616} which inhibits the formation of pIRS-1^{Tyr}. Cerebral insulin resistance is progressively developed and thereby causing the reduced level of pAkt^{S473}. The GSK3α/β become activated and may promote formation of Aβ oligomers and Tau phosphorylation. The accumulation of extracellular Aβ oligomers may induce M1 microglial reactivation and secretion of proinflammatory cytokines that associated with neuronal apoptosis and synaptic loss, and subsequently cognitive decline in aged APN-KO mice

glucose metabolism through p38MAPK activation or other insulin signaling responses.

We found that the insulin sensitivity was reduced by 9 months in the hippocampus and frontal cortex but were enhanced by 18 months in the hippocampus of APN-KO mice. It is possible that some unknown compensatory mechanisms might have been activated in the hippocampal neurons. One of the possible mechanisms is the overexpression of insulin receptor (IR) in the hippocampus, but not in the frontal cortex, to enhance insulin signaling as observed in 18-mth-old APN-KO mice (Additional file 2: Figure S2a & b). Overexpression of IR in the hippocampus may therefore induce Akt phosphorylation and inhibit GSK3. In addition to the Akt/GSK3 pathway, pErk1/2 was also increased solely in the hippocampus of 18-mth-old APN-KO mice. However, the improved insulin signaling could not reverse loss of synaptic proteins in aged APN-KO mice. Therefore, we observed cognitive impairments in the 18-mth-old APN-KO mice.

Inflammation is not only crucial in body defense mechanism but is also playing critical roles in neurodegeneration and T2DM. TNFα levels are increased in subjects with obesity and T2DM. Several studies have demonstrated the presence of proinflammatory cytokines and reactivated microglia in AD brains [46–48]. In this study, we showed that the number of activated microglia was increased in APN-KO mice and both cerebral IL-1β and TNFα levels were increased. Surveillance microglia is responsible to recognize and remove extracellular Aβ oligomers. Aβ oligomers in the cortex and hippocampus of APN-KO mice may induce microglial activation, leading to secretion of the proinflammatory cytokines. We believe that APN might directly regulate the activation state of microglia. Though there is still no information on whether APN can regulate microglia activation, a recent report has demonstrated that microglia expressed adiponectin receptors. Osmotin, plant homolog of adiponectin, inhibited Toll-like receptor 4 (TLR4) in microglia cell line BV2 through AdipoR1 to prevent LPS-induced inflammation [49]. Moreover, astrocytes and macrophages also possess APN receptors and being stimulated by APN, suggesting that APN can regulate both cerebral and peripheral inflammation [50, 51]. In addition to the increase of microglia-secreted cytokines, TNFα can also be secreted from adipocytes under APN deficient state or in APN-KO mice [42]. In contrast, increased APN production can suppress TNFα secretion from adipocytes [52]. Obese individuals and T2DM patients have increased TNFα levels in their circulation [53]. Plasma TNFα can cross the BBB and lead to cerebral insulin resistance by inhibiting IRS-1 phosphorylation at tyrosine residues [1, 6, 11]. Hence, peripheral inflammation due to chronic adiponectin deficiency may also contribute to AD pathologies.

Conclusion

In summary, the current study demonstrated that chronic APN deficiency might lead to cognitive decline and AD-like pathologies through insulin desensitization. It also raised the possibility that reduced CNS APN levels in T2DM and aging subjects could indeed be one of the causative factors of AD and cognitive impairment due to deregulated cerebral insulin signaling or cerebral insulin resistance. To our knowledge this is the first study to shed light on the role and molecular mechanism of APN on cognitive functions in mammals. This supports the use of adiponectin or adiponectin receptor agonists as target therapeutic agent in AD.

Methods

Animal

All mice were housed in a group of four to five per cage and maintained in the Laboratory Animal Unit of the University of Hong Kong. Mice were kept under 12 h-lights on/12 h-dark cycle provided with free access food and water. Heterozygous adiponectin mutants on C57BL/6 N genetic background [54] were intercrossed to generate APN-KO mice and wildtype littermate controls. Tail DNA was collected for genotyping by PCR amplification. Detail primer sequences and PCR conditions were used as described previously [54]. All experiments were performed with male mice only. All procedures were approved by the Committee on the Use of Live Animals in Teaching and Research of the University of Hong Kong.

Behavioral tests

Morris-Water-Maze test

All mice that subjected to behavioral studies were male. APN-KO and WT mice of two age groups (9-months and 18 months) were assessed for spatial reference memory in the Morris Water Maze as described previously [55]. Mice were subjected to visible platform training for 2 consecutive days (4 trials per day) with different platform location in each trial. Hidden platform tasks were carried out in 6 consecutive days 24 h after the last visible test trial. Memory retention was assessed by three probe tests which were performed at the beginning of the 5th, 7th and 9th day before the training was started. The platform was removed and the time spent in the target quadrant was recorded. Mice were allowed to freely swim in 1 min and the distance traveled and percent time spent in each quadrant were recorded using a video tracking system (EthoVision 3.0, Noldus Information Technology, Leesburg, VA, USA).

Open field test

APN-KO and WT mice of two age groups (9-months and 18 months) were put into a transparent plastic ($26 \times 26 \times 40$ cm^3) box and was allowed to freely explore the field in a single 60-min session under dim light. The center area was defined as 10×10 cm^2 in the center of the open field. Parameters including the velocity, time in movement, time in the central/marginal zone, and average distance toward the zone border or field center were recorded and analyzed by video tracking system (EthoVision 3.0, Noldus Information Technology, Leesburg, VA, USA).

Fear condition test

The experimental procedures were followed as described previously [56]. In brief, mice were placed individually into a conditioning chamber ($25 \times 25 \times 25$ cm^3) for 6 min of habituation in which the mice explored the context freely. This was followed by 3 pairs of conditioned stimulus (CS) (30 s, 4 Hz, 80 dB) and foot-shock which was applied to the floor grid of the chamber as the US (2 s, 0.5 mA). The inter-pair interval was 2 min with 2 min rest after the final CS pair. The chambers were cleaned with 70% alcohol between each training session. For contextual and cued tests, mice were placed at the same context for 8 min with no foot-shock and a new context with explicit cue in the absence of foot-shock respectively (Additional file 2). A video-tracking system EthoVision XT7 (Noldus, Wageningen, The Netherlands) was used for monitoring and recording throughout the training and memory test sessions. The videos were saved for later behavioral analysis.

Intracerebral injection

Mice were fasted overnight in cages and provided with free access of water. Mice were anesthetized by ketamine and xylazine, and then positioned in a stereotaxic frame. Deep anesthesia, breathing and body temperature were maintained throughout the surgical procedures. Mice were injected with insulin in a dose of 2 I.U/kg body weight. The skull was exposed by incising the scalp. Craniotomy was performed with a drill at (−2.5 mm, −2.2 mm) from the bregma line and midline respectively. Stainless syringe (Hamilton, Reno, NV) was inserted into 2.1 mm depth, in which the position corresponding to the right hippocampus. 2.0 μl of insulin solution or artificial cerebrospinal fluid (aCSF) was injected manually to the targeted tissue at a rate of 1.0 μl/min. Needle was left in place for an additional 5 min to prevent liquid backflow. Mice were sacrificed and decapitated 30 min after injection. Brains were dissected out and the hippocampi were collected for immunoblotting analysis.

Cell culture and RNAi transfection

Human neuroblastoma cell line (SH-SY5Y) was used in this study. To establish insulin resistance neuroblastoma cells (SH-SY5Y$_{IR}$), SH-SY5Y cells were pretreated with high concentration insulin (1000 nmol/L) for 48 h to induce intrinsic insulin resistance. Mammalian expressed trimeric Adiponectin (APN$_{Tri}$) was purified as described before. For cell overexpressing APP mutant, SH-SY5Y cells was stably transfected with Swedish mutant of APP (sw-APP) and cultured in DMEM/F12 with 10%FBS as described before [31]. Double sheath RNAi of scramble RNA, AdipoR1 and AdipoR2 were performed and the sequence of RNAi used as described previously [57]. Cells were pretreated with either APN$_{Tri}$ (10 μg/mL) or Compound C (Calbiochem, USA) 1 h before culturing with 10 nmol/L insulin. Cells were collected and lysed for immunoblotting analysis. Culture medium was collected for ELISA after culturing cells with APN for 48 h.

Aβ quantification

Sandwich enzyme-linked immunosorbent assay (ELISA) was performed as described previously [58] by mouse Beta Amyloid 42 and human Beta Amyloid 42 ELISA kits (Thermo Fisher Scientific, US).

CSF collection and dot blot immunoassay

Mice were deeply anesthetized with Ketamine/Xylazine. CSF was withdrawn by glass capillary from the cisterna magna as described previously [59]. For Dot Blot immunoassay, 1 μl of CSF was added onto a nitrocellulose membrane. Full length recombinant mouse Adiponectin protein was serially diluted and 1 μl of the serial diluted protein was added on the nitrocellulose membrane for standard curve. Membrane was dried in air for 1 h at room temperature and blocked by 5% non-fat milk/TBST. Membrane was then incubated with rabbit-anti-adiponectin (1:1000; AIS HKU, HK) at room temperature for 1 h followed by 30 min HRP conjugated Goat-anti-rabbit IgG antibody. Signal was developed by Westernbright Quantum HRP substrate (advansta, USA).

Cell lysis and immunoblotting

For Immunoblotting, mice were sacrificed and decapitated. Brains were dissected on ice. Frontal cortex and hippocampi were collected and homogenized in lysis buffer by sonication. Homogenates were centrifuged at 12,000 g for 10 min. Supernatants were aliquoted and kept at −80 °C. Protein concentration was determined by Bradford assay (Biorad, USA). 20 μg of the cell homogenates were subjected to 10% SDS polyacrylamide gels and transferred onto polyvinylidene fluoride (PVDF) membrane. Immunoblotting was performed as described previously [60]. Primary antibodies including rabbit-anti-IRS-1^{pS616} (Invitrogen, CA), mouse-anti-pGSK3α^{S21} (Cell Signaling Tech. Inc, USA), rabbit anti-GSK3α (Cell Signaling Tech. Inc, USA), rabbit anti-pGSK3β^{S9} (Cell Signaling Tech. Inc, USA), rabbit anti-GSK3β (Cell Signaling Tech. Inc, USA), rabbit anti-Erk1/2 (Cell Signaling Tech. Inc, USA), rabbit-anti-pErk1/2 (Cell Signaling Tech. Inc, USA), rabbit-anti-pAkt^{S473} (Cell Signaling Tech. Inc, USA), rabbit-anti-Akt (Cell Signaling Tech. Inc, USA), rabbit anti-AMPK (cell signaling Tech. Inc, USA), rabbit anti-pAMPK^{T172} (Cell Signaling Tech. Inc, USA), rabbit anti-IRS-1 (Cell Signaling Tech. Inc, USA), mouse anti-MHCII (AbDSerotec., UK), rabbit-anti-pTau^{pS199pS202} (Invitrogen, USA), and mouse-anti-Tau5 (Invitrogen, USA), mouse-anti-synaptophysin (Invitrogen, USA), and HRP-conjugated β-actin (Cell Signaling Tech. Inc, USA) were incubated at 4 °C overnight followed by stringent wash with TBS-Tween20. The PVDF membranes were incubated with HRP-conjugated secondary antibodies (goat anti-rabbit, 1:5000 or rabbit anti-mouse, 1:7000; Dako, Glostrup, Denmark).

Tissues processing, immunohistochemistry and immunofluorescence staining

For immunohistochemistry, mice were anesthetized with Ketamine/Xylazine. Dissected brains were fixed overnight in 4% paraformaldehyde at 4 °C. Fixed brains were dehydrated in gradient ethanol followed by xylene and embedded in paraffin wax. Sections were rehydrated by graded ethanol to water. Antigens retrieval was performed by incubating sections with 10 mM citrate buffer. Endogenous peroxidase was inactivated by hydrogen peroxide solution. Sections were incubated with primary antibodies, goat anti-GFAP (Santa Cruz, US), mouse monoclonal anti-Aβ (4G8, Biolegend), and rabbit anti-Iba-1 (Wako, Japan) at 4 °C overnight. Sections were incubated with either rabbit anti-mouse or rabbit anti-goat (1:200; Dako, Glostrup, Denmark). Brown color staining was developed and counterstained with hematoxylin. Quantification of staining was performed as described previously [58, 61]. For immunofluorescent staining, sections were incubated with rabbit anti-AdipoR1 (ab70362, Abcam, UK) at 4 °C overnight, followed by Donkey anti-rabbit IgG Alexa Fluor® 594-conjugated secondary antibody (Thermofisher, US) for 30 mins. Sections were mounted by slow fade® anti-fade DAPI reagent (Lifetech, US).

Thioflavin S staining

Brain sections were deparaffinized by xylene followed by gradient ethanol treatments (100, 95 70%, 50%) for 3 mins each. Sections were then incubated with 0.5% Thioflavin S in 50% ethanol for 30 min. Sections were then washed with 50% ethanol and dehydrated with gradient ethanol. Sections were mounted by DPX reagent.

Quantification of neuronal apoptotic cells

To detect neuronal apoptotic cells, sections were treated with 0.1 M citrate buffer at 90 °C (pH 6.0) for antigen retrieval. TUNEL assay was used with an *in-situ* cell death detection kit (Roche, Mannheim, Germany) followed by incubating with mouse monoclonal primary anti-NeuN antibody (MAB377; Millipore, US) at 4 °C overnight. Sections were then incubated with donkey anti-mouse IgG Alexa Fluor® 594-conjugated secondary antibody (Thermofisher, US) for 30 mins. Sections were mounted by slow fade® anti-fade DAPI reagent (Lifetech, US).

To quantify the degree of apoptotic cell death in the cortex and hippocampus, ten coronal sections from rostro-to-caudal region of the cortex and hippocampus were examined and TUNEL-positive cells were manually counted in a defined sampling region. One sampling region of interest from the hippocampal CA1 and two sampling regions in the cortex were defined. Only TUNEL-label cells colocalized with condensed nuclei staining were counted. The number of TUNEL-positive cells was the sum of apoptotic cell counts from all sample fields in the quantified sections of one embedded block. The number of TUNEL-positive cells reported was the mean of n number in each group.

Statistics

Dot blot immunoassay, western blot data and immunohistochemistry staining were quantified by ImageJ and presented as group mean ± S.E.M. Statistical analyses were performed by using unpaired Student *t*-test or one way ANOVAs followed by Newman-Keuls multiple comparison test. Behavioral tests data were analyzed by one-way ANOVA followed by Bonferroni's correction for multiple testing. Behavioral tests results were presented as mean ± S.E.M with $p < 0.05$ considered as statistically significant.

Additional files

Additional file 1: AdipoR1 expression in brain and dot-blot immunoassay of CSF adiponectin. **(a)** Immunofluorescent analysis of AdipoR1 in cortex and hippocampus of adult mouse. **(b)** Standard curve of full length mouse adiponectin (0-1000 ng/mL). **(c)** Representative dot-blot image of the serial diluted APN and CSF from 18-month old WT and APN-KO mice. **(d)** Dot-blot immunoassay of APN concentration in the CSF for both WT and APN-KO mice by 18 months. APN was undetectable in CSF of APN-KO mice. *$p < 0.05$; WT ($n = 4$) vs APN-KO ($n = 3$).

Additional file 2: Behavioral Tests. **(a)** Swim speeds of WT and APN-KO mice by 9-months and 18 months in Morris-Water-Maze tests displayed no significant difference ($p > 0.05$) indicating the escape latency observed was not due to locomotor defects. **(b)** Study design of fear-conditioning contextual and cue tests.

Additional file 3: Selected frame of the contextual test for wildtype (left) and APN-KO (right) mice. APN-KO mice froze significantly less than wildtype mice.

Additional file 4: Selected frame of the cue test for wildtype (left) and APN-KO (right) mice. The clip includes first section of 30-s tone and 30-s rest afterwards. Tone starts at 0" and ends at 30" in the clip. APN-KO mice froze significantly less than wildtype mice.

Additional file 5: Representative immunoblotting analysis of the levels of insulin signaling effectors (pErk1/2, pGSK3α^{21}, pGSK3α^{Y279}) in **(a)** 9-mth-old & **(b)** 18-mth-old WT and APN-KO mice. Densitometric analysis of the ratio of pErk1/2/Erk1/2, pGSK3α^{21}/GSK3α and pGSK3α^{Y279} / GSK3α in the hippocampus and frontal cortex of the APN-KO mice or WT mice by **(c)** 9-mths-of-age and **(d)** 18-mths-of-age. Mean ± S.E.M.; *$p < 0.05$, **$p < 0.01$, ***$p < 0.001$, *n.s. statistically not significant*; WT ($n = 3$) vs APN-KO ($n = 3$ or 4).

Additional file 6: **(a)** Immunoblotting analysis of IRβ in the hippocampus and frontal cortex of 18-month old wildtype and APN-KO mice. **(b)** Densitometric analysis of the ratio of IRβ. Mean ± S.E.M.; ***$p < 0.001$, *n.s. statistically not significant*; Scale bar: 100 μm.

Additional file 7: Cerebral insulin injection to the right hippocampus. **(a)** 2 μl of insulin (0.05I.U) or artificial cerebrospinal fluid were injected to the right hippocampus (coordination: 2.5 mm [D-V]; 2.2 mm [A-P]; 2.1 mm [Lateral] from Bregma) of 12-mth-old mice. **(b)** Trypan Blue dye was injected to the same coordination of the right hippocampus indicated successful injection.

Additional file 8: APN enhances insulin sensitivity in neuronal cells with insulin resistance. SH-SY5Y neuroblastoma cell pretreated with high concentration insulin (1 μmol/L) for 48 h to induce insulin resistance (SH-SY5Y$_{IR}$). Western blotting of pAMPK, pAkt and pGSK3β^{S9} levels of the SH-SY5Y$_{IR}$ cells that treated with 10 nmol/L insulin, 10 μg/mL APN^{Tri} & 10 nmol/L insulin with/without compound C (2 μM) for 24 h.

Abbreviations

Alzheimer's disease: AD; AMPK, APN: Adiponectin; Aβ: Amyloid-beta; CSF: cerebrospinal fluid; ELISA: Enzyme-linked immunosorbent assay; Erk: Extracellular signal-regulated kinase; GFAP: Glial fibrillary acidic protein; GSK3: Glycogen synthase kinase 3; Iba-1: Ionized calcium-binding adapter molecule 1; IL1β: Interleukin 1β; IR: Insulin receptor; IRS-1: Insulin receptor substrate 1; MHC: Major histocompatibility complex; NeuN: Neuronal nuclear antigen; TNFα: Tumor necrosis factor alpha; TUNEL: Terminal deoxynucleotidyl transferase dUTP Nick end labeling; WT: Wildtype

Acknowledgements

We thank Antibody and Immunoassay Services, LKS Faculty of Medicine, HKU to provide recombinant adiponectin proteins for the experiments. We also thank Dr. Qi Li, Department of Psychiatry, HKU, for providing the set-up of Cue and Contextual fear-conditioning tests.

Funding

This project was supported by UGC Matching Fund for Donation towards Research on Neuroinflammation, funding support from the Strategy Research Theme (SRT) on Neuroscience, and small project funding (201409176174), The University of Hong Kong.

Author contributions
R.C-L.N., performed most of the experiments, wrote the manuscript, conceived and designed the functional studies. O-Y.C. performed the MWM and OF tests. J.S-C.K. involved in IHC and WB experiments. P.W-L.H. collected mice samples. K.K-Y.C. and R.L-C.H. prepared mice for experiments. L.L.Z. and P.K-K.Y. assisted behavioral tests and analysis. A.Z. reviewed experimental results and advised on direction of study. S.K.C. supervised cognitive functions test, provided advice and edited the manuscript. K.S-L.L. proposed the hypothesis that adiponectin exerts neuroprotection in AD and edited the manuscript. K-H.C. gave comments on the manuscript, conceived and designed the functional studies. All authors agreed the data and the final manuscript.

Competing interests
The authors declare that they have no competing interests.

Author details
[1]Department of Medicine, LKS Faculty of Medicine, The University of Hong Kong, Hong Kong, Special Administrative Region, China. [2]Research Center of Heart, Brain, Hormone and Healthy Aging, LKS Faculty of Medicine, The University of Hong Kong, Hong Kong, Special Administrative Region, China. [3]Hong Kong University Alzheimer's Disease Research Network, LKS Faculty of Medicine, The University of Hong Kong, Hong Kong, Special Administrative Region, China. [4]Neuroimmunology and Neuroinflammation Research Laboratory, LKS Faculty of Medicine, The University of Hong Kong, Hong Kong, Special Administrative Region, China. [5]School of Biomedical Sciences, LKS Faculty of Medicine, The University of Hong Kong, Hong Kong, Special Administrative Region, China. [6]LKS Faculty of Medicine, The University of Hong Kong, Hong Kong, HKSAR, 8/F Department of Medicine, 21 Sassoon Road, Pofulam, China.

References

1. Talbot K, Wang H, Kazi H, Han L, Bakshi KP, Stucky A, Fuino RL, Kawaguchi KR, Samoyedny AJ, Wilson RS, Arvanitakis Z, Schneider J a, Wolf B a, Bennett D a, Trojanowski JQ, Arnold SE, Demonstrated brain insulin resistance in alzheimer's disease patients is assocaited with IGF-1 resisitance, IRS-1 dysregulation, and cogntive decline. J Clin Invest. 2012;122:1316–38.
2. Chen Y, Deng Y, Zhang B, Gong CX. Deregulation of brain insulin signaling in Alzheimer's disease. Neurosci Bull. 2014;30:282–94.
3. Yaffe K, Blackwell T, Kanaya A, Davidowitz N, Barrett-Connor E, Krueger K. Diabetes, impaired fasting glucose, and development of cognitive impairment in older women. Neurology. 2004;63:658–63.
4. Mushtag G, Khan J, Kamal M. Biological mechanisms linking Alzheimer's disease and type-2 diabetes mellitus. CNS Neurol Disord Drug Targets. 2014; 13:1192–201.
5. Willette A a, Bendlin BB, Starks EJ, Birdsill AC, Johnson SC, Christian BT, Okonkwo OC, La Rue A, Hermann BP, Koscik RL, Jonaitis EM, Sager M a, Asthana S. Association of insulin resistance with cerebral glucose uptake in late middle–aged adults at risk for Alzheimer disease. JAMA Neurol. 2015;53792:1–8.
6. Felice FG De. Science in medicine Alzheimer' s disease and insulin resistance: translating basic science into clinical applications. J Clin Invest. 2013;123:531–9.
7. Avrahami L, Farfara D, Shaham-Kol M, Vassar R, Frenkel D, Eldar-Finkelman H. Inhibition of glycogen synthase kinase-3 ameliorates β-amyloid pathology and restores lysosomal acidification and mammalian target of rapamycin activity in the alzheimer disease mouse model: In vivo and in vitro studies. J Biol Chem. 2013;288:1295–306.
8. Phiel CJ, Wilson CA, Lee VM, Klein PS. GSK-3 a regulates production of Alzheimer' s disease amyloid- b peptides. Nature. 2003;17(lane 2):435–40.
9. Son SM, Song H, Byun J, Park KS, Jang HC, Park YJ, Mook-Jung I. Altered APP processing in insulin-resistant conditions is mediated by autophagosome accumulation via the inhibition of mammalian target of rapamycin pathway. Diabetes. 2012;61:3126–38.
10. DaRocha-Souto B, Coma M, Pérez-Nievas BG, Scotton TC, Siao M, Sánchez-Ferrer P, Hashimoto T, Fan Z, Hudry E, Barroeta I, Serenó L, Rodríguez M, Sánchez MB, Hyman BT, Gómez-Isla T. Activation of glycogen synthase kinase-3 beta mediates β-amyloid induced neuritic damage in Alzheimer's disease. Neurobiol Dis. 2012;45:425–37.
11. Bomfim TR, Forny-germano L, Sathler LB, Brito-moreira J, Houzel J, Decker H, Silverman M a, Kazi H, Melo HM, Mcclean PL, Holscher C, Arnold SE, Talbot K, Klein WL, Munoz DP, Ferreira ST, De Felice FG. An anti-diabetes agent protects the mousebrain from defective insulin signalingcaused by Alzheimer's disease–associated Aβ oligomers. J Clin Invest. 2012;122:1339–53.
12. Gao C, Liu Y, Li L. New animal models of Alzheimer's disease that display insulin desensitization in the brain. Rev Neurosci. 2013;24:607–15.
13. Ramos-Rodriguez JJ, Ortiz O, Jimenez-Palomares M, Kay KR, Berrocoso E, Murillo-Carretero MI, Perdomo G, Spires-Jones T, Cozar-Castellano I, Lechuga-Sancho AM, Garcia-Alloza M. Differential central pathology and cognitive impairment in pre-diabetic and diabetic mice. Psychoneuroendocrinology. 2013;38:2462–75.
14. Grillo C, Piroli G, Lawrence R, Wrighten S, Green A, Wilson S, Sakai R, Kelly S, Wilson M, Molt D, Reagan L: Hippocampal Insulin Resistance Impairs Spatial Learning and Synaptic Plasticity. Diabetes. 2015;64:3927–36.
15. Adzovic L, Lynn AE, D'Angelo HM, Crockett AM, Kaercher RM, Royer SE, Hopp SC, Wenk GL. Insulin improves memory and reduces chronic neuroinflammation in the hippocampus of young but not aged brains. J Neuroinflammation. 2015;12:1–10.
16. Chen Y, Zhao Y, Dai C-L, Liang Z, Run X, Iqbal K, Liu F, Gong C-X. Intranasal insulin restores insulin signaling, increases synaptic proteins, and reduces Aβ level and microglia activation in the brains of 3xTg-AD mice. Exp Neurol. 2014;261:610–9.
17. Yamauchi T, Iwabu M, Okada-Iwabu M, Kadowaki T. Adiponectin receptors: a review of their structure, function and how they work. Best Pract Res Clin Endocrinol Metab. 2014;28:15–23.
18. Oh DK, Ciaraldi T, Henry RR. Adiponectin in health and disease. Diabetes Obes Metab. 2007;9:282–9.
19. Caselli C. Role of adiponectin system in insulin resistance. Mol Genet Metab. 2014;113:155–60.
20. Ruan H, Dong LQ. Adiponectin signaling and function in insulin target tissues. J Mol Cell Biol. 2016;8:1–40.
21. Anderson NJ, King MR, Delbruck L, Jolivalt CG. Role of insulin signaling impairment, adiponectin and dyslipidemia in peripheral and central neuropathy in mice. Dis Model Mech. 2014;7:625–33.
22. Cheng KKY, Lam KSL, Wang B, Xu A. Signaling mechanisms underlying the insulin-sensitizing effects of adiponectin. Best Pract Res Clin Endocrinol Metab. 2014;28:3–13.
23. Liu J, Guo M, Zhang D, Cheng S-Y, Liu M, Ding J, Scherer PE, Liu F, Lu X-Y. Adiponectin is critical in determining susceptibility to depressive behaviors and has antidepressant-like activity. Proc Natl Acad Sci. 2012;109:12248–53.
24. Thundyil J, Pavlovski D, Sobey CG, Arumugam TV. Adiponectin receptor signalling in the brain. Br J Pharmacol. 2012;165:313–27.
25. Kusminski CM, Mcternan PG, Schraw T, Kos K, O'Hare JP, Ahima R, Kumar S, Scherer PE. Adiponectin complexes in human cerebrospinal fluid: distinct complex distribution from serum. Diabetologia. 2007;50:634–42.
26. Zhang D, Guo M, Zhang W, Lu X. Adiponectin stimulates proliferation of adult hippocampal neural stem/progenitor cells through activation of p38 mitogen-activated protein kinase (p38MAPK)/glycogen synthase kinase 3β (GSK-3β)/β-catenin signaling cascade. J Biol Chem. 2011;12:44913–20.
27. Yau S-Y, Li A, Hoo RLC, Ching YP, Christie BR, Lee TMC, Xu A, So K-F. Physical exercise-induced hippocampal neurogenesis and antidepressant effects are mediated by the adipocyte hormone adiponectin. Proc Natl Acad Sci. 2014;2–7.
28. Mikesell R, Ryu J, Hsieh C, Cremasco V. Lack of adiponectin leads to increased lymphocyte activation and worse severity of a mouse model of multiple sclerosis. Eur J Immunol. 2013;43:2089–100.
29. Miao J, Shen LH, Tang YH, Wang YT, Tao MX, Jin KL, Zhao YJ, Yang GY. Overexpression of adiponectin improves neurobehavioral outcomes after focal cerebral ischemia in aged mice. CNS Neurosci Ther. 2013;19:969–77.
30. Masaki T, Anan F, Shimomura T, Fujiki M, Saikawa T, Yoshimatsu H. Association between hippocampal volume and serum adiponectin in patients with type 2 diabetes mellitus. Metabolism. 2012;61:1197–200.
31. Chan KH, Lam KSL, Cheng OY, Kwan JSC, Ho PWL, Cheng KKY, Chung SK, Ho JWM, Guo VY, Xu A. Adiponectin is Protective against Oxidative Stress Induced Cytotoxicity in Amyloid-Beta Neurotoxicity. PLoS One. 2012;7: e52354.
32. Yu Z, Li W, Hou D, Zhou L, Deng Y, Tian M, Feng X. Relationship between adiponectin gene polymorphisms and late-onset Alzheimer's disease. PLoS One. 2015;10:e0125186.

33. Khemka VK, Bagchi D, Bandyopadhyay K, Bir A, Chattopadhyay M, Biswas A, Basu D, Chakrabarti S. Altered serum levels of adipokines and insulin in probable Alzheimer's disease. J Alzheimer's Dis. 2014;41:1–9.
34. Teixeira AL, Diniz BS, Campos AC, Miranda AS, Rocha NP, Talib LL, Gattaz WF, Forlenza OV. Decreased levels of circulating adiponectin in mild cognitive impairment and alzheimer's disease. NeuroMolecular Med. 2013;15:115–21.
35. Une K, Takei Y a, Tomita N, Asamura T, Ohrui T, Furukawa K, Arai H. Adiponectin in plasma and cerebrospinal fluid in MCI and Alzheimer's disease. Eur J Neurol. 2011;18:1006–9.
36. Lesn SE, Sherman MA, Grant M, Kuskowski M, Schneider JA, Bennett DA, Ashe KH. Brain amyloid-b oligomers in ageing and Alzheimer's disease. Brain. 2013;136:1383–98.
37. Koh MT, Kotilinek L, Kayed R, Glabe CG, Yang A, LETTERS A specific amyloid-β protein assembly in the brain impairs memory. Nat. 2006;440:352–7.
38. Combs CK, Karlo JC, Kao SC, Landreth GE. beta-Amyloid stimulation of microglia and monocytes results in TNFalpha-dependent expression of inducible nitric oxide synthase and neuronal apoptosis. J Neurosci. 2001;21:1179–88.
39. Ferreira ST, Clarke JR, Bomfim TR, De Felice FG. Inflammation, defective insulin signaling, and neuronal dysfunction in Alzheimer's disease. Alzheimer's Dement. 2014;10(1 SUPPL):S76–83.
40. Wang C, Mao X, Wang L, Liu M, Wetzel MD, Guan KL, Dong LQ, Liu F. Adiponectin sensitizes insulin signaling by reducing p70 S6 kinase-mediated serine phosphorylation of IRS-1. J Biol Chem. 2007;282:7991–6.
41. Kadowaki T, Yamauchi T, Kubota N, Hara K, Ueki K, Tobe K. Review series adiponectin and adiponectin receptors in insulin resistance, diabetes, and the metabolic syndrome. J Clin Invest. 2006;116:1784–92.
42. Maeda N, Shimomura I, Kishida K, Nishizawa H, Matsuda M, Nagaretani H, Furuyama N, Kondo H, Takahashi M, Arita Y, Komuro R, Ouchi N, Kihara S, Tochino Y, Okutomi K, Horie M, Takeda S, Aoyama T, Funahashi T, Matsuzawa Y. Diet-induced insulin resistance in mice lacking adiponectin/ACRP30. Nat Med. 2002;8:731–7.
43. De Felice FG, Ferreira ST. Inflammation, defective insulin signaling, and mitochondrial dysfunction as common molecular denominators connecting type 2 diabetes to Alzheimer Disease. Diabetes. 2014;63:2262–72.
44. van Himbergen TM, Alexa SB, Ai M, Seshadri S, Otokozawa S, Au R, Thongtang N, Wolf PA, Schaefer EJ. Biomarkers for insulin resistance and inflammation and the risk for all-cause dementia and Alzheimer disease results from the framingham heart study. Arch Neurol. 2012;69:564–600.
45. Gao C, Hölscher C, Liu Y, Li L. GSK3: A key target for the development of novel treatments for type 2 diabetes mellitus and Alzheimer disease. Rev Neurosci. 2012;23:1–11.
46. Lue LF, Rydel R, Brigham EF, Yang LB, Hampel H, Murphy GM, Brachova L, Du Yan S, Walker DG, Shen Y, Rogers J. Inflammatory repertoire of Alzheimer's disease and nondemented elderly microglia in vitro. Glia. 2001;35:72–9.
47. Mosher KI, Wyss-Coray T. Microglial dysfunction in brain aging and Alzheimer's disease. Biochem Pharmacol. 2014;88:594–604.
48. Lue LF, Walker DG, Rogers J. Modeling microglial activation in Alzheimer's disease with human postmortem microglial cultures. Neurobiol Aging. 2001;22:945–56.
49. Badshah H, Ali T, Kim MO. Osmotin attenuates LPS-induced neuroinflammation and memory impairments via the TLR4/NFκB signaling pathway. Sci Rep. 2016;6:24493.
50. Wan Z, Mah D, Simtchouk S, Klegeris A, Little JP. Globular adiponectin induces a pro-inflammatory response in human astrocytic cells. Biochem Biophys Res Commun. 2014;446:37–42.
51. Mandal P, Pratt BT, Barnes M, Mcmullen MR, Nagy LE. Molecular mechanism for adiponectin-dependent m2 macrophage polarization link between the metabolic and innate immune activity of full-length adiponectin. J Biol Chem. 2011;286:13460–9.
52. Shibata R, Sato K, Pimentel DR, Takemura Y, Kihara S, Ohashi K, Funahashi T, Ouchi N, Walsh K. Adiponectin protects against myocardial ischemia-reperfusion injury through AMPK- and COX-2-dependent mechanisms. Nat Med. 2005;11:1096–103.
53. Hotamisligil GS, Arner P, Caro JF, Atkinson RL, Spiegelman BM. Increased adipose tissue expression of tumor necrosis factor-alpha in human obesity and insulin resistance. J Clin Invest. 1995;95:2409–15.
54. Fayad R, Pini M, Sennello J a, Cabay RJ, Chan L, Xu A, Fantuzzi G. Adiponectin deficiency protects mice from chemically induced colonic inflammation. Gastroenterology. 2007;132:601–14.
55. Durairajan SSK, Liu L-F, Lu J-H, Chen L-L, Yuan Q, Chung SK, Huang L, Li X-S, Huang J-D, Li M. Berberine ameliorates β-amyloid pathology, gliosis, and cognitive impairment in an Alzheimer's disease transgenic mouse model. Neurobiol Aging. 2012;33:2903–19.
56. Zhou IY, Ding AY, Li Q, Mcalonan GM, Wu EX. Magnetic resonance spectroscopy reveals N-acetylaspartate reduction in hippocampus and cingulate cortex after fear conditioning. Psychiatry Res Neuroimaging. 2012;204:178–83.
57. Kenneth KY, Karen SL. Adiponectin-Induced Endothelial Nitric Oxide Synthase Activation and … 2007(May).
58. Zhou L, Chan KH, Chu LW, Kwan JSC, Song YQ, Chen LH, Ho PWL, Cheng OY, Ho JWM, Lam KSL. Plasma amyloid-β oligomers level is a biomarker for Alzheimer's disease diagnosis. Biochem Biophys Res Commun. 2012;423: 697–702.
59. Liu L, Duff K. A technique for serial collection of cerebrospinal fluid from the cisterna magna in mouse. J Vis Exp. 2008;10–12.
60. Chan KH, Kwan JSC, Ho PWL, Ho SL, Chui WH, Chu a CY, Ho JWM, Zhang WY, Kung MHW. Aquaporin-4 water channel expression by thymoma of patients with and without myasthenia gravis. J Neuroimmunol. 2010;227: 178–84.
61. Gengler S, McClean PL, McCurtin R, Gault VA, Hölscher C. Val(8)GLP-1 rescues synaptic plasticity and reduces dense core plaques in APP/PS1 mice. Neurobiol Aging. 2012;33:265–76.

Induced pluripotent stem cells in Alzheimer's disease: applications for disease modeling and cell-replacement therapy

Juan Yang[2†], Song Li[1†], Xi-Biao He[4], Cheng Cheng[1] and Weidong Le[1,2,3*]

Abstract

Alzheimer's disease (AD) is the most common cause of dementia in those over the age of 65. While a numerous of disease-causing genes and risk factors have been identified, the exact etiological mechanisms of AD are not yet completely understood, due to the inability to test theoretical hypotheses on non-postmortem and patient-specific research systems. The use of recently developed and optimized induced pluripotent stem cells (iPSCs) technology may provide a promising platform to create reliable models, not only for better understanding the etiopathological process of AD, but also for efficient anti-AD drugs screening. More importantly, human-sourced iPSCs may also provide a beneficial tool for cell-replacement therapy against AD. Although considerable progress has been achieved, a number of key challenges still require to be addressed in iPSCs research, including the identification of robust disease phenotypes in AD modeling and the clinical availabilities of iPSCs-based cell-replacement therapy in human. In this review, we highlight recent progresses of iPSCs research and discuss the translational challenges of AD patients-derived iPSCs in disease modeling and cell-replacement therapy.

Keywords: Alzheimer's disease, Cell-replacement therapy, Disease modeling, Drugs screening, Induced pluripotent stem cells

Background

Alzheimer's disease (AD) is the most common form of dementia that begins with short-term memory deficits and culminates in total loss of cognition and executive functions. The formations of amyloid-β (Aβ) plaques and intracellular neurofibrillary tangles (NFTs), two important pathological hallmarks of AD, have been linked to the synapse loss, neuronal degeneration and subsequent dramatic brain atrophy of AD patients [1, 2]. Although these clinical features and pathological profiles of AD have been well documented and various animal models containing AD-related genetic backgrounds have been developed, the etiological mechanisms for AD are still far from being fully understood and effective therapeutic strategies for AD are still urgently needed.

Dozens of drugs and therapeutic strategies attempting to slow or halt neuronal loss and cognitive deficiency of AD are being investigated around the world [3]. However, only five pharmacological agents have been approved for clinical AD treatment by the Food and Drug Administration, including cholinesterase inhibitors tacrine, donepezil, galantamine, rivastigmine and N-methyl-D-aspartate (NMDA) receptor antagonist memantine [4]. Unfortunately, all these currently available pharmacological therapeutics only relieve symptoms without affecting the major pathological characteristics of AD. Moreover, the effectiveness of these agents varies from person to person as evidenced by a moderate efficiency in no more than 20 % of patients and tolerance, noncompliance and side-effects in more than 60 % of treated patients [5].

Several theoretical hypotheses have been raised for elucidating the pathological mechanisms of AD, including amyloid-cascade hypothesis [6], tau hypothesis [7],

* Correspondence: wdle@sibs.ac.cn
†Equal contributors
[1]Center for Translational Research on Neurological Diseases, the First Affiliated Hospital, Dalian Medical University, 116021 Dalian, China
[2]Key Laboratory of Stem Cell Biology, Institute of Health Sciences, Shanghai Institutes for Biological Sciences, Chinese Academy of Sciences/Shanghai Jiao Tong University School of Medicine, 200031 Shanghai, China
Full list of author information is available at the end of the article

mitochondrial cascade hypothesis [8], oxidative stress hypothesis [9] and neuroinflammation hypothesis [10]. Among them, amyloid-cascade hypothesis is widely accepted as the centerpiece of AD pathology, in which Aβ is recognized as the initiating factor in AD. Previous studies have reported that Aβ plaque deposition, an early critical event of AD, triggers the downstream features of AD including tangles formation, oxidative stress, neuroinflammation and neuronal loss. Several new candidates targeting Aβ have been tested in clinical trials in past years. Unfortunately, all of these therapeutic candidates failed to improve the cognitive and functional ability of AD patients, yet caused serious side-effects [11, 12]. Therefore, a better understanding of the upstream mechanisms of AD pathology is urgently required for the discovery of novel disease-modifying therapeutic strategies.

Till now, at least 3 causal genes and 22 risk genes have been identified to be involved in the pathogenesis of AD, including amyloid precursor protein (APP), presenilin-1/2 (PSEN1/2) [5, 13], apolipoprotein E (APOE) [14], ABCA7, BIN1, CASS4, CD33, CD2AP, CELF1, CLU, CR1, DSG2, EPHA1, FERMT2, HLA-DRB5-DBR1, INPP5D, MS4A, MEF2C, NME8, PICALM, PTK2B, SORL1, SLC24H4-RIN3, and ZCWPW1 [15]. However, genetic factors could only partially explain the risk of AD. The notion widely accepted to date is that the onset of AD is most likely the consequence of complicated interactions of multiple genetic and non-genetic factors (Fig. 1) [16]. Several non-genetic risk factors have been proposed, including aging, cerebro-cardiovascular diseases, metabolic disorders, traumatic brain injury, sleep disorders, chronic hypoxia and environmental toxins [3, 17–23]. However, the mechanisms underlying them still remain largely unknown, due to the lack of non-postmortem and AD patient-specific research models.

The identification of AD causal genes resulted in the generation of more than 150 transgenic AD mouse models, by over-expressing one or more mutated genes such as human APP, PSEN1/2, or Tau [24]. These transgenic models have greatly advanced the understanding of AD pathogenesis and promoted the findings of novel therapeutic targets and strategies for AD treatment. However, none of these transgenic models can reflect all pathogenic and clinical features of AD. Different combinations and extents of gene mutations led to a great variety of AD phenotypes [25, 26]. Although Aβ plaques and cognitive impairment were observed in almost all animal models, NFTs could only be generated by lines over-expressing human tau protein. Cholinergic neuronal loss can be observed in several lines, but massive neuronal loss in brain is rarely observed in these animal models. Based on these, in the current stage transgenic animal models cannot fully recapitulate the progress of human AD. In addition, the transgenic animals carrying autosomal dominant familial AD (FAD) genes may have limitations in modeling sporadic AD (SAD) [27, 28]. Therefore, more representative models are needed for facilitating the fundamental AD research and exploring more efficient therapeutic strategies for AD treatment.

The recently developed and optimized induced pluripotent stem cells (iPSCs) technology may provide an appealing access to overcome these challenges in AD research. iPSCs can be generated from somatic cells by using several key transcription factors for pluripotency. iPSCs are in general identical to embryonic stem cells (ESCs) with the ability to self-renew unlimitedly and differentiate into all cell types [29–31]. Additionally, human iPSCs derived from patients'own somatic cells may serve as a sufficient cell source for clinical transplantation therapy (also termed as cell-replacement therapy), which can efficiently prevent immunologic rejection and the ethical issues raised by the use of ESCs [32, 33]. More importantly, human iPSCs derived from either FAD or SAD patients' somatic cells contain a patient-specific pathogenic background, therefore, can provide a promising avenue for AD modeling, which bridges the gap between animal models and clinical testing. This strategy is extremely useful for the mechanism understanding of AD pathogenesis, clinical identifying of therapeutic targets and drug screening of the novel therapeutic candidates against AD (Fig. 2). In this review, we update the recent progress of iPSCs research, and discuss its potential applications, as well as the major challenges and future directions in disease modeling and cell-replacement therapy of AD.

Progress of iPSCs research

In 2006, Yamanaka and colleagues found mouse fibroblast cells can be reprogrammed into iPSCs by using 4 transcription factors including Octamer-binding transcription factor 4 (Oct4), sex determining region Y-box 2 (Sox2), Kruppel-like factor 4 and cMyc [30]. In 2007, this technology was successfully applied in human somatic cells [29]. Additionally, a combination of Oct4, Sox2, NANOG and LIN28 has also been demonstrated to induce iPSCs from human somatic cells [29, 31]. After the first discovery of mouse or human iPSCs, considerable efforts have been made to develop or optimize this technology, including reprogramming cells by using fewer or newly defined factors and more efficient delivery systems.

Oct4 inhibits the expression of differentiation-related genes in ESCs [34–36] and has been reported to be sufficient to direct the reprogramming of somatic cells into iPSCs [37, 38]. Moreover, Shu et al. have found that lineage specifiers, which act as pluripotency rivals to suppress ESCs identity, can induce mouse fibroblasts into iPSCs [39]. Lineage specifiers that are involved in

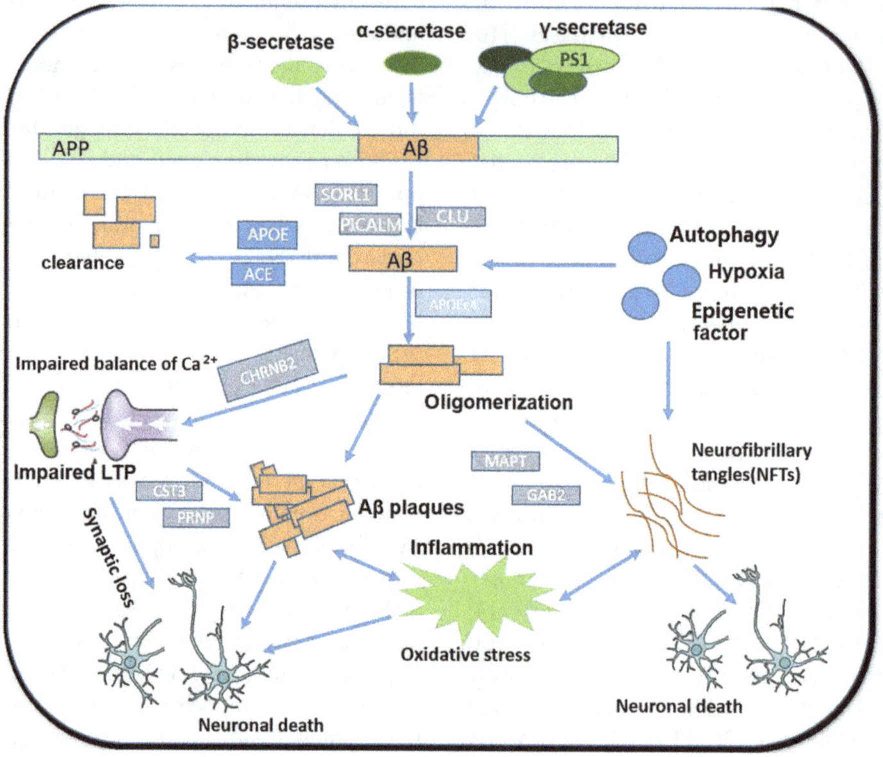

Fig. 1 Schematic diagram of causative or risk factors for AD pathogenesis

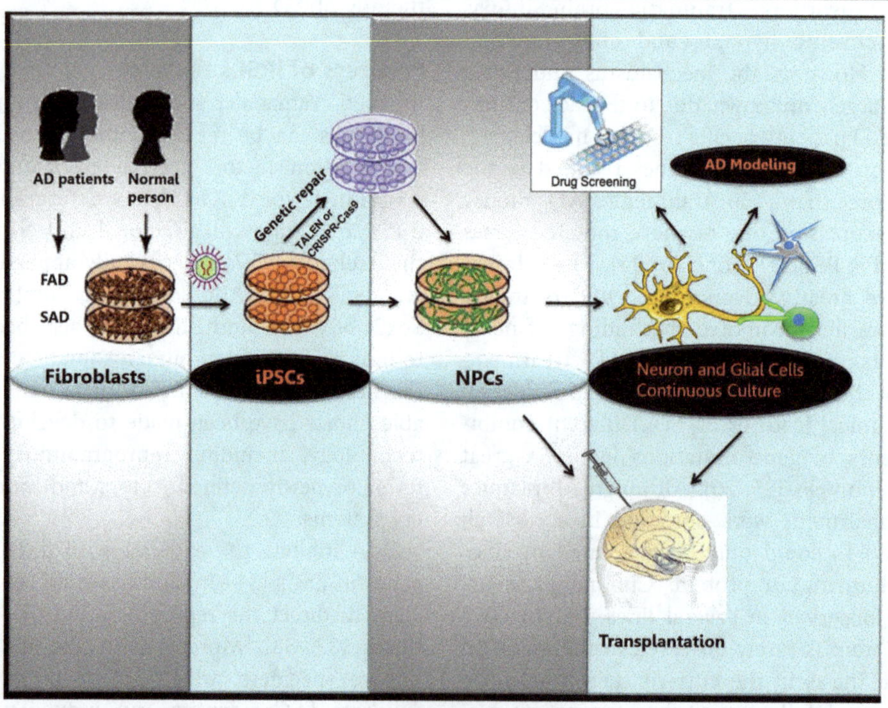

Fig. 2 Potential applications of iPSCs technology in AD modeling, drugs screening and cell-replacement therapy

mesendodermal specification (such as GATA3, GATA6, and SOX7) and ectodermal specification (such as SOX1, SOX3, and GMNN) can synergistically induce pluripotency in the absence of Oct4 and Sox2, suggesting a "see-saw effect" of the lineage specifiers in cell reprogramming. Additionally, more and more novel reprogramming factors have been identified as pluripotency-associated factors or maternal factors, such as PR domain-containing 14, Sall4, Esrrb, Utf1, Tet1, Tet2, Gli-similar protein 1 and inhibitors of differentiation 3 [40–48].

Manipulations of microRNAs (miRs), such as miR-291-3p, miR-294 and miR-295, have been reported to increase the efficiency of reprogramming without the presence of cMyc [49]. Anokye-Danso and colleagues have also found that miR-302-367 can replace traditional reprogramming factors to reprogram mouse and human somatic cells into iPSCs with higher efficiency [50].

Besides the utilization of pluripotency transcription factors, the induction of iPSCs has been extended to involve various kinds of donor cells, including fibroblasts, glias, neural progenitors, human keratinocytes, liver and stomach cells, pancreatic-β cells, mature B lymphocytes, human amniotic fluid-derived cells, as well as cells in blood and urine [51–56].

Additionally, the delivering strategies for inducing iPSCs have been improved. The retroviral or lentiviral vectors were routinely used to integrate the reprogramming genes into the host genome to induce iPSCs [30, 57]. Viral delivery system are efficient and reproducible in reprogramming, however, the random integration of transgenes into genome increases the risk of tumor formation and may cause mortality in chimeric and progeny mice derived from iPSCs [58]. Transfection of linear DNA by polycistronic vectors using liposomes or electroporation can avoid viral integration, but the reprogramming efficiency of these methods is much lower than viral delivery. The piggyBac transposon delivery system is less risky because the integration of non-viral constructsis more stable than virus vectors [59]. Furthermore, many viral integration-free systems for iPSCs generation have been established, such as adenovirus, Sendai virus, minicircle vector, episomal vectors, and direct protein delivery [60–65]. Importantly, Hou et al. have reported that small-molecules, such as VC6T plus FSK, can replace "master genes" Sox2 and Oct4 to induce cell reprogramming [65, 66]. This chemical reprogramming strategy is relatively simple and less time-consuming, and has promising potential in generating functional desirable cell types for clinical applications.

Application of iPSCs in AD modeling

The rapid development of iPSCs technology promotes the application of iPSCs in the research of neurodegenerative diseases. Since 2008, over 50 literatures have been published to demonstrate the neurodegenerative diseases modeling by using iPSCs, majorly generated from familial patients but a few from sporadic patients [32]. Among them, several research groups have reported the usage of iPSCs in AD modeling, which provide proof-of-principle for modeling patient-specific AD pathology by using iPSCs and recapitulate several pathological features of AD in vitro (Table 1).

Yagi et al. firstly generated iPSCs from AD patients carrying familial mutations in *PSEN1* (A246E) and *PSEN2* (N141I) and reported that these FAD-derived iPSCs had an increased $A\beta_{42}$ production and an elevated ratio of $A\beta_{42}/A\beta_{40}$ [67]. Then, Israel et al. generated iPSCs lines from two SAD patients (named as sAD1/sAD2) and two FAD patients with a duplication of APP (APP^{Dp}) [68]. They found that neurons derived from APP^{Dp}-iPSCs line and sAD2-iPSCs line have significantly higher levels of $A\beta_{40}$, increased phosphorylation of tau protein (at Thr 231) together with an elevated level of active glycogen synthase kinase-3β (aGSK-3β). Additionally, neurons from those AD-derived iPSCs (AD-iPSCs) accumulated large RAB5-positive early endosomes, which is consistent with the findings from the neurons of AD patients [69]. More interestingly, treatment of the neurons with β-secretase inhibitors (BSI), but not γ-secretase inhibitors, could significantly reduce the levels of phospho-tau (Thr 231) and aGSK-3β, while γ-secretase inhibitors only reduced the level of $A\beta_{40}$, suggesting that APP proteolytic processing, but not $A\beta_{40}$, had a direct relationship with GSK-3β activation and tau phosphorylation in human neurons. Consistent with these findings, Jang et al. and Shi et al. have also generated neurons from iPSCs derived from primary fibroblast of AD patients [70, 71] and found these cells could recapitulate AD pathogenic process such as $A\beta_{42}$ and hyperphosphorylated tau and could be used for screening new drugs and therapeutic regimens.

Sproul et al. also have found a higher $A\beta_{42}/A\beta_{40}$ ratio in the neural progenitor cells (NPCs) derived from AD-iPSCs harboring *PSEN1* A246E or M146L mutations [72]. Moreover, they identified 14 genes differentially-regulated in PSEN1 NPCs molecular profiling. Among these genes, *GFRA3*, *ISL1*, *DLX1*, *SEMA3B*, and *ERBB3* showed differential expression in late onset AD/Intermediate AD brains.

Kondo et al. generated seven AD-iPSCs lines, including three lines from a patient carrying APP E693 deletion (APP E693d), two lines from a patient harboring APP V717L mutation (APP V717L), and two lines from a SAD patient [73]. The authors found that Aβ oligomers accumulated in neurons derived from APP E693d-iPSCs and in neurons and astrocytes derived from one of the two SAD-iPSCs lines, which could be reduced by BSI. Furthermore, they found that the stress responses

Table 1 iPSCs-based AD modeling

Cell type	AD models	Phenotypes	Significance	Ref
FAD-iPSCs	Fibroblasts of FAD patient with mutations in PS1 and PS2	FAD-iPSCs-derived neurons have increased Aβ42 secretion; responds to γ-secretase inhibitors and modulators	Recapitulating the molecular pathogenesis of mutant PS; identification and validation of candidate drugs	[67]
FAD- and SAD-iPSCs	Fibroblasts of FAD patient with mutations in APP; sporadic AD	AD-iPSCs-derived neurons exhibited higher levels of Aβ, pTau, and active GSK-3β; β-secretase inhibitors caused significant reductions in pTau and active GSK-3β levels	The first SAD iPSC model; Demonstrating the direct relationship between APP processing in GSK-3β activation and tau phosphorylation	[68]
AD-iPSCs	Fibroblasts from AD patient	AD-specific iPSCs lines	Exploring AD pathologies; screening new drugs and therapeutic regimens	[70]
AD-iPSCs	Fibroblast of Down syndrome patients	Neurons generated from Down syndrome patients-iPSCs developed AD pathologies	Recapitulating AD pathogenic process including Aβ42 and hyperphosphorylated tau	[71]
FAD-iPSCs	PSEN1 mutant fibroblasts	produced greater ratios of Aβ42 to Aβ40; 14 genes differentially-regulated	Identify novel candidate genes during AD pathology	[72]
FAD-iPSCs SAD-iPSCs	Human dermal fibroblasts	Aβ oligomers accumulation; elevated endoplasmic reticulum (ER) and oxidative stress;	Illustrating how patient-specific iPSCs can be useful for analyzing AD pathogenesis and evaluating drugs.	[73]
FAD-iPSCs	Human fibroblast carrying APP mutation (V717I)	Increased APP expression and levels of APPsβ, Aβ; increased Aβ42 and Aβ38; increase in levels of total and phosphorylated Tau	Demonstrating the direct casual relationship between elevated Aβ and hyperphosphorylated tau using Aβ neutralizing antibodies, for the first time; Providing a model system for testing therapeutic strategies in the cell types most relevant to disease processes	[74]

in the AD neural cells were alleviated by BSI and docosahexaenoic acid treatment. This study illustrates the possible application of patient-specific iPSCs for screening anti-AD drugs and classifying AD patients.

Muratore et al. generated four iPSCs lines from two FAD patients carrying APP V717I mutation and differentiated them into neurons expressing forebrain neuron marker [74]. Both β- and γ-secretase cleavage of APP were affected by this mutation. Elevated β-secretase cleavage of APP led to an increased level of both sAPPβ and Aβ, while the alteration of the initial cleavage site of γ-secretase resulted in an increased $A\beta_{42}$ and $A\beta_{38}$. Moreover, they found that the levels of total and phosphorylated tau were increased in neurons derived from AD patient. Furthermore, Aβ-specific antibodies could reverse the phenotype of increased total tau in AD-iPSCs derived neurons. These findings indicate that the tau-related changes are relevant to Aβ phenotype and the increased tau might be a consequence of Aβ generation, which is consistent with the amyloid-cascade hypothesis of AD.

Furthermore, forebrain cholinergic neuron (FBCN) loss is directly relevant to the memory and cognition deficits in AD. Therefore, generation of FBCNs from AD patient-specific iPSCs is crucial for disease modeling in vitro and for the development of novel AD therapies. Based on this, Duan et al. have recently reported that FBCNs derived from SAD-iPSCs showed typical AD biochemical features as evidenced by an increased $A\beta_{42}/A\beta_{40}$ ratio and a higher susceptibility to glutamate-mediated cell death [75].

Down syndrome (DS) patients with early-onset dementia share similar neurodegenerative features with those of AD. Chang et al. have recently found that accumulated amyloid deposits, tau protein hyperphosphorylation and tau intracellular redistribution emerged rapidly in DS-iPSCs-derived neurons within 45 days but not in normal ESCs-derived neurons, suggesting DS-iPSC-derived neural cells can serve as an ideal cellular model of DS and AD and have potential for high-throughput screening of therapeutic candidates [76].

Challenges and future perspectives of iPSCs in AD disease modeling

The above mentioned research findings reveal several pathological features of AD, including Aβ generation and tau-phosphorylation, in AD-iPSCs derived from FAD and SAD patients, indicating the potential application of iPSCs technology in AD modeling and drug screening. However, there are still several concerns regarding AD-iPSCs models.

First of all, although iPSCs could serve as a promising avenue for disease modeling, the molecular principles for this technique, particularly in human cells, still remain poorly understood due to donor-to-donor variability and intercellular heterogeneity. In the study from Israel et al., only one of the two SAD-iPSCs lines has the same phenotypes as the APP^{Dp}-iPSCs line. Similarly, Kondo et al. have also found that seven AD-iPSCs lines with APP E693 deletion or APP V717L mutation or SAD did not always recapitulate the same phenotypes [73]. These inconsistencies might suggest that although there are similar mechanisms underlying the pathogenesis of FAD or SAD, a larger sample size is still required to investigate the comprehensive and robust heterogeneity of AD phenotypes in future study. In addition, although AD patient-derived human neurons have shown elevated levels of toxic Aβ species and phosphorylated tau, they also could not recapitulate Aβ plaques or tau tangles. One of the possible reasons for this might be the lack of a proper cell culture system, which mimics the in vivo condition and provides a better microenvironment to achieve enough pathogenic Aβ accumulation, as observed in human AD patients and transgenic AD mouse models. Recently, Kim et al. have found that robust Aβ and tau pathologies could be achieved in a 3-dimension human neural cell culture models [77]. Although this model was based on genetically engineered human neural stem cell line, not iPSCs, it may provide a promising tool for human AD iPSCs models.

Secondly, the neural cells differentiated from iPSCs displayed AD pathological hallmarks in less than two months, suggesting that disease-related cells may be more susceptible to display the hallmarks of disease in cell culture dishes than in patients' brains. However, there also remains the question that whether the one or two cell types differentiated from iPSCs can represent all complicate phenotypes of AD. In addition, the cells exhibited the pathological changes of AD, but synapse loss or neuronal degeneration was rarely observed. It has been reported that AD is a complex disease that affects both neuronal and glial activities and glia participates in Aβ clearance and inflammation in AD [78]. Therefore, further studies of glial cells derived from AD-iPSCs can facilitate the discovery of the exact mechanisms underling AD pathogenesis.

Thirdly, in these studies of AD-iPSCs, iPSCs derived from healthy individuals or family members were used as controls, which may have totally different genetic background from the AD-iPSCs. This kind of controls is not the most appropriate approach in disease modeling assays. Hence, isogenic iPSCs derived from AD-iPSCs, in which the mutations have been corrected to wild-type, are the most appropriate controls. Nowadays, isogenic, mutation-corrected control cell lines generated by transcription activator-like effector nucleases (TALENs) or clustered regularly interspaced short palindromic repeats (CRISPR)/CRISPR-associated protein (Cas) mediated genomic editing technology has been applied in human diseases, such as ALS, and tumors [79, 80].

Overall, AD-iPSC lines from more AD patients and further studies using both AD-iPSC-derived neuron and glial cells and isogenic controls can provide tools to discover more accurate features and mechanisms of AD.

iPSCs-based cell replacement therapy for AD: the mechanisms and rationales

iPSCs have great potential in cell transplantation therapy of neurodegenerative diseases including AD. Transplantable neural progenitors or neurons can be generated from ESCs and iPSCs [81, 82]. NPCs derived from ESCs or iPSCs can be further differentiated into neurons, astrocytes or oligodendrocytes, which provide promising aspect for cell-replacement therapy of various neurodegenerative disorders including AD.

The dysfunction of neurogenesis has been found in AD mouse models, indicating that the worsened imbalance between neurogenesis and neuronal loss may contribute to the pathogenesis of AD [83]. It is generally accepted that adult neurogenesis primarily occurs in two sites important for learning and memory, the subventricular zone (SVZ) of the lateral ventricles and the subgranular zone (SGZ) of the dentate gyrus (DG) of the hippocampus. Wang et al. have reported that AD transgenic mice harboring PSEN1P117L show a decreased survival of NPCs, leading to a reduced production of new neurons. In addition, the reduced adult neurogenesis in DG has been suggested to be correlated with an impaired contextual fear conditioning in mouse [84–87]. In APP V717F mice, an age-dependent decrease of cell proliferation in SGZ of DG was also observed [88]. Research reports suggest that neurogenesis was significantly enhanced as a self-repairing mechanism to compensate for the early onset of neurodegeneration; however, the survival of newly generated neurons was impaired following neurodegeneration progression [89]. Interestingly, although the cellular composition and morphological organization of the SVZ in human and non-human primates differ from those of rodents [90, 91], the proliferation and migration of NPCs in the SVZ of young APP transgenic mice have also been reported to be greatly decreased [92], suggesting that Aβ plaques might be involved in the impaired neurogenesis in AD mouse model. However, it has been reported that the decreased NPCs and neuroblasts as wells as severely impaired proliferation and differentiation of NPCs occurred preceding the onset of amyloid deposition and memory impairment in 2-month-old APPswe/PSEN1ΔE9 mice or triple transgenic mice carrying APPswe, PSEN1-M146V and tau-P301L mutations [93]. These findings suggest that progressive neuronal loss and impaired neurogenesis may be important pathological events of AD.

Previous studies have found that transplanted NSCs differentiate into mature cell types and improve cognitive ability of AD animal models via various mechanisms, with or without the involvement of Aβ or tau pathologies. For instance, NSCs have been reported to rescue cognitive functions and promote synaptogenesis without altering Aβ or tau pathologies in AD mouse models [94–96]. Moreover, NSCs have also been found to attenuate the expression of proinflammatory cytokines and neuronal loss in AD model [97]. In contrast to these research reports, Lee et al. have revealed that human NSCs transplantation reduced tau phosphorylation, down-regulated BACE1 expression and Aβ production via Akt/GSK3β signaling, and decreased the expression of inflammatory mediators through deactivation of microglia [98]. As a primary source of NSCs, iPSCs, especially human-derived iPSCs, may provide a promising strategy for cell-replacement therapy of AD.

It is likely that the transplantation of NSCs can provide not only a direct cell-replacing strategy for AD therapy, but also can be used as vehicles for the delivery of potential therapeutic agents, including neprilysin, insulin-degrading enzyme, plasmin and cathepsin B, to reverse AD pathologies [99, 100]. It is suggested that the future NSCs- or iPSCs-based cell therapy in AD should focus on such indirect mechanisms [101–103].

iPSCs-based cell replacement therapy for AD: hints from other CNS disorders

iPSCs have great potential as cell source in cell transplantation therapy of neurodegenerative diseases [104, 105]. One of the main purposes of iPSCs-based cell replacement therapy in AD and other neurodegenerative diseases is to produce new neurons to replace those lost or function-deficient cells during disease progression or to produce glial cells to protect neurons from ongoing degeneration. Data from in vivo studies suggest that iPSCs-derived neurospheres were able to survive and differentiate into neurons, astrocytes, and oligodendrocytes, after transplantation into injured mouse spinal cord [106]. In addition, previous research report has also indicated that after transplantation into the fetal mouse brain, NPCs derived from mouse iPSCs migrate into various brain regions and differentiate into glia and neurons [107], and thus are capable to integrate into preexisting functional neuronal circuitries in the CNS or compensate the degenerative neurons. Electrophysiological experiments and morphological observations demonstrate that the grafted neurons display normal neuronal activity and are functionally integrated into the host brain. All these findings support the notion that iPSCs- or iPSCs derivatives-based cell replacement therapy could be efficiently used to treat neurodegenerative diseases. Indeed, several lines of studies have tested this idea in experimental models of Parkinson's disease (PD) and amyotrophic lateral sclerosis (ALS).

It has been reported that transplanted neural stem cells in parkinsonian rat striatum can release and re-uptake dopamine and alleviate PD symptoms [108]. Human iPSCs-derived neurons can improve the functional defects of rotational asymmetry in PD rat model after transplantation [109]. Autologous iPSCs-derived dopamine neurons can provide long-term functional recovery in monkey model of PD [84]. In addition, glial-rich neural progenitors derived from human iPSCs can improve lifespan of ALS mice after being transplanted into the lumbar spinal cord [85].

As for AD, Fujiwara et al. have reported that the spatial memory of AD mice was improved significantly after grafted with human iPSCs-derived neural progenitors [110]. In addition, Huang's group has found that after transplantation of the embryonic medial ganglionic eminence (MGE)-derived interneuron progenitors into the hippocampal hilus of aged apoE4-KI mice, the transplanted cells developed into mature interneurons, and the neurons functionally integrated into the hippocampal circuitry and rescued learning and memory [111]. Moreover, Nicholas et al. found that MGE-like progenitors derived from both ESCs and iPSCs could be induced to differentiate into GABAergic interneurons and displayed mature physiological properties in mouse brain up to 7 months post-transplantation [112]. These research findings indicate that transplanted human iPSCs-derived cells can functionally rescue pathological changes in the brains of AD patients. All these preclinical progresses in the investigation of cell transplantation in neurodegenerative diseases may provide proof-of-concept for the final clinical translation of iPSCs in therapy of AD.

Although great achievements have been made for iPSCs-based cell replacement therapy, one major challenge is teratoma formation. It has been demonstrated in the mouse system that iPSCs-derived chimeras frequently develop tumors, which should be carefully evaluated after transplantation before clinical application. Takahashi et al. calculated that approximately 20 % of the mice derived from iPSCs develop tumors [113]. Transgene reactivation and incomplete reprogramming are considered as the primary causes of tumorigenesis [114]. In order to reduce the risk of tumor formation that limits the clinic application of iPSCs, many studies have provided strategies. Wang et al. have introduced a mifepristone-regulated caspase-1 expression system to selectively eliminate tumor cells derived from undifferentiated ESCs but not differentiated dopamine neurons [115]. Cui et al. have identified that the suppression of canonical wingless-type MMTV integration site family (WNT) signaling pathway can reduce the tumorigenicity and substantially improved retinal integration of ESCs-derived retinal progenitor cells transplanted in mice [116]. In addition, Nori et al. have recently suggested that integration-free iPSCs should be chosen to avoid tumorigenesis [117]. Overall, these progresses of iPSCs research can provide new avenue for the clinical translation of cell transplantation therapy against various neurodegenerative diseases including AD.

Conclusion

AD patient-specific iPSCs-derived neurons or glia cells can recapture not only familial, but also sporadic form of AD. Moreover, iPSCs provide unique platforms to detect the early-disease phenotypes during neurogenesis or neurodegeneration which may point towards underlying pathogenic mechanisms of AD. In addition, isogenic iPSCs of AD-iPSCs can be obtained by TALEN- or CRISPR/Cas-mediated genetic repairing technology. Genetically repaired AD-iPSCs can serve as more appropriate control cells for disease modeling and cells transplantation. Altogether, even though there are several challenges in the clinical usage of iPSCs technology, the recent promising achievements in this field will contribute significantly for exploring molecular mechanisms of AD and promoting clinical AD therapy.

Abbreviations

BSI: β-secretase inhibitor; aGSK-3β: active glycogen synthase kinase-3β; AD: Alzheimer's disease; Aβ: Amyloid-β (Aβ); APP: Amyloid precursor protein; APOE: Apolipoprotein E; CRISPR: Clustered regularly interspaced short palindromic repeats; Cas: CRISPR-associated protein; DG: Dentate gyrus; DS: Down syndrome; APP^{Dp}: Duplication of APP; ESCs: Embryonic stem cells; FAD: Familial AD; FBCN: Forebrain cholinergic neuron; iPSCs: Induced pluripotent stem cells; miRs: microRNAs; NMDA: N-methyl-D-aspartate; NPCs: Neural progenitor cells; NFTs: Neurofibrillary tangles; Oct4: Octamer-binding transcription factor 4; PSEN1/2: Presenilin-1/2; Sox: Sex determining region Y-box; SAD: Sporadic AD; TALENs: Transcription activator-like effector nucleases; SGZ: Subgranular zone; SVZ: Subventricular zone.

Competing interests

The authors declare no competing interests.

Authors' contributions

WL proposed the writing of the review paper. JY, SL and CC wrote and revised the manuscript. JY and SL constructed the schematic diagrams. XBH, SL and WL discussed and revised the manuscript. All authors read and approved the final manuscript.

Acknowledgments

This work was supported by grants from the National Natural Sciences Foundation of China (81430021 and 81370470), the Program for Liaoning Innovative Research Team in University (LT2015009).

Author details

[1]Center for Translational Research on Neurological Diseases, the First Affiliated Hospital, Dalian Medical University, 116021 Dalian, China. [2]Key Laboratory of Stem Cell Biology, Institute of Health Sciences, Shanghai Institutes for Biological Sciences, Chinese Academy of Sciences/Shanghai Jiao Tong University School of Medicine, 200031 Shanghai, China. [3]Collaborative Innovation Center for Brain Science, the First Affiliated Hospital, Dalian Medical University, 116011 Dalian, China. [4]Shanghai University of Medicine and Health Sciences, Shanghai 201318, China.

References

1. Braak H, Braak E. Neuropathological stageing of Alzheimer-related changes. Acta Neuropathol. 1991;82(4):239–59.
2. Robakis NK. Cell signaling abnormalities may drive neurodegeneration in familial Alzheimer disease. Neurochem Res. 2014;39(3):570–5.
3. Roberson ED, Mucke L. 100 years and counting: prospects for defeating Alzheimer's disease. Science. 2006;314(5800):781–4.
4. Kumar A, Singh A, Ekavali. A review on Alzheimer's disease pathophysiology and its management: an update. Pharmacol Rep. 2015;67(2):195–203.
5. Serretti A, Olgiati P, De Ronchi D. Genetics of Alzheimer's disease. A rapidly evolving field. J Alzheimers Dis. 2007;12(1):73–92.
6. Hardy JA, Higgins GA. Alzheimer's disease: the amyloid cascade hypothesis. Science. 1992;256(5054):184–5.
7. Maccioni RB, Farias G, Morales I, Navarrete L. The revitalized tau hypothesis on Alzheimer's disease. Arch Med Res. 2010;41(3):226–31.
8. Swerdlow RH, Burns JM, Khan SM. The Alzheimer's disease mitochondrial cascade hypothesis: progress and perspectives. Biochim Biophys Acta. 2014;1842(8):1219–31.
9. Praticò D. Oxidative stress hypothesis in Alzheimer's disease: a reappraisal. Trends Pharmacol Sci. 2008;29(12):609–15.
10. Heppner FL, Ransohoff RM, Becher B. Immune attack: the role of inflammation in Alzheimer disease. Nat Rev Neurosci. 2015;16(6):358–72.
11. Salloway S, Sperling R, Fox NC, Blennow K, Klunk W, Raskind M, Sabbagh M, Honig LS, Porsteinsson AP, Ferris S, Reichert M, Ketter N, Nejadnik B, Guenzler V, Miloslavsky M, Wang D, Lu Y, Lull J, Tudor IC, Liu E, Grundman M, Yuen E, Black R, Brashear HR. Bapineuzumab 301 and 302 Clinical Trial Investigators. Two phase 3 trials of bapineuzumab in mild-to-moderate Alzheimer's disease. N Engl J Med. 2014;370(4):322–33.
12. Doody RS, Thomas RG, Farlow M, Iwatsubo T, Vellas B, Joffe S, Kieburtz K, Raman R, Sun X, Aisen PS, Siemers E, Liu-Seifert H, Mohs R, Alzheimer's Disease Cooperative Study Steering Committee; Solanezumab Study Group. Phase 3 trials of solanezumab for mild-to-moderate Alzheimer's disease. N Engl J Med. 2014;370(4):311–21.
13. Lippa CF, Swearer JM, Kane KJ, Nochlin D, Bird TD, Ghetti B, Nee LE, St George-Hyslop P, Pollen DA, Drachman DA. Familial Alzheimer's disease: site of mutation influences clinical phenotype. Ann Neurol. 2000;48(3): 376–9.
14. Michaelson DM. APOE epsilon4: the most prevalent yet understudied risk factor for Alzheimer's disease. Alzheimers Dement. 2014;10(6):861–8.
15. Karch CM, Goate AM. Alzheimer's disease risk genes and mechanisms of disease pathogenesis. Biol Psychiatry. 2015;77(1):43–51.
16. Gatz M, Reynolds CA, Fratiglioni L, Johansson B, Mortimer JA, Berg S, Fiske A, Pedersen NL. Role of genes and environments for explaining Alzheimer disease. Arch Gen Psychiatry. 2006;63(2):168–74.
17. Sleegers K, Van Duijn CM. Alzheimer's Disease: Genes Pathogenesis and Risk Prediction. Community Genet. 2001;4(4):197–203.
18. Willette AA, Bendlin BB, Starks EJ, Birdsill AC, Johnson SC, Christian BT, Okonkwo OC, La Rue A, Hermann BP, Koscik RL, Jonaitis EM, Sager MA, Asthana S.. Association of insulin resistance with cerebral glucose uptake in late middle-aged adults at risk for Alzheimer Disease. JAMA Neurol. 2015;72(9):1013–20.
19. Hernandez-Zimbron LF, Rivas-Arancibia S. Oxidative stress caused by ozone exposure induces beta-amyloid 1–42 overproduction and mitochondrial accumulation by activating the amyloidogenic pathway. Neuroscience. 2015; 304:340–8.
20. Liu H, Qiu H, Yang J, Ni J, Le W. Chronic hypoxia facilitates Alzheimer's disease through demethylation of gamma-secretase by downregulating DNA methyltransferase 3b. Alzheimers Dement. 2016; 12(2):130–43.
21. Coupland KG, Kim WS, Halliday GM, Hallupp M, Dobson-Stone C, Kwok JB. Effect of PSEN1 mutations on MAPT methylation in early-onset Alzheimer's disease. Curr Alzheimer Res. 2015;12(8):745–51.
22. Li L, Zhang S, Zhang X, Li T, Tang Y, Liu H, Yang W, Le W. Autophagy enhancer carbamazepine alleviates memory deficits and cerebral amyloid-beta pathology in a mouse model of Alzheimer's disease. Curr Alzheimer Res. 2013;10(4):433–41.

23. Ju YE, Lucey BP, Holtzman DM. Sleep and Alzheimer disease pathology–a bidirectional relationship. Nat Rev Neurol. 2014;10(2):115–9.
24. Webster SJ, Bachstetter AD, Nelson PT, Schmitt FA, Van Eldik LJ. Using mice to model Alzheimer's dementia: an overview of the clinical disease and the preclinical behavioral changes in 10 mouse models. Front Genet. 2014;5:88.
25. Bilkei-Gorzo A. Genetic mouse models of brain ageing and Alzheimer's disease. Pharmacol Ther. 2014;142(2):244–57.
26. Kim TK, Lee JE, Park SK, Lee KW, Seo JS, Im JY, Kim ST, Lee JY, Kim YH, Lee JK, Han PL. Analysis of differential plaque depositions in the brains of Tg2576 and Tg-APPswe/PS1dE9 transgenic mouse models of Alzheimer disease. Exp Mol Med. 2012;44(8):492–502.
27. Kitazawa M, Medeiros R, Laferla FM. Transgenic mouse models of Alzheimer disease: developing a better model as a tool for therapeutic interventions. Curr Pharm Des. 2012;18(8):1131–47.
28. Kuhn HG, Cooper-Kuhn CM, Boekhoorn K, Lucassen PJ. Changes in neurogenesis in dementia and Alzheimer mouse models: are they functionally relevant? Eur Arch Psychiatry Clin Neurosci. 2007;257(5):281–9.
29. Yu J, Vodyanik MA, Smuga-Otto K, Antosiewicz-Bourget J, Frane JL, Tian S, Nie J, Jonsdottir GA, Ruotti V, Stewart R, Slukvin II, Thomson JA. Induced pluripotent stem cell lines derived from human somatic cells. Science. 2007; 318(5858):1917–20.
30. Takahashi K, Yamanaka S. Induction of pluripotent stem cells from mouse embryonic and adult fibroblast cultures by defined factors. Cell. 2006;126(4): 663–76.
31. Takahashi K, Tanabe K, Ohnuki M, Narita M, Ichisaka T, Tomoda K, Yamanaka S. Induction of pluripotent stem cells from adult human fibroblasts by defined factors. Cell. 2007;131(5):861–72.
32. Hargus G, Ehrlich M, Hallmann AL, Kuhlmann T. Human stem cell models of neurodegeneration: a novel approach to study mechanisms of disease development. Acta Neuropathol. 2014;127(2): 151–73.
33. Bellin M, Marchetto MC, Gage FH, Mummery CL. Induced pluripotent stem cells: the new patient? Nat Rev Mol Cell Biol. 2012;13(11):713–26.
34. Kim JB, Zaehres H, Wu G, Gentile L, Ko K, Sebastiano V, Arauzo-Bravo MJ, Ruau D, Han DW, Zenke M, Scholer HR. Pluripotent stem cells induced from adult neural stem cells by reprogramming with two factors. Nature. 2008; 454(7204):646–50.
35. Pardo M, Lang B, Yu L, Prosser H, Bradley A, Babu MM, Choudhary J. An expanded Oct4 interaction network: implications for stem cell biology, development, and disease. Cell Stem Cell. 2010;6(4):382–95.
36. Chen SM, Lee MS, Chang CY, Lin SZ, Cheng EH, Liu YH, Pan HC, Lee HC, Su HL. Prerequisite OCT4 maintenance potentiates the neural induction of differentiating human embryonic stem cells and induced pluripotent stem cells. Cell Transplant. 2015;24(5):829–44.
37. Krohne TU, Westenskow PD, Kurihara T, Friedlander DF, Lehmann M, Dorsey AL, Li W, Zhu S, Schultz A, Wang J, Siuzdak G, Ding S, Friedlander M. Generation of retinal pigment epithelial cells from small molecules and OCT4 reprogrammed human induced pluripotent stem cells. Stem Cells Transl Med. 2012;1(2):96–109.
38. Li Y, Zhang Q, Yin X, Yang W, Du Y, Hou P, Ge J, Liu C, Zhang W, Zhang X, Wu Y, Li H, Liu K, Wu C, Song Z, Zhao Y, Shi Y, Deng H. Generation of iPSCs from mouse fibroblasts with a single gene, Oct4, and small molecules. Cell Res. 2011;21(1):196–204.
39. Shu J, Wu C, Wu Y, Li Z, Shao S, Zhao W, Tang X, Yang H, Shen L, Zuo X, Yang W, Shi Y, Chi X, Zhang H, Gao G, Shu Y, Yuan K, He W, Tang C, Zhao Y, Deng H.. Induction of pluripotency in mouse somatic cells with lineage specifiers. Cell. 2013;153(5):963–75.
40. Nakagawa M, Koyanagi M, Tanabe K, Takahashi K, Ichisaka T, Aoi T, Okita K, Mochiduki Y, Takizawa N, Yamanaka S. Generation of induced pluripotent stem cells without Myc from mouse and human fibroblasts. Nat Biotechnol. 2008;26(1):101–6.
41. Aoi T. Advance in study of induced pluripotent stem cells (iPS cells). Nihon Rinsho. 2008;66(5):850–6.
42. Buganim Y, Jaenisch R. Transdifferentiation by defined factors as a powerful research tool to address basic biological questions. Cell Cycle. 2012;11(24):4485–6.
43. Chia NY, Chan YS, Feng B, Lu X, Orlov YL, Moreau D, Kumar P, Yang L, Jiang J, Lau MS, Huss M, Soh BS, Kraus P, Li P, Lufkin T, Lim B, Clarke ND, Bard F, Ng HH. A genome-wide RNAi screen reveals determinants of human embryonic stem cell identity. Nature. 2010;468(7321):316–20.
44. Doege CA, Inoue K, Yamashita T, Rhee DB, Travis S, Fujita R, Guarnieri P, Bhagat G, Vanti WB, Shih A, Levine RL, Nik S, Chen EI, Abeliovich A. Early-stage epigenetic modification during somatic cell reprogramming by Parp1 and Tet2. Nature. 2012;488(7413):652–5.
45. Maherali N, Ahfeldt T, Rigamonti A, Utikal J, Cowan C, Hochedlinger K. A high-efficiency system for the generation and study of human induced pluripotent stem cells. Cell Stem Cell. 2008;3(3):340–5.
46. Hu X, Zhang L, Mao SQ, Li Z, Chen J, Zhang RR, Wu HP, Gao J, Guo F, Liu W, Xu GF, Dai HQ, Shi YG, Li X, Hu B, Tang F, Pei D, Xu GL. Tet and TDG mediate DNA demethylation essential for mesenchymal-to-epithelial transition in somatic cell reprogramming. Cell Stem Cell. 2014;14(4):512–22.
47. Moon JH, Heo JS, Kwon S, Kim J, Hwang J, Kang PJ, Kim A, Kim HO, Whang KY, Yoon BS, You S. Two-step generation of induced pluripotent stem cells from mouse fibroblasts using Id3 and Oct4. J Mol Cell Biol. 2012;4(1):59–62.
48. Chen J, Gao Y, Huang H, Xu K, Chen X, Jiang Y, Li H, Gao S, Tao Y, Wang H, Zhang Y, Wang H, Cai T, Gao S. The combination of Tet1 with Oct4 generates high-quality mouse-induced pluripotent stem cells. Stem Cells. 2015;33(3):686–98.
49. Judson RL, Babiarz JE, Venere M, Blelloch R. Embryonic stem cell-specific microRNAs promote induced pluripotency. Nat Biotechnol. 2009;27(5):459–61.
50. Anokye-Danso F, Trivedi CM, Juhr D, Gupta M, Cui Z, Tian Y, Zhang Y, Yang W, Gruber PJ, Epstein JA, Morrisey EE. Highly efficient miRNA-mediated reprogramming of mouse and human somatic cells to pluripotency. Cell Stem Cell. 2011;8(4):376–88.
51. Tsai SY, Clavel C, Kim S, Ang YS, Grisanti L, Lee DF, Kelley K, Rendl M.. Oct4 and klf4 reprogram dermal papilla cells into induced pluripotent stem cells. Stem Cells. 2010;28(2):221–8.
52. Watanabe S, Hirai H, Asakura Y, Tastad C, Verma M, Keller C, Dutton JR, Asakura A.. MyoD gene suppression by Oct4 is required for reprogramming in myoblasts to produce induced pluripotent stem cells. Stem Cells. 2011; 29(3):505–16.
53. Montserrat N, Ramirez-Bajo MJ, Xia Y, Sancho-Martinez I, Moya-Rull D, Miquel-Serra L, Yang S, Nivet E, Cortina C, Gonzalez F, Izpisua Belmonte JC, Campistol JM. Generation of induced pluripotent stem cells from human renal proximal tubular cells with only two transcription factors, OCT4 and SOX2. J Biol Chem. 2012;287(29):24131–8.
54. Meng X, Neises A, Su RJ, Payne KJ, Ritter L, Gridley DS, Wang J, Sheng M, Lau KH, Baylink DJ, Zhang XB. Efficient reprogramming of human cord blood CD34+ cells into induced pluripotent stem cells with OCT4 and SOX2 alone. Mol Ther. 2012;20(2):408–16.
55. Zhou T, Benda C, Duzinger S, Huang Y, Li X, Li Y, Guo X, Cao G, Chen S, Hao L, Chan YC, Ng KM, Ho JC, Wieser M, Wu J, Redl H, Tse HF, Grillari J, Grillari-Voglauer R, Pei D, Esteban MA. Generation of induced pluripotent stem cells from urine. J Am Soc Nephrol. 2011;22(7):1221–8.
56. Stadtfeld M, Brennand K, Hochedlinger K. Reprogramming of pancreatic beta cells into induced pluripotent stem cells. Curr Biol. 2008;18(12):890–4.
57. Sommer AG, Rozelle SS, Sullivan S, Mills JA, Park SM, Smith BW, Iyer AM, French DL, Kotton DN, Gadue P, Murphy GJ, Mostoslavsky G. Generation of human induced pluripotent stem cells from peripheral blood using the STEMCCA lentiviral vector. J Vis Exp. 2012;(68). doi: 10.3791/4327
58. Okita K, Ichisaka T, Yamanaka S. Generation of germline-competent induced pluripotent stem cells. Nature. 2007;448(7151):313–7.
59. Urschitz J, Kawasumi M, Owens J, Morozumi K, Yamashiro H, Stoytchev I, Marh J, Dee JA, Kawamoto K, Coates CJ, Kaminski JM, Pelczar P, Yanagimachi R, Moisyadi S. Helper-independent piggyBac plasmids for gene delivery approaches: strategies for avoiding potential genotoxic effects. Proc Natl Acad Sci U S A. 2010;107(18):8117–22.
60. Fink KD, Rossignol J, Lu M, Leveque X, Hulse TD, Crane AT, Nerriere-Daguin V, Wyse RD, Starski PA, Schloop MT, Dues DJ, Witte SJ, Song C, Vallier L, Nguyen TH, Naveilhan P, Anegon I, Lescaudron L, Dunbar GL. Survival and differentiation of adenovirus-generated induced pluripotent stem cells transplanted into the rat striatum. Cell Transplant. 2014;23(11):1407–23.
61. Stadtfeld M, Nagaya M, Utikal J, Weir G, Hochedlinger K. Induced pluripotent stem cells generated without viral integration. Science. 2008; 322(5903):945–9.
62. Woltjen K, Michael IP, Mohseni P, Desai R, Mileikovsky M, Hamalainen R, Cowling R, Wang W, Liu P, Gertsenstein M, Kaji K, Sung HK, Nagy A. piggyBac transposition reprograms fibroblasts to induced pluripotent stem cells. Nature. 2009;458(7239):766–70.
63. Li M, Izpisua Belmonte JC. No factor left behind: generation of transgene-free induced pluripotent stem cells. Am J Stem Cells. 2011;1(1):75–80.

64. Piao Y, Hung SS, Lim SY, Wong RC, Ko MS. Efficient generation of integration-free human induced pluripotent stem cells from keratinocytes by simple transfection of episomal vectors. Stem Cells Transl Med. 2014;3(7):787–91.
65. Zhou H, Wu S, Joo JY, Zhu S, Han DW, Lin T, Trauger S, Bien G, Yao S, Zhu Y, Siuzdak G, Schöler HR, Duan L, Ding S. Generation of induced pluripotent stem cells using recombinant proteins. Cell Stem Cell. 2009;4(5):381–4.
66. Hou P, Li Y, Zhang X, Liu C, Guan J, Li H, Zhao T, Ye J, Yang W, Liu K, Ge J, Xu J, Zhang Q, Zhao Y, Deng H. Pluripotent stem cells induced from mouse somatic cells by small-molecule compounds. Science. 2013;341(6146):651–4.
67. Yagi T, Ito D, Okada Y, Akamatsu W, Nihei Y, Yoshizaki T, Yamanaka S, Okano H, Suzuki N. Modeling familial Alzheimer's disease with induced pluripotent stem cells. Hum Mol Genet. 2011;20(23):4530–9.
68. Israel MA, Yuan SH, Bardy C, Reyna SM, Mu Y, Herrera C, Hefferan MP, Van Gorp S, Nazor KL, Boscolo FS, Carson CT, Laurent LC, Marsala M, Gage FH, Remes AM, Koo EH, Goldstein LS. Probing sporadic and familial Alzheimer's disease using induced pluripotent stem cells. Nature. 2012;482(7384):216–20.
69. Cataldo AM, Peterhoff CM, Troncoso JC, Gomez-Isla T, Hyman BT, Nixon RA. Endocytic pathway abnormalities precede amyloid beta deposition in sporadic Alzheimer's disease and Down syndrome: differential effects of APOE genotype and presenilin mutations. Am J Pathol. 2000;157(1):277–86.
70. Jang J, Yoo JE, Lee JA, Lee DR, Kim JY, Huh YJ, Kim DS, Park CY, Hwang DY, Kim HS, Kang HC, Kim DW. Disease-specific induced pluripotent stem cells: a platform for human disease modeling and drug discovery. Exp Mol Med. 2012;44(3):202–13.
71. Shi Y, Kirwan P, Smith J, MacLean G, Orkin SH, Livesey FJ. A human stem cell model of early Alzheimer's disease pathology in Down syndrome. Sci Transl Med. 2012;4(124):124ra29.
72. Sproul AA, Jacob S, Pre D, Kim SH, Nestor MW, Navarro-Sobrino M, Santa-Maria I, Zimmer M, Aubry S, Steele JW, Kahler DJ, Dranovsky A, Arancio O, Crary JF, Gandy S, Noggle SA. Characterization and molecular profiling of PSEN1 familial Alzheimer's disease iPSC-derived neural progenitors. PLoS One. 2014;9(1):e84547.
73. Kondo T, Asai M, Tsukita K, Kutoku Y, Ohsawa Y, Sunada Y, Imamura K, Egawa N, Yahata N, Okita K, Takahashi K, Asaka I, Aoi T, Watanabe A, Watanabe K, Kadoya C, Nakano R, Watanabe D, Maruyama K, Hori O, Hibino S, Choshi T, Nakahata T, Hioki H, Kaneko T, Naitoh M, Yoshikawa K, Yamawaki S, Suzuki S, Hata R, Ueno S, Seki T, Kobayashi K, Toda T, Murakami K, Irie K, Klein WL, Mori H, Asada T, Takahashi R, Iwata N, Yamanaka S, Inoue H.. Modeling Alzheimer's disease with iPSCs reveals stress phenotypes associated with intracellular Abeta and differential drug responsiveness. Cell Stem Cell. 2013;12(4):487–96.
74. Muratore CR, Rice HC, Srikanth P, Callahan DG, Shin T, Benjamin LN, Walsh DM, Selkoe DJ, Young-Pearse TL. The familial Alzheimer's disease APPV717I mutation alters APP processing and Tau expression in iPSC-derived neurons. Hum Mol Genet. 2014;23(13):3523–36.
75. Duan L, Bhattacharyya BJ, Belmadani A, Pan L, Miller RJ, Kessler JA. Stem cell derived basal forebrain cholinergic neurons from Alzheimer's disease patients are more susceptible to cell death. Mol Neurodegener. 2014;9:3.
76. Chang CY, Chen SM, Lu HE, Lai SM, Lai PS, Shen PW, Chen PY, Shen CI, Harn HJ, Lin SZ, Hwang SM, Su HL.. N-butylidenephthalide attenuates Alzheimer's disease-like cytopathy in Down syndrome induced pluripotent stem cell-derived neurons. Sci Rep. 2015;5:8744.
77. Choi SH, Kim YH, Hebisch M, Sliwinski C, Lee S, D'Avanzo C, Chen H, Hooli B, Asselin C, Muffat J, Klee JB, Zhang C, Wainger BJ, Peitz M, Kovacs DM, Woolf CJ, Wagner SL, Tanzi RE, Kim DY. A three-dimensional human neural cell culture model of Alzheimer's disease. Nature. 2014;515(7526):274–8.
78. Solito E, Sastre M. Microglia function in Alzheimer's disease. Front Pharmacol. 2012;3:14.
79. Chen H, Qian K, Du Z, Cao J, Petersen A, Liu H, Blackbourn LW, Huang CL, Errigo A, Yin Y, Lu J, Ayala M, Zhang SC. Modeling ALS with iPSCs reveals that mutant SOD1 misregulates neurofilament balance in motor neurons. Cell Stem Cell. 2014;14(6):796–809.
80. Chen S, Sanjana NE, Zheng K, Shalem O, Lee K, Shi X, Scott DA, Song J, Pan JQ, Weissleder R, Lee H, Zhang F, Sharp PA. Genome-wide CRISPR screen in a mouse model of tumor growth and metastasis. Cell. 2015;160(6):1246–60.
81. Klincumhom N, Pirity MK, Berzsenyi S, Ujhelly O, Muenthaisong S, Rungarunlert S, Tharasanit T, Techakumphu M, Dinnyes A. Generation of neuronal progenitor cells and neurons from mouse sleeping beauty transposon-generated induced pluripotent stem cells. Cell Reprogram. 2012;14(5):390–7.
82. Sareen D, Gowing G, Sahabian A, Staggenborg K, Paradis R, Avalos P, Latter J, Ornelas L, Garcia L, Svendsen CN. Human induced pluripotent stem cells are a novel source of neural progenitor cells (iNPCs) that migrate and integrate in the rodent spinal cord. J Comp Neurol. 2014;522(12):2707–28.
83. Haughey NJ, Liu D, Nath A, Borchard AC, Mattson MP. Disruption of neurogenesis in the subventricular zone of adult mice, and in human cortical neuronal precursor cells in culture, by amyloid beta-peptide: implications for the pathogenesis of Alzheimer's disease. Neuromolecular Med. 2002;1(2):125–35.
84. Hallett PJ, Deleidi M, Astradsson A, Smith GA, Cooper O, Osborn TM, Sundberg M, Moore MA, Perez-Torres E, Brownell AL, Schumacher JM, Spealman RD, Isacson O. Successful function of autologous iPSC-derived dopamine neurons following transplantation in a non-human primate model of Parkinson's disease. Cell Stem Cell. 2015;16(3):269–74.
85. Kondo T, Funayama M, Tsukita K, Hotta A, Yasuda A, Nori S, Kaneko S, Nakamura M, Takahashi R, Okano H, Yamanaka S, Inoue H. Focal transplantation of human iPSC-derived glial-rich neural progenitors improves lifespan of ALS mice. Stem Cell Reports. 2014;3(2):242–9.
86. Wang R, Dineley KT, Sweatt JD, Zheng H. Presenilin 1 familial Alzheimer's disease mutation leads to defective associative learning and impaired adult neurogenesis. Neuroscience. 2004;126(2):305–12.
87. Wen PH, Hof PR, Chen X, Gluck K, Austin G, Younkin SG, Younkin LH, DeGasperi R, Gama Sosa MA, Robakis NK, Haroutunian V, Elder GA. The presenilin-1 familial Alzheimer disease mutant P117L impairs neurogenesis in the hippocampus of adult mice. Exp Neurol. 2004;188(2):224–37.
88. Donovan MH, Yazdani U, Norris RD, Games D, German DC, Eisch AJ. Decreased adult hippocampal neurogenesis in the PDAPP mouse model of Alzheimer's disease. J Comp Neurol. 2006;495(1):70–83.
89. Chen Q, Nakajima A, Choi SH, Xiong X, Sisodia SS, Tang YP. Adult neurogenesis is functionally associated with AD-like neurodegeneration. Neurobiol Dis. 2008; 29(2):316–26.
90. Brus M, Keller M, Levy F. Temporal features of adult neurogenesis: differences and similarities across mammalian species. Front Neurosci. 2013;7:135.
91. Sanai N, Berger MS, Garcia-Verdugo JM, Alvarez-Buylla A. Comment on "Human neuroblasts migrate to the olfactory bulb via a lateral ventricular extension". Science. 2007;318(5849):393.
92. Veeraraghavalu K, Choi SH, Zhang X, Sisodia SS. Presenilin 1 mutants impair the self-renewal and differentiation of adult murine subventricular zone-neuronal progenitors via cell-autonomous mechanisms involving notch signaling. J Neurosci. 2010;30(20):6903–15.
93. Demars M, Hu YS, Gadadhar A, Lazarov O. Impaired neurogenesis is an early event in the etiology of familial Alzheimer's disease in transgenic mice. J Neurosci Res. 2010;88(10):2103–17.
94. Blurton-Jones M, Kitazawa M, Martinez-Coria H, Castello NA, Muller FJ, Loring JF, Yamasaki TR, Poon WW, Green KN, LaFerla FM. Neural stem cells improve cognition via BDNF in a transgenic model of Alzheimer disease. Proc Natl Acad Sci U S A. 2009;106(32):13594–9.
95. Ager RR, Davis JL, Agazaryan A, Benavente F, Poon WW, LaFerla FM, Blurton-Jones M. Human neural stem cells improve cognition and promote synaptic growth in two complementary transgenic models of Alzheimer's disease and neuronal loss. Hippocampus. 2015;25(7):813–26.
96. Zhang W, Wang PJ, Sha HY, Ni J, Li MH, Gu GJ. Neural stem cell transplants improve cognitive function without altering amyloid pathology in an APP/PS1 double transgenic model of Alzheimer's disease. Mol Neurobiol. 2014; 50(2):423–37.
97. Ryu JK, Cho T, Wang YT, McLarnon JG. Neural progenitor cells attenuate inflammatory reactivity and neuronal loss in an animal model of inflamed AD brain. J Neuroinflammation. 2009;6:39.
98. Lee IS, Jung K, Kim IS, Lee H, Kim M, Yun S, Hwang K, Shin JE, Park KI. Human neural stem cells alleviate Alzheimer-like pathology in a mouse model. Mol Neurodegener. 2015;10:38.
99. Kim SU, Lee HJ, Kim YB. Neural stem cell-based treatment for neurodegenerative diseases. Neuropathology. 2013;33(5):491–504.
100. Martinez-Morales PL, Revilla A, Ocana I, Gonzalez C, Sainz P, McGuire D, Liste I. Progress in stem cell therapy for major human neurological disorders. Stem Cell Rev. 2013;9(5):685–99.
101. Tong LM, Fong H, Huang Y. Stem cell therapy for Alzheimer's disease and related disorders: current status and future perspectives. Exp Mol Med. 2015;47:e151.
102. Yu DX, Marchetto MC, Gage FH. Therapeutic translation of iPSCs for treating neurological disease. Cell Stem Cell. 2013;12(6):678–88.
103. Hermann A, Storch A. Induced neural stem cells (iNSCs) in neurodegenerative diseases. J Neural Transm (Vienna). 2013;120 Suppl 1:S19–25.

104. Hargus G, Ehrlich M, Arauzo-Bravo MJ, Hemmer K, Hallmann AL, Reinhardt P, Kim KP, Adachi K, Santourlidis S, Ghanjati F, Fauser M, Ossig C, Storch A, Kim JB, Schwamborn JC, Sterneckert J, Schöler HR, Kuhlmann T, Zaehres H. Origin-dependent neural cell identities in differentiated human iPSCs in vitro and after transplantation into the mouse brain. Cell Rep. 2014;8(6): 1697–703.
105. Hicks AU, Lappalainen RS, Narkilahti S, Suuronen R, Corbett D, Sivenius J, Hovatta O, Jolkkonen J. Transplantation of human embryonic stem cell-derived neural precursor cells and enriched environment after cortical stroke in rats: cell survival and functional recovery. Eur J Neurosci. 2009; 29(3):562–74.
106. Tsuji O, Miura K, Okada Y, Fujiyoshi K, Mukaino M, Nagoshi N, Kitamura K, Kumagai G, Nishino M, Tomisato S, Higashi H, Nagai T, Katoh H, Kohda K, Matsuzaki Y, Yuzaki M, Ikeda E, Toyama Y, Nakamura M, Yamanaka S, Okano H. Therapeutic potential of appropriately evaluated safe-induced pluripotent stem cells for spinal cord injury. Proc Natl Acad Sci U S A. 2010;107(28):12704–9.
107. Wernig M, Zhao JP, Pruszak J, Hedlund E, Fu D, Soldner F, Broccoli V, Constantine-Paton M, Isacson O, Jaenisch R. Neurons derived from reprogrammed fibroblasts functionally integrate into the fetal brain and improve symptoms of rats with Parkinson's disease. Proc Natl Acad Sci U S A. 2008;105(15):5856–61.
108. Kang X, Xu H, Teng S, Zhang X, Deng Z, Zhou L, Zuo P, Liu B, Liu B, Wu Q, Wang L, Hu M, Dou H, Liu W, Zhu F, Li Q, Guo S, Gu J, Lei Q, Lü J, Mu Y, Jin M, Wang S, Jiang W, Liu K, Wang C, Li W, Zhang K, Zhou Z. Dopamine release from transplanted neural stem cells in Parkinsonian rat striatum in vivo. Proc Natl Acad Sci U S A. 2014;111(44):15804–9.
109. Han F, Wang W, Chen B, Chen C, Li S, Lu X, Duan J, Zhang Y, Zhang YA, Guo W, Li G. Human induced pluripotent stem cell-derived neurons improve motor asymmetry in a 6-hydroxydopamine-induced rat model of Parkinson's disease. Cytotherapy. 2015;17(5):665–79.
110. Fujiwara N, Shimizu J, Takai K, Arimitsu N, Saito A, Kono T, Umehara T, Ueda Y, Wakisaka S, Suzuki T, Suzuki N. Restoration of spatial memory dysfunction of human APP transgenic mice by transplantation of neuronal precursors derived from human iPS cells. Neurosci Lett. 2013;557 Pt B:129–34.
111. Tong LM, Djukic B, Arnold C, Gillespie AK, Yoon SY, Wang MM, Zhang O, Knoferle J, Rubenstein JL, Alvarez-Buylla A, Huang Y. Inhibitory interneuron progenitor transplantation restores normal learning and memory in ApoE4 knock-in mice without or with Abeta accumulation. J Neurosci. 2014;34(29): 9506–15.
112. Nicholas CR, Chen J, Tang Y, Southwell DG, Chalmers N, Vogt D, Arnold CM, Chen YJ, Stanley EG, Elefanty AG, Sasai Y, Alvarez-Buylla A, Rubenstein JL, Kriegstein AR. Functional maturation of hPSC-derived forebrain interneurons requires an extended timeline and mimics human neural development. Cell Stem Cell. 2013;12(5):573–86.
113. Abdullah AI, Pollock A, Sun T. The path from skin to brain: generation of functional neurons from fibroblasts. Mol Neurobiol. 2012;45(3):586–95.
114. Nakamura M, Okano H. Cell transplantation therapies for spinal cord injury focusing on induced pluripotent stem cells. Cell Res. 2013;23(1):70–80.
115. Wang Y, Yang D, Song L, Li T, Yang J, Zhang X, Le W. Mifepristone-inducible caspase-1 expression in mouse embryonic stem cells eliminates tumor formation but spares differentiated cells in vitro and in vivo. Stem Cells. 2012; 30(2):169–79.
116. Cui L, Guan Y, Qu Z, Zhang J, Liao B, Ma B, Qian J, Li D, Li W, Xu GT, Jin Y. WNT signaling determines tumorigenicity and function of ESC-derived retinal progenitors. J Clin Invest. 2013;123(4):1647–61.
117. Nori S, Okada Y, Nishimura S, Sasaki T, Itakura G, Kobayashi Y, Renault-Mihara F, Shimizu A, Koya I, Yoshida R, et al. Long-term safety issues of iPSC-based cell therapy in a spinal cord injury model: oncogenic transformation with epithelial-mesenchymal transition. Stem Cell Reports. 2015;4(3):360–73.

10

Quantification of plasma phosphorylated tau to use as a biomarker for brain Alzheimer pathology: pilot case-control studies including patients with Alzheimer's disease and down syndrome

Harutsugu Tatebe[1,2], Takashi Kasai[1], Takuma Ohmichi[1], Yusuke Kishi[3], Tomoshi Kakeya[3], Masaaki Waragai[4], Masaki Kondo[1], David Allsop[5] and Takahiko Tokuda[1,6*]

Abstract

Background: There is still a substantial unmet need for less invasive and lower-cost blood-based biomarkers to detect brain Alzheimer's disease (AD) pathology. This study is aimed to determine whether quantification of plasma tau phosphorylated at threonine 181 (p-tau181) is informative in the diagnosis of AD.

Methods: We have developed a novel ultrasensitive immunoassay to quantify plasma p-tau181, and measured the levels of plasma p-tau181 in three cohorts.

Results: In the first cohort composed of 20 AD patients and 15 age-matched controls, the plasma levels of p-tau181 were significantly higher in the AD patients than those in the controls (0.171 ± 0.166 pg/ml in AD versus 0.0405 ± 0.0756 pg/ml in controls, $p = 0.0039$). The percentage of the subjects whose levels of plasma p-tau181 exceeded the cut-off value (0.0921 pg/ml) was significantly higher in the AD group compared with the control group (60% in AD versus 16.7% in controls, $p = 0.0090$). In the second cohort composed of 20 patients with Down syndrome (DS) and 22 age-matched controls, the plasma concentrations of p-tau181 were significantly higher in the DS group (0.767 ± 1.26 pg/ml in DS versus 0.0415 ± 0.0710 pg/ml in controls, $p = 0.0313$). There was a significant correlation between the plasma levels of p-tau181 and age in the DS group ($R^2 = 0.4451$, $p = 0.0013$). All of the DS individuals showing an extremely high concentration of plasma p-tau181 (> 1.0 pg/ml) were older than the age of 40. In the third cohort composed of 8 AD patients and 3 patients with other neurological diseases, the levels of plasma p-tau181 significantly correlated with those of CSF p-tau181 ($R^2 = 0.4525$, $p = 0.023$).

Conclusions: We report for the first time quantitative data on the plasma levels of p-tau181 in controls and patients with AD and DS, and these data suggest that the plasma p-tau181 is a promising blood biomarker for brain AD pathology. This exploratory pilot study warrants further large-scale and well-controlled studies to validate the usefulness of plasma p-tau181 as an urgently needed surrogate marker for the diagnosis and disease progression of AD.

Keywords: Plasma biomarker, Tau phosphorylated at threonine 181 (p-tau181), Simoa, Alzheimer's disease, Down syndrome

* Correspondence: ttokuda@koto.kpu-m.ac.jp
[1]Department of Neurology, Kyoto Prefectural University of Medicine, Kyoto 602-0841, Japan
[6]Department of Molecular Pathobiology of Brain Diseases, Kyoto Prefectural University of Medicine, Kyoto 602-0841, Japan
Full list of author information is available at the end of the article

Background

Alzheimer's disease (AD) is the most common cause of dementia and one of the major medical problems to be resolved throughout the world. The pathognomonic brain pathologies characteristic of AD consist of senile plaques containing amyloid β (Aβ) peptide, and neurofibrillary tangles (NFT) composed of hyperphosphorylated tau protein. The same pathological changes are also present in the brains of aged people with Down syndrome (DS) [1] and so adults with DS can be regarded as a cohort of preclinical AD [2]. Accurate and sensitive biomarkers are needed urgently to aid in the diagnosis of AD, especially in those with preclinical AD, not least to facilitate the development of new disease-modifying treatments. Numerous previous studies searching for useful AD-biomarkers have reported the value of measuring levels of Aβ1–42, total (t-tau) and phosphorylated tau (p-tau) in cerebrospinal fluid (CSF), or visualizing plaques and tangles by means of positron emission tomography (PET) brain imaging using specific probes for Aβ or tau [3–6]. The current consensus is that these CSF and PET biomarkers can differentiate AD from normal aging and from other dementing disorders, and changes in these biomarkers can also facilitate detection of AD many years before any overt clinical symptoms become clear [7–10]. However, these CSF and PET biomarkers are, respectively, invasive and costly, and so they have not been utilized widely in routine clinical practice. Thus, there is still a substantial unmet need for less invasive and lower-cost alternatives, particularly for high-throughput screening of people at risk of developing AD. For this reason, there have been many studies of blood-based molecular markers, including plasma Aβ species, as a potential alternative and less invasive method for the diagnosis of AD. However, the reported results have been very contradictory [11–15] and so the prevailing view is that AD (or preclinical AD) cannot be distinguished from controls without AD pathology on the basis of plasma levels of Aβ40 and Aβ42 [16].

In the last few years a new method has become available for measuring levels of plasma t-tau by using an ultrasensitive digital enzyme-linked immunosorbent assay (ELISA) technique, and this has been studied as a potential diagnostic biomarker for AD. However, a substantial overlap was found in levels of plasma t-tau between patients with AD and age-matched controls [17]. Here, we report the development of a new assay using this type of ultrasensitive technique to quantify plasma p-tau phosphorylated at threonine 181 (p-tau181), instead of t-tau. There are no previous reports on quantification of plasma p-tau181 in patients with AD or in those with DS. In this small-scale pilot study, we have quantified levels of plasma p-tau181 in patients with AD and DS as well as control cases, and have compared levels between these groups.

Methods

Study design, subject characterization, and sample collection

To determine usefulness of p-tau181 for the diagnosis of AD pathology, we measured levels of p-tau181 in plasma and CSF samples obtained from 3 cohorts; 1) plasma samples obtained from 20 Caucasian patients with AD (ages 60–89, mean ± SD of 77.4 ± 7.7) and 15 age-matched Caucasian controls (ages 71–84, mean ± SD of 76.3 ± 3.2) (purchased from ProteoGenex, Inc., CA, USA via KAC Co. Ltd., Tokyo, Japan), 2) plasma samples from 20 patients with DS (ages 19–57, mean ± SD of 34.0 ± 11.5) and 22 age-matched healthy controls (ages 14–56, mean ± SD of 37.4 ± 12.0) recruited at outpatient clinic of Department of Neurology, Kyoto Prefectural University of Medicine, Kyoto, Japan and 3) plasma and CSF samples obtained simultaneously from 8 patients with AD and other neurological diseases (1 Parkinson's disease (PD), 2 vascular dementia (VaD)) recruited at outpatient clinic of Department of Neurology, Higashi Matsudo Municipal Hospital, Chiba, Japan.

In the cohort 2, we enrolled 20 adult patients with DS from the registration for DS in Kyoto Prefectural University of Medicine and Hananoki Medical Welfare Center, from February 2013 to January 2017. Plasma of 22 age-matched healthy controls was obtained from another registration of Kyoto Prefectural University of Medicine during the aforementioned period. Social maturity in the DS patients was estimated as 'social ages' using the social maturity scale revised (S-M) (Nihonbunkakagakusha, Tokyo), which is a social maturity scale developed for the Japanese based on the Vineland Social Maturity Scale [18]. In 6 out of 20 patients with DS, 'social ages' were longitudinally evaluated twice, approximately 1 year apart, and calculated the changes of the social ages of the patient during that period (named as Δsocial ages). Brain Aβ-amyloid burden was evaluated with positron emission tomography (PET) using *N*-methyl-[11C]-2-(4′-methylamino-phenyl)-6-hydroxy-benzothiazole ([11C]PiB) in 6 DS patients as described previously [19]. A mean cortical PiB retention measurement was also computed across cortical regions of interest (ROIs) without including the cerebellum. The PiB retention outcomes were evaluated based on the standardized uptake value (SUV) measures. The SUVs were determined over 50–70 min post injection intervals and normalized to injected dose and body mass. SUV ratio (SUVR) was generated using the cerebellum as reference. In the cohort 3, patients were diagnosed based on clinical and neuroimaging findings; patients with AD were diagnosed using the National Institute of Neurological and Communication Disorders and Stroke-Alzheimer's Disease and Related Disorders Association criteria for probable AD [20]; those with VaD were diagnosed according to NINDS (the National Institute of Neurological Disorders and Stroke)-AIREN (Association Internationale pour la Recherche et l'Enseignement en Neurosciences) clinical criteria for the diagnosis of VaD [21]; a patient with PD was diagnosed according to the UK PD Society Brain Bank criteria [22].

In the cohort 2 and 3, plasma samples were taken through venous puncture, and a total of 8 ml of blood was collected in EDTA-containing tubes. After collection, plasma was separated by centrifugation for 15 min at 2000 g and distributed in polypropylene vials, then stored at −80 °C until analysis. In the cohort 3, plasma and CSF samples were simultaneously taken. The CSF samples were centrifuged for 10 min at 400 g, aliquoted and stored at −80 °C, the plasma samples were processed as described above.

Ethics, consent and permissions

All subjects including patients with DS provided written informed consent to participate in the study, which was approved by the University Ethics Committee (Kyoto Prefectural University of Medicine, Kyoto, Japan; the reference number RBMR-C-1027-2). The study procedures were designed and performed in accordance with the Declaration of Helsinki.

Immunoassay protocols

For the CSF samples of cohort 3, the levels of CSF p-tau181 were measured using INNOTEST® PHOSPHO-TAU(181P) (FUJIREBIO Inc., Tokyo, Japan) according to the manufacturer's instruction. The plasma levels of p-tau181 were analyzed with a novel ultrasensitive immunoassay specific for p-tau181 using digital array technology [23, 24]. To develop this novel p-tau181 immunoassay, we modified the Human Total Tau kit (Simoa™ Tau 2.0 Kit, Quanterix, Lexington, MA) on the Simoa HD-1 analyzer (Quanterix). This kit is an updated version of the assay reported previously [25] that uses a monoclonal capture antibody that reacts with a linear epitope in the midregion of all tau isoforms and a detection antibody that reacts with an epitope in the N-terminal region of t-tau. Instead of this detection antibody against t-tau, we employed anti-human PHF-tau monoclonal antibody AT270 (Thermo Fisher Scientific, Rockford, IL, USA) as the detection antibody for our novel p-tau181 immunoassay. This set of capture and detection antibodies specifically reacts with p-tau181 without reacting with unphosphorylated tau [26]. The other immunoassay reagents used in our p-tau181 assay were the same as those in the Simoa™ Tau 2.0 Kit, except for the calibrator to make the standard curve for the assay. We used Hu Tau [pT181] Standard in Human Tau [pT181] phosphoELISA™ ELISA kit (Invitrogen, Thermo Fisher Scientific) as the calibrator for our p-tau181 assay. The standard curve for our p-ta181 assay was carried out with duplicate measurements using the Hu Tau [pT181] Standard at different concentrations (0, 0.039, 0.15, 0.625, 2.5 and 10 pg/ml) of the p-tau181 protein diluted in Tau 2.0 Sample Diluent (contained in Simoa™ Tau 2.0 Kit). Regarding the assay procedure for plasma p-tau181, we followed that of the Simoa™ Tau 2.0 Kit except for changing the detection antibody and the calibrator as mentioned above. All plasma samples were diluted 4 times with the Tau 2.0 Sample Diluent prior to the assays, to minimize matrix effects. To eliminate inter-assay variability as a confounding factor, all plasma samples belonging to the same cohort were run in duplicate on the same day with the same lot of standards. The relative concentration estimates of plasma p-tau181 were calculated according to the standard curve. We assumed the levels of plasma p-tau to be 0 in samples in which we could not detect p-tau with our ultrasensitive assay in order to compare the patient and control groups.

The details of the procedures for method validation of our novel p-tau181 immunoassay are described in Additional file 1.

Statistical analysis

Regarding differences between the patients with AD or DS and controls, the groups were compared using Mann–Whitney U test. Tau elevation profiles were also analyzed for area-under-the-curve (AUC) and receiver operating characteristics (ROC) in the cohort 1 (AD and controls). We tested associations between the levels of plasma p-tau181 and demographic factors in the cohort 2 (patients with DS and controls) as well as associations between levels of plasma and CSF p-tau181 in the cohort 3 (patients with DS and other neurological diseases) using Spearman correlation. All analyses were carried out using GraphPad Prism software (version 6.0, GraphPad software, San Diego, USA). The level of significance was set at $p < 0.05$. The characteristics of the patients in the cohort 3, including clinically diagnosed patients with AD (n = 8), VaD.

Results

Patient characteristics

Cohort 1 was a set of purchased samples consisting of plasma from 20 clinically diagnosed patients with AD and 15 controls (Table 1). Mean ages were matched for these two groups (mean ± standard deviation (SD: range), AD: 77.4 ± 7.7 (60–89), 76.3 ± 3.2 (71–84)).

Table 1 Characteristics of patients with AD and controls of cohort 1

Diagnosis	Number	M/F	Ages Mean ± SD (range)	MMSE scores Mean ± SD (range)
AD	20	8/12	77.4 ± 7.7 (60–89)	12.8 ± 5.0 (2–19)
Control	15	1/14	76.3 ± 3.2 (71–84)	N/A

M/F Male/female, *AD* Alzheimer's disease, *MMSE* Mini-mental state examination, *N/A* not available

Cohort 2 consisted of 20 patients with DS (Table 2) and 22 healthy controls, and mean ages were matched for these two groups as mentioned above. Estimated social ages (18 out of 20 patients), the changes of social age during the 1-year follow-up period (6 out of 20), and the mean cortical SUVR values in PIB-PET study of the DS patients are shown in Table 2. Cohort 3 consisted of 8 AD, 2 VaD and 1 PD patients (Table 3), whose CSF and plasma samples were collected simultaneously in each patient to determine the correlation between CSF and plasma levels of p-tau181 as measured with our novel immunoassay.

Standard curve for the novel p-tau181 immunoassay and assay method validation

Figure 1 shows the standard curve for our novel p-tau181 immunoassay, demonstrating that p-tau181 was detected with high sensitivity. The goodness of fit was 0.9999. The repeatability of the standard curve was determined in separate experiments (Additional file 1), and showed permissible repeatability of the standard curve with CV values of assay signal intensities (quantified by units of average number of enzyme labels per bead (AEB) in Simoa assay) such as 22.0, 11.3, 8.5, and 2.8% for standard p-tau solutions of 0, 0.039, 0.15 and 0.625 pg/ml, respectively. The limit of detection (LOD) of the assay, which requires 50 μl of plasma, is 0.0090 pg/ml (determined as described in Additional file 1). The LOD of our novel p-tau assay is accordingly ~1000-fold more sensitive than conventional ELISAs, for example, the above-mentioned INNOTEST® PHOSPHO-TAU(181P) (LOD = 13 pg/ml). Intra-assay precision was determined (Additional file 1), and it was robust with coefficient of variations (CVs) between 2.8 and 11.2% (Additional file 2). To eliminate inter-assay variability, all plasma samples of the same cohort were analyzed on the same day. In quality control experiments (Additional file 1), mean and CV values of the plasma p-tau were calculated in each sample (n = 6), which determined CV values ranging 3.8 to 10.4% (Additional file 3). In spike recovery and parallelism experiments (Additional file 1), the mean recovery rates were calculated to be 121.6 ± 3.5% after subtraction of the endogenous p-tau concentration. Parallelism of serially diluted plasma samples is also demonstrated in Additional file 4, which showed that plasma samples diluted 1:4 to 1:16 gave reliable results.

Comparison of the plasma levels of p-tau181 in cohort 1

The plasma levels of p-tau181 were significantly higher in the AD group (mean ± SD 0.171 ± 0.166 pg/ml, 95%

Table 2 Characteristics of patients with DS of the cohort 2

Case	Sex	Age (years)	Social Age[a] (years), BL	ΔSocial Age[b] (years)	Mean cortical SUVR (PiB-PET)	Plasma p-tau181 (pg/ml)
1	M	36	8.75	1.10	1.553	0.0000
2	F	26	4.17	N/A	N/A	0.0000
3	F	19	4.50	2.00	1.400	0.0000
4	M	26	4.92	0.19	1.536	0.0000
5	F	22	7.42	−0.10	1.142	0.0000
6	F	31	N/A	N/A	N/A	0.0000
7	F	24	10.0	N/A	N/A	0.1494
8	F	25	7.00	N/A	N/A	0.0000
9	M	48	4.42	N/A	N/A	0.2040
10	M	25	7.08	−1.00	1.578	0.1408
11	F	45	1.92	N/A	N/A	2.0731
12	M	26	6.50	−1.10	N/A	0.2787
13	M	57	4.08	N/A	N/A	1.3516
14	M	31	2.33	N/A	N/A	0.2382
15	F	55	2.42	N/A	1.828	4.0296
16	F	42	4.17	N/A	N/A	2.7619
17	M	43	6.08	N/A	N/A	3.3685
18	M	25	N/A	N/A	N/A	0.3256
19	M	29	4.67	N/A	N/A	0.4112
20	F	45	8.33	N/A	N/A	0.0000

BL Baseline, SUVR standardized uptake value ratio, N/A not available

[a]Social ages were estimated using social maturity scale revised (S-M). Although data were calculated as units of years and months on this buttery [18], we recalculated those into unit of years for statistical analysis. Social ages in this figure were represented as unit of years

[b]"ΔSocial Age" represents the changes of the social age in individual DS patients who can be evaluated twice, approximately 1 year apart

Table 3 Characteristics of subjects of the cohort 3

Case	Sex	Age (years)	Clinical diagnosis	MMSE	CSF p-tau181 (pg/ml)	Plasma p-tau181 (pg/ml)
1	M	86	AD	17	63.5	0.1057
2	F	70	AD	23	96.0	0.3785
3	F	88	AD	20	51.7	0.1063
4	F	86	VaD	18	39.3	0.0783
5	F	75	AD	18	103.0	0.2774
6	M	76	AD	5	117.0	0.1797
7	F	76	AD	4	88.0	0.1057
8	F	85	AD	12	57.0	0.1162
9	F	68	PD	30	28.8	0.0629
10	F	82	VaD	18	71.8	0.0763
11	F	76	AD	24	67.6	0.1636

MMSE Mini-mental state examination, AD Alzheimer's disease, VaD Vascular dementia, PD Parkinson's disease

confidence interval (95% CI) of the mean 0.0934–0.248, $n = 20$) than those in the age-matched controls (0.0405 ± 0.0756 pg/ml, 95% CI of the mean − 0.00311 – 0.0842, $n = 15$) ($p = 0.0039$, Mann–Whitney U test; Fig. 2a). Figure 2b shows the ROC curve for the classification of patients with AD and controls based on the levels of plasma p-tau181 measured in Cohort 1. The AUC for the ROC analysis was 0.786. From the ROC curve analysis, when the cut-off value of the plasma p-tau181 used to discriminate those two groups was set at 0.0921 pg/ml, we obtained the highest likelihood ratio of the classification belonging to the AD or control group. Among the 20 patients with AD and 15 controls, there were 12 patients (60.0%) and 2 controls (16.7%) with levels of plasma p-tau181 higher than this cut-off value (i.e. more than 0.0921 pg/ml, Table 1, Fig. 2a). Thus, the percentage of the subjects whose levels of plasma p-tau181 exceeded the cut-off value was significantly higher in the AD group compared with the control group ($p = 0.0090$, Fisher's exact test).

Plasma levels of p-tau181 in patients with DS

The plasma levels of p-tau181 were significantly higher in the DS group (mean ± SD 0.767 ± 1.26 pg/ml, 95% CI of the mean 0.178–1.355, $n = 20$) than those in the age-matched controls (0.0415 ± 0.0710 pg/ml, 95% CI of the mean 0.0100–0.0729, $n = 22$) ($p = 0.0313$, Mann–Whitney U test; Fig. 3a). When the cut-off value to discriminate those two groups was set to 0.0921 pg/ml, that is the value obtained for Cohort 1 (AD vs. Control), 12 out of 20 patients with DS (60.0%) and 6 out of 22 controls (27.3%)

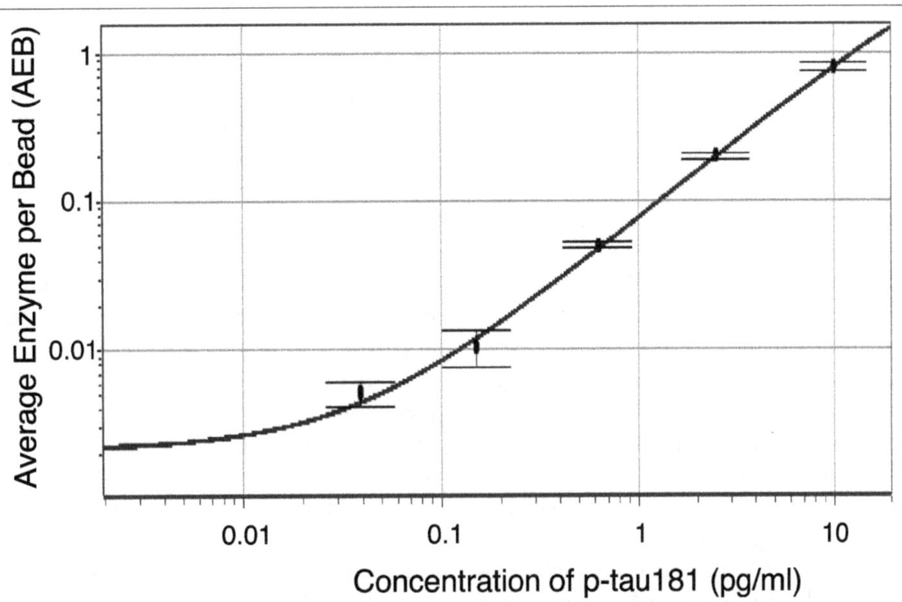

Fig. 1 Standard curve for the plasma p-tau181 immunoassay (ultrasensitive digital array technology, Simoa™ system, Quanterix). Data represent the mean ± SD of duplicate readings. The goodness of fit was 0.9999. The limit of detection of the assay is 0.0090 pg/ml

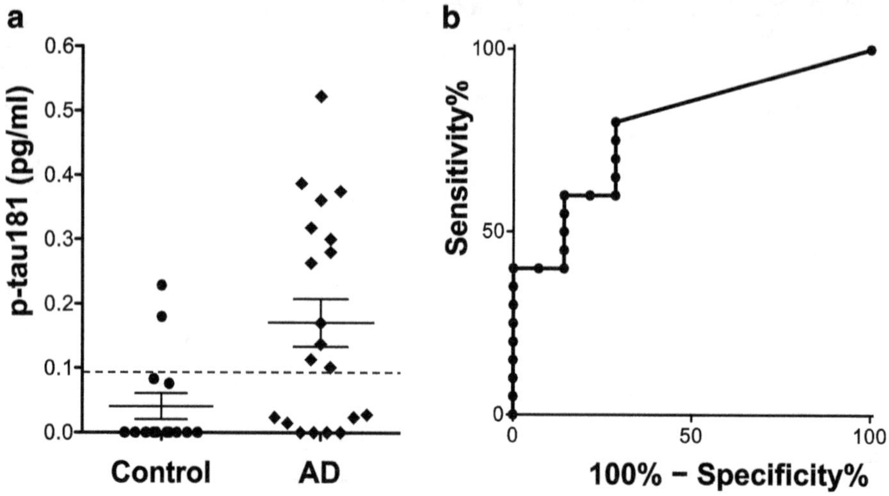

Fig. 2 a Plots for the concentrations of plasma p-tau181 in the control patients (n = 15) and the clinically diagnosed patients with AD (n = 20) of Cohort 1. The solid lines represent the mean value ± standard errors (SE) of the concentrations of each group. The concentration of plasma p-tau181 in the AD group was significantly higher than that in the age-matched control subjects (p = 0.0039, Mann–Whitney U test). The dashed line corresponds to the cut-off value of the plasma p-tau181 to discriminate those two groups (0.0921 pg/ml). **b** ROC analysis of the levels of plasma p-tau181 for the discrimination between AD and control groups (AUC = 0.786, sensitivity = 60.0%, specificity = 85.7%)

had levels of plasma p-ta181 higher than the cut-off value (i.e. more than 0.0921 pg/ml, Fig. 3a). The percentage of the subjects whose levels of plasma p-tau181 exceeded the cut-off value was significantly higher in the DS group compared with the control group (p = 0.0332, Fisher's exact test).

Individuals with DS develop dementia at a much lower age, and also have a shorter life expectancy in general. Thus, age-matched controls mentioned above may not possibly be the right control group. As a result, we have made another comparison between the levels of plasma p-tau in the DS group and those in the controls for the AD group in our cohort 1. We found that there is still a significant difference in the plasma p-tau levels between those two groups (p = 0.0116, Mann–Whitney U test).

A significant correlation between the plasma levels of p-tau181 and age was observed in the DS group (R^2 = 0.4451, p = 0.0013, Pearson correlation; Fig. 3b), but not in the control group (R^2 = 0.0317, p = 0.4275, data not shown). All of the DS patients showing an extremely high concentration of plasma p-tau181 (> 1.0 pg/ml) were older than the age of 40 (Fig. 3b). Plasma p-tau181 levels in patients with DS were weakly, but not significantly, correlated negatively with their social ages (p = 0.0563, n = 18; Fig. 3c). In the DS patients whose social ages were longitudinally evaluated (n = 6; Table 2), 2 patients who exhibited a decrease in social age, suggesting that their cognitive function had started to decline, had abnormally high levels of p-tau181. Meanwhile, those whose social ages remained unchanged showed much lower values of plasma p-tau181 around 0 pg/ml (Fig. 3d).

We performed a PiB-PET study in 6 individuals with DS aged 19 to 55 years (Table 2). The level of plasma p-tau181 was increased in a patient of 55 years who had a clear positive Aβ-amyloid burden in the cerebral cortices (mean cortical SUVR = 1.828), while the levels of p-tau181 were lower (around 0 pg/ml) in the other patients whose mean cortical SUVRs were less than 1.6 (Fig. 3e).

Correlation between the levels of p-tau181 in CSF and plasma

We next examined any correlation between the CSF and plasma levels of p-tau181 in the patients in Cohort 3 (n = 11) in which matched CSF and plasma samples were taken from each patient. In this small cohort, the levels of plasma p-tau181 significantly correlated with those of CSF p-tau181 (R^2 = 0.4525, p = 0.023, n = 11, Pearson correlation; Fig. 4).

Discussion

To our knowledge, this is the first study to report an immunoassay method that can specifically quantify the levels of p-tau181 in human plasma and to present quantitative data on the plasma levels of p-tau181 in patients with AD and DS as well as in control subjects. We used a recently developed digital array technology (Simoa™ system, Quanterix) that can be applied to development of unprecedented biomarkers for brain diseases due to its ultra-high sensitivity. Even in the control subjects of Cohorts 1 and 2, we were able to obtain values for plasma p-tau181 concentrations due to the ultra-high sensitivity of this assay to detect minute amounts of p-tau181 in human plasma. The determined mean levels of plasma p-tau181 in the

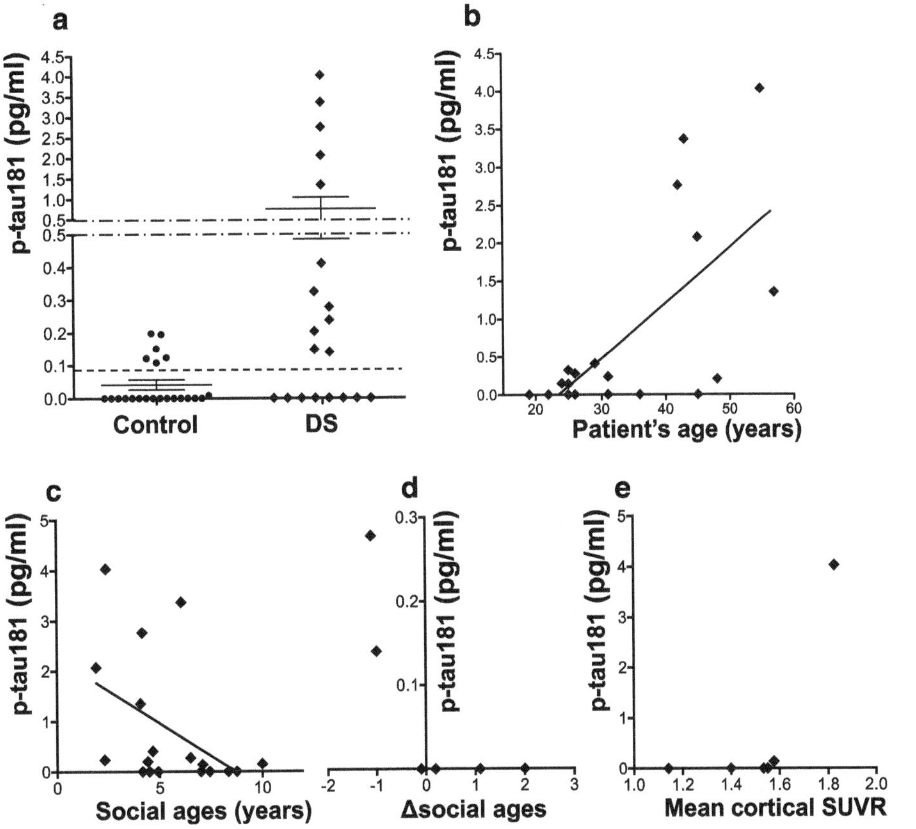

Fig. 3 a Plots for the concentrations of plasma p-tau181 in the control patients (n = 22) and the clinically diagnosed patients with DS (n = 20) of Cohort 2. The solid lines represent the mean value ± standard errors (SE) of the concentrations of each group. The concentration of plasma p-tau181 in the DS group was significantly higher than that in the age-matched controls (p = 0.0313, Mann–Whitney U test). The dashed line corresponds to the cut-off value of the plasma p-tau181 to discriminate AD from control (0.0921 pg/ml) derived from the ROC analysis of AD and control groups in Cohort 1 (Fig. 2a). **b** A scatter plot of the levels of plasma p-tau181 versus the patient age of the DS patients (n = 20) and a linear regression line for the correlation of those two parameters. There is a significant correlation between the levels of plasma p-tau181 and the age of the DS patients (R^2 = 0.4451, p = 0.0013, Pearson correlation). **c** A scatter plot of the levels of plasma p-tau181 versus the social ages of the DS patients (n = 18) indexed by social maturity scale developed for the Japanese (S-M) [18] that represents the intellectual ability of each DS patient. The solid lines represent the linear regression line between those two parameters. The levels of plasma p-tau181 were weakly correlated negatively with the social ages of DS patients, but the correlation was not significant (p = 0.0563, n = 18). **d** A scatter plot of the levels of plasma p-tau181 versus the Δsocial ages of the DS patients (n = 6), which indicates the changes of the social ages of the patient during the ~1-year follow-up period. The larger negative values of Δsocial ages means the more cognitive decline the patient had. **e** A scatter plot of the levels of plasma p-tau181 versus the mean cortical SUVR in PiB-PET study of the DS patients (n = 6), which represents the severity of cerebral Aβ-amyloid burden

control subjects were similar between Cohort 1 and Cohort 2 (mean ± SD 0.0405 ± 0.0756 pg/ml, 95% CI of the mean – 0.00311 – 0.0842 in the controls of Cohort 1; mean ± SD 0.0415 ± 0.0710 pg/ml, 95% CI of the mean 0.0100–0.0729 in those of Cohort 2), suggesting that our p-tau181 immunoassay is reliable. Ours is the first study to suggest that the plasma level of p-tau181 is a promising blood biomarker for brain AD pathology in patients with AD and DS. Although the AUC value (0.786) for the ROC analysis using Cohort 1 (AD vs. Control) was not so high, this could be mainly due to the nature of this pilot study which involved only a small number of subjects. As shown in Fig. 2a, discrimination between AD and controls based on the levels of plasma p-tau181 was fairly good when the cut-off value was set at 0.0921 pg/ml, because the percentage of subjects with levels of plasma p-tau181 above this cut-off was significantly higher in the AD group (60.0%) than the control group (16.7%) (p = 0.0090). We also confirmed a significant discrimination ability of the levels of plasma p-tau181 between the DS and control group in Cohort 2 by using the same cut-off value as for Cohort 1 (0.0921 pg/ml) (p = 0.0332, Fig. 3a). Interestingly, all of the DS patients who showed extremely high concentrations of plasma p-tau181 (> 1.0 pg/ml) were older than the age of 40, which is around the age when tau pathology begins to develop in the brains of DS individuals [1]. Regarding the relevance to brain AD pathology, among the 6 patients with DS who underwent PiB-PET, the level of plasma p-tau181 was not increased in the 5 patients whose mean cortical SUVRs were less than 1.6,

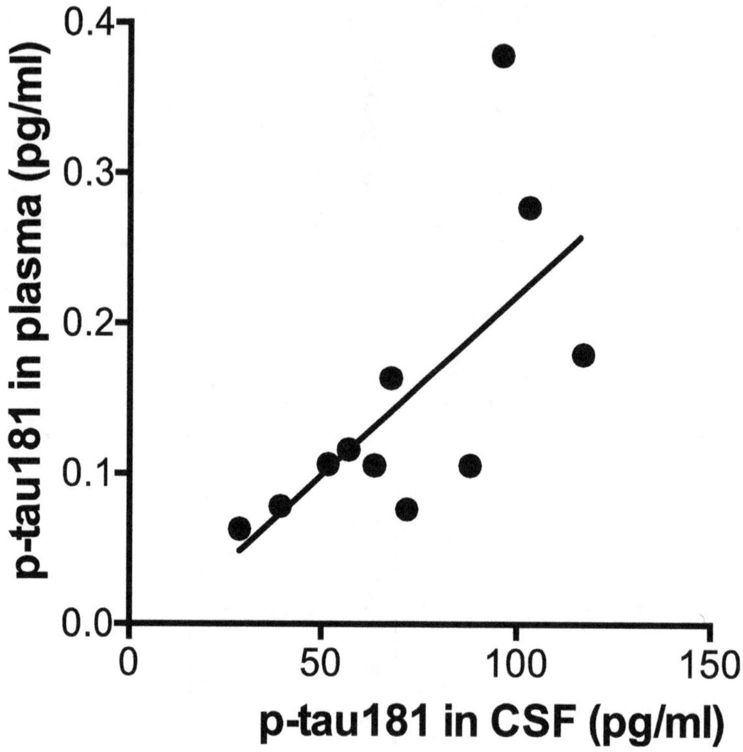

Fig. 4 A scatter plot of the levels of plasma p-tau181 versus those of CSF p-tau181 in the patients of Cohort 3 (n = 11) and a linear regression line for the correlation of those two parameters. There is a significant correlation between the levels of plasma and CSF p-tau181 in this small cohort ($R^2 = 0.4525$, $p = 0.023$, $n = 11$, Pearson correlation)

but increased only in the patient with an obviously positive amyloid burden (mean cortical SUVR = 1.828) (Fig. 3e). Further, we consider that the levels of plasma p-tau181 might correlate with cognitive status in the DS cohort. Plasma p-tau181 levels in patients with DS had a tendency to correlate negatively with their social ages (Fig. 3c), and were increased only in the 2 patients who started to suffer from cognitive decline with a decrement in their social age during the ~1-year follow-up period (Fig. 3d).

Our aim was to develop a novel ultrasensitive assay for p-tau181 and to use it as a possible blood biomarker for the diagnosis of brain AD pathology. Although the value of the three core CSF biomarkers (Aβ42, t-tau, and p-tau) has been established in numerous studies, including meta-analyses that have used a huge number of subjects [3–6], these CSF biomarkers have serious limitations because of their invasiveness and the considerable care and skill needed to collect CSF samples, and so these markers have not found their way into routine clinical use. Regarding potential blood biomarkers for AD, plasma Aβ40 and/or Aβ42 have been studied, but contradictory results were reported [11–15]. Thus, at the present time, patients with AD pathology cannot be distinguished from controls by measuring the levels of plasma Aβ species [16]. Since t-tau is another reasonable candidate plasma biomarker for AD pathology, there have been several studies that have explored the levels of plasma t-tau in patients with AD and related disorders in comparison with healthy controls [17, 27–33]. Using a recently-developed ultrasensitive digital ELISA method and plasma samples obtained from large cohort studies, Zetterberg et al. reported levels of plasma t-tau in large numbers of patients with AD and controls [17, 28]. Because the overlap between normal aging and AD was large in their studies, they concluded that their results do not support plasma t-tau as an AD biomarker in individual people, despite group-level differences in plasma levels between those two groups. One possible reason for the failure of plasma Aβ species and t-tau as specific biomarkers for AD pathology is that these molecules can have a peripheral source outside of the brain, for example plasma Aβ species may originate from platelets [34, 35] and t-tau from peripheral nerves [36, 37]. We have focused on the development of a novel immunoassay to quantify plasma p-tau181, because high CSF t-tau is not only found in AD but also in other brain disorders with neuronal damage, while high CSF p-tau is more specific for brain AD pathology [5, 38, 39]. In our assay, we used an established set of capture and detection antibodies that have been validated already in previous studies, including large cohort studies such as the Alzheimer's Disease Neuroimaging Initiative (ADNI) study; the capture antibody is the same as that used in the Simoa™ Tau

2.0 Kit (Quanterix) which can determine exact levels of plasma t-tau in samples from AD and control cases; the detection antibody (AT270) has been used in the international standard ELISA to quantify CSF p-tau181 (INNOTEST® PHOSPHO-TAU(181P), FUJIREBIO Inc.) in many previous studies [40, 41].

We also demonstrated a significant positive correlation between plasma and CSF p-tau181 levels in Cohort 3. This finding suggests that the level of plasma p-tau181 is likely to reflect the concentration of p-tau181 in the interstitial and extracellular compartments within the brain, and therefore p-tau181 in plasma should be of brain origin. Regarding the correlation of plasma and CSF levels of t-tau, a recent large-scale study demonstrated that the levels of t-tau in plasma were positively associated with those in CSF, but this association was weak and differed according to the examined cohort; the association was not significant in the ADNI cohort, but significant in the other cohort [17]. Considering this previous report and our results together, we consider that the differences between plasma-CSF correlations of p-tau181 and t-tau could mainly reflect their different sources from within and outside of the brain, as mentioned above; t-tau can have both a brain and peripheral origin [36, 37], whereas p-tau181 should be exclusively of brain origin [5, 38, 39].

This is the first study to quantify at an ultrasensitive level the amount of p-tau181 in human plasma and to show the value of this measure for the diagnosis of brain AD pathology, but it is not without limitations. Firstly, this is a small-scale exploratory pilot study, and the data presented are still preliminary. Thus, we need to confirm whether or not plasma p-tau181 will be useful as a diagnostic biomarker for brain AD pathology as well as a biomarker to evaluate disease severity in large-scale studies. Blood-based biomarkers are required for early/preclinical diagnosis and for selection of appropriate subjects for clinical trials of disease-modifying therapies, and we consider that plasma p-tau181 is a promising candidate for an AD blood biomarker. Another limitation is that we only used plasma and CSF samples from clinically diagnosed patients not proven by autopsy. It has been reported that more than 20% of patients diagnosed clinically and recruited by dementia specialists do not have any cerebral amyloid burden in amyloid PET studies [42], suggesting that the diagnosis of AD based only on clinical symptoms, without objective biomarkers, is flawed. In Cohort 1 of the present study, 8 out of 20 AD patients who had been diagnosed based on clinical symptoms showed levels of plasma p-tau181 lower than the cut-off value differentiating between AD and control groups (Fig. 2a). One of the reasons for this finding is the possibility that some of those patients with lower plasma p-tau181 could be non-AD dementia, misdiagnosed as AD. Supporting this possibility, in Cohort 2, all of the 7 DS patients aged over 40 (except a 45-year-old female), which is around the age when tau pathology starts in DS, showed substantially and extremely elevated levels of plasma p-tau181 compared to those of the controls (Fig. 3a).

Conclusions

By using a newly developed ultrasensitive immunoassay, we report for the first time quantitative data on the plasma levels of p-tau181 in patients with AD and DS as well as control subjects. Our results provide highly valuable information that the plasma p-tau181 is a promising blood biomarker for the detection of brain AD pathology, since there is still a great unmet need for less invasive and lower-cost blood-based biomarkers to detect brain AD pathology. This small-scale pilot study warrants further large-scale and well-controlled studies with strict protocols, especially those including patients with AD who have brain AD pathologies proven by autopsy and/or PET studies for detection of cerebral amyloid and tau burden, to validate the usefulness of plasma p-tau181 as an urgently needed blood biomarker for the diagnosis and disease progression of AD.

Abbreviations

[11C]PiB: *N*-methyl-[11C]-2-(4′-methylamino-phenyl)-6-hydroxy-benzothiazole; 95% CI: 95% confidence interval; AD: Alzheimer's disease;; ADNI: Alzheimer's Disease Neuroimaging Initiative; AUC: area under the curve; BL: baseline; CSF: cerebrospinal fluid; CV: coefficient of variation; DS: Down syndrome; ELISA: enzyme-linked immunosorbent assay; LOD: the limit of detection; M/F: male/female; MMSE: mini-mental state examination; N/A: not available; NFT: neurofibrillary tangles; NINDS-AIREN: the National Institute of Neurological Disorders and Stroke-Association Internationale pour la Recherche et l'Enseignement en Neurosciences; PD: Parkinson's disease; PET: positron emission tomography; p-tau181: tau phosphorylated at threonine 181; ROC: receiver operating characteristics; SD: standard deviation; SE: standard errors; S-M: social maturity scale revised; SUV: standardized uptake value; SUVR: standardized uptake value ratio; t-tau: total tau; VaD: vascular dementia

Acknowledgements

We thank the Tokuda lab members (R. Ishii, N. Sori and W.T.E Yeung) for experimental support.

Funding

This study was funded by the Japan Society for the Promotion of Science (JSPS) Grant-in-Aid for Scientific Research (KAKENHI: 15 K09322 to T.T.); and Agency for Research and Medical Development (AMED) (16dk0207030h0001; to T.T.).

Author's contributions

TT, TKasai and HT designed the study. HT, TT, TO, MW and MK performed the research. TKasai, YK, TKakeya and DA supported experimental design and data analysis. TT, TKasai and DA wrote the manuscript. All authors read and approved the final manuscript.

Author details
[1]Department of Neurology, Kyoto Prefectural University of Medicine, Kyoto 602-0841, Japan. [2]Department of Zaitaku (Homecare) Medicine, Kyoto Prefectural University of Medicine, Kyoto 602-0841, Japan. [3]Strategic Marketing Division, SCRUM Inc, Tokyo 130-0021, Japan. [4]Department of Neurology, Higashi Matsudo Municipal Hospital, Matsudo 270-2222, Japan. [5]Division of Biomedical and Life Sciences, Faculty of Health and Medicine, Lancaster University, Lancaster LA1 4YQ, UK. [6]Department of Molecular Pathobiology of Brain Diseases, Kyoto Prefectural University of Medicine, Kyoto 602-0841, Japan.

References

1. Mann DM. Cerebral amyloidosis, ageing and Alzheimer's disease; a contribution from studies on Down's syndrome. Neurobiol Aging. 1989;10: 397–9.
2. Dubois B, Feldman HH, Jacova C, Hampel H, Molinuevo JL, Blennow K, et al. Advancing research diagnostic criteria for Alzheimer's disease: the IWG-2 criteria. Lancet Neurol. 2014;13:614–29. https://doi.org/10.1016/S1474-4422(14)70090-0.
3. Shaw LM, Vanderstichele H, Knapik-Czajka M, Clark CM, Aisen PS, Petersen RC, et al. Cerebrospinal fluid biomarker signature in Alzheimer's disease neuroimaging initiative subjects. Ann Neurol. 2009;65:403–13. https://doi.org/10.1002/ana.21610.
4. Skillbäck T, Farahmand BY, Rosén C, Mattsson N, Nägga K, Kilander L, et al. Cerebrospinal fluid tau and amyloid-β1-42 in patients with dementia. Brain. 2015;138:2716–31. https://doi.org/10.1093/brain/awv181.
5. Blennow K, Dubois B, Fagan AM, Lewczuk P, de Leon MJ, Hampel H. Clinical utility of cerebrospinal fluid biomarkers in the diagnosis of early Alzheimer's disease. Alzheimers Dement. 2015;11:58–69. https://doi.org/10.1016/j.jalz.2014.02.004.
6. Olsson B, Lautner R, Andreasson U, Öhrfelt A, Portelius E, Bjerke M, et al. CSF and blood biomarkers for the diagnosis of Alzheimer's disease: a systematic review and meta-analysis. Lancet Neurol. 2016;15:673–84. https://doi.org/10.1016/S1474-4422(16)00070-3.
7. Bateman RJ, Xiong C, Benzinger TL, Fagan AM, Goate A, Fox NC, et al. Dominantly inherited Alzheimer network.. Clinical and biomarker changes in dominantly inherited Alzheimer's disease. N Engl J Med. 2012;367:795–804. https://doi.org/10.1056/NEJMoa1202753.
8. Roe CM, Fagan AM, Grant EA, Hassenstab J, Moulder KL, Maue Dreyfus D, et al. Amyloid imaging and CSF biomarkers in predicting cognitive impairment up to 7.5 years later. Neurology. 2013;80:1784–91. https://doi.org/10.1212/WNL.0b013e3182918ca6.
9. Villemagne VL, Burnham S, Bourgeat P, Brown B, Ellis KA, Salvado O, et al. Amyloid β deposition, neurodegeneration, and cognitive decline in sporadic Alzheimer's disease: a prospective cohort study. Lancet Neurol. 2013;12:357–67. https://doi.org/10.1016/S1474-4422(13)70044-9.
10. Vos SJ, Xiong C, Visser PJ, Jasielec MS, Hassenstab J, Grant EA, et al. Preclinical Alzheimer's disease and its outcome: a longitudinal cohort study. Lancet Neurol. 2013;12:957–65. https://doi.org/10.1016/S1474-4422(13)70194-7.
11. Mehta PD, Pirttilä T, Mehta SP, Sersen EA, Aisen PS, Wisniewski HM. Plasma and cerebrospinal fluid levels of amyloid beta proteins 1-40 and 1-42 in Alzheimer disease. Arch Neurol. 2000;57:100–5.
12. Mayeux R, Honig LS, Tang MX, Manly J, Stern Y, Schupf N, et al. Plasma Aβ40 and Aβ42 and Alzheimer's disease: relation to age, mortality, and risk. Neurology 2003;61:1185–1190.
13. Lui JK, Laws SM, Li QX, Villemagne VL, Ames D, Brown B, et al. Plasma amyloid-beta as a biomarker in Alzheimer's disease: the AIBL study of aging. J Alzheimers Dis. 2010;20:1233–42. https://doi.org/10.3233/JAD-2010-090249.
14. Poljak A, Crawford JD, Smythe GA, Brodaty H, Slavin MJ, Kochan NA, et al. The relationship between plasma Aβ levels, cognitive function and brain Volumetrics: Sydney memory and ageing study. Curr Alzheimer Res. 2016; 13:243–55.
15. Lövheim H, Elgh F, Johansson A, Zetterberg H, Blennow K, Hallmans G, et al. Plasma concentrations of free amyloid β cannot predict the development of Alzheimer's disease. Alzheimers Dement. 2017; https://doi.org/10.1016/j.jalz.2016.12.004.
16. Wood H. Alzheimer disease: biomarkers of AD risk - the end of the road for plasma amyloid-β? Nat Rev Neurol. 2016;12:613. https://doi.org/10.1038/nrneurol.2016.160.
17. Mattsson N, Zetterberg H, Janelidze S, Insel PS, Andreasson U, Stomrud E, et al. Plasma tau in Alzheimer disease. Neurology. 2016;87:1827–35. https://doi.org/10.1212/WNL.0000000000003246.
18. Suzuki H, Kobayashi C, Ikeda Y, Kanno A, Hashimoto S, Hosokawa K. The developmental characteristics of scoial maturity on children with down syndrome -using scial maturity scale -revised (S-M). Bull Spec Educ. 1997;21:139–47.
19. Kondo M, Tokuda T, Itsukage M, Kuriyama N, Matsushima S, Yamada K, et al. Distribution of amyloid burden differs between idiopathic normal pressure hydrocephalus and Alzheimer's disease. Neuroradiol J. 2013;26:41–6. https://doi.org/10.1177/197140091302600107.
20. McKhann G, Drachman D, Folstein M, Katzman R, Price D, Stadlan EM. Clinical diagnosis of Alzheimer's disease: report of the NINCDS-ADRDA work group under the auspices of Department of Health and Human Services Task Force on Alzheimer's disease. Neurology. 1984;34:939–44.
21. Román GC, Tatemichi TK, Erkinjuntti T, Cummings JL, Masdeu JC, Garcia JH, et al. Vascular dementia: diagnostic criteria for research studies. Report of the NINDS-AIREN international workshop. Neurology. 1993;43:250–60.
22. Gibb WR, Lees AJ. The relevance of the Lewy body to the pathogenesis of idiopathic Parkinson's disease. J Neurol Neurosurg Psychiatry. 1988;51:745–52.
23. Rissin DM, Kan CW, Campbell TG, Howes SC, Fournier DR, Song L, et al. Single-molecule enzyme-linked immunosorbent assay detects serum proteins at subfemtomolar concentrations. Nat Biotechnol. 2010;28:595–9. https://doi.org/10.1038/nbt.1641.
24. Rissin DM, Fournier DR, Piech T, Kan CW, Campbell TG, Song L, et al. Simultaneous detection of single molecules and singulated ensembles of molecules enables immunoassays with broad dynamic range. Anal Chem. 2011;83:2279–85. https://doi.org/10.1021/ac103161b.
25. Randall J, Mörtberg E, Provuncher GK, Fournier DR, Duffy DC, Rubertsson S, et al. Tau proteins in serum predict neurological outcome after hypoxic brain injury from cardiac arrest: results of a pilot study. Resuscitation. 2013; 84:351–6. https://doi.org/10.1016/j.resuscitation.2012.07.027.
26. Goedert M, Jakes R, Crowther RA, Cohen P, Vanmechelen E, Vandermeeren M, et al. Epitope mapping of monoclonal antibodies to the paired helical filaments of Alzheimer's disease: identification of phosphorylation sites in tau protein. Biochem J. 1994;301:871–7.
27. Sparks DL, Kryscio RJ, Sabbagh MN, Ziolkowski C, Lin Y, Sparks LM, et al. Tau is reduced in AD plasma and validation of employed ELISA methods. Am J Neurodegener Dis. 2012;1:99–106.
28. Zetterberg H, Wilson D, Andreasson U, Minthon L, Blennow K, Randall J, et al. Plasma tau levels in Alzheimer's disease. Alzheimers Res Ther. 2013;5:9. https://doi.org/10.1186/alzrt163.
29. Chiu MJ, Yang SY, Horng HE, Yang CC, Chen TF, Chieh JJ, et al. Combined plasma biomarkers for diagnosing mild cognition impairment and Alzheimer's disease. ACS Chem Neurosci. 2013;4:1530–6. https://doi.org/10.1021/cn400129p.
30. Chiu MJ, Chen YF, Chen TF, Yang SY, Yang FP, Tseng TW, et al. Plasma tau as a window to the brain-negative associations with brain volume and memory function in mild cognitive impairment and early Alzheimer's disease. Hum Brain Mapp. 2014;35:3132–42. https://doi.org/10.1002/hbm.22390.
31. Krishnan S, Rani P. Evaluation of selenium, redox status and their association with plasma amyloid/tau in Alzheimer's disease. Biol Trace Elem Res. 2014; 158:158–65. https://doi.org/10.1007/s12011-014-9930-x.
32. Tzen KY, Yang SY, Chen TF, Cheng TW, Horng HE, Wen HP, et al. Plasma Aβ but not tau is related to brain PiB retention in early Alzheimer's disease. ACS Chem Neurosci. 2014;5:830–6. https://doi.org/10.1021/cn500101j.
33. Wang T, Xiao S, Liu Y, Lin Z, Su N, Li X, et al. The efficacy of plasma biomarkers in early diagnosis of Alzheimer's disease. Int J Geriatr Psychiatry. 2014;29:713–9. https://doi.org/10.1002/gps.4053.
34. Li QX, Whyte S, Tanner JE, Evin G, Beyreuther K, Masters CL. Secretion of Alzheimer's disease Abeta amyloid peptide by activated human platelets. Lab Investig. 1998;78:461–9.
35. Skovronsky DM, Lee VM, Praticò D. Amyloid precursor protein and amyloid beta peptide in human platelets. Role of cyclooxygenase and protein kinase C. J Biol Chem. 2001;276:17036–43. https://doi.org/10.1074/jbc.M006285200.
36. Couchie D, Mavilia C, Georgieff IS, Liem RK, Shelanski ML, Nunez J. Primary

structure of high molecular weight tau present in the peripheral nervous system. Proc Natl Acad Sci U S A. 1992;89:4378–81.

37. Jin K, Takeda A, Shiga Y, Sato S, Ohnuma A, Nomura H, et al. CSF tau protein: a new prognostic marker for Guillain-Barré syndrome. Neurology. 2006;67:1470–2. https://doi.org/10.1212/01.wnl.0000240119.29939.c7.
38. Hesse C, Rosengren L, Andreasen N, Davidsson P, Vanderstichele H, Vanmechelen E, et al. Transient increase in total tau but not phospho-tau in human cerebrospinal fluid after acute stroke. Neurosci Lett. 2001;297:187–90.
39. Blennow K. Cerebrospinal fluid protein biomarkers for Alzheimer's disease. NeuroRx. 2004;1:213–25. https://doi.org/10.1602/neurorx.1.2.213.
40. Andreasen N, Minthon L, Davidsson P, Vanmechelen E, Vanderstichele H, Winblad B, et al. Evaluation of CSF-tau and CSF-Abeta42 as diagnostic markers for Alzheimer disease in clinical practice. Arch Neurol. 2001;58:373–9.
41. Hansson O, Zetterberg H, Buchhave P, Londos E, Blennow K, Minthon L. Association between CSF biomarkers and incipient Alzheimer's disease in patients with mild cognitive impairment: a follow-up study. Lancet Neurol. 2006;5:228–34. https://doi.org/10.1016/S1474-4422(06)70355-6.
42. Salloway S, Sperling R, Fox NC, Blennow K, Klunk W, Raskind M, et al. Two phase 3 trials of bapineuzumab in mild-to-moderate Alzheimer's disease. N Engl J Med. 2014;370:322–33. https://doi.org/10.1056/NEJMoa1304839.

11

Targeting psychologic stress signaling pathways in Alzheimer's disease

Hunter S. Futch[1,2,4], Cara L. Croft[1,2,4], Van Q. Truong[1,2,4], Eric G. Krause[3,4] and Todd E. Golde[1,2,4*]

Abstract

Alzheimer's Disease (AD) is the most prevalent progressive neurodegenerative disease; to date, no AD therapy has proven effective in delaying or preventing the disease course. In the search for novel therapeutic targets in AD, it has been shown that increased chronic psychologic stress is associated with AD risk. Subsequently, biologic pathways underlying psychologic stress have been identified and shown to be able to exacerbate AD relevant pathologies. In this review, we summarize the literature relevant to the association between psychologic stress and AD, focusing on studies investigating the effects of stress paradigms on transgenic mouse models of Amyloid-β (Aβ) and tau pathologies. In recent years, a substantial amount of research has been done investigating a key stress-response mediator, corticotropin-releasing hormone (CRH), and its interactions with AD relevant processes. We highlight attempts to target the CRH signaling pathway as a therapeutic intervention in these transgenic mouse models and discuss how targeting this pathway is a promising avenue for further investigation.

Keywords: Alzheimer's disease, Corticotropin-releasing hormone, Psychologic distress, Chronic stress, Neurodegeneration

Background

Alzheimer's Disease (AD) is a progressive neurodegenerative process that is currently the sixth leading cause of death in the United States [1]. The AD brain is characterized by the aggregation of misfolded proteins and marked neuronal loss [2]. The hallmark pathologic features of AD, intracellular neurofibrillary tau tangles (NFT's), extracellular Amyloid-β (Aβ) plaques, synaptic and neuronal loss and reactive gliosis, have all been extensively studied. Despite this enormous scientific effort, many aspects of the disease remain poorly understood [3]. Although genetic factors clearly play a role in AD, studies of monozygotic twins have suggested that non-genetic risk factors are also involved [4, 5]. As non-genetic risk factors may be more easily modifiable than genetic risk factors, it is worthwhile to explore these pathways in search of therapeutic strategies for the treatment or prevention of AD. One non-genetic risk factor that has been associated with increased risk for AD is increased chronic psychologic stress. Epidemiologic studies have shown that individuals predisposed to experiencing psychologic stress, and those affected with diseases associated with chronic stress such as Major Depression and Post-traumatic Stress Disorder (PTSD), have an increased risk of developing AD (Table 1) [6–12].

Although these studies associating psychologic stress and AD are intriguing, like most epidemiologic studies of AD these studies are subject to many confounds that could dampen enthusiasm for further research let alone for guiding a therapeutic development program. Indeed, unless based on autopsy proven AD or other modalities such as amyloid imaging that are now available to enable more accurate diagnosis of AD in living patients, most epidemiologic studies likely included a relatively high percentage of individuals (20% or more) with other forms of dementia and even the control group (>20%), if over age 65, is likely to have amyloid pathology [13, 14]. Thus, these studies are conservatively viewed as epidemiologic associations with dementia and not necessarily AD. Further, epidemiologic studies of psychologic stress are particularly challenging, as it is difficult to quantify stress in a way that is potentially reflective of the biological processes associated with this relatively subjective

* Correspondence: tgolde@ufl.edu
[1]Department of Neuroscience, University of Florida, Gainesville, FL 32610, USA
[2]Center for Translational Research in Neurodegenerative Disease, University of Florida, Gainesville, FL 32610, USA
Full list of author information is available at the end of the article

Table 1 Relevant epidemiologic studies associating stress with increased risk of developing AD

Epidemiologic studies	Description	Results	Comments
Andel et al. (2012) [11]	Prospective study. Occupation used as a surrogate for stress level	Correlation between markers of Job Stress (Low job control, High demands, Low social support, High job strain) in risk of developing any type of dementia (OR 1.06–1.23) or AD (OR 1.04–1.23)	Study used only occupation of participant as surrogate for stress but did not survey participants directly about their stress levels. Clinical Diagnosis (Dx) of AD
Kaup et al. (2016) [7]	Prospective study. Elderly participants (Mean age 74) were assessed for depressive symptoms yearly for 5 years and then observed for an additional 11 years for onset of dementia	Patients found to have High and increasing symptoms were significantly more likely to develop any type of dementia (OR 1.94)	Clinical Dx of AD
Tsolaki et al. (2010) [12]	Retrospective Case–control study of patients with dementia and without.	Found that 78% of those with dementia had a stressful life event prior to onset of dementia while only 55% of the control subjects encountered a stressful life event. AD (OR 2.24)	Clinical Dx of AD
Wilson et al. (2003) [8]	Prospective study as part of the larger Religious Orders study of catholic nuns and priests, measuring stress proneness and incident AD.	Participants receiving the highest scores in the neuroticism scale used for a marker of stress proneness were twice as likely to develop AD within the 4.9 year average follow-up.	
Johansson et al. (2014) [9]	Prospective study examining stress levels of women at three examinations over 35 years.	Hazard ratio for incident dementia were 1.1 (.71–1.71) reporting stress at 1/3 examinations, 1.73 (1.01–2.95) at 2/3 examinations, and 2.51 (1.33–4.77) at 3/3 examinations.	Clinical Dx of AD

phenotype. Finally, in a disease like AD with a long prodromal state, it can be challenging to link early or midlife risk factors with development of the disease late in life.

Given these and other potential confounds, epidemiologic data likely needs to be combined with biological or genetic data to serve as a basis for developing novel AD therapies. In this review we will evaluate the biological underpinnings that suggest the association between AD and stress may be strong enough to warrant investigation as a possible avenue for AD therapy. The course of molecular research into stress and AD began largely with investigation into stress-steroids, namely cortisol, but more recently has shifted towards Corticotropin-Releasing Hormone (CRH), a neuropeptide which exerts its effects primarily through activation of the CRHR1 receptor [15]. These data have shown that stress mediators are able to regulate AD relevant processes and provide converging evidence that activation of the stress response pathway may be able to exacerbate AD pathologies.

Main text

Stress signaling

When approaching the biology underlying the stress response, it is important to consider all of the potential contributors if we are to determine what pathways mediate the effects of stress on AD relevant processes. CRH and the CRH family peptides urocortin (UCN) 1, 2, and 3 are the main coordinators of the response to psychologic stress. These peptides exert their effects through binding and activating the CRHR1 and CRHR2 receptors in the central nervous system (CNS) and the periphery [15–17]. The classical stress response pathway begins with the perception of stress leading to the release of CRH from the paraventricular nuclei (PVN) of the hypothalamus, binding to CRHR1 Receptors in the anterior pituitary and causing the release of Adrenocorticotropic Hormone (ACTH) into the systemic circulation. ACTH then binds to MC_2 receptors in the adrenal cortices, inducing glucocorticoid release [18]. This cascade is known as the Hypothalamic-Pituitary-Adrenal (HPA) axis [18, 19].

In addition to the CRHR1 present in the anterior pituitary, the CRHR1 is also widely expressed throughout the brain (Fig. 1). Its signaling in these locations is thought to cause many of the psychologic effects of stress and is also implicated in learning and memory [20–22]. Indeed, CRHR1 is expressed on both glutamatergic and dopaminergic neurons and can have either anxiogenic or anxiolytic effects depending on the brain region [23]. It appears that stress, up to a certain threshold, is stimulating and induces rapid memory formation; above that threshold, stress becomes overwhelming and deleterious [23, 24]. CRH expressing neurons are

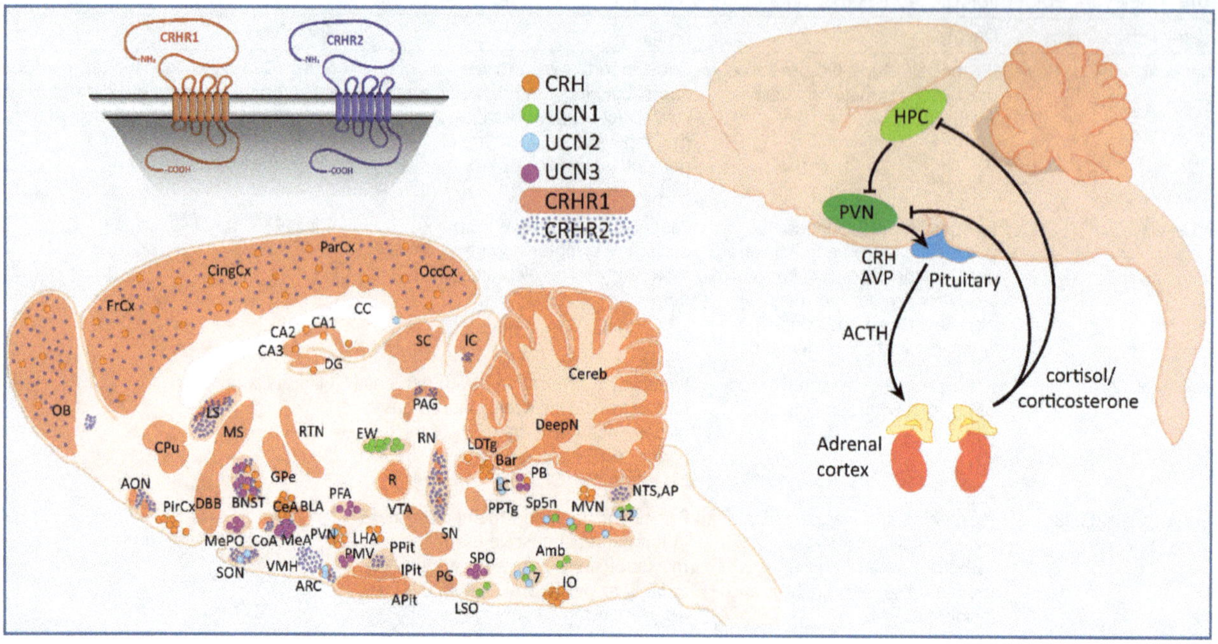

Fig. 1 CRH-family expression and HPA axis. Adapted from [23, 67]

distributed throughout the CNS. Of special relevance in AD is the expression of CRH in the cortex and hippocampal-amygdalar complex, areas which also express the CRHR1 receptor [15]. The role of the CRHR2 receptor is not yet fully understood; it has been implicated in the anorexic effects of stress, and theories as to its role vary from functioning as a counterbalance to CRHR1 stress signaling, to being a part of a different stress pathway that responds to inescapable and unpredictable stressors [16]. The CRHR2 is expressed in discrete areas of the brain, but is widely expressed in the periphery (Fig. 1) [25]. The urocortins, similarly to the CRHR2, are expressed discretely within the brain. Both CRHR1 and CRHR2 are G-Protein Coupled Receptors that signal primarily through the G_s, G_q, and MAPK/ERK pathways [15]. Activation of these pathways can lead to increased intracellular calcium levels [26], an effect that may be worthwhile to explore considering the hypothesized role of calcium dyshomeostasis in AD [27]. In terms of specificity towards CRHR1 and 2, i) CRH has specificity for the CRHR1, ii) urocortin 1 can activate both CRHR1 and CRHR2, and iii) urocortin 2 and 3 are unique in that they show specificity for CRHR2 and do not appear to have affinity for CRHR1 at physiologic concentrations [15, 28] (Fig. 2). Overall, CRH and the urocortins are proposed to act as neuromodulators within the CNS to orchestrate various components of the psychologic stress response [17].

Cortisol and AD

In the 1990's and early 2000's, an appreciable amount of study focused on the role of cortisol and corticosteroids

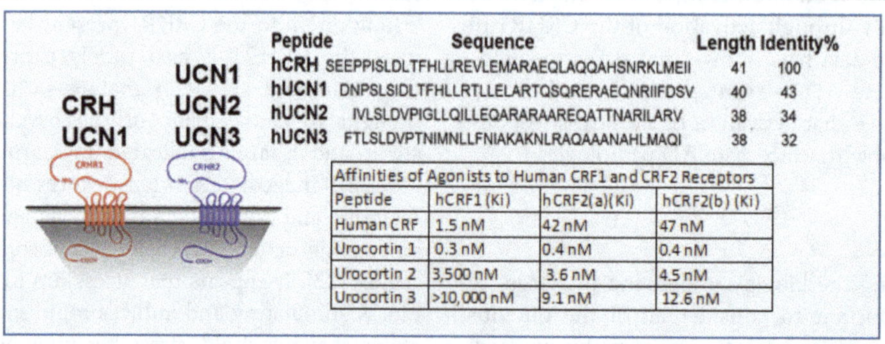

Affinities of Agonists to Human CRF1 and CRF2 Receptors

Peptide	hCRF1 (Ki)	hCRF2(a)(Ki)	hCRF2(b) (Ki)
Human CRF	1.5 nM	42 nM	47 nM
Urocortin 1	0.3 nM	0.4 nM	0.4 nM
Urocortin 2	3,500 nM	3.6 nM	4.5 nM
Urocortin 3	>10,000 nM	9.1 nM	12.6 nM

Fig. 2 CRH-family peptides and receptor affinities [17]

in AD; this was largely driven by several observations. One of the direct effects of psychologic stress is an increased level of circulating glucocorticoids, mainly cortisol in humans and corticosterone in mice [18]. Cushing's syndrome, a state of excess glucocorticoids seen in patients with pituitary tumors or those who have received large amounts of exogenous steroids, is associated with atrophy of the hippocampus, a feature shared with both conditions of chronic stress and AD [29–31]. The hypothesized role that glucocorticoids play in AD has been reviewed elsewhere [31–33], but we will make note of the most critical data. AD patients have been shown to have mildly increased levels of cortisol when compared to controls (Table 2) [34, 35] and corticosteroids have been shown to be able to induce Aβ plaque load and hyperphosphorylated tau levels in APP overexpressing mouse models [36–39], effects that were able to be reduced with a glucocorticoid receptor (GR) antagonist [40].

The hippocampus is a key negative regulator of the HPA axis, with increased glucocorticoid levels causing increased GR signaling in the hippocampus leading to inhibition of CRH release from the hypothalamus [18]. One hypothesis for the increased levels of glucocorticoids found in AD is that hippocampal damage may cause a loss of negative feedback on hypothalamic CRH release. AD patients have also been found to have altered responses to a CRH stimulation test, with higher levels of cortisol than controls [41, 42], suggesting that AD patients may have a more complex alteration in HPA axis activity.

CRH and AD

In the early 2000's, investigation into the stress response and AD began to branch into the CRH signaling pathway. This occurred simultaneously with a large effort to target CRH signaling in various stress related disorders (Major Depression, PTSD, addiction). Since this time, a substantial amount of data implicating CRH signaling in both Aβ production and tau phosphorylation has been produced.

Aβ

An increasing amount of evidence shows that stress and specifically CRH-CRHR1 signaling can increase Aβ peptide production. In primary neuronal cultures (PNC's), CRH treatment was shown to increase levels of total secreted Aβ peptide, an effect that was partially blocked by the small molecule CRHR1 antagonists Antalarmin and R121919 [43]. Our group was able to replicate the CRH-induced increases in Aβ in both PNC's and a CRHR1 overexpressing SH-SY5Y cell line, but we saw similar increases upon treatment with the peptide CRHR1 antagonist Astressin as were seen with CRH treatment [44]. Recent work showing that adrenergic GPCR's are able to affect APP processing led to our hypothesis that the CRHR1 may also be able to directly regulate these processes [45]. An in vitro γ-secretase assay showed that CRH treatment can modulate γ-secretase activity towards increased Aβ42 production [44] and that upon CRH treatment, CRHR1 is internalized by a β-arrestin 2 mediated interaction, where it then colocalized with γ-secretase intracellularly. This fit well with previous data that has shown that β-arrestin regulates Aβ production via γ-secretase [46]. Furthermore, we showed that the peptide CRHR1 antagonists Astressin and α-helical CRH were able to induce rapid internalization of cells overexpressing the CRHR1. This data led to the hypothesis that CRHR1 antagonists may modulate γ-secretase activity towards increased Aβ production through inducing internalization of the receptor. Evaluation of the G_s coupled pathway of CRHR1 has shown that pretreatment with the Protein Kinase A (PKA) inhibitor H-89 was able to significantly reduce Aβ40 and Aβ42 production in a CRH treated PNC model [43]. Through these investigations, a picture begins to form that

Table 2 Relevant stress biomarker studies in AD

Biomarker studies	Description	Results	Comments
Bernardi et al. (2000) [42]	Serum levels of Cortisol and two neurosteroids, Allopregnanolone and dehydroepiandrosterone (DHEA), were compared in AD patients and controls	AD patients had significantly higher levels of cortisol and lower levels of Allopregnanolone compared to age matched controls	Clinical Dx of AD *N* = 12
Popp et al. (2015) [34]	Longitudinal prospective study examining serum and CSF levels of cortisol and Aβ in age matched controls, patients with mild cognitive impairment (MCI), and AD patients.	CSF cortisol levels are elevated in subjects with AD and MCI. Elevated CSF cortisol levels were associated with faster cognitive decline in MCI of the AD type.	Clinical Dx of AD
Ennis et al. (2016) [35]	Prospective trial measuring once yearly a 24 h urinary cortisol level, over an average interval of 10.56 years	Elevated urinary cortisol level was related with a 1.31 times increase in AD risk, predicting increased AD risk an average of 6 years before onset.	Clinical Dx of AD. Participants that went on to be grouped in the "Future AD" group were 10 years older on average than control group

includes three possible mechanisms for CRH induced Aβ increases.

1. **CRHR1 interactions with β-arrestin 2 and γ-secretase:** demonstrated by the data that CRHR1 antagonists do not stimulate the receptor, but do induce its internalization and increase Aβ40 and Aβ42 production in vitro [44].
2. **CRH directly modulating γ -secretase activity:** demonstrated by data that CRH treatment increases Aβ42 production in an in vitro γ–secretase assay [44].
3. **Classical CRHR1 G_s/G_q pathway signaling:** demonstrated by data that treatment with PKA inhibitor H-89 is able to reduce CRH induced increases in Aβ40 and Aβ42 in vitro [43].

Multiple stress paradigms have been able to induce increases in Aβ40 and Aβ42 levels and plaque load in the brains of wild type (WT) and mutant APP overexpressing transgenic mouse models (Table 3).

Studies investigating the mechanisms through which stress mediates these effects on Aβ have focused mainly on CRHR1 and GR signaling. While acute restraint stress was able to induce increases in total soluble Aβ levels in the brain interstitial fluid (ISF) of Tg2576 mice, these increases were not reproduced with administration of corticosterone to the mice. These increases *were* able to be induced by the administration of CRH and blocked by administration of the CRHR1 antagonist α-helical CRH [47]. These findings suggest that acute stress-induced increases in Aβ40 and Aβ42 in the brain may be due to a CRH-mediated effect, which agrees with previous data showing that corticosteroid-induced increases in brain Aβ40 and Aβ42 levels take place 48–72 h after administration [36]. In addition, it was found that chronic isolation stress caused increases in both GR and CRHR1 expression in the cortex and hippocampus, along with increased corticosterone levels and plaque burden in the Tg2576 mouse model [48]. In a double transgenic Tg2576 and CRH overexpressing mouse model, it was shown that overexpression of CRH was related with large increases in brain Aβ40 and Aβ42 levels along with increased plaque burden in the cortex [49].

While the role of the urocortins in stress-induced Aβ production has been largely unexplored, one study found that injection of urocortin 1 (an agonist for both CRHR1 and CRHR2) into the amygdala of male Wistar rats induced increases in amygdalar Aβ40 levels, while 5 h of acute restraint stress in the rats showed increases in both Aβ40 and Aβ42 [50]. A double transgenic Tg2576 and homozygous CRHR1 knockout mouse line (supplemented with corticosterone for health maintenance) showed highly significant decreases (>60%) in basal levels of Aβ40, Aβ42, and APP C-Terminal Fragment (α and β) levels in the brain, suggesting that a CRHR1-mediated mechanism contributes to an appreciable amount of Aβ processing [51].

Tau

While there is a substantial amount of evidence that CRH signaling can affect Aβ production and Aβ plaque deposition, most data connecting the CRH signaling

Table 3 Studies involving stress paradigms and Aβ production

Studies on Aβ	Model	Stress paradigm	Effect	Comments
Kang et al. (2007) [47]	Tg2576 [82]	3 months isolation	↑	
Dong et al. (2008) [48]	Tg2576	6 months isolation	↑	
Lee et al. (2009) [83]	Tg2576	2 h restraint daily for 16 days	↑	Measured ISF, soluble Aβ
Ray et al. (2011) [50]	Wistar rat	5 h restraint or bilateral UCN1 injection in amygdala	↑	
Huang et al. (2011) [84]	APP/PS1 [85]	4 months isolation	↑	
Rothman et al. (2012) [86]	3xTg AD [87]	Cage switched for 6 h/day for 2–3 days/week for 6 weeks	↑	
Dong et al. (2012) [49]	Tg2576/ CRH overexpressing [88]	CRH overexpressing transgenic	↑	
Rothman et al. (2013) [53]	3xTg AD	6 h sleep restriction for 6 weeks	-	Aβ and tau measures trending upward but non-significant
Dong et al. (2014) [43]	Tg2576	One week or 10 months of isolation	↑	
Baglietto-Vargas et al. (2015) [89]	3xTg AD	5 h of multimodal stress. Brief restraint, shaker plate with bright lights and noise	↑	
Park et al. (2015) [44]	C57BL/6 J	3 h restraint	↑	
Justice et al. (2015) [90]	APP/PS1	PTSD-like induction for two hours followed by a trigger	↑	

Studies in WT mice or rats observed levels of soluble Aβ42 and Aβ40 in brain homogenate, studies in transgenic mice included measurements of plaque load and insoluble Aβ unless noted otherwise pathway with tau-related processes is shown through studies on tau phosphorylation and not aggregate deposition. The neurofibrillary tangles found in the AD brain are composed of hyperphosphorylated, cleaved, and conformationally altered tau protein [52]. Phosphorylation of tau at certain residues causes its dissociation from microtubules and enables aggregates to form [52].

Multiple stress paradigms have been able to increase tau phosphorylation in mice [53–60] (Table 4) and it was shown that a CRH KO mouse model did not show the stress induced increases in hyperphosphorylated tau that were seen in WT mice [57].

Furthermore, it was shown that stress induced tau phosphorylation could not be replicated by administration of corticosterone and that CRHR1 antagonist NBI27914 was able to decrease the effect of stress on tau phosphorylation [54] at certain phospho-epitopes. Mice that had undergone adrenalectomy also replicated the stress-induced increases in tau phosphorylation. These data provide several pieces of evidence pointing away from a glucocorticoid mediated mechanism and towards one mediated by CRH [55]. It was also shown that a CRHR1 knockout mouse line did not replicate these increases in stress induced tau phosphorylation, while their CRHR2 knockout counterparts actually had a hyperactive response to stress when compared to WT mice, lending evidence to the hypothesis that the CRHR2 may have a regulatory role over CRHR1 signaling [55]. A CRHR1 and CRHR2 double knockout mouse maintained the lack of response seen with the CRHR1 single knockout mouse [59]. Lastly, a CRH overexpressing mouse model showed increased tau phosphorylation at multiple sites when compared with controls [56]. Unfortunately, the vast majority of these studies on stress and tau pathology have used WT mice and only measure tau phosphorylation and not aggregate formation. While increased phosphorylation of tau frequently correlates with increased aggregation and neurodegeneration in models of tau pathology, further evaluation of the CRH signaling pathway in deposit-forming models of tau pathology is necessary. As transgenic models of tau aggregation are actually models of Frontotemporal Dementia (FTD), these studies could additionally link stress to other dementias or neurodegenerative processes.

Interventions targeting the CRH signaling pathway

With evidence showing that both CRH and glucocorticoids can exacerbate AD pathology in the brains of transgenic mouse models, it follows that abnormalities in the HPA axis may play a role in the development and progression of AD. Targeting CRH could be the most efficacious single intervention within the HPA axis, as an intervention blocking the effects of CRH would decrease downstream glucocorticoid release, potentially blocking both CRH-mediated and glucocorticoid-mediated effects on Aβ production and tau phosphorylation.

Overactive CRH signaling has been implicated in anxiety, major depression, and inflammatory disorders and an effective intervention targeting the CRH signaling pathway is highly sought in these fields [16, 17, 61, 62]. Despite preclinical studies demonstrating their potential efficacy, for unknown reasons, the CRHR1 antagonists GSK511679 and Pexacerfont were not shown to be effective in clinical trials investigating their effects in alcoholism and generalized anxiety disorder [63]. While there has yet to be a clinical trial investigating an anti-CRH therapy in any neurodegenerative disease, there has been substantial effort to implement CRHR1 antagonists preclinically in mouse models of Aβ and tau pathologies (Table 5). CRHR1 antagonists have shown some efficacy in decreasing stress induced Aβ pathologies, with no effect in an acute stress paradigm [44], but alleviating effects in chronic stress paradigms [43] as well as in unstressed APP overexpressing mice [64]. Studies have utilized both peptide and small molecule CRHR1 antagonists (Astressin, Antalarmin, α-helical CRH, R121919, NBI27914) in the various aforementioned stress paradigms. One study found that even in

Table 4 Studies involving stress paradigms and tau phosphorylation/aggregation

Studies on Tau	Model	Stress paradigm	Effect	Comments
Rissman et al. (2007) [55]	C57BL/6 J, multiple CRHR knockouts	Acute restraint at multiple time points up to two hours. Also done in adrenalectomized mice.	↑	
Carroll et al. (2011) [54]	PS19 [91]	Variable stressor once per day for 4 weeks, or restraint six hours/day and isolation for one month	↑	Variable stress paradigm not consistent in elevating tau measures
Rissman et al. (2012) [59]	CRHR Knockouts	Half hour restraint one time or daily for 14 days	↑	
Filipcik et al. (2012) [57]	C57BL/6 J	30 min or 120 min restraint	↑	
Campbell et al. (2015) [51]	CRH overexpressing		↑	
Le et al. (2016) [58]	Primary Neuronal Culture from C57BL/6 J	Treatment with CRH	↑	

Studies utilizing WT mice observed tau phosphorylation at various phospho-epitopes. Study utilizing PS19 mice quantified inclusions

Table 5 Studies testing CRHR1 antagonists in mouse models and in vitro models relevant to AD

CRHR1 antagonist	Studies	Dosage	Outcome	Comments
Antalarmin	Rissman et al. (2012) [59], Dong et al. (2014) [43], Park et al. (2015) [44],	20 mg/kg	Rissman (2012) - Able to block acute stress induced tau phosphorylation but not that induced by chronic stress [59]. Dong (2014) - Able to decrease Aβ levels and plaque load in a chronic stress paradigm [43]. Park (2015) - Unable to block rises in Aβ in response to acute stress [44].	Dong (2014) measured PBS soluble Aβ, which represents roughly 5% of total Aβ.
A-helical CRH	Park et al. (2015) [44]	5 & 10 μM	Unable to block CRH induced Aβ increases in vitro.	
Astressin	Park et al. (2015) [44]	5 & 10 μM	Unable to block CRH induced Aβ increases in vitro.	
NBI 30775/R121919	Rissman et al. (2012) [59], Campbell et al. (2015) [51], Dong et al. (2014) [43], Zhang et al. (2016) [64]	20 mg/kg. Zhang (2016) utilized osmotic mini pump	Campbell (2015) [51] – able to decrease AT8 and PHF-1 phosphorylation in CRH overexpressing mice but not at S262 and S422. Rissman (2012) [59] – Able to decrease stress induced AT8 and PHF-1 increases in phosphorylation	
NBI27914	Park et al. (2015) [44], Lee et al. (2009) [83], Carroll et al. (2011) [54]	10 mg/kg	Carroll (2011) [54] - NBI27914 rescued freezing and decreased AT8 phosphorylation and decreased neurodegeneration in PS1 tau transgenic mice. Lee (2009) [83] – NBI27914 reduced stress induced increases in Aβ levels and plaque load. Park (2015) [44] – NBI27914 increased secreted Aβ42/ Aβ40 ratio in vitro	

unstressed mice, the CRHR1 antagonist R121919 was able to significantly decrease amyloid deposits in the brain. The effects of the CRHR1 inhibitors on tau showed either decreased tau inclusions in the cortex of PS19 tau mice [54] or decreased tau phosphorylation [43, 59], but, in contrast to the work done in various APP overexpressing mouse models, the investigation into stress and tau aggregation is limited to a single study.

Although there has been some proof of efficacy for CRHR1 antagonists in decreasing AD pathology in mouse models, one should question the probability of their success in human trials, as these antagonists have a history of having promising effects in rodent models and then failing in the clinic [61, 62, 65, 66]. In addition, CRHR1 antagonists can induce the internalization of CRHR1 and cause increases in Aβ40 and Aβ42 in in vitro models of the human CRHR1, drawing some concern to their use as an AD prevention. We believe that the strength of the literature shows that the CRH signaling pathway is an interesting target that merits further investigation into possible therapeutic interventions, but we posit that direct targeting of CRH will provide stronger and more worthwhile effects than receptor-based interventions. Direct targeting of CRH could be accomplished through several methods including, but not limited to, CRISPR-CAS9, antisense oligonucleotides, or direct immunotargeting of the CRH peptide. Any investigator attempting to develop one of these methods can do so with the knowledge that the creation of a therapy able to effectively downregulate CRH signaling would have broad impact in many conditions of chronic stress and possibly AD.

Impact of psychologic stress on other neurodegenerative diseases

In addition to AD, psychologic stress has been explored as a risk factor and exacerbating component in Parkinson's Disease, Huntington's Disease and vascular dementia. There are several comprehensive reviews available on the impact of psychologic stress and Major Depression on neurodegenerative disease [32, 67, 68], and it is likely that stress acts through unique mechanisms in each disease. Similarly to AD, increased psychologic stress has been associated epidemiologically with an increased risk of Parkinson's Disease [69, 70]. Stress paradigms have been shown to exacerbate the phenotype of several mouse and rat models of Parkinson's [71–76], yet there do not appear to be studies attempting to target stress pathways therapeutically within these models. Furthermore, early reports have shown that stress paradigms have a detrimental effect on the phenotype of the R6/1 mouse model of Huntington's [77, 78]. Further investigation into the mechanisms of how stress signaling affects these proteinopathies is needed, and should also grow to include other neurodegenerative proteinopathies such as Amyotrophic Lateral Sclerosis (ALS) and FTD. Indeed, as mentioned earlier some of the work already done on tau mouse models may be applicable to FTD. Lastly, it is pertinent to mention that the risk of both stroke and vascular dementia have also been associated with increased psychologic stress levels [11, 79, 80]. As patients with all of the neurodegenerative conditions mentioned suffer from stressful neuropsychiatric comorbidities [67, 81], interventions targeting stress signaling pathways could have both preventative and therapeutic effects on these diseases.

Conclusions

Considerable epidemiologic data suggests that chronic psychologic stress can be a risk factor in AD, or at least dementia. Studies in animal and cell models provide biological underpinnings to support this association and identify CRH as the logical therapeutic target. Based on current data, successful antagonism of CRH may result in beneficial effects on both Aβ amyloid and tau pathology, an effect that would be predicted to have a major impact on AD. More speculatively, such therapies could improve the harmful negative behavioral symptoms that accompany chronic stress. Indeed, normal stress-signaling is not always deleterious and plays a role in learning and memory. Empirical studies will need to be carried out in order to determine if one can target CRH directly in a manner that has beneficial effects and avoids side effects due to under-stimulation of the pathway. Given the need for novel targets in AD, we believe that additional preclinical studies that explore the potential impact of targeting CRH could pave the way for increased interest in this pathway as a target in AD.

Abbreviations

ACTH: Adrenocorticotropic Hormone; AD: Alzheimer's Disease; ALS: Amyotrophic Lateral Sclerosis; Aβ: Amyloid β; CRH: Corticotropin-releasing hormone; CRHR1: Corticotropin-Releasing Hormone Receptor 1; CRHR2: Corticotropin-Releasing Hormone Receptor 2; FTD: Frontotemporal Dementia; GR: Glucocorticoid Receptor; HPA: Hypothalamic-Pituitary-Adrenal; NFT: Neurofibrillary tangles; PKA: Protein Kinase A; PTSD: Post-traumatic Stress Disorder; PVN: Paraventricular nuclei; UCN: Urocortin; WT: Wild type

Acknowledgements

Hyo-Jin Park (University of Florida) provided the basis for this work within the lab.

Funding

NIH U01AG046139, R01AG018454, P50AG047266

Authors' contributions

HF did the majority of the appropriate literature search and manuscript production. VT edited the manuscript and provided illustrations. CC edited the manuscript providing tau protein expertise. EK edited the manuscript providing HPA axis expertise. TG extensively edited the manuscript providing AD expertise. All authors read and approved the final manuscript.

Competing interests

The authors declare that they have no competing interests.

Author details

[1]Department of Neuroscience, University of Florida, Gainesville, FL 32610, USA. [2]Center for Translational Research in Neurodegenerative Disease, University of Florida, Gainesville, FL 32610, USA. [3]Department of Pharmacodynamics, College of Pharmacy, University of Florida, Gainesville, USA. [4]McKnight Brain Institute, University of Florida, 1149 Newell Drive, PO Box 1000015, Gainesville, FL 32610, USA.

References

1. 2016 Alzheimer's disease facts and figures. Alzheimers Dement. 2016;12:459–509.
2. Aguzzi A, O'Connor T. Protein aggregation diseases: pathogenicity and therapeutic perspectives. Nat Rev Drug Discov. 2010;9:237–48.
3. Golde TE, Borchelt DR, Giasson BI, Lewis J. Thinking laterally about neurodegenerative proteinopathies. J Clin Invest. 2013;123:1847–55.
4. Gatz M, Reynolds CA, Finkel D, Pedersen NL, Walters E. Dementia in Swedish twins: predicting incident cases. Behav Genet. 2010;40:768–75.
5. Iacono D, Volkman I, Nennesmo I, Pedersen NL, Fratiglioni L, Johansson B, et al. Neuropathologic assessment of dementia markers in identical and fraternal twins: AD and non-AD pathologies in older twins. Brain Pathol. 2014;24:317–33.
6. Byers AL, Yaffe K. Depression and risk of developing dementia. Nat Rev Neurol. 2011;7:323–31.
7. Kaup AR, Byers AL, Falvey C, Simonsick EM, Satterfield S, Ayonayon HN, et al. Trajectories of depressive symptoms in older adults and risk of dementia. JAMA Psychiatry. 2016;73:525.
8. Wilson RS, Evans DA, Bienias JL, De Leon CM, Schneider JA, Bennett DA. Proneness to psychological distress is associated with risk of Alzheimer's disease. Neurology. 2003;61:1479–85.
9. Johansson L, Guo X, Duberstein PR, Hällström T, Waern M, Östling S, et al. Midlife personality and risk of Alzheimer disease and distress a 38-year follow-up. Neurology. 2014;83:1538–44.
10. Xu W, Tan L, Wang H-F, Jiang T, Tan M-S, Tan L, et al. Meta-analysis of modifiable risk factors for Alzheimer's disease. J. Neurol. Neurosurg. Psychiatry. 2015;jnnp-2015-310548.
11. Andel R, Crowe M, Hahn EA, Mortimer JA, Pedersen NL, Fratiglioni L, et al. Work-related stress may increase the risk of vascular dementia. J Am Geriatr Soc. 2012;60:60–7.
12. Tsolaki M, Papaliagkas V, Kounti F, Messini C, Boziki M, Anogianakis G, et al. Severely stressful events and dementia: a study of an elderly Greek demented population. Psychiatry Res. 2010;176:51–4.
13. Bangen KJ, Clark AL, Werhane M, Edmonds EC, Nation DA, Evangelista N, et al. Cortical amyloid burden differences across empirically-derived mild cognitive impairment subtypes and interaction with APOE ε4 genotype. Brandt J, editor. J. Alzheimers Dis. 2016;52:849–61.
14. Loring DW, Goldstein FC, Chen C, Drane DL, Lah JJ, Zhao L, et al. False-positive error rates for reliable digit span and auditory verbal learning test performance validity measures in amnestic mild cognitive impairment and early Alzheimer disease. Arch Clin Neuropsychol. 2016;31:313–31.
15. Dautzenberg FM, Hauger RL. The CRF peptide family and their receptors: yet more partners discovered. Trends Pharmacol Sci. 2002;23:71–7.
16. Hauger RL, Risbrough V, Oakley RH, Olivares-Reyes JA, Dautzenberg FM. Role of CRF receptor signaling in stress vulnerability, anxiety, and depression. Ann N Y Acad Sci. 2009;1179:120–43.
17. Hauger RL, Risbrough V, Brauns O, Dautzenberg FM. Corticotropin releasing factor (CRF) receptor signaling in the central nervous system: new molecular targets. CNS Neurol. Disord.-Drug targets former. Curr. Drug targets-CNS Neurol. Disord. 2006;5:453–79.

18. Herman JP, McKlveen JM, Ghosal S, Kopp B, Wulsin A, Makinson R, et al. Regulation of the Hypothalamic-Pituitary-Adrenocortical Stress Response. In: Terjung R, editor. Compr. Physiol. [Internet]. Hoboken, NJ, USA: John Wiley & Sons, Inc.; 2016 [cited 2016 Sep 30]. p. 603–21. Available from: http://doi.wiley.com/10.1002/cphy.c150015.
19. Rivier C, Vale W. Modulation of stress-induced ACTH release by corticotropin-releasing factor, catecholamines and vasopressin. Nature. 1983;305:325–7.
20. Potter E, Sutton S, Donaldson C, Chen R, Perrin M, Lewis K, et al. Distribution of corticotropin-releasing factor receptor mRNA expression in the rat brain and pituitary. Proc Natl Acad Sci U S A. 1994;91:8777–81.
21. Chalmers DT, Lovenberg TW, De Souza EB. Localization of novel corticotropin-releasing factor receptor (CRF2) mRNA expression to specific subcortical nuclei in rat brain: comparison with CRF1 receptor mRNA expression. J Neurosci. 1995;15:6340–50.
22. Van Pett K, Viau V, Bittencourt JC, Chan RK, Li HY, Arias C, et al. Distribution of mRNAs encoding CRF receptors in brain and pituitary of rat and mouse. J Comp Neurol. 2000;428:191–212.
23. Refojo D, Schweizer M, Kuehne C, Ehrenberg S, Thoeringer C, Vogl AM, et al. Glutamatergic and dopaminergic neurons mediate Anxiogenic and anxiolytic effects of CRHR1. Science. 2011;333:1903–7.
24. Sapolsky RM. Stress and the brain: individual variability and the inverted-U. Nat Neurosci. 2015;18:1344–6.
25. Bamberger CM, Bamberger A. The peripheral CRH/urocortin system. Ann N Y Acad Sci. 2000;917:290–6.
26. Inda C, dos Santos Claro PA, Bonfiglio JJ, Senin SA, Maccarrone G, Turck CW, et al. Different cAMP sources are critically involved in G protein–coupled receptor CRHR1 signaling. J Cell Biol. 2016;214:181–95.
27. Agostini M, Fasolato C. When, where and how? Focus on neuronal calcium dysfunctions in Alzheimer's Disease. Cell Calcium [Internet]. 2016 [cited 2016 Oct 11]; Available from: http://linkinghub.elsevier.com/retrieve/pii/S0143416016300999.
28. Hoare SRJ, Sullivan SK, Schwarz DA, Ling N, Vale WW, Crowe PD, et al. Ligand affinity for amino-terminal and Juxtamembrane domains of the Corticotropin releasing factor type I receptor: Regulation by G-protein and Nonpeptide antagonists. Biochemistry (Mosc). 2004;43:3996–4011.
29. Höschl C, Hajek T. Hippocampal damage mediated by corticosteroids—a neuropsychiatric research challenge. Eur Arch Psychiatry Clin Neurosci. 2001;251:81–8.
30. Sousa N, Lukoyanov NV, Madeira MD, Almeida OFX, Paula-Barbosa MM. Reorganization of the morphology of hippocampal neurites and synapses after stress-induced damage correlates with behavioral improvement. Neuroscience. 2000;97:253–66.
31. Lupien SJ, McEwen BS, Gunnar MR, Heim C. Effects of stress throughout the lifespan on the brain, behaviour and cognition. Nat Rev Neurosci. 2009;10:434–45.
32. Pardon M-C, Rattray I. What do we know about the long-term consequences of stress on ageing and the progression of age-related neurodegenerative disorders? Neurosci Biobehav Rev. 2008;32:1103–20.
33. Landfield PW, Blalock EM, Chen K-C, Porter NM. A new glucocorticoid hypothesis of brain aging: implications for Alzheimer's disease. Curr Alzheimer Res. 2007;4:205–12.
34. Popp J, Wolfsgruber S, Heuser I, Peters O, Hüll M, Schröder J, et al. Cerebrospinal fluid cortisol and clinical disease progression in MCI and dementia of Alzheimer's type. Neurobiol Aging. 2015;36:601–7.
35. Ennis GE, An Y, Resnick SM, Ferrucci L, O'Brien RJ, Moffat SD. Long-term cortisol measures predict Alzheimer disease risk. Neurology. 2016:10–1212.
36. Green KN. Glucocorticoids increase amyloid-beta and tau pathology in a mouse model of Alzheimer's disease. J Neurosci. 2006;26:9047–56.
37. Catania C, Sotiropoulos I, Silva R, Onofri C, Breen KC, Sousa N, et al. The amyloidogenic potential and behavioral correlates of stress. Mol Psychiatry. 2009;14:95–105.
38. Pinheiro S, Silva J, Mota C, Vaz-Silva J, Veloso A, Pinto V, et al. Tau Mislocation in glucocorticoid-triggered hippocampal pathology. Mol Neurobiol. 2016;53:4745–53.
39. Sotiropoulos I, Catania C, Pinto LG, Silva R, Pollerberg GE, Takashima A, et al. Stress acts cumulatively to precipitate Alzheimer's disease-like tau pathology and cognitive deficits. J Neurosci. 2011;31:7840–7.
40. Baglietto-Vargas D, Medeiros R, Martinez-Coria H, LaFerla FM, Green KN. Mifepristone alters amyloid precursor protein processing to preclude amyloid Beta and Also reduces tau pathology. Biol Psychiatry. 2013;74:357–66.
41. Näsman B, Olsson T, Fagerlund M, Eriksson S, Viitanen M, Carlström K. Blunted adrenocorticotropin and increased adrenal steroid response to human corticotropin-releasing hormone in Alzheimer's disease. Biol Pyschiatry. 1996;39:311–8.
42. Bernardi F, Lanzone A, Cento RM, Spada RS, Pezzani I, Genazzani AD, et al. Allopregnanolone and dehydroepiandrosterone response to corticotropin-releasing factor in patients suffering from Alzheimer's disease and vascular dementia. Eur J Endocrinol. 2000;142:466–71.
43. Dong H, Wang S, Zeng Z, Li F, Montalvo-Ortiz J, Tucker C, et al. Effects of corticotrophin-releasing factor receptor 1 antagonists on amyloid-β and behavior in Tg2576 mice. Psychopharmacology. 2014;231:4711–22.
44. Park H-J, Ran Y, Jung JI, Holmes O, Price AR, Smithson L, et al. The stress response neuropeptide CRF increases amyloid- production by regulating -secretase activity. EMBO J. 2015;34:1674–86.
45. Chen Y, Peng Y, Che P, Gannon M, Liu Y, Li L, et al. α_{2A} adrenergic receptor promotes amyloidogenesis through disrupting APP-SorLA interaction. Proc. Natl. Acad. Sci. 2014;111:17296–301.
46. Thathiah A, Horré K, Snellinx A, Vandewyer E, Huang Y, Ciesielska M, et al. β-arrestin 2 regulates Aβ generation and γ-secretase activity in Alzheimer's disease. Nat. Med. 2012;19:43–9.
47. Kang JE, Cirrito JR, Dong H, Csernsnsky JG, Holtzman DM. Acute stress increases interstitial fluid amyloid-beta via corticotropin-releasing factor and neuronal activity. Proc Natl Acad Sci. 2007;104:10673–8.
48. Dong H, Yuede CM, Yoo H-S, Martin MV, Deal C, Mace AG, et al. Corticosterone and related receptor expression are associated with increased β-amyloid plaques in isolated Tg2576 mice. Neuroscience. 2008;155:154–63.
49. Dong H, Murphy KM, Meng L, Montalvo-Ortiz J, Zeng Z, Kolber BJ, et al. Corticotrophin releasing factor accelerates neuropathology and cognitive decline in a mouse model of Alzheimer's disease. J Alzheimers Dis. 2012;28:579–92.
50. Ray B, Gaskins DL, Sajdyk TJ, Spence JP, Fitz SD, Shekhar A, et al. Restraint stress and repeated corticotrophin-releasing factor receptor activation in the amygdala both increase amyloid-β precursor protein and amyloid-β peptide but have divergent effects on brain-derived neurotrophic factor and pre-synaptic proteins in the prefrontal cortex of rats. Neuroscience. 2011;184:139–50.
51. Campbell SN, Zhang C, Roe AD, Lee N, Lao KU, Monte L, et al. Impact of CRFR1 ablation on amyloid-β production and accumulation in a mouse model of Alzheimer's disease. J Alzheimers Dis. 2015;45:1175–84.
52. Iqbal K, Liu F, Gong C-X. Tau and neurodegenerative disease: the story so far. Nat Rev Neurol. 2015;12:15–27.
53. Rothman SM, Herdener N, Frankola KA, Mughal MR, Mattson MP. Chronic mild sleep restriction accentuates contextual memory impairments, and accumulations of cortical Aβ and pTau in a mouse model of Alzheimer's disease. Brain Res. 2013;1529:200–8.
54. Carroll JC, Iba M, Bangasser DA, Valentino RJ, James MJ, Brunden KR, et al. Chronic stress exacerbates tau pathology, neurodegeneration, and cognitive performance through a Corticotropin-releasing factor receptor-dependent mechanism in a transgenic mouse model of Tauopathy. J Neurosci. 2011;31:14436–49.
55. Rissman RA, Lee K-F, Vale W, Sawchenko PE. Corticotropin-releasing factor receptors differentially regulate stress-induced tau phosphorylation. J Neurosci. 2007;27:6552–62.
56. Campbell SN, Zhang C, Monte L, Roe AD, Rice KC, Taché Y, et al. Increased tau phosphorylation and aggregation in the hippocampus of mice overexpressing corticotropin-releasing factor. J Alzheimers Dis. 2015;43:967–76.
57. Filipcik P, Novak P, Mravec B, Ondicova K, Krajciova G, Novak M, et al. Tau protein phosphorylation in diverse brain areas of normal and CRH deficient mice: up-Regulation by stress. Cell Mol Neurobiol. 2012;32:837–45.
58. Le MH, Weissmiller AM, Monte L, Lin PH, Hexom TC, Natera O, et al. Functional Impact of Corticotropin-Releasing Factor Exposure on Tau Phosphorylation and Axon Transport. Ryabinin AE, editor. PLOS ONE. 2016;11:e0147250.
59. Rissman RA, Staup MA, Lee AR, Justice NJ, Rice KC, Vale W, et al. Corticotropin-releasing factor receptor-dependent effects of repeated stress on tau phosphorylation, solubility, and aggregation. Proc Natl Acad Sci. 2012;109:6277–82.
60. Kvetnansky R, Novak P, Vargovic P, Lejavova K, Horvathova L, Ondicova K, et al. Exaggerated phosphorylation of brain tau protein in CRH KO mice exposed to repeated immobilization stress. Stress. 2016;19:395–405.
61. Kehne JH, Cain CK. Therapeutic utility of non-peptidic CRF1 receptor

antagonists in anxiety, depression, and stress-related disorders: evidence from animal models. Pharmacol Ther. 2010;128:460–87.
62. Lowery EG, Thiele TE. Pre-clinical evidence that corticotropin-releasing factor (CRF) receptor antagonists are promising targets for pharmacological treatment of alcoholism. CNS Neurol. Disord.-Drug targets former. Curr. Drug targets-CNS Neurol. Disord. 2010;9:77–86.
63. Kwako LE, Spagnolo PA, Schwandt ML, Thorsell A, George DT, Momenan R, et al. The corticotropin releasing hormone-1 (CRH1) receptor antagonist pexacerfont in alcohol dependence: a randomized controlled experimental medicine study. Neuropsychopharmacology. 2015;40:1053–63.
64. Zhang C, Kuo C-C, Moghadam SH, Monte L, Campbell SN, Rice KC, et al. Corticotropin-releasing factor receptor-1 antagonism mitigates beta amyloid pathology and cognitive and synaptic deficits in a mouse model of Alzheimer's disease. Alzheimers Dement. 2016;12:527–37.
65. Contoreggi C, Lee MR, Chrousos G. Addiction and corticotropin-releasing hormone type 1 receptor antagonist medications: Antistress drugs as treatments for addiction. Ann N Y Acad Sci. 2013;1282:107–18.
66. Spierling SR, Zorrilla EP. Don't stress about CRF: assessing the translational failures of CRF1antagonists. Psychopharmacology (Berl.) [Internet]. 2017 [cited 2017 Mar 12]; Available from: http://link.springer.com/10.1007/s00213-017-4556-2.
67. Réus GZ, Titus SE, Abelaira HM, Freitas SM, Tuon T, Quevedo J, et al. Neurochemical correlation between major depressive disorder and neurodegenerative diseases. Life Sci. 2016;158:121–9.
68. Bao A-M, Meynen G, Swaab DF. The stress system in depression and neurodegeneration: focus on the human hypothalamus. Brain Res Rev. 2008;57:531–53.
69. Austin KW, Ameringer SW, Cloud LJ. An integrated review of psychological stress in Parkinson's disease: biological mechanisms and symptom and health outcomes. Park Dis. 2016;2016:1–15.
70. Hou G, Tian R, Li J, Yuan T-F. Chronic stress and Parkinson's disease. CNS Neurosci Ther. 2014;20:1–2.
71. Smith LK, Jadavji NM, Colwell KL, Katrina Perehudoff S, Metz GA. Stress accelerates neural degeneration and exaggerates motor symptoms in a rat model of Parkinson's disease. Eur J Neurosci. 2008;27:2133–46.
72. Lauretti E, Di Meco A, Merali S, Praticò D. Chronic behavioral stress exaggerates motor deficit and neuroinflammation in the MPTP mouse model of Parkinson's disease. Transl Psychiatry. 2016;6:e733.
73. Kibel A, Drenjančević-Perić I. Impact of glucocorticoids and chronic stress on progression of Parkinson's disease. Med Hypotheses. 2008;71:952–6.
74. Wu Q, Yang X, Zhang Y, Zhang L, Feng L. Chronic mild stress accelerates the progression of Parkinson's disease in A53T α-synuclein transgenic mice. Exp Neurol. 2016;285:61–71.
75. Sugama S, Kakinuma Y. Loss of dopaminergic neurons occurs in the ventral tegmental area and hypothalamus of rats following chronic stress: possible pathogenetic loci for depression involved in Parkinson's disease. Neurosci Res. 2016;111:48–55.
76. Sugama S, Sekiyama K, Kodama T, Takamatsu Y, Takenouchi T, Hashimoto M, et al. Chronic restraint stress triggers dopaminergic and noradrenergic neurodegeneration: possible role of chronic stress in the onset of Parkinson's disease. Brain Behav Immun. 2016;51:39–46.
77. Mo C, Renoir T, Pang TYC, Hannan AJ. Short-term memory acquisition in female Huntington's disease mice is vulnerable to acute stress. Behav Brain Res. 2013;253:318–22.
78. Mo C, Renoir T, Hannan AJ. Effects of chronic stress on the onset and progression of Huntington's disease in transgenic mice. Neurobiol Dis. 2014;71:81–94.
79. Kronenberg G, Schöner J, Nolte C, Heinz A, Endres M, Gertz K. Charting the perfect storm: emerging biological interfaces between stress and stroke. Eur. Arch. Psychiatry Clin. Neurosci. [Internet]. 2017 [cited 2017 May 13]; Available from: http://link.springer.com/10.1007/s00406-017-0794-x.
80. Stuller KA, Jarrett B, DeVries AC. Stress and social isolation increase vulnerability to stroke. Exp Neurol. 2012;233:33–9.
81. van der Linde RM, Dening T, Stephan BCM, Prina AM, Evans E, Brayne C. Longitudinal course of behavioural and psychological symptoms of dementia: systematic review. Br J Psychiatry. 2016;209:366–77.
82. Hsiao K, Chapman P, Nilsen S, Eckman C, Harigaya Y, Younkin S, et al. Correlative memory deficits, Aβ elevation, and amyloid plaques in transgenic mice. Science. 1996;274:99–102.
83. Lee K-W, Kim J-B, Seo J-S, Kim T-K, Im J-Y, Baek I-S, et al. Behavioral stress accelerates plaque pathogenesis in the brain of Tg2576 mice via generation of metabolic oxidative stress. J Neurochem. 2009;108:165–75.
84. Huang H-J, Liang K-C, Ke H-C, Chang Y-Y, Hsieh-Li HM. Long-term social isolation exacerbates the impairment of spatial working memory in APP/PS1 transgenic mice. Brain Res. 2011;1371:150–60.
85. Borchelt DR, Ratovitski T, Van Lare J, Lee MK, Gonzales V, Jenkins NA, et al. Accelerated amyloid deposition in the brains of transgenic mice coexpressing mutant presenilin 1 and amyloid precursor proteins. Neuron. 1997;19:939–45.
86. Rothman SM, Herdener N, Camandola S, Texel SJ, Mughal MR, Cong W-N, et al. 3xTgAD mice exhibit altered behavior and elevated Aβ after chronic mild social stress. Neurobiol. Aging. 2012;33:830.e1–830.e12.
87. Oddo S, Caccamo A, Shepherd JD, Murphy MP, Golde TE, Kayed R, et al. Triple-transgenic model of Alzheimer's disease with plaques and tangles: intracellular Aβ and synaptic dysfunction. Neuron. 2003;39:409–21.
88. Stenzel-Poore MP, Heinrichs SC, Rivest S, Koob GF, Vale WW. Overproduction of corticotropin-releasing factor in transgenic mice: a genetic model of anxiogenic behavior. J Neurosci. 1994;14:2579–84.
89. Baglietto-Vargas D, Chen Y, Suh D, Ager RR, Rodriguez-Ortiz CJ, Medeiros R, et al. Short-term modern life-like stress exacerbates Aβ-pathology and synapse loss in 3xTg-AD mice. J Neurochem. 2015;134:915–26.
90. Justice NJ, Huang L, Tian J-B, Cole A, Pruski M, Hunt AJ, et al. Posttraumatic stress disorder-like induction elevates -amyloid levels, which directly activates Corticotropin-releasing factor neurons to exacerbate stress responses. J Neurosci. 2015;35:2612–23.
91. Yoshiyama Y, Higuchi M, Zhang B, Huang S-M, Iwata N, Saido TC, et al. Synapse loss and microglial activation precede tangles in a P301S Tauopathy mouse model. Neuron. 2007;53:337–51.

12

Amelioration of amyloid-β-induced deficits by DcR3 in an Alzheimer's disease model

Yi-Ling Liu[1], Wei-Ting Chen[2], Yu-Yi Lin[1], Po-Hung Lu[1], Shie-Liang Hsieh[4,5,6,7*] and Irene Han-Juo Cheng[1,2,3*]

Abstract

Background: Microglia mediate amyloid-beta peptide (Aβ)-induced neuroinflammation, which is one of the key events in the pathogenesis of Alzheimer's disease (AD). Decoy receptor 3 (DcR3)/TNFRSF6B is a pleiotropic immunomodulator that promotes macrophage differentiation toward the M2 anti-inflammatory phenotype. Based on its role as an immunosupressor, we examined whether DcR3 could alleviate neuroinflammation and AD-like deficits in the central nervous system.

Method: We crossed human APP transgenic mice (line J20) with human DcR3 transgenic mice to generate wild-type, APP, DcR3, and APP/DcR3 mice for pathological analysis. The Morris water maze, fear conditioning test, open-field, and elevated-plus maze were used to access their cognitive behavioral changes. Furthermore, the pathological and immune profiles were examined by immunostaining, ELISA, Q-PCR, and IP. In vitro assays were designed to examine DcR3-mediated innate cytokine profile alteration and the potential protective mechanism.

Results: We reported that DcR3 ameliorates hippocampus-dependent memory deficits and reduces amyloid plaque deposition in APP transgenic mouse. The protective mechanism of DcR3 mediates through interacting with heparan sulfate proteoglycans and activating IL-4^{+}YM1^{+} M2a-like microglia that reduces Aβ-induced proinflammatory cytokines and promotes phagocytosis ability of microglia.

Conclusion: The neuroprotective effect of DcR3 is mediated via modulating microglia activation into anti-inflammatory M2a phenotype, and upregulating DcR3 expression in the brain may be a potential therapeutic approach for AD.

Keywords: Alzheimer's Disease, Neuroinflammation, Decoy Receptor 3, M2a microglia

Background

Alzheimer's disease (AD) is the most common incurable neurodegenerative disease. One of the pathological hallmarks of AD is the extracellular amyloid plaques composed of amyloid-beta peptide (Aβ) which is generated by proteolytic cleavage of amyloid precursor protein (APP). The abnormal accumulation of Aβ is considered to be a critical factor in AD pathogenesis [1, 2]. The aggregation of Aβ into small oligomers and fibrillar plaques triggers neuroinflammation that contributes to the neuronal loss and cognitive decline [1, 3]. Although suppression of chronic inflammation has been proposed as a new direction for AD intervention, the therapeutic effects of anti-inflammatory drugs in current clinical trials are far from satisfactory [4]. Therefore, a novel strategy is necessary to protect neurons from Aβ-induced neurotoxicity and neuroinflammation to preserve memory.

Microglia serve as the first line of host defense in the brain. Microglia activation can be beneficial or detrimental in AD pathogenesis via removing Aβ by phagocytosis or producing pro-inflammatory cytokines that damage neurons [5, 6]. The activated microglia are classified into M1 inflammatory (classical) and M2 anti-inflammatory (alternative) phenotypes [7]. The M1 phenotype can be triggered by lipopolysaccharides, interferon-γ, and Aβ. They produce pro-inflammatory cytokines, such as IL-1β and TNF-α [8, 9], to kill pathogens and induce cytotoxicity [10]. In contrast, the M2 microglia reduce Aβ plaque deposition and alleviate memory impairments in an AD mouse model [11]. Therefore, modulation of microglia activation and differentiation is a potential approach to regulate neuroinflammation in AD [11, 12].

* Correspondence: slhsieh@gate.sinica.edu.tw; hjcheng@ym.edu.tw
[4]Genomics Research Center, Academia Sinica, Taipei, Taiwan
[1]Institute of Brain Science, National Yang-Ming University, Taipei, Taiwan
Full list of author information is available at the end of the article

M2 phenotype microglia can be divided into M2a-d subtypes according to the surface and intracellular markers [13, 14]. The M2a subtype microglia ($YM1^+$, $FIZZ1^+$, $CCL17^+$, arginase-1^+) are induced by IL-4, IL-13, fungal and helminth infections and are capable of suppressing inflammation [15]. However, the functions of these microglia subtypes are still controversial assayed in different in vitro systems [16–18].

Decoy receptor 3 (DcR3)/TNFRSF6B is a soluble decoy receptor which can neutralize the biological functions of three members of tumor necrosis factor superfamily: Fas ligand (FasL) LIGHT, and TL1A to reduce cell death [19–21]. In addition to its neutralizing effect, DcR3 interacts with heparan sulfate proteoglycans (HSPGs) to promote the differentiation of M2-like macrophages through epigenetic regulation [22–24]. DcR3 upregulates the expression of M2 macrophage markers (mannose receptor/CD206, arginase-I, YM-1, CD86, MMP7 and MMP-9) and downregulates the expression of M1 markers (iNOS, CD80, FcγR, IL-6, and TNF-α) [24, 25]. DcR3 transgenic mice are resistant to type-I diabetes and Th17-mediated autoimmune diseases [23]. However, the role of DcR3 in Aβ-mediated neuroinflammation in the brain has not yet been identified.

Given that DcR3 exerts anti-apoptotic and immune-modulatory effects via neutralizing FasL and non-deoy functions we asked whether DcR3 ameliorates AD-like functional deficits and pathological changes using both in vivo and in vitro systems. Here, we demonstrated that Aβ-induced cognitive deficits and neurodegeneration were improved by DcR3 in transgenic mice overexpressing a mutated human APP minigene (hAPP/J20 line). DcR3 skewed microglia differentiation to IL-$4^+$$YM1^+$ M2a-like subtype, modulated neuroinflammation, conserved synaptic density, and reduced Aβ. Our observations suggest that DcR3 may become a promising reagent for the treatment of AD in the future.

Methods

Mice

Hemizygous hAPP transgenic mice (line J20) express an alternatively spliced human APP minigene with the Swedish and Indiana familial AD mutations driven by the PDGF promoter [26]. Hemizygous DcR3 transgenic mice express human DcR3 driven from the CD68 promoter in macrophages/microglia/monocytes [25]. Female DcR3 transgene mice were crossed with male APP transgenic mice to obtain wild-type DcR3 single transgenic, APP single transgenic, and APP/DcR3 double transgenic mice. The littermates of these mice were examined in behavioral tests at 6 months of age and sacrificed for pathological examinations at 6 or 12 months of age.

Morris Water Maze

The water maze consisted of a water pool (122 cm in diameter) containing opaque water and a platform (10 cm in diameter) submerged 1 cm below the water surface. The hidden platform test consisted of 10 sessions over 5 days and each session comprised three 60-s trials with 15-min inter-trial intervals. The platform location remained constant during the hidden platform sessions, and the entry points were changed semi-randomly between days. One day after the final day of hidden platform training section, a probe trial was conducted by removing the platform and allowing mice to explore in the pool for 1 min. The quadrant in which the platform was previously located was defined as the target quadrant, and the proportion of time (as a percentage) that the each mouse spent in the target quadrant was used to measure memory retention. The number of platform crossings and swim speed were recorded and analyzed with the EthoVision video tracking system (Version 3.1 Noldus Wageningen, Netherlands).

Fear conditioning

During the day 1 training section mice were habituated in a conditioning box (Graphic State 2.101 Contents, Coulbourn Instruments, PA, USA) for 5 min and then received five pairs of an 8-s tone and a 2-s shock (0.4 mA) followed by a 2-min resting interval. On day 2 testing sections, the trained mice were placed back to the same testing box, and their freezing time was scored for 5 min to measure the contextual conditioned fear response. The cued test was conducted 5 min after the contextual test. Mice were habituated for 5 min in a novel-shaped box and then exposed to three 10-s auditory cues followed with a 2-min resting interval. The freezing times of each mouse were scored during all testing sessions.

Open field

To detect spontaneous locomotor activity mice were placed in an open chamber (24.32 × 24.32 cm^2). Their horizontal movement was detected by a 16 × 16 infrared photo-beam arrays placed 1.5 cm above the bottom of the chamber for 15 min (Version 2.0, TRU Scan Photo-beam LINC, Coulbourn Instruments, PA, USA).

Elevated plus maze

The elevated plus-shaped maze consisted of two open arms and two closed arms. All mice were individually placed at the center of the maze and allowed to explore for 10 min. The time spent and distances traveled on each arm were calculated with the Etho Vision video tracking system.

Immunofluorescence and thioflavin-S staining

Paraformaldehyde-fixed brains were sliced coronally by using a microtome (Leica SM2010R Heidelberg, Germany) and were stored in cryoprotectant medium (30% glycerol, 30% ethylene glycol in PBS) at -20 °C. For immunohistochemistry (IHC) staining, brain slices were blocked in a TBS-buffered solution containing 1% glycine, 0.4% Triton X-100, 10% FBS (FBL01, Caisson labs, USA), 0.1% sodium azide (13412, Sigma, MO, USA) and 3% serum bovine albumin for 2 h and then incubated for 24 h at 4 °C with anti-Iba1 (019–19741, Wako), anti-YM1 (01404, Stem Cell technology), anti-synaptophysin (04–1019, Millipore), anti-MAP2 (MAB378, Millipore) and anti-Aβ (SIG-39320, 6E10, Covance) to measure the distribution of microglia, M2a activated microglia, pre-synaptic density, neuronal density and the total level of Aβ. After incubation, the slices were incubated for 2 h with Alexa594-labeled (111–585–003, Jackson ImmunoResearch) and Alexa488-labeled secondary antibodies (115–546–003, Jackson ImmunoResearch) at room temperature.

For thioflavin-S staining brain slices were incubated with 0.015% thioflavin-S (T1892; Sigma MO, USA) for 15 min at room temperature. All chemicals unless otherwise stated were purchased from Bio Basic Inc. (Canada).

For immunocytochemistry staining primary cells were fixed with 4% paraformaldehyde to measure the degeneration of primary neurons and the morphology changes of microglia in responses to different treatment conditions. Fixed cells were stained with anti-MAP2 or anti-Iba1 antibody to visualize the structure changes. The stained slices or cells were imaged with a fluorescence microscope (Axio Observer A1; Zeiss Germany) or a confocal microscope (Fluoview FV10i; Olympus USA). Images were analyzed with MetaMorph® Microscopy Automation & Image Analysis Software (Molecular Devices, CA, USA).

To quantify the total or M2a microglia surrounding plaques slices were double stained with 6E10 and anti-Iba1 or anti-YM1 antibodies. Plaque areas were circled to determine the centers. The circles were then enlarged 10 μm in radius from the center, which was considered to be the periphery area for measuring the microglia or secreted YM1 coverage.

Enzyme-linked immunosorbent assays (ELISAs)

For DcR3 measurement up to 500 μl of blood was collected from the facial vein at the submandibular area and was centrifuged at 1,000 g for 15 min to isolate the serum. Serum DcR3 concentrations were measured with a human DcR3 Duo Set (DY142, R&D, USA).

For Aβ measurement the hippocampus of each mouse was homogenized in 5 M guanidine/5 mM Tris (pH 8.0) buffer and diluted with 0.25% casein blocking buffer to a final concentration of 0.5 M guanidine with protease inhibitor (04693116001, Roche, Basel, Switzerland). The levels of total Aβ and Aβ42 were quantified using Aβ ELISA kits (27729 and 27711, IBL, Hamburg, Germany).

For cytokines measurement diluted hippocampus lysates and conditioned media were applied to TNF-α, IL-1β, and IL-6 ELISA kits (555268, 559603, 555240, BD System, NJ, USA). For YM1 measurement, the hippocampus was homogenized in diluting reagent provided by ELISA kit at the concentration of 20 μg tissue/μl, and YM1 concentration were measured using mouse YM1/Chitinase 3-like 3 DuoSet ELISA (DY2446, R&D, USA).

Quantitative real-time PCR (Q-PCR)

The RNA from the hippocampus and the primary microglia were purified using the Total RNA Mini Kit (Geneaid Taiwan) or TRI reagent (T9424, Sigma, MO, USA), and then immediately reverse transcribed into cDNA by MMLV high-performance reverse transcriptase (RT80125K, Epicentre, WI, USA). The mRNA expression levels were analyzed by using primers (listed in Additional file 1: Table S1) mixed with SYBR Green PCR Master Mix (10476600, Roche, Penzberg, Germany). A StepOnePlus Real-Time PCR System (Applied Biosystem, ABI, MA, USA) was used to monitor the changes of fluorescence intensity from PCR products. GAPDH was used as internal control. The data were analyzed using StepOne software version 2.0.

Immunoprecipitation (IP)

Cortexes from 12-month-old mice were homogenized with a pestle at the concentration of 1 μg tissue /9 μl HEPES buffer (1% CHAPS 50 mM HEPES, 10 mM EDTA, 150 mM NaCl, pH 7.4). Tissue lysates were centrifuged at 600 × g for 5 mins and supernatants were collected. 200 μl samples were pre-cleared with 50 μl protein G bead (LSKMAGG02, Millipore, Germany) rotating at room temperature for 30 mins. Pre-cleared lysates were incubated with anti-DcR3 (33302, Biolegend, CA, USA), anti-syndecan-1 (10593–1-AP, ProteinTech, IL, USA), anti-glypican-1 (sc-66910, Santa Cruz biotechnology, TX, USA), or anti-Aβ (6E10, SIG-39320, COVANCE, NJ, USA) antibodies at 4 °C overnight, and were then mixed with protein G beads rotating at room temperature for 1 h. The beads were washed with 0.1% Tween 20 in PBS for 20 mins and were eluted by SDS-sample buffer (87.5 mM Tris-HCl, 1% SDS, 30% glycerol, 0.6 M DTT, 180 μM bromphenol blue, pH 6.8) at 95 °C, 10 mins. The eluted samples and input controls were monitored by Western blot.

Gel electrophoresis and Western blotting analysis

Proteins were separated via 10% or 15% Tris-glycine SDS-polyacrylamide gel electrophoresis and transferred to nitrocellulose membranes. The membranes

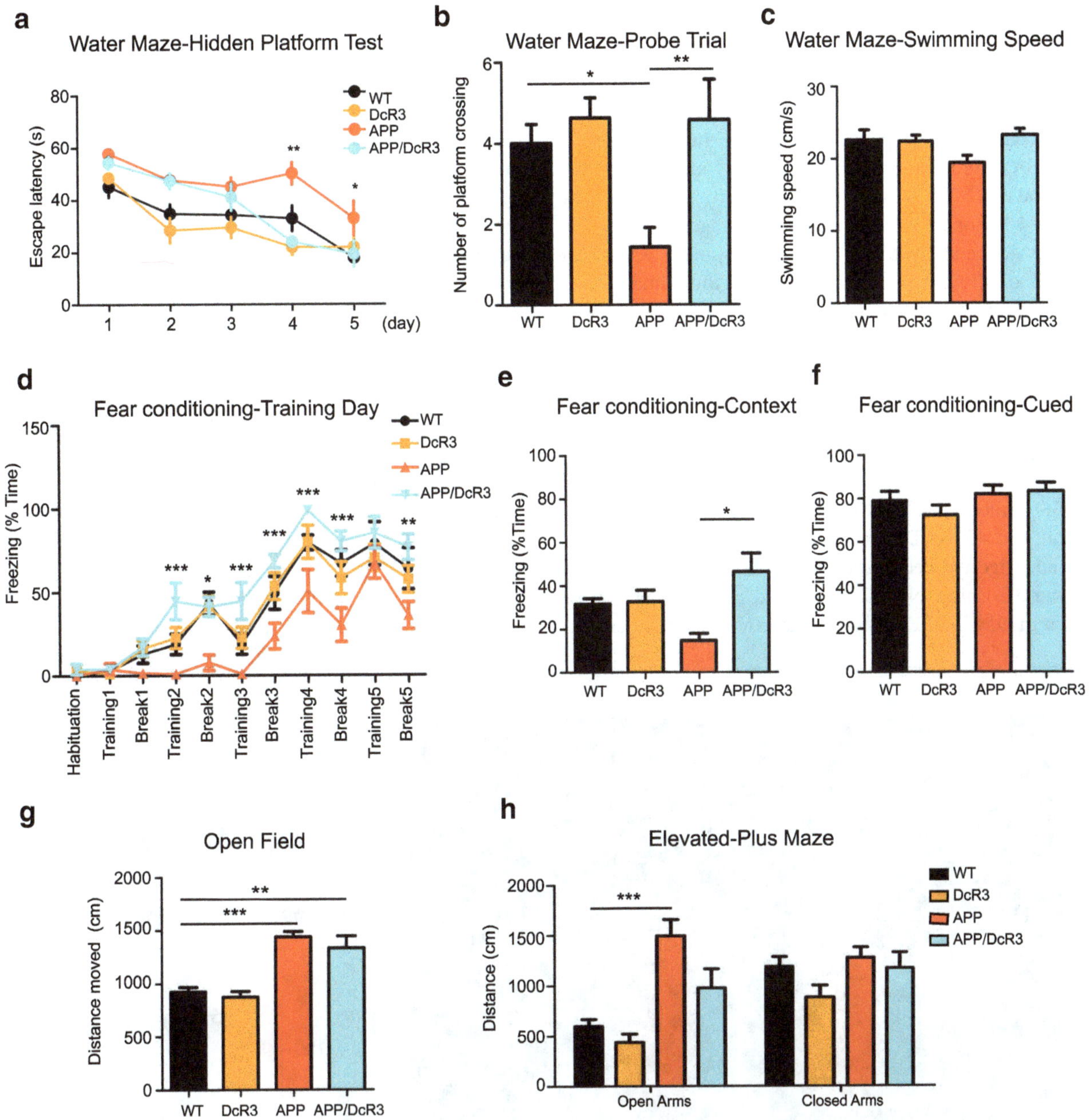

Fig. 1 DcR3 improved the hippocampus-related cognitive deficits in APP mice. Mice were subjected to **a**-**c** the Morris water maze test and **d**-**f** the fear conditioning test. **a** The mean daily escape latencies calculated from six trials per day in the hidden platform test. **b** The number of times that the mice crossed the original platform location in the probe trial. **c** Swimming speed during probe trials. **d** Freezing behavior during training day of fear conditioning test. **e**, **f** Percent of time freezing in the **e** contextual test and **f** cued test on the second day. **g** Distance moved in the open field test during 15 min. **h** Distance traveled in the open or closed arms of the elevated plus test during 10 min. $N = 5$-11 mice per genotype. $^{*}P \leq 0.05$, $^{**}P \leq 0.01$, $^{***}P \leq 0.001$

were probed with rabbit anti-PSD95 (3450 Cell Signaling, MA, USA), mouse anti-DcR3 (33302, Biolegend, CA, USA), rabbit anti-syndecan-1 (10593–1-AP, ProteinTech, IL, USA), rabbit anti-glypican-1 (sc-66910, Santa Cruz biotechnology, TX, USA), mouse anti-Aβ (6E10, SIG-39320, COVANCE, NJ, USA), anti-YM1 (01404, Stem Cell technology, Vancouver, Canada), mouse anti-GAPDH (60004-1-Ig, ProteinTech, IL, USA), and mouse anti-actin (MAB1501, Millipore, MA, USA) antibodies. The membranes were washed and probed with the HRP-conjugated goat anti-mouse IgG and goat anti-rabbit IgG (12–349, AP132P, Millipore, MA, USA). Protein signals were developed by using a chemiluminescent substrate ECL detection system (WBKLS0500, Millipore,

MA, USA) and quantified by using a luminescence imaging system (LAS-4000, Fujifilm, Japan).

Oligomeric Aβ (oAβ) fibrillar Aβ (fAβ) and DcR3 preparation

HFIP-treated Aβ1-42 peptides (rPeptide Inc. A–1163–2, GA, USA) were dissolved in 10% DMSO at 100 μM and stored at −80 °C. Before the experiment, the stock was aged at 4 °C for 24 h to generate oAβ or aged at 37 °C for 18 days to generate fAβ. A DcR3-SAS and Vector-SAS stable line were generated by transfecting the human DcR3 gene or control vector into SAS cells. Culture medium was collected after 24 h of DcR3-SAS and Vector-SAS growth for the conditioned medium experiment.

Primary neuron and microglia preparation and conditioned medium (CM) stimulation

Primary microglia were prepared from postnatal day 0–5 C57B6/J mice. The cortexes were digested with 100 U papain and 400 U DNase I in HBSS buffer at 37 °C for 30 min. Digested cells were passed through a 70-μm cell strainer (Corning NY, USA). Mixed cortical cells were grown in DMEM-F12. After 21 days incubation, microglia were isolated from a 30:37:70% Percoll (P4937, Sigma. MO, USA) gradient and were seeded in 25-T flasks for 24 h.

Primary cortical neuron cultures were prepared from postnatal day 0–1 C57B6/J mice as primary microglia but seeded at a density of $4x10^5$ per well for 7 days in the neurobasal medium.

To obtain conditioned medium (CM) microglial culture were stimulated with the DcR3-SAS medium before, together or after incubating with Aβ for 72 h and their media were collected as pre-, co- or post-treatment Aβ/DcR3-CM. Aβ-CM was collected from microglial culture stimulated with Vector-SAS medium and Aβ for 72 h, and control-CM was collected from microglial culture stimulated with the vector-SAS medium. For the DcR3 immune-depletion control, the DcR3-SAS medium was incubated with anti-DcR3 (33302, Biolegend, CA, USA) and protein G bead (LSKMAGG02, Millipore, Germany) rotating at 4 °C overnight. DcR3 depleted SAS medium was collected for microglia treatment. For the competition assay, microglia were co-treated with DcR3 and 30 μg/ml heparin sulfate (HS) to interfere the DcR3-HSPG interaction for 8 h and then incubated with Aβ

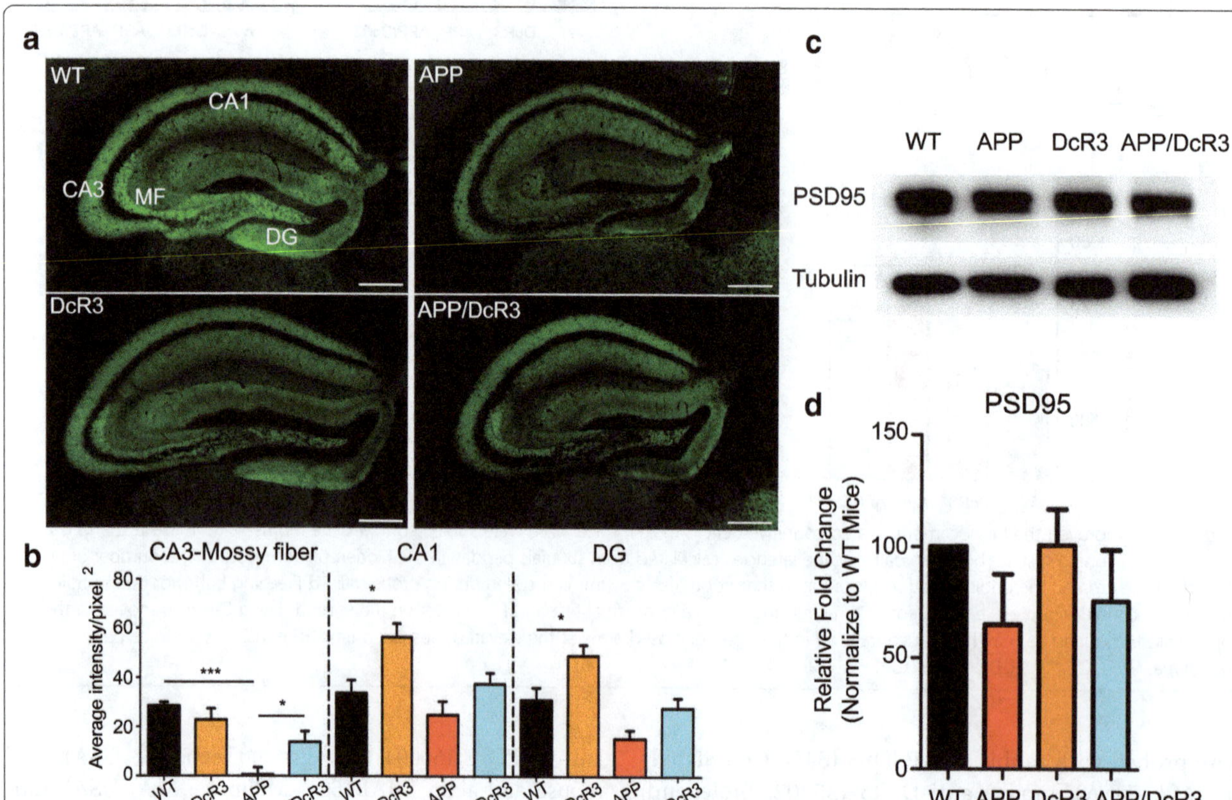

Fig. 2 DcR3 restored the pre-synapse marker expression in APP mice. **a** Representative immunofluorescence synaptophysin images in the hippocampus. MF: mossy fiber; DG: dentate gyrus. *Scale bar: 100 μm.* **b** Quantification of synaptophysin intensity in CA3-mossy fibers, CA1, and the DG regions. $N = 7\text{-}14$ slices from at least 3 mice per genotype. **c** Representative Western blot imaging of PSD95 among four genotypes of mice and **d** averaged intensity of PSD95. $N = 5$ mice per genotype. $^*P \leq 0.05$, $^{**}P \leq 0.01$, $^{***}P \leq 0.001$

for 72 h. These conditioned media were collected and applied to primary neurons for 72 h.

Cell survival

Neuronal survival rate after different CM treatment was assessed using MTT (3006 Biotium Inc., CA, USA) and propidium iodide (PI) staining assays according to the manufacturer's instructions. For the MTT assay, formazan was solubilized in lysis buffer (10% SDS and 20 mM HCl), and the concentration was determined according to the optical density at 570 nm with a Sunrise™ absorbance reader with Magellan™ data analysis software (Version 6; Tecan Switzerland).

For PI staining neurons were incubated with 10 μg/ml PI in PBS for 20 min and were fixed in 4% paraformaldehyde for immunofluorescence staining with the MAP2 antibody. The staining results were quantified as the ratio of PI^+ neurons to total $MAP2^+$ neurons by using MetaMorph® Microscopy Automation & Image Analysis Software (Molecular Devices, CA, USA).

Mouse cytokine array

The cytokines in the primary microglia conditioned medium were detected by using the mouse cytokine array C1000 (AAM-CYT-1000 RayBiotech, GA, USA). Membranes were incubated with control CM, Aβ-CM or Aβ/DcR3-CM (pre-treatment condition) for 16 h and detected with a Biotin-Streptavidin system. Signals were scanned by using a Fujinon LAS-4000 system and quantified by using Multi Gauge V3.0 software (Fujifilm Corporation, Tokyo, Japan). The level of each cytokine in the control group was set as 100.

Microglial phagocytosis assay

Purified microglia were seeded at a density of $1x10^5$ cells/well on poly-D-lysine coated coverslips. Attached microglia were treated with oAβ or oAβ + DcR3 for 72 h. Their phagocytic ability was examined by incubating with red fluorescent carboxylated microspheres (F8821 1 μm in diameter, Polysciences Life Technologies, USA) coated with fetal calf serum at 37 °C for 30 min. After three PBS washes, microglia were fixed with 4% paraformaldehyde and stained with anti-Iba1 antibody to visualize the number of engulfed microspheres in the microglia.

Statistical analysis

Data are presented as the mean ± s.e.m. from at least three independent experiments and were analyzed using Prism software (GraphPad). Differences between data sets were analyzed by unpaired two-tailed Student's *t*-tests or one-way ANOVA followed by the Bonferroni post hoc test. During multiple contrast analysis, the alpha was set as 0.05 (95% confidence intervals). All the precise numbers of samples and their statistical analysis methods of each experiment are listed in Additional file 2: Table S2. A *p* value less than 0.05 was considered to be statistically significant.

Results

DcR3 protects against Aβ-induced cognitive deficits and synaptic loss

To investigate the effects of DcR3 on the functional and pathological features of AD transgenic mice overexpressing mutated human APP (line J20) and human DcR3 were crossed to generate APP/DcR3 double transgenic mice. The levels of the full-length APP (FL-APP) in APP and DcR3/APP mice did not change, and nor did the level of DcR3 in DcR3 and DcR3/APP mice (Additional file 3: Figure S1). Because this line of APP mice develops memory impairments and Aβ plaques at the age of 4 months and 5 months, respectively [26, 27], we followed the behavioral changes and Aβ plaque formation in APP/DcR3, APP, DcR3, and wild-type (WT) littermates, respectively, to determine whether DcR3 modulates the pathogenesis of AD at 6 months after birth.

The Morris water maze was used to assess the spatial learning and memory deficits among these four genotypes of mice (Fig. 1a & b). During the 5 days of the hidden platform test the APP transgenic mice spent more time than WT mice to locate the platform, indicating their deficits in memory acquisition. In contrast, the APP/DcR3 double transgenic mice use less time than the APP transgenic mice to reach the platform at last two days (Fig. 1a). At the 6th day of the probe trial, deficits in memory retention were observed in the APP transgenic mice but not in the APP/DcR3 double transgenic mice (Fig. 1b) compared with WT mice. No significant difference in swimming speeds was found among the 4 genotypes of mice (Fig. 1c). This observation suggested that overexpression of DcR3 rescued spatial learning and memory deficits in 6-month-old APP transgenic mice.

Contextual fear conditioning and auditory-cued fear conditioning tests were further applied to evaluate hippocampus-dependent and amygdala-dependent emotional memory respectively. During the training day, impaired learning was observed in the APP transgenic mice but not in the APP/DcR3 double transgenic mice (Fig. 1d). On day 2 of testing, the APP/DcR3 mice displayed a longer freezing time than the APP mice in the contextual fear conditioning test (Fig. 1e), suggesting that DcR3 reversed the hippocampus-dependent fear memory deficits. In contrast, there was no difference in the amygdala-dependent cued fear conditioning test among the 4 genotypes of mice (Fig. 1f). This observation suggests that DcR3 could ameliorate Aβ-induced hippocampus-related memory deficits.

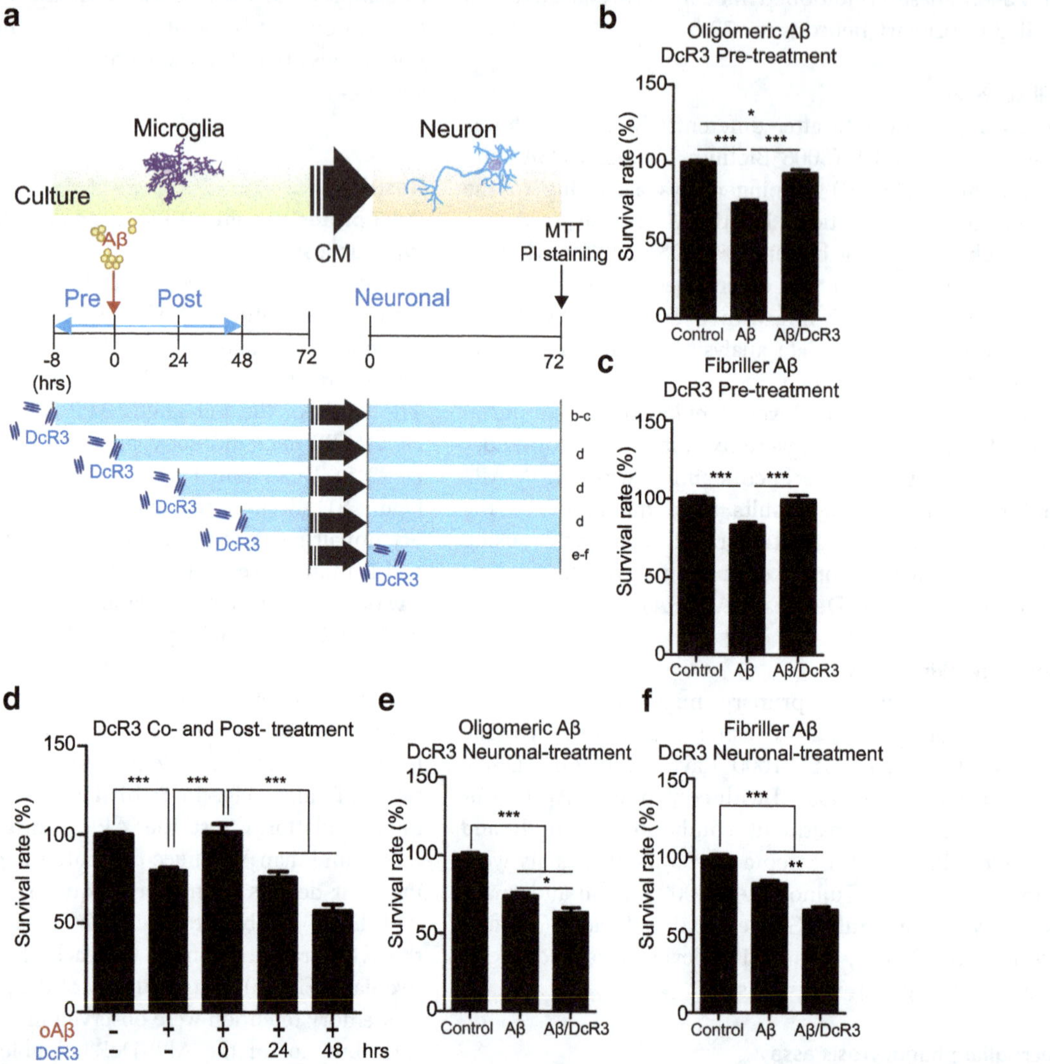

Fig. 3 DcR3 suppressed Aβ-induced neurotoxicity in primary neuronal cultures. **a** Schematic of in vitro Aβ and DcR3 treatment conditions. Microglia were stimulated with **b**, **d**, **e** oligomeric and **c**, **f** fibrillar Aβ for 72 h with the addition of DcR3 at different time points, and their conditioned media (CM) were collected for treating onto primary neurons. The survival rates of primary neurons after 72 h incubating with different CM were determined by MTT assay. **b-c** The survival rate of primary neuron treated with CM from microglia exposing to DcR3 at 8 h before stimulating with Aβ. **d** The survival rate of primary neuron treated with CM from microglia exposing to DcR3 at 0, 24 and 48 h after stimulating with Aβ. **e**, **f** The survival rate of primary neuron treated with Aβ-CM in addition with DcR3. N ≥ 3 independent experiments. $^{*}P \leq 0.05$, $^{**}P \leq 0.01$, $^{***}P \leq 0.001$

We further examined the spontaneous motor activity and anxiety levels of these mice in the open field test and in the elevated plus maze. Consistent with previous findings [27] the APP mice traveled a longer distance in the open field and spent more time in the open arm of the elevated plus maze. In these two tests, the APP/DcR3 mice also had higher locomotor activity and lower anxiety-like behavior similar to the APP mice (Fig. 1g and h). These observations suggest that DcR3 reverses hippocampus-dependent memory impairment without changing locomotion- and anxiety-related behaviors.

The decline in the cognitive functions in AD patients or mouse models is accompanied by a loss of synaptic markers such as synaptophysin and PSD95 [26, 28, 29]. We thus investigated whether DcR3 prevented the loss of synapses by examining the synaptophysin and PSD95 density (Fig. 2a-d). Compared with WT littermates, significant loss of synaptophysin in the mossy fiber-CA3 pathway was observed in the APP mice as revealed by immunohistochemistry (IHC) staining (Fig. 2a, b & Additional file 4: Figure S2a), while synaptophysin expression level was reversed in the APP/DcR3 mice (Fig. 2a, b & Additional file 4: Figure S2a). Moreover, the synaptophysin intensity in the CA1 area and the dentate gyrus of DcR3 mice was higher than that of WT littermates, suggesting DcR3 is able to upregulate synaptophysin expression even without the presence of Aβ plaques. However, the levels of post-synaptic marker PSD95 and MAP2$^+$ neuron had no significant difference among all 4 genotypes of mice (Fig. 2c & d and Additional file 4: Figure S2b & S2c). Because the mossy fiber pathway is critical for memory formation [30], the reversal of synaptophysin loss in this area suggests that DcR3 could preserve synapses to improve spatial memory in the APP mice [31].

DcR3 mediates neuronal protection via microglia

Because microglia are the major players in Aβ-induced neurotoxicity we asked whether microglia are involved in DcR3-mediated neuronal protection. To address this question, primary microglia were pre-incubated with recombinant DcR3 or control medium for 8 h, followed by exposing to oligomeric or fibrillar Aβ (oAβ or fAβ) for 72 h (DcR3 pre-treatment condition). These Aβ/DcR3-stimulated conditioned media (CM) were harvested and incubated with primary neuronal cells for 72 h (Fig. 3a). The survival rate of the neuronal cells was determined by MTT assay (Fig. 3b & c) and PI staining (Additional file 5: Figure S3a & S3b). Compare with the Aβ-CM, the survival rate was significantly increased in the Aβ/DcR3-CM-treated neurons. To further observe neurotic dystrophy in these CM-treated neurons, the anti-MAP2 antibody was used to detect the morphology of neurons. More dystrophic neurites and swelling structure (arrow) were observed in the Aβ-CM than Aβ/DcR3-CM treated neurons (Additional file 5: Figure S3c), suggesting DcR3 modulated-CM prevented the loss of synaptic process in response to Aβ-induced stress.

We further examined the protective effect of DcR3 by incubating neurons with DcR3-CM simultaneously or after exposure to Aβ respectively (Fig. 3a, DcR3 co- and post-treatment). Compared with the Aβ-CM, the survival rate was significantly increased in neurons co-treated, but not post-treated, with DcR3-CM (Fig. 3d). These results suggested that DcR3-CM-mediated protection is via preventing but not reversing Aβ-induced neurotoxic effect (Fig. 3b-d & Additional file 5: Figure S3a & S3b). To further distinguish whether the neuroprotective effect of DcR3 was contributed from microglia or neuron, primary neurons were incubated with Aβ-CM and recombinant DcR3 for 72 h (Fig. 3a, neuronal treatment). Under this condition, DcR3 failed to protect primary neuron against Aβ-induced neurotoxicity (Fig. 3e & f). These observations suggest that the DcR3-mediated neuronal protection is via modulating microglia activation, rather than promoting neuronal resistance to Aβ-CM.

To examine the quality of oAβ and fAβ structures western blot was applied to examine the aggregation states of Aβ before, after microglial treatment, and after neuronal treatment. The oligomeric (10-72 kDa) and

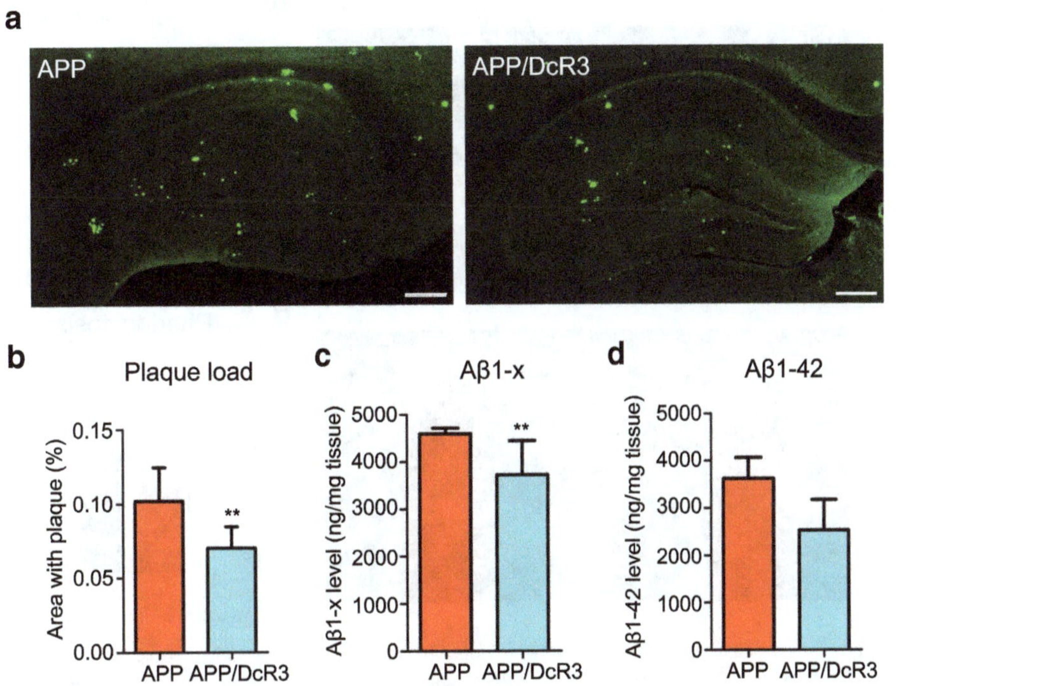

Fig. 4 DcR3 reversed amyloid pathology in APP mice. **a** Representative thioflavin-S staining images in coronal brain sections from 12-month-old APP and APP/DcR3 mice. *Scale bar: 100 μm.* **b** Quantification of the percentage of area covered by amyloid plaques in the hippocampi of APP and APP/DcR3 mice. $N = 24$–34 slices from 4–6 mice per genotype. **c, d** The hippocampal levels of guanidine soluble **c** total Aβ1-x and **d** Aβ1-42 in APP and APP/DcR3 mice were measured via ELISA. $N = 6$ mice per genotype. $^{**}P \leq 0.01$ versus APP mice

fibrillar (in the stacking gel) structures remain the major species in oAβ and fAβ group respectively (Additional file 6: Figure S4a-c). To further confirm the importance of DcR3 in neuroprotection, DcR3 in the SAS medium were removed by the anti-DcR3 conjugated protein G beads before treating onto microglia (Additional file 6: Figure S4d). While we treated the neuron with the DcR3-depleted CM, the neuronal survival rate was not returned to normal, which indicated a critical role of DcR3 on modulating innate-related cytokine-induced cytotoxicity (Additional file 6: Figure S4e).

DcR3 reduces amyloid plaque deposition and enhances of Aβ uptake

Next, we investigated whether DcR3 improves pathological changes by measuring the amyloid plaque deposition and Aβ levels in mice. Compared with APP mice, less β-sheet amyloid plaques were observed in the hippocampus of APP/DcR3 mice as determined by thioflavin-S staining (Fig. 4a & b). In contrast, total Aβ deposition had no significant difference between APP and APP/DcR3 mice as determined by the 6E10 antibody (Additional file 7: Figure S5a-c). Furthermore, the guanidine-soluble total Aβ and Aβ1–42, which play major synaptotoxic roles in AD [26], were decreased in the hippocampus of APP/DcR3 mice as determined by ELISA (Fig. 4c & d). All the evidence indicated that DcR3 reduces amyloid with β-sheet structure and guanidine-soluble Aβ in APP mice.

We further examined the Aβ phagocytic activity of microglia which are first recruited to amyloid plaques before being activated to engulf Aβ to clear amyloid plaques in vivo [32]. We observed that clusters of Iba1-positive microglia (green) were found adjacent to the amyloid plaques (red) in the hippocampi of the APP mice. Interestingly, DcR3 enhanced microglia recruitment (Fig. 5a). Reconstruction analysis showed a higher percentage of microglia and amyloid plaques colocalization in APP/DcR3 than that in the APP mice (Fig. 5b). This observation supports the argument that DcR3 enhances the recruitment of activated microglia to clear amyloid plaques.

We further asked whether DcR3 directly promotes the Aβ-induced phagocytic ability of primary microglia by in vitro culture system. To determine phagocytic ability oAβ- or oAβ + DcR3-treated primary microglia were incubated with fluorescence labeled microspheres. In the presence of DcR3, the phagocytic activities of the microglia were upregulated significantly (Fig. 5c & d). These observations suggest that DcR3 enhances the phagocytosis of microglia, which may enhance Aβ-clearance ability.

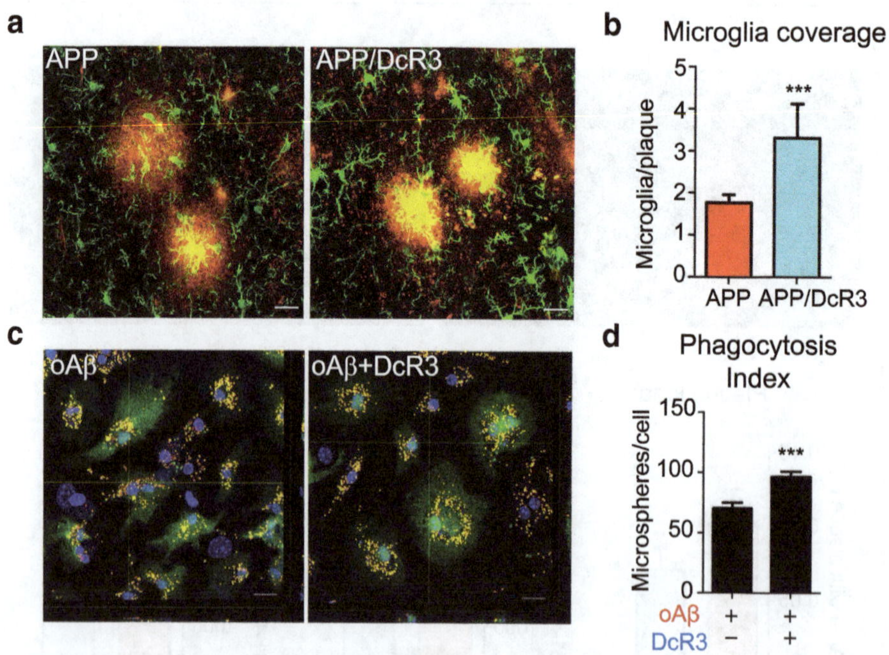

Fig. 5 DcR3 modulated the phagocytic ability of microglia. **a** Representative confocal IHC images of Iba1+ microglia (*green*) and Aβ plaques (*red*) in APP and APP/DcR3 mice. *Scale bar: 20 μm.* **b** Quantification of colocalization of activated microglia and plaques. The ratio is calculated as (area of microglia)/(area of plaque) in the region of interest. Number of plaques analyzed: APP = 342, APP/DcR3 = 324 from at least 3 mice per genotype. ***$P < 0.001$ versus APP. **c** Representative confocal images of oAβ- or oAβ + DcR3-treated primary microglia with engulfed microspheres. *Scale bar: 10 μm.* **d** The number of microspheres engulfed per cell was quantified by using MetaMorph. $N = 74$–76 cells per condition. ***$P \leq 0.001$ versus oAβ group

DcR3 enhances the IL-4⁺YM1⁺ M2a-like microglia population and anti-inflammatory signaling through binding with HSPGs

Although no change in microglia survival rate was found there was an obvious difference in the morphology of primary microglia at 72 h after Aβ or Aβ/DcR3 treatment in vitro. The morphology of microglia without any treatment is in fusiform and ramified shape, which are characteristics of resting microglia. After oAβ treatment for 72 h, microglia enlarged and became an amoeboid shape. In oAβ/DcR3 treated microglia, the size of amoeboid shape microglia is smaller than the oAβ group (Additional file 8: Figure S6). These observations demonstrated the potent modulatory effect of DcR3 to attenuate oAβ-induced microglia activation.

Because the change of microglial population can be detrimental or beneficial in neuroinflammation we further investigated the phenotype of microglia activated by Aβ and DcR3 in vivo and in vitro. The expression of cytokines was determined by ELISA, while the markers of type I and type II microglia and components of inflammasome-related proteins were measured by qPCR (Fig. 6a-c and Additional file 9: Figure S7). Compared with APP mice, the expression of TNF-α and IL-1β, which are secreted by activated M1 microglia, were downregulated in APP/DcR3 mice (Fig. 6a & b). In

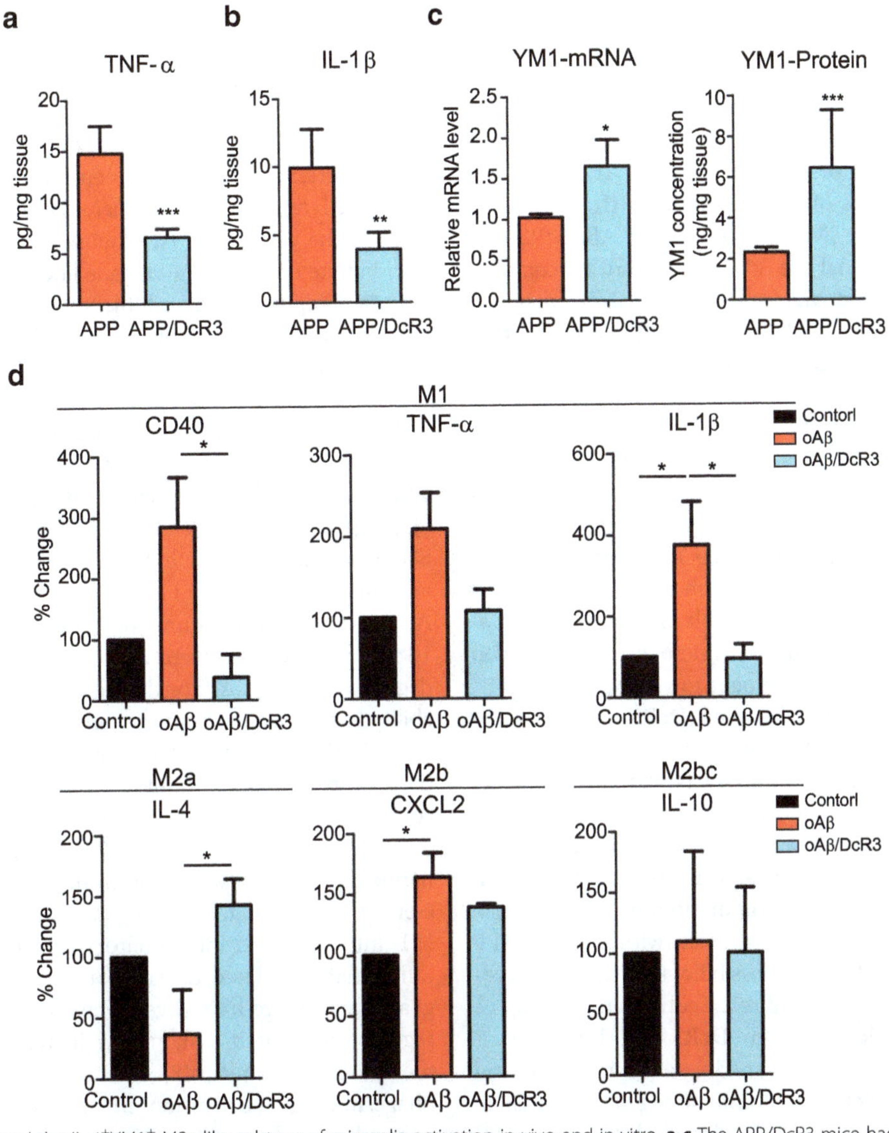

Fig. 6 DcR3 enhanced the IL-4⁺YM1⁺ M2a-like subtype of microglia activation in vivo and in vitro. **a-c** The APP/DcR3 mice had lower **a** TNF-α and **b** IL-1β levels but higher **c** YM1 mRNA and protein level than APP mice in the hippocampus. $N = 6–16$ mice per genotype. $^{***}P \le 0.001$; $^{**}P \le 0.01$; $^{*}P \le 0.05$ versus APP mice. **d** Cytokine array determined the cytokine levels in the conditioned medium. Levels of each cytokine in the control CM was arbitrarily set as 100%. $N = 3$ per group. $^{*}P \le 0.05$

contrast, the expression of YM1 and CCL17, the surface markers for M2a microglia [9], was upregulated by DcR3 (Fig. 6c & Additional file 9: Figure S7a & Additional file 10: Figure S8a-b). Nevertheless, the expression of other inflammatory markers, including the innate immune markers of M2b (IL-6, IL-10), M2c (IL-10, TGF-β, arganise1, CD206) [9, 16], and inflammasome (NLRP3, ASC, IL-18) [11], were similar (Additional file 9: Figure S7b-i). Furthermore, YM1 intensity near the plaques was higher and became more condensed in the APP/DcR3 mice than that in APP mice (Additional file 10: Figure S8a & S8b), indicating that microglia recruited to the plaques are polarized toward M2a-like subtype.

Since the sources of TNF-α and IL-1β in the brain are not only from microglia we confirmed the role of DcR3 to modulate the secretion of cytokines from microglia by using in vitro culture system. The cytokine profiles in the Aβ-CM or Aβ/DcR3-CM (from Fig. 3a, pre-treatment condition) were analyzed by cytokine array (Fig. 6d). Compared with Aβ-CM, lower levels of pro-inflammatory mediators (CD40, TNF-α, IL-1β, IL-12) with higher the levels of the M2a inducer (IL-4) and the M2a marker (YM1) were observed in Aβ/DcR3-CM (Fig. 6d and Additional file 11: Figure S9a). In contrast, the levels of M2b and M2c markers (CXCL2 and IL-10) were not altered by DcR3 (Fig. 6d). All these observations suggest that DcR3 has the potent effect to modulate cytokine secretion by modulating the activation and differentiation of microglia. It is interesting to note that DcR3 did not alter the expression of MMP9, which contributes to plaque clearance in the brain [33], suggesting MMP9-dependent proteolytic degradation of Aβ was not influenced by DcR3 (Additional file 11: Figure S9b). The complete list of all the changes from this cytokines array is listed in Additional file 12: Table S3. Thus, we concluded that DcR3 is able to skew microglia differentiation into IL-4$^+$YM1$^+$ M2a-like microglia in vivo and in vitro.

Because the interaction between DcR3 and HSPG is critical for modulating macrophage activation in vitro [24] we asked whether DcR3 also interacts with glypicans and syndecans, which are the most abundant HSPGs to modulate myeloid cell differentiation in the brain [22, 34, 35]. We found that DcR3 interacts with glypican-1 (Fig. 7a) and syndecan (Fig. 7b) by co-immunoprecipitation assay. In contrast, DcR3 did not interact with Aβ or APP (Fig. 7c), thus excluding the possibility that the neuroprotective effect of DcR3 is via direct neutralization of Aβ or APP. The interaction between DcR3 and HSPGs suggested that human DcR3 may modulate the activation and differentiation of microglia via interacting with HSPGs in vivo. To further confirm the role of HSPG in DcR3-mediated protection against Aβ-induced neurotoxicity, heparin sulfate (HS) was used to block DcR3-HSPG interaction by a competition assay as described in Fig. 4a [22]. In the presence of HS, DcR3-mediated neuroprotective effect against Aβ was attenuated (Fig 7d), suggesting DcR3-HSPG interaction contributes partially against Aβ-induced toxicity [36].

Discussion

In this study a human secreted protein DcR3 prevented Aβ-induced functional and pathological deficits in both in vivo and in vitro AD models. Three potential mechanisms involve in DcR3 neuroprotective effect against amyloid pathogenesis (Fig. 8). First, under Aβ stress, DcR3 induces IL-4$^+$YM1$^+$ M2a-like microglia that reduce the pro-inflammation cytokines to prevent neurotoxicity. Second, DcR3 enhances microglia recruitment to plaques and phagocytic efficiency to clear Aβ. Finally, DcR3 interacts with surface HSPGs. This interaction may eliminate Aβ-HSPGs downstream cytotoxicity or inhibit the HSPGs-mediated inflammatory responses [37, 38].

DcR3 promotes anti-inflammatory effect

The importance of microglia-neuron interaction has been implicated in many neuroinflammatory-related disorders [39]. In the pre-plaque AD mouse oAβ and complement C1q initiate complement cascade and recruit microglia via CR3 to eliminate synapses [40]. Manipulation of the innate immune system into alternatively M2 activated microglia has been considered as a promising therapeutic strategy for AD [11, 41]. For example, intracerebral injections of IL-4/IL-13 or IL-33 reverse memory deficits and reduce Aβ plaque load in AD mouse models [41, 42]. In addition, YM1$^+$ cells could protect neurons during acute brain injury [43, 44]. We found that DcR3-triggered IL-4$^+$YM1$^+$ M2a-like microglia contribute to anti-inflammatory response and functional recovery in vitro and in vivo. DcR3 reduces Aβ – induced pro-inflammatory cytokines, TNF-α and IL-1β [45], to prevent severe neuroinflammation and neurodegeneration [5]. Although DcR3 has been shown its' ability to polarize macrophage differentiation in the periphery [24, 25], this study first presents that DcR3 modulates the complex innate immunity profiles and is able to counter Aβ-induced neuroinflammation in the brain.

In disease-related models microglia activation has dynamic, multidimensional and mosaic signatures [46]. Generally speaking, switching activated microglia from M1 into M2 anti-inflammatory spectrum can reverse inflammatory-related diseases [12, 47]. However, microglia/ macrophage have diverse characteristics in different regions and switch dynamically in response to environmental changes [46, 48]. Studies focusing on macrophage/microglia activation in specific tissues or using particular cytokine stimulation in vitro might not reveal the complex profiles of innate immunity environment [49, 50]. In addition, the M1/M2 microglia classification has been questioned on modulating neurotrophic factors

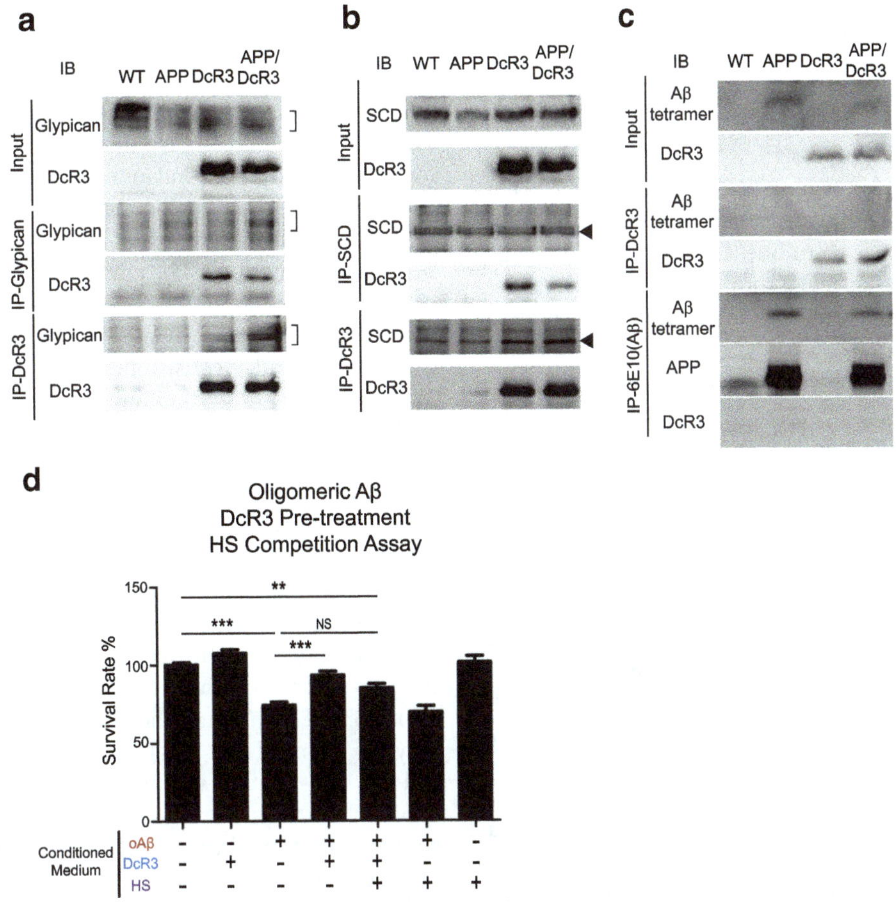

Fig. 7 DcR3 interacted with HSPG to protect neuron under Aβ stress. **a-c** Co-immunoprecipitation to determine the interaction between DcR3 with **a** glypican, **b** syndecan (SCD), and **c** Aβ or APP. **d** Heparan sulfate (HS) competition treatment to block the protective function of DcR3 against Aβ stress in vitro. $N = 3$ per group. ***$P \leq 0.001$; **$P \leq 0.01$; NS, not significant

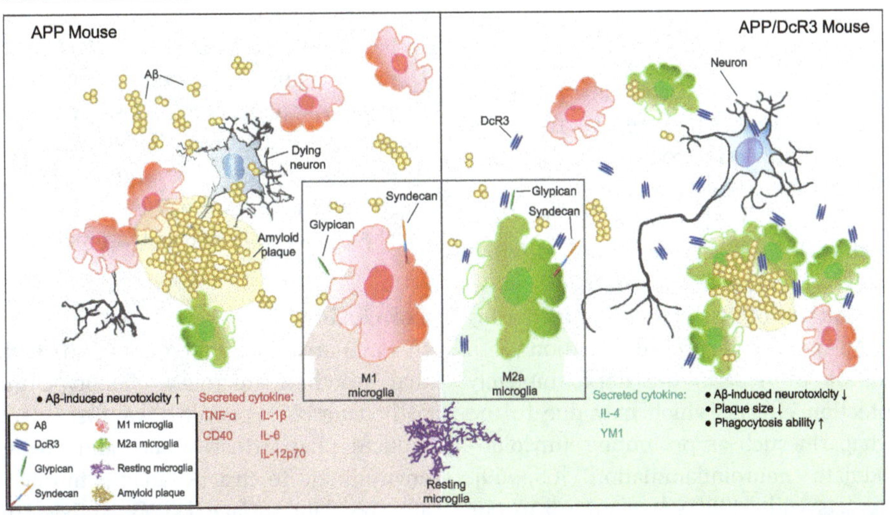

Fig. 8 Working model: In the presence of Aβ, microglia polarize toward the M1 phenotype and secrete pro-inflammatory cytokines, which trigger neurodegeneration. DcR3 interacts with HSPGs and drives microglia polarization to the IL-4^{+}YM1^{+} M2a-like subtype that secrete more anti-inflammatory cytokines. This change enhances Aβ phagocytosis, thereby reducing amyloid plaques and cognitive deficits in APP mice

to regulate synaptic plasticity and memory [48, 51, 52]. Therefore, more evidence are needed to better understand the roles of microglia populations toward AD pathogenesis.

DcR3 promotes phagocytosis

To remove plaque via phagocytosis activated microglia are recruited to the site of plaques in AD animal models and patients [32, 53]. This recruitment is important for engulfing amyloids or tissue debris through lysosome-dependent manner or for constituting a barrier to prevents neurotoxic protofibrillar Aβ42 [32, 54, 55]. Although both astrocyte and microglia could be found near the plaques, only microglia have the ability to degrade Aβ [32]. Inefficient phagocytosis ability of microglia has been reported in AD animal models, and down-regulating phagocytosis-related gene expression has been found in AD subjects [56, 57]. This deficit could be caused by Aβ aggregates, reactive oxygen species (ROS), and pro-inflammatory mediators such as TNF-α, IL-1β, IL-6, and IL-18 [58, 59]. Regulating microglia phagocytosis is considered as a detrimental way to prevent tissue damage in the brain [60]. We found that DcR3 induces more microglia activation near plaque regions (Fig. 5a-b) and enhances microglia phagocytosis to remove Aβ in vivo and in vitro (Fig. 4 & Fig. 5c-d). The enhanced phagocytic ability of Aβ + DcR3-stimulated microglia may reverse the deficit of reducing phagocytic cells in AD patients or AD mice models [61, 62]. Altogether, our results suggest a potential beneficial role of DcR3 on modulating microglia into anti-inflammatory phagocytosis status.

DcR3 interacts with HSPG to regulate neuronal survival

We found that DcR3 interacts with mouse surface HSPGs glypican-1 and syndecan-1 (Fig. 7a & b), and DcR3 neuroprotective effect can be shaded by heparin in vitro (Fig. 7d). The HSPGs on the microglia and oligodendrocytes near lesions could modulate the accumulation of senile plaques and neurofibrillary tangles. [63, 64]. Glypican-1 can bind to Aβ aggregates to upregulate ER stress and to stimulate microglia activation that results in enhanced cytotoxicity [34, 65]. Syndecans are involved in the production of Aβ [66], ROS [35], and inflammatory cytokines [35, 67]. Furthermore, deletion of HSPGs accelerates Aβ clearance in APP/PS1 mice, suggesting that inhibition of Aβ-HSPG interaction is able to suppress Aβ-induced neuroinflammation [64]. However, the addition of heparin did not completely reverse DcR3 protection effects, which may due to the multiple roles of heparin such as promoting amyloidogenesis and modulate neuroinflammation [68, 69]. Because DcR3 interacts with HSPGs but not Aβ in our AD mouse model (Fig. 7a-c), DcR3-mediated neuronal protection may compete Aβ binding to HSPG or suppress HSPGs-CD14/TLR4 mediated inflammation [38]. The functions of HSPGs binding domain in DcR3 and its contributions to innate systems requires further analysis.

The anti-inflammatory treatments using cytokines and DcR3

Several clinical studies have shown contradictory evidence for non-steroidal anti-inflammatory drugs (NSAIDs) in the treatment or prevention of AD [70]. These NSAIDs cannot be used in high doses or for a long period of time because of potential side effects in the cardiovascular or gastrointestinal systems [71]. In all NSAID clinical trials, cognitive performance had no significant improvements, and inconsistent results were reported for indomethacin [72, 73], ibuprofen [74, 75], celecoxib [76], rofecoxib [77, 78], and naproxen treatments [76]. A potential reason for the failure of anti-inflammatory approaches is that different anti-inflammatory cytokines induce diverse responses. For example, one anti-inflammatory cytokine, IL-10, facilitates Aβ aggregation, inhibits microglial phagocytic ability, and causes cognitive dysfunction in APP mice [79, 80]. In contrast, the other anti-inflammatory cytokine, IL-4, triggers microglia phagocytosis to reduce Aβ deposition [15, 81]. Thus, the IL-10 induced microglia may be harmful but IL-4$^+$ microglia may be beneficial to AD-related symptoms. For novel treatment approaches, it is important to identify the microglia subtypes that ameliorates AD pathogenesis.

In comparison to other anti-inflammatory treatments DcR3 is a non-cytokine that induces an anti-inflammatory response, neutralizes FasL-induced cell death, and reduces ROS production [82]. Therefore, DcR3 may be an alternative agent for designing the future treatment. DcR3 concentration in our transgenic mouse serum is 268.6 ± 59.2 pg/ml (Additional file 3: Figure S1), which is slightly higher than healthy human (63.7 ± 21.9 pg/ml) but similar to the asthma patients (266.1 ± 60.6 pg/mL) [83]. Because DcR3 is highly expressed in the endometrium during pregnancy, it appears to be a safe natural immunomodulator to suppress neuronal inflammation in the presence of dangerous endogenous signals [84]. These findings suggested that DcR3 may be a safe therapeutic agent for early AD and other neuroinflammation-related diseases.

Conclusions

In summary, our findings are in line with the current idea that switching microglia phenotype modulates amyloid pathogenesis. Especially, we first identified that DcR3 induces phagocytosis ability and creates an IL-4$^+$YM1$^+$ environment to clear Aβ plaque in the brain. DcR3 might also regulate surface HSPGs activity that mediates Aβ-related neurodegeneration and pro-inflammatory signalings (Fig. 8). Taken together, the DcR3-induced specific IL-4$^+$YM1$^+$ innate response could broaden our views on

AD early-intervention and bring a novel thinking on medical development.

Additional files

Additional file 1: Table S1. List of the real-time PCR primers sets (5'-3') for the target genes.

Additional file 2: Table S2. Statement on sample size and statistical measures.

Additional file 3: Figure S1. Full-length APP and DcR3 expression in four genotypes of mice at 6 months of age. (a, b) Levels of full-length APP did not change between the APP and APP/DcR3 mice (c) Levels of DcR3 did not change between the DcR3 and APP/DcR3 mice ($N = 18$-22 mice per genotype). $^*P \leq 0.05$. NS, not significant.

Additional file 4: Figure S2. Synaptophysin and MAP2 immunostaining in the hippocampus. (a)Enlarged view of synaptophysin staining in Fig. 2a. *Scale bar: 100 μm.* (b)Representative immunofluorescence images labeled with neuronal marker MAP2 in the mouse brain slice. *Scale bar: 100 μm.* (c) Quantification graph comparing the average intensity in CA3-mossy fibers, CA1, and DG region ($N = 7$-13 mice per genotype).

Additional file 5: Figure S3. DcR3 protected neurons against Aβ stress in vitro. (a) Representative illustrations of PI staining used to measure the number of dead neurons after CM treatment. Red: dead cells (PI); Blue: nucleus (DAPI). *Scale bar: 20 μm.* (b) The ratio of PI/DAPI indicates the change in the number of dead neurons after treatment with the conditioned medium. (c) Primary neurons were labeled with neuronal markers (MAP2, Green), and nucleus (DAPI, Blue). Arrow indicated broken and swelling neurites. *Scale bar: 20 μm*

Additional file 6: Figure S4. Aβ aggregation status and DcR3 immuno-depletion control for the conditioned media experiment. (a-c) Western blotting were applied to determine the aggregation state of Aβ peptide in (a) fresh prepared oAβ or fAβ, (b) after 72 h incubating with microglia, (c) after 72 h incubating with neuron. (d) Representative Western blotting image of DcR3 protein levels after immuno-depletion. (e) DcR3 depletion conditioned treatment had no protective function on neuronal survival under Aβ stress ($n = 4$). $^*P \leq 0.05$,$^{***}P \leq 0.001$. The neuronal survival rate of DcR3 Depletion conditioned media treatment was reduced compared to oAβ/DcR3 treatment.

Additional file 7: Figure S5. Effect of DcR3 on Aβ deposition in the hippocampus. (a) Immunostaining of total Aβ (6E10, Red) and nucleus (DAPI, Blue) of the hippocampus. *Scale bar: 200 μm.* (b, c) Quantification data of (b) total numbers of Aβ plaques and (c) plaque coverage ($N = 4$ mice per genotype, $N = 8$ brain slices per mouse).

Additional file 8: Figure S6. Morphological changes of primary microglia in vitro under Aβ or Aβ/DcR3 treatment. The representative fluorescent images were labeled with microglia marker (Iba1, red) and nucleus (DAPI, blue) in microglia culture. *Scale bar: 20 μm.*

Additional file 9: Figure S7. Expression inflammatory-related genes in mice of four genotypes. The mRNA levels of (a) M2a, (b, c) M2b, (c-f) M2c, and (g-i) inflammasome related proteins were examined by using qPCR. $^*P \leq 0.05$.

Additional file 10: Figure S8. DcR3 induced more M2a microglia surrounded plaques and more YM1 expression in vivo. (a) The representative confocal images were labeled with M2a activated microglia marker (YM1, green) and Aβ (6E10, red) in the mouse brain slices. *Scale bar: 20 μm.* ($N = 13$-14 slices per genotype) (b) Quantification of the YM1 positive signal intensity surrounded plaques. The quantification method for Fig. 5b and Additional file 10: Figure S8 is showen in Additional file 13: Figure S10. $^{***}P \leq 0.001$ vs. APP mice.

Additional file 11: Figure S9. Identifying protein expression patterns in primary microglia lysates and CM. (a) DcR3 promoted more YM1 secretion in the Aβ treated primary microglia culture according to the immunoblotting analysis. GAPDH was used as a loading control. (b) The changes in pro-MMP9 levels in the cytokine array analysis.

Additional file 12: Table S3. List of the C3 cytokine array data.

Additional file 13: Figure S10. Illustration of the quantification method of microglia or YM1 around each plaque in Fig. 5b and Additional file 10: Figure S8. Plaque areas were circled to determine the centers. The circles were then enlarged 10 μm in radius from the center, which was considered to be the region of interest for measuring the microglia or secreted YM1 coverage.

Abbreviations

AD: Alzheimer's disease; ANOVA: Analysis of variance; APP: Amyloid precursor protein; Aβ: Amyloid-beta peptide; CM: Conditioned medium; DcR3: Decoy receptor 3; ELISAs: Enzyme-linked immunosorbent assays; fAβ: Fibrillar Aβ; FL-APP: Full-length amyloid precursor protein; HS: Heparan sulfate; HSPGs: Heparan sulfate WT, Wild-type; IHC: Immunohistochemistry; IL: Interleukin; NSAIDs: Non-steroidal anti-inflammatory drugs; oAβ: Oligomeric Aβ; PAGE: Polyacrylamide gel electrophoresis; Q-PCR: Quantitative real-time Polymerase Chain Reaction; ROS: Reactive oxygen species; TNFR: Tumor necrosis factor receptor; TNF-α: Tumor necrosis factor alpha

Acknowledgments

We thank Drs. Ding-I Yang, Young-Ji Shiao, Nien-Jung Chen, Li-Chung Hsu, and Cheng-Chang Lien for the comments on this work. We also thank Po-Han Wei, Chih-Wei Sung, Ming-Ting Huang, Chien-Chun Chen, Yen-Ching Huang, and Yen-Chen Lin for experimental assistance. Behavioral studies were carried out at the Animal Behavioral Core at Brain Research Center, National Yang-Ming University. The technical services of confocal images were provided by Imaging Core Facility of Nanotechnology of the UST-NYMU. We are also grateful to the Transgenic Mouse Model Core Facility of the National Core Facility Program for Biotechnology, National Science Council and the Gene Knockout Mouse Core Laboratory of National Taiwan University Center of Genomic Medicine for technical services.

Funding

This work was supported by Taiwan Ministry of Science and Technology grant (MOST-104-2320-B-010-027 for IHC and MOST 105-2321-B-001-053, MOST 105-2811-B-001-0998 for SLH), Summit and Thematic Research Project (MOST-104-210-01-09-02, MOST-105-0210-01-13-01) of Academia Sinica, National Health Research Institutes (NHRI-EX103-10338NI, NHRI-EX106-10614NI), Cheng Hsin General Hospital (105F003C27), Yen Tjing Ling Medical Foundation (CI-106-2), Taipei Veterans General Hospital grant (V103E4-002), and Taiwan Ministry of Education Aim for Top University Grant.

Authors' contributions

YLL, SLH and IHC wrote the manuscript. YLL, SLH and IHC participated in experimental design, execution and data interpretation. YLL was responsible for conducting all the studies; WTC undertook co-immunoprecipitation; YYL assisted in DcR3 depletion assay and PSD95 immunoblotting; PHL assisted in primary culture and took confocal images. IHC and SLH conceived the study. All authors read and approved the final manuscript.

Authors' information

Not applicable.

Competing interests

The authors declare that they have no competing interests.

Author details
[1]Institute of Brain Science, National Yang-Ming University, Taipei, Taiwan. [2]Brain Research Center, National Yang-Ming University, Taipei, Taiwan. [3]Infection and Immunity Research Center, National Yang-Ming University, Taipei, Taiwan. [4]Genomics Research Center, Academia Sinica, Taipei, Taiwan. [5]Institute of Clinical Medicine, School of Medicine, National Yang-Ming University, Taipei, Taiwan. [6]Institute of Microbiology and Immunology, National Yang-Ming University, Taipei, Taiwan. [7]Department of Medical Research and Education, Taipei Veterans General Hospital, Taipei, Taiwan.

References

1. Querfurth HW, LaFerla FM. Alzheimer's disease. N Engl J Med. 2010;362:329–44.
2. Ashe KH, Zahs KR. Probing the biology of Alzheimer's disease in mice. Neuron. 2010;66:631–45.
3. Wright AL, Zinn R, Hohensinn B, Konen LM, Beynon SB, Tan RP, Clark IA, Abdipranoto A, Vissel B. Neuroinflammation and neuronal loss precede Abeta plaque deposition in the hAPP-J20 mouse model of Alzheimer's disease. PLoS One. 2013;8:e59586.
4. ADAPT-FS Research Group. Follow-up evaluation of cognitive function in the randomized Alzheimer's disease anti-inflammatory prevention trial and its follow-up study. Alzheimers Dement. 2015;11:216–25. e211.
5. Wang WY, Tan MS, Yu JT, Tan L. Role of pro-inflammatory cytokines released from microglia in Alzheimer's disease. Ann Transl Med. 2015;3:136.
6. Koenigsknecht J, Landreth G. Microglial phagocytosis of fibrillar beta-amyloid through a beta1 integrin-dependent mechanism. J Neurosci. 2004;24:9838–46.
7. Kigerl KA, Gensel JC, Ankeny DP, Alexander JK, Donnelly DJ, Popovich PG. Identification of two distinct macrophage subsets with divergent effects causing either neurotoxicity or regeneration in the injured mouse spinal cord. J Neurosci. 2009;29:13435–44.
8. Jang E, Lee S, Kim JH, Seo JW, Lee WH, Mori K, Nakao K, Suk K. Secreted protein lipocalin-2 promotes microglial M1 polarization. FASEB J. 2013;27:1176–90.
9. David S, Kroner A. Repertoire of microglial and macrophage responses after spinal cord injury. Nat Rev Neurosci. 2011;12:388–99.
10. Hu X, Li P, Guo Y, Wang H, Leak RK, Chen S, Gao Y, Chen J. Microglia/macrophage polarization dynamics reveal novel mechanism of injury expansion after focal cerebral ischemia. Stroke. 2012;43:3063–70.
11. Heneka MT, Kummer MP, Stutz A, Delekate A, Schwartz S, Vieira-Saecker A, Griep A, Axt D, Remus A, Tzeng TC, et al. NLRP3 is activated in Alzheimer's disease and contributes to pathology in APP/PS1 mice. Nature. 2013;493:674–8.
12. Tang Y, Le W. Differential roles of M1 and M2 microglia in neurodegenerative diseases. Mol Neurobiol. 2016;53:1181–94.
13. Roszer T. Understanding the mysterious M2 macrophage through activation markers and effector mechanisms. Mediators Inflamm. 2015;2015:816460.
14. Orme J, Mohan C. Macrophage subpopulations in systemic lupus erythematosus. Discov Med. 2012;13:151–8.
15. Pepe G, Calderazzi G, De Maglie M, Villa AM, Vegeto E. Heterogeneous induction of microglia M2a phenotype by central administration of interleukin-4. J Neuroinflammation. 2014;11:211.
16. Chhor V, Le Charpentier T, Lebon S, Ore MV, Celador IL, Josserand J, Degos V, Jacotot E, Hagberg H, Savman K, et al. Characterization of phenotype markers and neuronotoxic potential of polarised primary microglia in vitro. Brain Behav Immun. 2013;32:70–85.
17. Hickman SE, Kingery ND, Ohsumi TK, Borowsky ML, Wang LC, Means TK, El Khoury J. The microglial sensome revealed by direct RNA sequencing. Nat Neurosci. 2013;16:1896–905.
18. Cherry JD, Olschowka JA, O'Banion MK. Arginase 1+ microglia reduce Abeta plaque deposition during IL-1beta-dependent neuroinflammation. J Neuroinflammation. 2015;12:203.
19. Hsu TL, Chang YC, Chen SJ, Liu YJ, Chiu AW, Chio CC, Chen L, Hsieh SL. Modulation of dendritic cell differentiation and maturation by decoy receptor 3. J Immunol. 2002;168:4846–53.
20. Zhang J, Salcedo TW, Wan X, Ullrich S, Hu B, Gregorio T, Feng P, Qi S, Chen H, Cho YH, et al. Modulation of T-cell responses to alloantigens by TR6/DcR3. J Clin Invest. 2001;107:1459–68.
21. Yang CR, Hsieh SL, Teng CM, Ho FM, Su WL, Lin WW. Soluble decoy receptor 3 induces angiogenesis by neutralization of TL1A, a cytokine belonging to tumor necrosis factor superfamily and exhibiting angiostatic action. Cancer Res. 2004;64:1122–9.
22. Chang YC, Chan YH, Jackson DG, Hsieh SL. The glycosaminoglycan-binding domain of decoy receptor 3 is essential for induction of monocyte adhesion. J Immunol. 2006;176:173–80.
23. Lin WW, Hsieh SL. Decoy receptor 3: a pleiotropic immunomodulator and biomarker for inflammatory diseases, autoimmune diseases and cancer. Biochem Pharmacol. 2011;81:838–47.
24. Chang YC, Chen TC, Lee CT, Yang CY, Wang HW, Wang CC, Hsieh SL. Epigenetic control of MHC class II expression in tumor-associated macrophages by decoy receptor 3. Blood. 2008;111:5054–63.
25. Tai SK, Chang HC, Lan KL, Lee CT, Yang CY, Chen NJ, Chou TY, Tarng DC, Hsieh SL. Decoy receptor 3 enhances tumor progression via induction of tumor-associated macrophages. J Immunol. 2012;188:2464–71.
26. Mucke L, Masliah E, Yu GQ, Mallory M, Rockenstein EM, Tatsuno G, Hu K, Kholodenko D, Johnson-Wood K, McConlogue L. High-level neuronal expression of abeta 1-42 in wild-type human amyloid protein precursor transgenic mice: synaptotoxicity without plaque formation. J Neurosci. 2000;20:4050–8.
27. Cheng IH, Scearce-Levie K, Legleiter J, Palop JJ, Gerstein H, Bien-Ly N, Puolivali J, Lesne S, Ashe KH, Muchowski PJ, Mucke L. Accelerating amyloid-beta fibrillization reduces oligomer levels and functional deficits in Alzheimer disease mouse models. J Biol Chem. 2007;282:23818–28.
28. Sinclair LI, Tayler HM, Love S. Synaptic protein levels altered in vascular dementia. Neuropathol Appl Neurobiol. 2015;41:533–43.
29. Shao CY, Mirra SS, Sait HB, Sacktor TC, Sigurdsson EM. Postsynaptic degeneration as revealed by PSD-95 reduction occurs after advanced Abeta and tau pathology in transgenic mouse models of Alzheimer's disease. Acta Neuropathol. 2011;122:285–92.
30. Ramirez-Amaya V, Balderas I, Sandoval J, Escobar ML, Bermudez-Rattoni F. Spatial long-term memory is related to mossy fiber synaptogenesis. J Neurosci. 2001;21:7340–8.
31. Gilbert PE, Brushfield AM. The role of the CA3 hippocampal subregion in spatial memory: a process oriented behavioral assessment. Prog Neuropsychopharmacol Biol Psychiatry. 2009;33:774–81.
32. Bolmont T, Haiss F, Eicke D, Radde R, Mathis CA, Klunk WE, Kohsaka S, Jucker M, Calhoun ME. Dynamics of the microglial/amyloid interaction indicate a role in plaque maintenance. J Neurosci. 2008;28:4283–92.
33. Yan P, Hu X, Song H, Yin K, Bateman RJ, Cirrito JR, Xiao Q, Hsu FF, Turk JW, Xu J, et al. Matrix metalloproteinase-9 degrades amyloid-beta fibrils in vitro and compact plaques in situ. J Biol Chem. 2006;281:24566–74.
34. Watanabe N, Araki W, Chui DH, Makifuchi T, Ihara Y, Tabira T. Glypican-1 as an Abeta binding HSPG in the human brain: its localization in DIG domains and possible roles in the pathogenesis of Alzheimer's disease. FASEB J. 2004;18:1013–5.
35. Kaur C, Sivakumar V, Yip GW, Ling EA. Expression of syndecan-2 in the amoeboid microglial cells and its involvement in inflammation in the hypoxic developing brain. Glia. 2009;57:336–49.
36. Pitti RM, Marsters SA, Lawrence DA, Roy M, Kischkel FC, Dowd P, Huang A, Donahue CJ, Sherwood SW, Baldwin DT, et al. Genomic amplification of a decoy receptor for Fas ligand in lung and colon cancer. Nature. 1998;396:699–703.
37. Sandwall E, O'Callaghan P, Zhang X, Lindahl U, Lannfelt L, Li JP. Heparan sulfate mediates amyloid-beta internalization and cytotoxicity. Glycobiology. 2010;20:533–41.
38. O'Callaghan P, Li JP, Lannfelt L, Lindahl U, Zhang X. Microglial heparan sulfate proteoglycans facilitate the cluster-of-differentiation 14 (CD14)/toll-like receptor 4 (TLR4)-dependent inflammatory response. J Biol Chem. 2015; 290:14904–14.
39. Zhan Y, Paolicelli RC, Sforazzini F, Weinhard L, Bolasco G, Pagani F, Vyssotski AL, Bifone A, Gozzi A, Ragozzino D, Gross CT. Deficient neuron-microglia signaling results in impaired functional brain connectivity and social behavior. Nat Neurosci. 2014;17:400–6.
40. Hong S, Beja-Glasser VF, Nfonoyim BM, Frouin A, Li S, Ramakrishnan S, Merry KM, Shi Q, Rosenthal A, Barres BA, et al. Complement and microglia mediate early synapse loss in Alzheimer mouse models. Science. 2016;352:712–6.
41. Simard AR, Soulet D, Gowing G, Julien JP, Rivest S. Bone marrow-derived microglia play a critical role in restricting senile plaque formation in Alzheimer's disease. Neuron. 2006;49:489–502.
42. Fu AK, Hung KW, Yuen MY, Zhou X, Mak DS, Chan IC, Cheung TH, Zhang B, Fu WY, Liew FY, Ip NY. IL-33 ameliorates Alzheimer's disease-like pathology and cognitive decline. Proc Natl Acad Sci U S A. 2016;113:2705-2713.

43. Perego C, Fumagalli S, De Simoni MG. Temporal pattern of expression and colocalization of microglia/macrophage phenotype markers following brain ischemic injury in mice. J Neuroinflammation. 2011;8:174.
44. Ohtaki H, Ylostalo JH, Foraker JE, Robinson AP, Reger RL, Shioda S, Prockop DJ. Stem/progenitor cells from bone marrow decrease neuronal death in global ischemia by modulation of inflammatory/immune responses. Proc Natl Acad Sci U S A. 2008;105:14638–43.
45. Ye L, Huang Y, Zhao L, Li Y, Sun L, Zhou Y, Qian G, Zheng JC. IL-1beta and TNF-alpha induce neurotoxicity through glutamate production: a potential role for neuronal glutaminase. J Neurochem. 2013;125:897–908.
46. Martinez FO, Gordon S. The M1 and M2 paradigm of macrophage activation: time for reassessment. F1000Prime Rep. 2014;6:13.
47. Dong W, Embury CM, Lu Y, Whitmire SM, Dyavarshetty B, Gelbard HA, Gendelman HE, Kiyota T. The mixed-lineage kinase 3 inhibitor URMC-099 facilitates microglial amyloid-beta degradation. J Neuroinflammation. 2016;13:184.
48. Ransohoff RM. A polarizing question: do M1 and M2 microglia exist? Nat Neurosci. 2016;19:987–91.
49. Fujisaka S, Usui I, Bukhari A, Ikutani M, Oya T, Kanatani Y, Tsuneyama K, Nagai Y, Takatsu K, Urakaze M, et al. Regulatory mechanisms for adipose tissue M1 and M2 macrophages in diet-induced obese mice. Diabetes. 2009;58:2574–82.
50. Jablonski KA, Amici SA, Webb LM, Ruiz-Rosado Jde D, Popovich PG, Partida-Sanchez S, Guerau-de-Arellano M. Novel markers to delineate murine M1 and M2 macrophages. PLoS One. 2015;10:e0145342.
51. Schafer DP, Lehrman EK, Kautzman AG, Koyama R, Mardinly AR, Yamasaki R, Ransohoff RM, Greenberg ME, Barres BA, Stevens B. Microglia sculpt postnatal neural circuits in an activity and complement-dependent manner. Neuron. 2012;74:691–705.
52. Parkhurst CN, Yang G, Ninan I, Savas JN, Yates 3rd JR, Lafaille JJ, Hempstead BL, Littman DR, Gan WB. Microglia promote learning-dependent synapse formation through brain-derived neurotrophic factor. Cell. 2013;155:1596–609.
53. Wisniewski HM, Wegiel J, Wang KC, Lach B. Ultrastructural studies of the cells forming amyloid in the cortical vessel wall in Alzheimer's disease. Acta Neuropathol. 1992;84:117–27.
54. Ma Y, Bao J, Zhao X, Shen H, Lv J, Ma S, Zhang X, Li Z, Wang S, Wang Q, Ji J. Activated cyclin-dependent kinase 5 promotes microglial phagocytosis of fibrillar beta-amyloid by up-regulating lipoprotein lipase expression. Mol Cell Proteomics. 2013;12:2833–44.
55. Condello C, Yuan P, Schain A, Grutzendler J. Microglia constitute a barrier that prevents neurotoxic protofibrillar Abeta42 hotspots around plaques. Nat Commun. 2015;6:6176.
56. Marsh SE, Abud EM, Lakatos A, Karimzadeh A, Yeung ST, Davtyan H, Fote GM, Lau L, Weinger JG, Lane TE, et al. The adaptive immune system restrains Alzheimer's disease pathogenesis by modulating microglial function. Proc Natl Acad Sci U S A. 2016;113:E1316–1325.
57. Zhang B, Gaiteri C, Bodea LG, Wang Z, McElwee J, Podtelezhnikov AA, Zhang C, Xie T, Tran L, Dobrin R, et al. Integrated systems approach identifies genetic nodes and networks in late-onset Alzheimer's disease. Cell. 2013;153:707–20.
58. Ritzel RM, Patel AR, Pan S, Crapser J, Hammond M, Jellison E, McCullough LD. Age- and location-related changes in microglial function. Neurobiol Aging. 2015;36:2153–63.
59. Pan XD, Zhu YG, Lin N, Zhang J, Ye QY, Huang HP, Chen XC. Microglial phagocytosis induced by fibrillar beta-amyloid is attenuated by oligomeric beta-amyloid: implications for Alzheimer's disease. Mol Neurodegener. 2011;6:45.
60. Wang Y, Cella M, Mallinson K, Ulrich JD, Young KL, Robinette ML, Gilfillan S, Krishnan GM, Sudhakar S, Zinselmeyer BH, et al. TREM2 lipid sensing sustains the microglial response in an Alzheimer's disease model. Cell. 2015;160:1061–71.
61. Bhattacharjee S, Zhao Y, Lukiw WJ. Deficits in the miRNA-34a-regulated endogenous TREM2 phagocytosis sensor-receptor in Alzheimer's disease (AD); an update. Front Aging Neurosci. 2014;6:116.
62. Kiyota T, Gendelman HE, Weir RA, Higgins EE, Zhang G, Jain M. CCL2 affects beta-amyloidosis and progressive neurocognitive dysfunction in a mouse model of Alzheimer's disease. Neurobiol Aging. 2013;34:1060–8.
63. van Horssen J, Otte-Holler I, David G, Maat-Schieman ML, van den Heuvel LP, Wesseling P, de Waal RM, Verbeek MM. Heparan sulfate proteoglycan expression in cerebrovascular amyloid beta deposits in Alzheimer's disease and hereditary cerebral hemorrhage with amyloidosis (Dutch) brains. Acta Neuropathol. 2001;102:604–14.
64. Liu CC, Zhao N, Yamaguchi Y, Cirrito JR, Kanekiyo T, Holtzman DM, Bu G. Neuronal heparan sulfates promote amyloid pathology by modulating brain amyloid-beta clearance and aggregation in Alzheimer's disease. Sci Transl Med. 2016;8:332ra344.
65. O'Callaghan P, Sandwall E, Li JP, Yu H, Ravid R, Guan ZZ, van Kuppevelt TH, Nilsson LN, Ingelsson M, Hyman BT, et al. Heparan sulfate accumulation with Abeta deposits in Alzheimer's disease and Tg2576 mice is contributed by glial cells. Brain Pathol. 2008;18:548–61.
66. Schulz JG, Annaert W, Vandekerckhove J, Zimmermann P, De Strooper B, David G. Syndecan 3 intramembrane proteolysis is presenilin/gamma-secretase-dependent and modulates cytosolic signaling. J Biol Chem. 2003;278:48651–7.
67. Zhang X, Wu C, Song J, Gotte M, Sorokin L. Syndecan-1, a cell surface proteoglycan, negatively regulates initial leukocyte recruitment to the brain across the choroid plexus in murine experimental autoimmune encephalomyelitis. J Immunol. 2013;191:4551–61.
68. Zhang X, Li JP. Heparan sulfate proteoglycans in amyloidosis. Prog Mol Biol Transl Sci. 2010;93:309–34.
69. Simard JM, Tosun C, Ivanova S, Kurland DB, Hong C, Radecki L, Gisriel C, Mehta R, Schreibman D, Gerzanich V. Heparin reduces neuroinflammation and transsynaptic neuronal apoptosis in a model of subarachnoid hemorrhage. Transl Stroke Res. 2012;3:155–65.
70. Imbimbo BP, Solfrizzi V, Panza F. Are NSAIDs useful to treat Alzheimer's disease or mild cognitive impairment? Front Aging Neurosci. 2010;2:19.
71. Solomon SD, Wittes J, Finn PV, Fowler R, Viner J, Bertagnolli MM, Arber N, Levin B, Meinert CL, Martin B, et al. Cardiovascular risk of celecoxib in 6 randomized placebo-controlled trials: the cross trial safety analysis. Circulation. 2008;117:2104–13.
72. Rogers J, Kirby LC, Hempelman SR, Berry DL, McGeer PL, Kaszniak AW, Zalinski J, Cofield M, Mansukhani L, Willson P, et al. Clinical trial of indomethacin in Alzheimer's disease. Neurology. 1993;43:1609–11.
73. de Jong D, Jansen R, Hoefnagels W, Jellesma-Eggenkamp M, Verbeek M, Borm G, Kremer B. No effect of one-year treatment with indomethacin on Alzheimer's disease progression: a randomized controlled trial. PLoS One. 2008;3:e1475.
74. Morihara T, Teter B, Yang F, Lim GP, Boudinot S, Boudinot FD, Frautschy SA, Cole GM. Ibuprofen suppresses interleukin-1beta induction of pro-amyloidogenic alpha1-antichymotrypsin to ameliorate beta-amyloid (Abeta) pathology in Alzheimer's models. Neuropsychopharmacology. 2005;30:1111–20.
75. Pasqualetti P, Bonomini C, Dal Forno G, Paulon L, Sinforiani E, Marra C, Zanetti O, Rossini PM. A randomized controlled study on effects of ibuprofen on cognitive progression of Alzheimer's disease. Aging Clin Exp Res. 2009;21:102–10.
76. Group AR, Martin BK, Szekely C, Brandt J, Piantadosi S, Breitner JC, Craft S, Evans D, Green R, Mullan M. Cognitive function over time in the Alzheimer's Disease Anti-inflammatory Prevention Trial (ADAPT): results of a randomized, controlled trial of naproxen and celecoxib. Arch Neurol. 2008;65:896–905.
77. Reines SA, Block GA, Morris JC, Liu G, Nessly ML, Lines CR, Norman BA, Baranak CC, Rofecoxib Protocol 091 Study G. Rofecoxib: no effect on Alzheimer's disease in a 1-year, randomized, blinded, controlled study. Neurology. 2004;62:66–71.
78. Thal LJ, Ferris SH, Kirby L, Block GA, Lines CR, Yuen E, Assaid C, Nessly ML, Norman BA, Baranak CC, et al. A randomized, double-blind, study of rofecoxib in patients with mild cognitive impairment. Neuropsychopharmacology. 2005;30:1204–15.
79. Chakrabarty P, Li A, Ceballos-Diaz C, Eddy JA, Funk CC, Moore B, DiNunno N, Rosario AM, Cruz PE, Verbeeck C, et al. IL-10 alters immunoproteostasis in APP mice, increasing plaque burden and worsening cognitive behavior. Neuron. 2015;85:519–33.
80. Guillot-Sestier MV, Doty KR, Gate D, Rodriguez Jr J, Leung BP, Rezai-Zadeh K, Town T. Il10 deficiency rebalances innate immunity to mitigate Alzheimer-like pathology. Neuron. 2015;85:534–48.
81. Latta CH, Sudduth TL, Weekman EM, Brothers HM, Abner EL, Popa GJ, Mendenhall MD, Gonzalez-Oregon F, Braun K, Wilcock DM. Determining the role of IL-4 induced neuroinflammation in microglial activity and amyloid-beta using BV2 microglial cells and APP/PS1 transgenic mice. J Neuroinflammation. 2015;12:41.
82. Wang Y, Shen D, Wang VM, Yu CR, Wang RX, Tuo J, Chan CC. Enhanced apoptosis in retinal pigment epithelium under inflammatory stimuli and oxidative stress. Apoptosis. 2012;17:1144–55.

13

Soluble oligomeric amyloid-β induces calcium dyshomeostasis that precedes synapse loss in the living mouse brain

Michal Arbel-Ornath[1†], Eloise Hudry[1†], Josiah R. Boivin[1], Tadafumi Hashimoto[1,2], Shuko Takeda[1], Kishore V. Kuchibhotla[1,3], Steven Hou[1], Carli R. Lattarulo[1], Arianna M. Belcher[1], Naomi Shakerdge[1], Pariss B. Trujillo[1], Alona Muzikansky[4], Rebecca A. Betensky[4], Bradley T. Hyman[1] and Brian J. Bacskai[1*]

Abstract

Background: Amyloid-β oligomers (oAβ) are thought to mediate neurotoxicity in Alzheimer's disease (AD), and previous studies in AD transgenic mice suggest that calcium dysregulation may contribute to these pathological effects. Even though AD mouse models remain a valuable resource to investigate amyloid neurotoxicity, the concomitant presence of soluble Aβ species, fibrillar Aβ, and fragments of amyloid precursor protein (APP) complicate the interpretation of the phenotypes.

Method: To explore the specific contribution of soluble oligomeric Aβ (oAβ) to calcium dyshomeostasis and synaptic morphological changes, we acutely exposed the healthy mouse brain, at 3 to 6 months of age, to naturally occurring soluble oligomers and investigated their effect on calcium levels using in vivo multiphoton imaging.

Results: We observed a dramatic increase in the levels of neuronal resting calcium, which was dependent upon extracellular calcium influx and activation of NMDA receptors. Ryanodine receptors, previously implicated in AD models, did not appear to be primarily involved using this experimental setting. We used the high resolution cortical volumes acquired in-vivo to measure the effect on synaptic densities and observed that, while spine density remained stable within the first hour of oAβ exposure, a significant decrease in the number of dendritic spines was observed 24 h post treatment, despite restoration of intraneuronal calcium levels at this time point.

Conclusions: These observations demonstrate a specific effect of oAβ on NMDA-mediated calcium influx, which triggers synaptic collapse in vivo. Moreover, this work leverages a method to quantitatively measure calcium concentration at the level of neuronal processes, cell bodies and single synaptic elements repeatedly and thus can be applicable to testing putative drugs and/or other intervention methodologies.

Keywords: Alzheimer's disease, Amyloid β oligomers, Calcium, In vivo imaging

Background

Alzheimer's disease (AD) is a devastating age-related neurological disorder characterized by the accumulation of extracellular amyloid β (Aβ) peptides and intraneuronal neurofibrillary tangles. Fibrillar amyloid plaques constitute a major diagnostic hallmark of the disease and correlate with deleterious local effects including gliosis, neuritic dystrophies and synapse loss [1, 2]. However, accumulating data suggest that small soluble aggregates of Aβ (oligomers, oAβ) mainly contribute to neuronal toxicity [3–7], accumulating in the vicinity of senile plaques and at the synapse [8]. Despite these important findings, no direct evidence has specifically linked the presence of oligomers in their natural form with neuronal dysfunction and spine morphological changes in vivo. While synthetic Aβ peptides have been extensively used in the past, they showed a relatively weak potency as compared with "native" oligomers from AD brains in physiological concentrations. In transgenic mice, the

* Correspondence: bbacskai@partners.org
Dr. Arbel-Ornath and Dr. Hudry are co-first authors.
†Equal contributors
[1]Alzheimer Research Unit, Department of Neurology, Massachusetts General Hospital and Harvard Medical School, 114, 16th St., Charlestown, MA 02129, USA
Full list of author information is available at the end of the article

concomitant presence of full-length human APP and its downstream catalytic fragments has prevented us from specifically addressing oAβ-related neurotoxicity. We therefore developed an assay to directly examine the consequences of naturally occurring oAβ on the intact mouse brain using longitudinal multiphoton calcium imaging, and observed acute changes in calcium homeostasis, followed by synaptic loss.

The calcium hypothesis of AD argues that Aβ peptides impact neuronal calcium homeostasis, leading to synaptic failure, spine loss, neural network disruption and cognitive deficits [9–11]. Indirect evidence suggests that calcium alterations may be an early neuropathological change associated with mild cognitive impairment in AD patients [12–14]. Aβ-induced stress has been experimentally linked with abnormal activation of calcium dependent molecular cascades [5, 15], alteration of long term potentiation [16] and memory deficits [16, 17]. The development of new calcium sensors and their combination with in vivo two-photon imaging has further allowed a direct evaluation of calcium changes in AD mouse models, demonstrating in particular a dramatic increase in resting calcium levels in a subset of neurites surrounding amyloid deposits [18]. Increased proportions of hypoactive and hyperactive neurons have been reported in transgenic animals, the latter being found in clusters near amyloid plaques [19]. At the network level, a gradual decline in visual sensory performances has been observed in APP mice, a phenomenon correlated with the amyloid load [20–22]. Intriguingly, most of these studies did not detect changes before amyloid deposition, with only one previous work reporting hyperactivity associated with synthetically cross-linked dimers in vivo [6]. Taken together, testing the hypothesis that physiologically relevant oAβ causes local neuritic calcium elevation in the intact brain has not been achieved.

In the present study, we investigated the effect of naturally occurring soluble oAβ on neuronal calcium homeostasis in adult wild type animals. Acute application of oAβ, prepared from conditioned media isolated from transgenic primary neurons (TgCM), to the mouse brain surface dramatically increased neuronal resting calcium levels, whereas no change could be observed when conditioned media collected from the wild-type littermates cultures (WtCM) was used. This effect was abolished after immunodepletion of Aβ, thus specifically linking the presence of neurotoxic oAβ with intraneuronal calcium dysregulation. Because MK-801 efficiently blocked oAβ-induced Ca^{2+} increase, we also concluded that calcium dysregulation was primarily mediated through NMDA receptors, whereas antagonists of intracellular calcium channels were ineffective. In this regard, the current work addresses a long-standing controversy about whether oAβ activates the release of internal calcium stores or opens cell surface receptors. In addition, while the calcium rise was rapidly buffered, synapse loss was only detected after 24 h, demonstrating that oAβ-induced functional alterations precede morphological changes in vivo. Lastly, the approach used here to repeatedly measure calcium concentrations in vivo in the different neuronal compartments, including soma, dendrites and synaptic elements, may find broad applications to evaluate modulators of oAβ neurotoxicity and investigate the impact of various soluble neurotoxic species relevant in other neurodegenerative diseases.

Methods

Animals

Tg2576 males (Taconic Farms), which heterozygously overexpress human APPswe under the PrP promoter, were mated with wild-type females (B6;SJL) for preparation of primary cortical neurons. In vivo imaging experiments were performed using wild-type C57BL/6 males (3–6 months of age, Charles River). Each experimental group consisted of 3 to 6 animals.

Preparation of wild type and transgenic neuronal conditioned media and Aβ immunodepletion

Cortical neurons were prepared as previously described [15] and plated on 35-mm culture dishes coated with poly-D-lysine (Sigma-Aldrich) and maintained in Neurobasal/B-27 media. Tissue from each embryo was collected and used for genotyping using PCR. Conditioned media was collected at 14 days in vitro (DIV) from either transgenic cultures (TgCM) or their wild-type littermates (WtCM). The concentrations of Aβ40 and Aβ42 were quantified by a mouse/human ELISA kit (Wako).

Immunodepletion of human Aβ from TgCM was performed overnight using the mAb 6E10 (Covance) and protein G sepharose beads (Sigma-Aldrich). Briefly, to avoid non-specific binding, protein G beads were washed with cold Neurobasal medium and incubated with 1 ml of TgCM for 30 min at 4 °C while shaking. The mixture was then centrifuged and the beads were discarded. The supernatant was further incubated with 100 μl pre-washed protein G beads and 9 μg of 6E10 antibody for 5 h at 4 °C while shaking. The supernatant was then collected and Aβ content was measured using a human/mouse ELISA kit (Wako).

Size exclusion chromatography of condition media

Size exclusion chromatography (SEC) was performed as previously described [5]. Briefly, TgCM or WtCM was collected from 14 DIV neurons and centrifuged at 3,000 g at 4 °C in Amicon Ultra-15ML 3 K to concentrate proteins approximately fivefold. Concentrated TgCM or WtCM was separated by tandem Superdex 75 10/300 GL columns in 50 mM ammonium acetate, pH 8.5, with AKTA purifier 10 and dialyzed against PBS. Aβ40 content within the different fractions was measured after dialysis of the fractions with PBS using mouse/human ELISA kit (Wako). Fractions were also subjected to oligomer-specific ELISA kit (IBL). Assay was performed according to the manufacture instructions.

Viral vector construction and production

The YC3.6 cDNA was cloned into an AAV2 backbone, under a hybrid cytomegalovirus (CMV) immediate-early enhancer/chicken β-actin promoter/exon1/intron and before the woodchuck hepatitis virus posttranscriptional regulatory element (WPRE). High titers of AAV serotype 8 were produced using the triple transfection protocol by both the Harvard and UPENN Vector Cores. Viruses were tittered by quantitative PCR and the final concentrations of these AAV viral stocks reached $4x10^{12}$ vg/ml.

Stereotactic intraparenchymal injection of AAV-CBA-YC3.6

Stereotactic intracortical injections of AAV-CBA-YC3.6 were performed as described previously [23]. Briefly, animals were anesthetized by intraperitoneal injection of ketamine/xylazine (100 mg/kg and 50 mg/kg body weight, respectively) and positioned on a stereotactic frame (Kopf Instruments). Injections of vector were performed in the somatosensory cortex with 3 μl of viral suspension using a 33-gauge sharp needle attached to a 10-μl Hamilton syringe (Hamilton Medical), at a rate of 0.1 μl/min. Stereotactic coordinates of the injection sites were calculated from bregma (anteroposterior −1 mm, mediolateral ± 1 mm and dorsoventral – 1 mm).

Cranial window implantation

One month after injection of AAV-CBA-YC3.6, mice were anesthetized with isoflurane (1–1.5%) and a cranial window was implanted by removing a piece of skull above the somatosensory cortex and replacing it with a 8 mm diameter cover glass (as described previously [24]). For all experiments, the dura mater was removed prior to window installation. Texas Red dextran (70 kDa; 12.5 mg/ml in PBS; Molecular Probes) was injected into a lateral tail vein before imaging to provide a fluorescent angiogram. Mice were imaged first to determine resting calcium at baseline. The window was then opened and closed again along with either WtCM, TgCM or depleted-TgCM diluted 1:1 with PBS (final volume applied was 50 μl). The window, containing the applied solution, was then resealed with dental cement. One hour later, each animal was reimaged at the same fields of view to determine the relative changes in $[Ca^{2+}]$ $(\Delta R/Ri)_i$. To test the effect of different calcium channel inhibitors, both dantrolene (5 μM) and MK-801 (5 μM) were incubated on the brain for 10 min before topical application with TgCM and each inhibitor mixed together for another hour.

In vitro resting calcium imaging and measurements

To evaluate the effect of calcium channel antagonists in vitro using Tg2576 primary neurons, we used two different ratiometric calcium indicators, indo-1 AM (Life technologies) and YC3.6. For indo 1- experiments, 10–12 DIV cultures were incubated with 5 μM indo-1 AM for 45 min before imaging. For YC3.6 experiments, cells were transfected at 7 DIV with a pAAV-CBA-YC3.6 plasmid, using Lipofectamine 2000 (Life technologies), and imaged 2–3 days later. In both cases, hAPPsw transgenic neurons were imaged before and after bath application of an antagonist to calcium channels, using an LSM510 confocal microscope (Zeiss) with an environmental chamber that maintains constant conditions of 37 °C and 5% CO_2. In the case of indo-1, a chameleon laser (Coherent, Inc) generated two photon excitation at 750 nm and emitted light was collected at 390–465 nm and 468–533 nm corresponding to the calcium bound and unbound dye, respectively. For YC3.6 experiments, single photon excitation was used at 458 nm using an argon laser, and emitted light was collected using the 435–485 BP and 505 LP filters for detection of CFP and YFP fluorescence, respectively. We tested the effect of the following agents on resting calcium levels in transgenic neurons: $NiCl_2$ (100 μM), nifedipine (5 μM), ω-conotoxin (1 μM), MK-801 (5 μM), 2-APB (100 μM) and dantrolene (10 μM). All pharmacological agents were purchased from Sigma-Aldrich and dissolved either in double distilled water (ddw) or DMSO according to the manufacturer instructions. For indo-1 AM experiments, 5–6 fields of view were imaged randomly before and 10–15 min after bath application of the inhibitor. During culture experiments with YC3.6, a limited number of neurons were transfected, allowing us to reimage the same cells before and after treatment and thus to calculate the relative change in YFP/CFP ratio for each cell (ΔR/Ri). Each experiment was repeated over 3–4 independent trials.

In vivo multiphoton imaging

For in vivo calcium imaging, an Olympus FluoView FV1000MPE multiphoton laser-scanning system mounted on an Olympus BX61WI microscope and an Olympus 25× dipping objective (NA = 1.05) were used. A DeepSee Mai Tai Ti:sapphire mode-locked laser (Mai Tai; Spectra-Physics) generated two-photon excitation at 860 nm, and detectors containing three photomultiplier tubes (Hamamatsu, Ichinocho) collected emitted light in the range of 460–500, 520–560 and 575–630 nm. Mice were placed on the microscope stage and heated using a heating pad with feedback regulation from a rectal temperature probe (Harvard apparatus). Four to six cortical volumes (Z-series, 127 μm × 127 μm, 2 μm slices, depth of 200–300 μm) were taken per mouse, before and after topical application of conditioned media, at a resolution of 512 × 512 pixels. Because of those imaging settings (small field of view and slow scan speed) we mostly did not record any type of neuronal oscillations (1.66 s per frame > 1Hz). CFP and YFP PMTs settings remained unchanged throughout the different imaging sessions. Laser power was adjusted as needed.

Image processing and analysis

Cell cultures

Cells were imaged using a confocal Zeiss LSM510 system. Images were processed and analyzed using ImageJ software (https://imagej.nih.gov/ij/). For indo-1 experiments, single plane images of channels corresponding to calcium bound and unbound dye were obtained. For each channel, the background, corresponding to the mode of the image, was subtracted and a median filter with radius 2 was applied before dividing the emitted fluorescence intensity of the calcium bound channel by the unbound dye channel, thus creating a ratio-image. For YC3.6 experiments, single channels corresponding to CFP and YFP fluorescence were processed in the same way described for indo-1, creating a YFP/CFP ratio image. In both cases, cell bodies were manually selected using the free hand tool, before and after application of an antagonist. The selected regions of interest were then placed on the ratio image and measured. To convert the measured ratios, either for indo-1 or YC3.6, into calcium concentrations, calibration experiments were performed in CHO cells using each calcium indicator and solutions with either zero or 39 μM calcium in the presence of ionomycin (20 μM, Life Technologies). This allowed the determination of the Rmin and Rmax for each indicator (indo-1: Rmin = 0.54, Rmax = 3.04, YC3.6: Rmin = 0.19, Rmax = 1.618). Ratios were then converted to actual calcium concentration using the indo-1 K_D (250nM) and the K_D of YC3.6 (278nM) with standard ratiometric equations [25, 26]:

$$[Ca2+]i = Kd'\left(\frac{R-Rmin}{Rmax-R}\right)^{1/n};\ Kd' = Kd\left(\frac{Sf2}{Sb2}\right)^{1/n}$$

Sf2 and *Sb2* represent the intensities at calcium free and calcium bound of the denominator (i.e. YFP or Indo-1 at 400 nm).

Pseudocolored images presented were created in Matlab based on each indicator ratio, which was then converted to calcium concentration using the empirical Rmin and Rmax and assigned to the jet colormap. We used the ratio values to supply the Hue and Saturation (color) and the reference image to supply the Value (intensity).

In vivo

Image stacks were processed in Image J as follows: the background of CFP and YFP channels, corresponding to the mode of the deepest slice of the z-stack, was subtracted, and a median filter (radius 2) was applied before dividing the emitted fluorescence intensity of YFP by CFP, thus creating a ratio image. Neurites, cell bodies and dendritic spines were identified and selected using the YFP images. The YFP/CFP ratio was then measured for each ROI using the ratio images. YFP/CFP ratios were converted to $[Ca^{2+}]_i$ with standard ratiometric equations (see above) using the in situ K_D and Hill coefficient of YC3.6 we have previously determined [18]. We established the dynamic range of the indicator in-vivo, using the same in vivo experimental settings as all our in vivo experiments. Rmin and Rmax were calculated using the lowest 2.5% of plaque-associated neuritic dystrophies (in AD transgenic mice) and the upper 2.5% of neurites in a dying mouse, respectively (Rmin = 0.79, Rmax = 4.5).

Dendritic Spine analysis

2D projections of YFP-filled neurites were obtained in ImageJ. Dendrites of at least 20 μm long with prominent dendritic spine protrusions, were considered for analysis. Spines were selected manually and the relative changes in spine density were calculated for each neurite as compared with the average spine density before treatment for each animal. The nature of the treatment was kept blinded until statistical analyses.

Statistical analyses

To assess whether ΔR/Ri values were different between the treatment groups in Neurite, Soma and Spines, a linear mixed effects model was fitted with treatment group as fixed effect and mouse as random effect. The same model was used for the analysis of Spine density.

To assess whether there was a difference between before vs. after CM application measurements in each group separately, a linear mixed effect model was fitted for each treatment group predicting the difference (after-before) with a fixed effect of an intercept only and a random effect of mouse.

YFP/CFP ratios were pooled and presented in histograms. Histograms for each group before treatment was fitted with a normal distribution curve using the Graph Pad curve fitting tool. Fisher exact test was used for comparison of calcium overload before and after treatment within each group. For the cell culture data, one way ANOVA with post hoc Dunn's multiple comparison test was used for comparison of ΔR/Ri for each group and its vehicle treatment group (ddw or DMSO).

Results

Acute exposure of naturally occurring oAβ to the healthy living brain disrupts intraneuronal calcium homeostasis and synaptic integrity in vivo

Previous works have established that resting calcium levels and neuronal function are affected in transgenic mice with plaques, whereas no change was observed before amyloid deposition in most studies [18–21]. We have previously observed that TgCM treatment of wild type cortical neurons in vitro induced AD-like morphological changes that include calcium dyshomeostasis, calcineurin activation [15], dendritic spine loss and neuritic simplification [5].

To appreciate the specific contribution of soluble oAβ species to calcium dysregulation, we designed an acute in vivo assay of Aβ neurotoxicity by topically applying oAβ-enriched medium on the cortical surface of wild-type C57BL/6 mice. Culture medium from primary cortical neurons derived from Tg2576 embryos was used as a source of soluble oAβ (termed TgCM), which mainly contains low molecular weight oligomers (dimers to tetramers) as evidence from size exclusion chromatography (SEC) followed by Aβ40 ELISA (Additional file 1: Figure S1) [5, 15, 27]. To validate the presence of oAβ in the TgCM, the different SEC fractions were also subjected to oligomeric Aβ ELISA (IBL) that utilizes the same antibody for capture and detection. Additional file 1: Figure S1B shows the presence of oAβ (at much lower levels compared to total Aβ40 signal) in both the high and low molecular weight fractions. Higher levels were detected between fractions 11 and 16, which corresponds to 13.7 kDa and smaller, very low levels were detected at fractions 25–28, which correspond to 6.5 kDa and lower. However, the signal at these fractions was very close to the limit of the ELISA kit sensitivity. This data suggest that that most Aβ oligomers within the TgCM are of low molecular weight.

Conditioned media from non-Tg neurons (termed WtCM) and Aβ immunodepleted TgCM were used as controls. Within different batches of TgCM, Aβ40 and Aβ42 concentration respectively reached 4-8nM and 130–260pM, which corresponds to the levels detected in human cerebral spinal fluid [28]. Additionally, the concentration of oAβ in the TgCM reached 400pM to 600pM, representing 7.5–10% of the total amount of $A\beta_{40}$. The content of murine Aβ40 in several batches of WtCM ranged from 200pM to 500pM while murine Aβ42 could not be detected.

To quantify absolute calcium levels in the brain, mice were injected with an AAV8 encoding the ratiometric calcium indicator yellow-cameleon YC3.6 [29]. Four weeks later, a craniotomy was performed above the somatosensory cortex and CFP and YFP fluorescent signals were measured. After evaluating the baseline neuronal resting calcium, the cranial window was reopened and either TgCM or WtCM, diluted 1:1 in PBS (final concentration of Aβ40 of 2nM in TgCM and 180pM in WtCM), was directly applied to the brain surface. Using the labeled brain vasculature as a guide, we were able to reimage the same field of view and calculate the relative changes in intracellular calcium. We imaged the first 300 μm of the cortical surface, which consist of neurites and cell bodies located in layers II/III (Figs. 1a and 2a).

Using the YC3.6 K_D (278nM) previously calculated in cultures [18] and the dynamic range of the indicator (Rmin and Rmax) obtained from the in-vivo data acquired using the same microscope under the same settings (see Methods), we converted YFP/CFP ratios into absolute calcium concentrations. Our measurements indicate that $[Ca^{2+}]$ i is tightly regulated in wild type mice and reaches 70 ± 4nM on average. The values of $[Ca^{2+}]$ i in neurites in wild type brain generally follow a normal distribution (Fig. 1c, $r^2 = 0.99$). As expected, only rare neurites would be classified as having calcium overload at baseline (threshold defined as $[Ca^{2+}]$ i greater than two SD above the mean of all neurites in the first imaging session, 90nM). Topical application of TgCM to the healthy brain progressively increased the YFP/CFP ratios and thus $[Ca^{2+}]$ i, which reached a peak after an hour before returning to baseline levels by 5 h (Additional file 2: Figure S2). One-hour exposure with TgCM induced a dramatic elevation of intraneuronal calcium, as evident in the pseudocolored images and the right shift of the calcium distribution curves towards higher YFP/CFP ratio values (Fig. 1b, c). TgCM incubation resulted in a greater number of calcium-overloaded neurites (threshold for calcium overload is represented by a black line; $n = 295$ neurites in 5 mice, calcium overload: before = 3.09%, after = 25.82%, $p < 0.0001$ Fisher exact test). Conversely, when mice were incubated with WtCM, no significant change in calcium levels was observed ($n = 409$ neurites in 5 mice, calcium overload: before = 3.8%, after = 1.38%, $p = 0.643$ Fisher exact test). To demonstrate that TgCM-induced elevation of $[Ca^{2+}]_I$ was directly related to the presence of Aβ peptides in the medium, we immunodepleted human Aβ from the TgCM and followed the same experimental settings. Immunodepletion of Aβ with 6E10 antibody effectively removed about 80% of Aβ present in TgCM (initial concentration of Aβ40 in TgCM: 4.1nM, after immunodepletion: 0.8nM). The effect of TgCM was abolished after immunodepletion and only a modest non-significant trend of calcium overload was detected ($n = 206$ neurites in 3 mice, calcium overload: before = 1.9%, after = 5.8%, $p = 0.07$ Fisher exact test, comparison of before and after YFP/CFP ratios $p < 0.2847$).

Comparing resting calcium before and after treatment within the same neuronal processes, we observed that

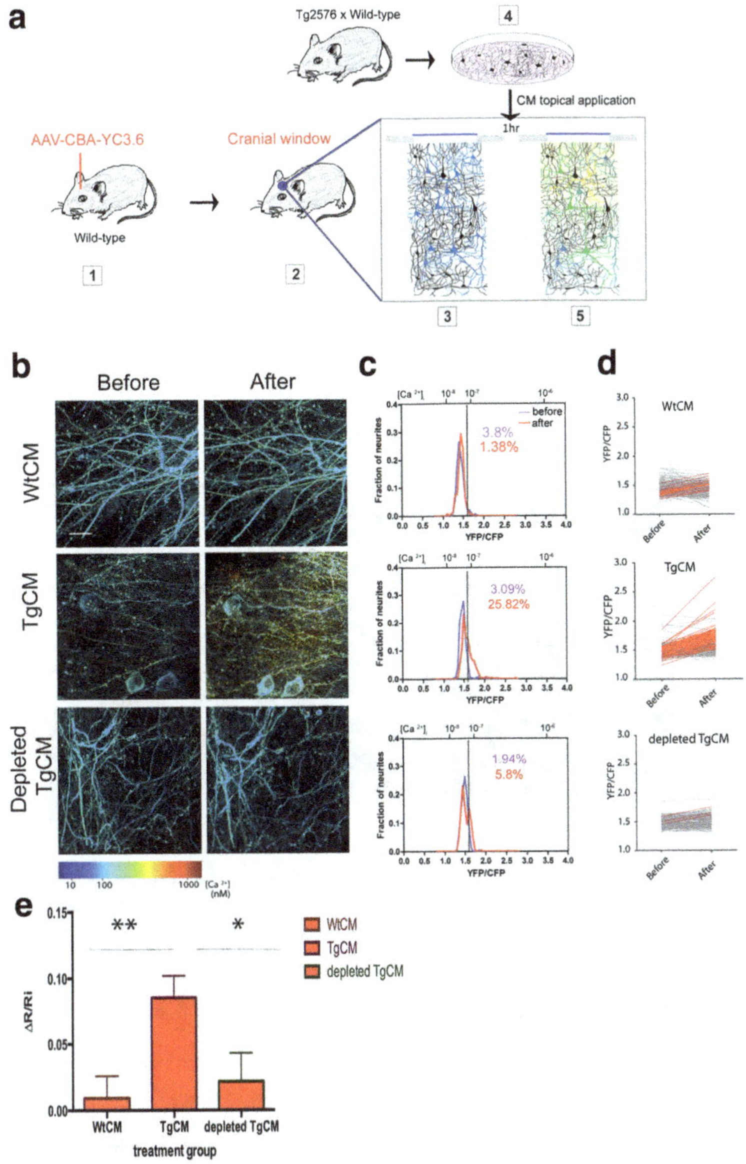

Fig. 1 Oligomeric Aβ induces calcium overload in the healthy mouse brain. **a** A new experimental setting was designed to specifically address the effect of oAβ on calcium homeostasis in vivo. Wild-type C57BL/6 mice were injected with an AAV-CBA-YC3.6 and a cranial window was installed 4 weeks later. After a first imaging session at baseline, the window was opened and WtCM, TgCM or depleted TgCM was topically applied for 1 hour before reimaging again the exact same fields of view. **b** Neurites, consisting of dendrites and axons, filled with YC3.6 were imaged before and after treatment with TgCM, WtCM or depleted-TgCM. Images were pseudocolored according to calcium concentration (Scale bar = 20 μm). **c** Individual neurites were selected for measuring YFP and CFP ratio and calculating resting calcium levels. Distribution curves of $[Ca^{2+}]_i$ (YFP/CFP ratio on the lower x-axis and $[Ca^{2+}]_i$ on the upper x-axis) are presented before (*purple curve*) and after treatment (*red curve*) for each experimental group. Acute exposure to TgCM, but not to WtCM or immunodepleted-TgCM, resulted in a shift in the $[Ca^{2+}]_i$ distribution towards higher ratio values, i.e. higher calcium concentrations. The *black* line indicates the threshold for calcium overload which represents 2 SD above the mean of ratios measured from all mice before treatment. The percentage of neurites with calcium overload before (*purple*) and after (*red*) treatment is noted on the graphs. Calcium overload was only significantly increased in the TgCM treated group from 3.09 to 25.82% ($p < 0.0001$ Fisher exact test). **d** YFP/CFP ratios before and after treatment with WtCM, TgCM or depleted TgCM represented for each neurite. The *red* traces account for the neurites that showed an increase of ≥10% in YFP/CFP ratio after topical application of CM. **e** The relative change in ratio was calculated for each neurite and the mean + SEM of each group is presented (linear mixed effects model fitted with treatment group as fixed effect and mouse as random effect ** $p = 0.0012$, *$p = 0.0183$)

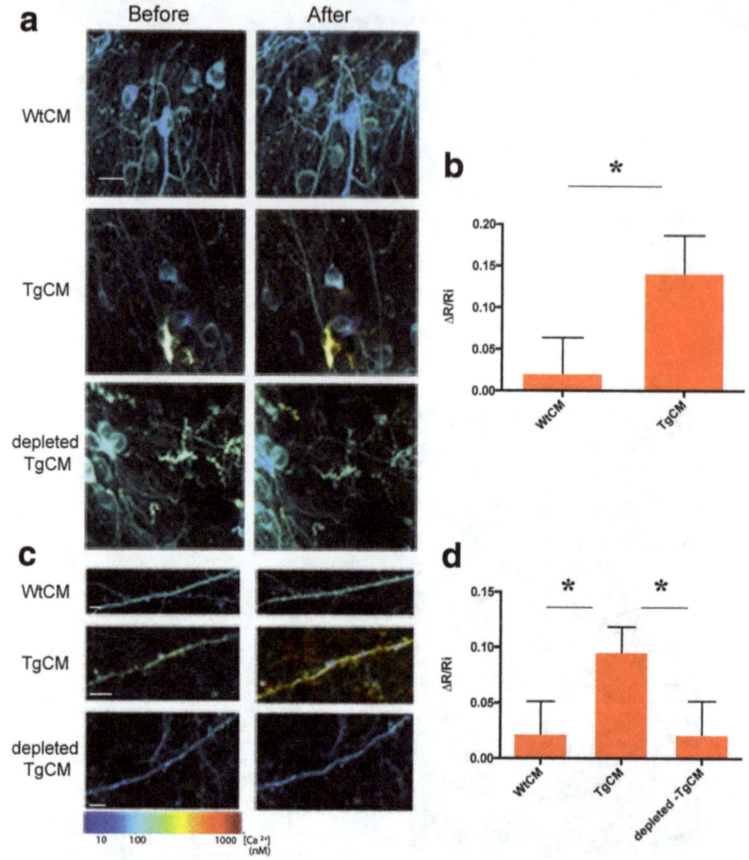

Fig. 2 Oligomeric Aβ induces calcium overload in neuronal cell bodies and dendritic spines. Neuronal cell bodies (**a**,**b**) or dendritic spines (**c**,**d**) were imaged before and 1 h after treatment with conditioned media, and the YFP/CFP ratio and resting calcium were calculated for each compartment. Images were pseudocolored according to calcium concentrations. **b** In cell bodies, TgCM, but not WtCM, induced an increase in resting calcium. (TgCM: $n = 165$ cells, WtCM: $n = 157$ cells, in 5 mice, pair-wise comparison of the relative change in YC ratio, * $p = 0.0458$). **d** TgCM effect on YC ratio in dendritic spines followed the same trend as neurites and was significantly different from that of WtCM and depleted-TgCM (pair-wise analysis TgCM vs. WtCM * $p = 0.0466$; TgCM vs. depleted-TgCM * $p = 0.0494$; WtCM vs. depleted-TgCM $p = 0.9916$). Scale bars = 20 μm in (**a**) and 5 μm in (**c**)

the YFP/CFP ratios were increased by 10% or more for the vast majority of TgCM-treated neurites, whereas such a change was only occasionally observed after WtCM and depleted-TgCM incubation (Fig. 1d). From these values we calculated the relative change in YFP/CFP ratio for each neurite (ΔR/Ri, Fig. 1e) and showed that TgCM induced an average increase in the YFP/CFP ratio of 8.5 ± 1.6% (from 70nM to about 85nM). Application of TgCM was significantly different from that of WtCM and depleted-TgCM while the later two groups were not different from each other (Fig. 1e, linear mixed effect model. Overall change between the groups $p = 0.0029$, post hoc comparisons between every 2 groups: $p = 0.0012$ TgCM vs. WtCM; $p = 0.0183$ TgCM vs. depleted TgCM; $p = 0.6507$ WtCM vs. depleted-TgCM. $n = 295$ neurites within 5 mice for TgCM, 405 neurites within 5 mice for WtCM and 206 neurites picked from 3 mice for depleted-TgCM).

When only the overloaded neurites after TgCM treatment were analyzed, the average reached a mean change of 16.9 ± 4.8% (from 70nM to 100nM). Reimaging the same fields and analyzing the YFP/CFP ratios in the same neurites 5 h post treatment did not show any change from baseline (Additional file 2: Figure S2), suggesting that elevation in $[Ca^{2+}]_i$ was a transient event rapidly buffered in the healthy brain of wild type mice.

When cell bodies were selected (Fig. 2a and b), resting calcium concentration at baseline was lower than the level measured in neurites, averaging at 58nM. Exposure with oligomeric Aβ also disrupted calcium homeostasis in the neuronal soma as compared with WtCM treatment (ΔR/Ri : TgCM 14.4 ± 4.25%, WtCM 2.09 ± 4.2%, pair-wise comparison, $p = 0.0458$). However, we could not analyze the depleted –TgCM as we could trace cell bodies only in one of 3 mice tested. TgCM treatment effect was significantly different from that of WtCM.

Dendritic spines showed indistinguishable $[Ca^{2+}]_i$ from that of the neurites (Fig. 2c, d; YFP/CFP ratios corresponding to about 72 ± 10nM and 70 ± 4nM in spines and neurites, respectively). Similarly to our observations in neurites, TgCM application led to a 9.6% ± 2.3% increase in calcium levels (comparison before and after TgCM: $p = 0.0268$). WtCM and depleted-TgCM application did not have any effect (before vs. after comparison; WtCM: $p = 0.3736$, depleted-TgCM: $p = 0.5552$). The effect of TgCM on the relative change in calcium was significantly different from that of WtCM and depleted TgCM, which did not differ from each others (pair-wise comparisons; TgCM vs. WtCM $p = 0.0466$, TgCM vs. depleted TgCM $p = 0.0494$, WtCM vs. depleted TgCM $p = 0.9916$). In contrast with the acute and dramatic impact of oAβ on intraneuronal calcium, no change in spine density was detected 1 h after treatment with TgCM (relative change compared with the average spine density before treatment: −0.2% ± 4.1%, $p = 0.9502$, 760 spines counted in 4 mice) or with WtCM (relative change compared with the average spine density before treatment: 2.2% ± 5.3%, $p = 0.708$ 578 spines counted within 3 mice, Fig. 3). However, a robust decrease in the density of dendritic spines was observed 24 h after TgCM application (relative change compared with the average spine density before treatment: −28.7% ± 4.3%, $p < 0.0001$, $n = 635$ spines within 3 mice, Fig. 3), at a time when the calcium levels were restored to baseline (Additional file 2: Figure S2). By contrast, non-significant change in spine density was observed 24 h post application of WtCM (relative change compared with the average spine density before treatment (8.9% ± 4%, $p = 0.0555$, 1382 spines counted within 3 mice, Fig. 3), suggesting that this observation did not derive from the surgical procedure itself. Pair-wise analysis between the two groups (TgCM/WtCM) showed no difference at 1 h ($p = 0.7463$) and significant change in spine density at 24 h ($p < 0.0001$) after treatment.

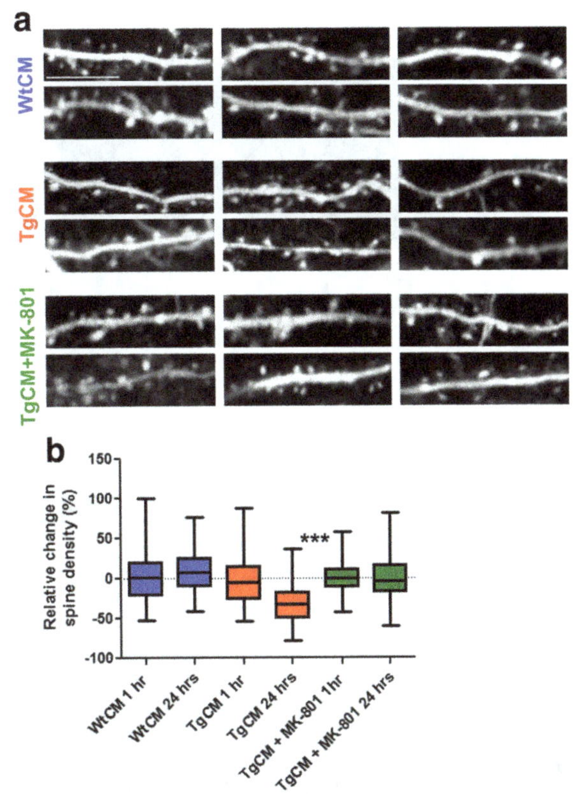

Fig. 3 Oligomeric Aβ decreases spine density at 24 h. **a** Representative images of YFP-filled neurites and dendritic spines before and after 1 h or 24 h treatment with WtCM, TgCM and TgCM + MK-801 (Scale bar = 10 μm). **b** Box plots showing the relative changes in percentage of spine densities after treatment accordingly to the mean spine density calculated for each animal before treatment. Whiskers represent the minimal and maximal values of each experimental group ($n = 3$–4 mice per group. For WtCM: $n = 58$ neurites and 578 spines evaluated after 1 h and $n = 91$ neurites and 1382 spines evaluated after 24 h. For TgCM: $n = 68$ neurites and 760 spines evaluated after 1 h and $n = 69$ neurites and 635 spines evaluated after 24 h. For TgCM + Mk-801: $n = 152$ neurites and 854 spines evaluated after 1 h and $n = 174$ neurites and 1044 spines evaluated after 24 h. Linear mixed effects model was fitted with treatment group and time of imaging (as outlined in the graph) as fixed effect and mouse as random effect. (pair-wise comparisons: TgCM 1 h vs. 24 h: *** $p < 0.0001$, Wtcm 1 h vs. 24 h $p = 0.3897$, TgCM + MK-801 1 h vs. 24 h $p = 0.6667$)

NMDA receptors mediate oAβ-induced increase in resting calcium

Intracellular changes in neuronal $[Ca^{2+}]_i$ can result from increased entry of extracellular calcium, leakage of intracellular calcium stores or loss of buffering capacity. To determine the molecular mechanisms underlying TgCM-induced calcium dysregulation, we examined these possibilities in vitro and in vivo.

As a preliminary approach, we used cortical primary neurons cultured from Tg2576 embryos to perform an initial screen of various calcium channel inhibitors. These neurons chronically secrete human Aβ that oligomerize to form predominantly species from dimers to tetramers after 14DIV (Additional file 1: Figure S1). We have previously demonstrated that, similarly to wild type neurons treated with TgCM, Tg2576 neurons also exhibit spine loss and decreased neurite arborization [5, 15]. We assessed the calcium levels with two different calcium probes: YC3.6 and the small molecule ratiometric indicator indo-1/AM. To explore the contribution of the extracellular calcium pool and the role of voltage gated calcium channels (VGCC), we incubated the cells with indo-1 AM and imaged before and 10 min after exposure to 0.5 mM $NiCl_2$. Transgenic neurons in culture presented a wide distribution of calcium concentrations (Fig. 4a, note the right tail of the distribution curve). Before treatment, 21.3% of transgenic neurons showed

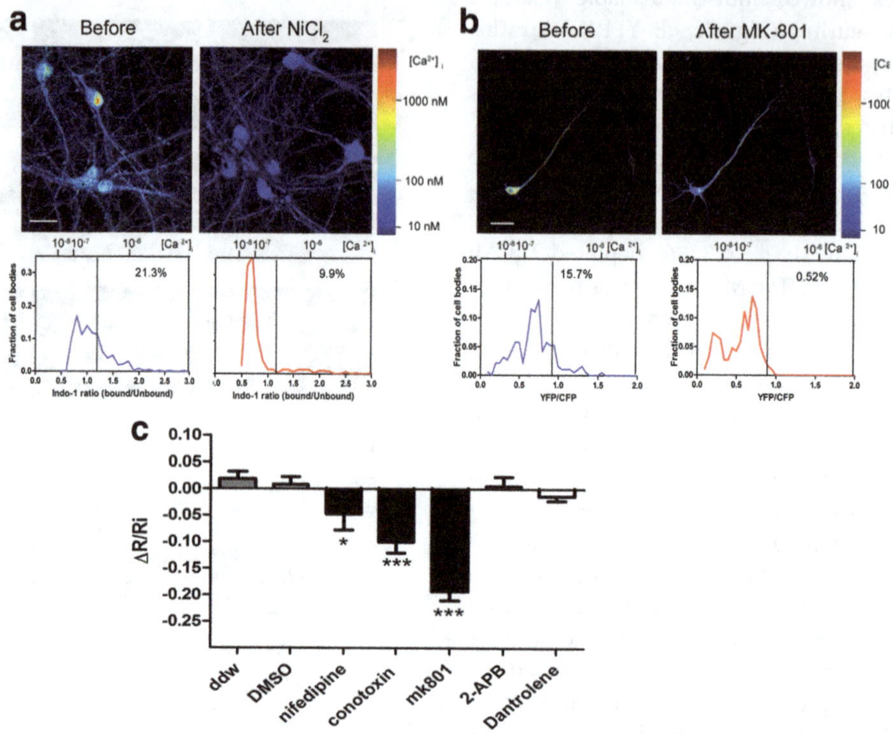

Fig. 4 Extracellular calcium is the source of calcium overload in primary neurons expressing human APP. **a** Tg2576 neurons were incubated with the ratiometric calcium indicator indo-1 AM and then imaged before and after application of $NiCl_2$ to block all voltage gate calcium channels. The ratios of bound vs. unbound indo-1 were calculated, converted to calcium concentration and pseudocolored using the jet color map. Distribution curves of $[Ca^{2+}]_i$ (bound/unbound ratio on the lower x-axis and $[Ca^{2+}]_i$ on the upper x-axis) are presented in the lower panel showing a wider distribution at baseline, which became more narrow and was shifted to the left after application of $NiCl_2$. The *black* line indicates the threshold for calcium overload. The percentage of neurons with calcium overload, noted on the graphs before and after treatment, is significantly reduced by $NiCl_2$ from 21.3 to 9.9% ($n = 366$ neurons before treatment and 321 after treatment in three separate experiments, Fisher exact test, $p < 0.0001$). **b** Neurons were transfected with YC3.6 and imaged before and after application of the NMDA receptor antagonist, MK-801. Ratios were converted to calcium levels and pseudocolored as in A. Upper panel shows resting calcium measured in the same neuron before and after inhibition of NMDA receptors. Distribution curves of $[Ca^{2+}]_i$ (YFP/CFP on the lower x-axis and $[Ca^{2+}]_i$ on the upper x-axis) are shown on the lower panel. Again, the wide distribution of calcium initially observed in transgenic neurons was shifted to the left after treatment with MK-801, dramatically reducing calcium overload from 15.7 to 0.5% ($n = 189$ neurons in 4 separate experiments, Fisher exact test $p < 0.0001$). **c** Summary bar graph for experiments with antagonists for different calcium channel measured with YC3.6 as described in B. The relative change in ratio (ΔR/Ri) after exposure with each inhibitor was calculated for individual cells and presented here as the group mean + SEM (each inhibitor was tested in three independent experiments: vehicles: ddw – $n = 243$, DMSO – $n = 161$; inhibitors: Nifedipine (L-type voltage channels) – $n = 158$, ω-conotoxin (N-type channels) – $n = 141$, 2-APB (IP_3R) – 173, dantrolene (RyR) – 208). The effect of the treatment was tested by comparing each inhibitor to its appropriate vehicle using one way ANOVA with post hoc Dunn's Multiple comparison test (* $p < 0.05$, ** $p < 0.01$, *** $p < 0.0001$). (Scale bar = 50 μm)

calcium overload (marked by a black line, R = 1.32, 467nM), similar to our previous in vivo observations using this APP mouse model [18]. A 10-min incubation with $NiCl_2$ significantly decreased the resting calcium levels and reduced the percentage of calcium overloaded cells from 21.3% to 9.9% (Tg before: $n = 366$ neurons in 3 experiments. Tg after $NiCl_2$: $n = 321$ neurons in 3 experiments, $p < 0.0001$, Fisher exact test). We then performed similar experiments with specific pharmacological blockers of several calcium channels (nifedipine for L-type VGCC, ω-conotoxin for N-type VGCC and MK-801 for NMDA-R), as well as inhibitors of intracellular calcium release from the ER (2-APB for IP_3 receptors and dantrolene for ryanodine receptors). These experiments were performed in transgenic neurons transfected with YC3.6 and the sparse expression of YC3.6 allowed us to re-visit each cell after application and thus appreciate the relative change in ratio for each neuron (ΔR/Ri). As evident in Fig. 4c, vehicles alone (water or DMSO) did not affect the resting calcium in cells. We observed that N-type, L-type VGCC and NMDA receptor antagonist were effective in reducing $[Ca^{2+}]_i$ in the presence of oAβ by 4.7%, 10.05% and 19.31%, respectively (One way ANOVA with post hoc Dunn's multiple comparison test for comparison across all groups: Nifedipine vs. DMSO: $p < 0.05$, ω-conotoxin vs. ddw: $p < 0.0001$, MK-801 vs. ddw: $p < 0.0001$). MK-801 led to the most dramatic effect (Fig. 4*b*, *c*), shifting the distribution curve to the left and reducing calcium overload from 15.7 to 0.52% ($p < 0.0001$ Fisher exact test). Dantrolene and 2-APB, ryanodine and IP_3 receptors antagonists that block calcium release from the ER, did not alter the resting calcium levels of Tg primary neurons. The moderate decrease in $[Ca^{2+}]_i$ observed when nifedipine or ω-conotoxin along with the more dramatic effect of MK-801 strongly support a major role for extracellular calcium as the source for calcium overload.

To test if oAβ-induced calcium dysregulation also relies on extracellular stores and NMDAR activation in vivo, MK-801 (5 μM) was applied on the surface of the brain for 10 min before and along with the application of TgCM. As shown in Fig. 5, TgCM failed to affect resting calcium in mice pretreated with MK-801 (ΔR/Ri comparing before and after MK-801 + TgCM treatment: $p = 0.7719$). The percentage of calcium overloaded neurites also remained unchanged after MK-801/TgCM application (1.67 to 3.5%, $n = 656$ neurites from 7 mice, $p = 0.0548$ Fisher exact test), while TgCM alone resulted in 25.8% of neurites showing calcium overload ($p < 0.0001$, Fisher exact test). Additionally, we did not see any significant spine loss 1 h or 24 h after topical application of MK-801/TgCM (relative change compared with the average spine density before treatment: at 1 h: 0.4% ± 3.3%, $p = 0.9123$, and at 24 h: 2.4% ± 3.3; $n = 4$ mice), implying that the presence of MK-801 also counteracted the deleterious impact of oligomeric Aβ species on synapse loss previously observed with TgCM alone at 24 h. Importantly, MK-801 alone did not significantly changed calcium overload (2.79% to 2.4% overload before and after, $p = 0.37$, fisher exact test, $n = 322$ neurites in 3 mice Fig. 5e), thus demonstrating that the impact of this inhibitor was directly associated with oAβ-dependent activation of NMDAR in the first place. In contrast, treatment with dantrolene (5 μM) did not counteract the effect of TgCM (ΔR/Ri comparing before and after dntrolene + TgCM treatment: $p = 0.0003$).As evident by the change in the shape of the neurite distribution curve and the increased percentage of calcium overloaded neurites (from 2.07 to 21.23%; $n = 674$ neurites from 4 mice, $p < 0.0001$ Fisher

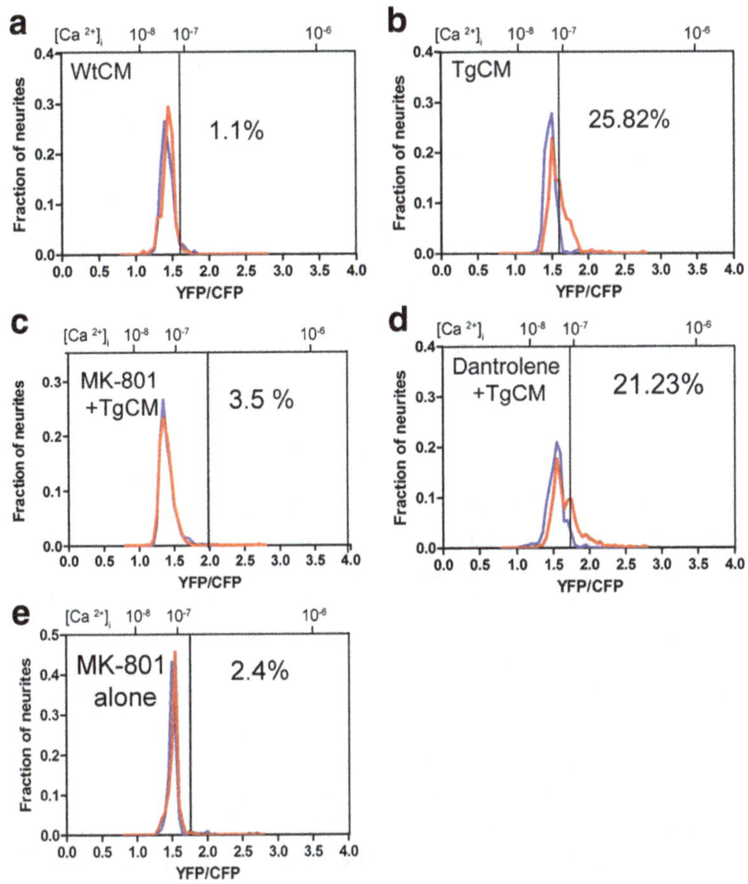

Fig. 5 Oligomeric Aβ induces calcium overload through activation of NMDA receptors in vivo. The antagonists MK-801 and Dantrolene were applied 10-min before and during TgCM application. Distribution curves of $[Ca^{2+}]_i$ (YFP/CFP ratio on the lower x-axis and $[Ca^{2+}]_i$ on the upper x-axis) are presented before (*purple curve*) and after treatment (*red curve*) for mice treated with WtCM (**a**) TgCM (**b**) MK-801 + TgCM (**c**), dantrolene + TgCM (**d**) and MK-801 alone (**e**). The *black* line indicates the threshold for calcium overload. The percent of overloaded neurites is noted on each graph. Treatment with MK-801, but not of dantrolene, abolished the effect of TgCM on resting calcium (pair-wise comparisons of the relative change in YC ratio: TgCM vs. TgCM + MK-801 $p = 0.0221$; TgCM vs. TgCM + Dantrolene $p = 0.7656$; TgCM + MK-801 vs. TgCM + Dantrolene $p = 0.0077$)

exact). To conclude, MK-801 and dantrolene led to an opposite effect on resting calcium once applied to the brain along with TgCM (pair-wise comparison TgCM + MK-801 vs. TgCM + dantrolene: $p = 0.0077$), suggesting that extracellular soluble amyloid species initially act through activation of these calcium channels in vivo, while the calcium retained in the ER does not seem to play a primary role.

Discussion

Disruption of intracellular calcium balance has been invoked as a potential mechanism of physiological and pathophysiological changes associated with normal aging [30] and, to a greater extent, with a variety of neurologic disorders including schizophrenia [31], bipolar disorder [32], autism spectrum disorder [33], Parkinson's disease [34, 35], Huntington disease [36] and AD [10, 11, 37–39]. The relationship between the pathological hallmarks of AD and abnormal calcium homeostasis has been a focus of investigation, and while neurofibrillary tangles seemed to affect neither resting $[Ca^{2+}]_i$ [40] nor neuronal responses to stimuli [41], the amyloid pathology has been linked to increased resting calcium [18], neuronal hyperactivity [19] and a gradual decline in neuronal performance in response to visual stimuli [20, 21].

Accumulating evidence suggests that soluble oAβ are more potent neurotoxic species than Aβ fibrils, leading to synaptic and neural network dysfunction [3, 4, 42–44]. Though the effect of different species of oAβ has been tested in culture models, studying their relevance in vivo has been challenging because of the concomitant presence of amyloid plaques [8, 45]. In this study, we specifically investigated the effect of naturally secreted soluble species of Aβ, primarily oAβ, on calcium homeostasis in the healthy living brain. We utilized conditioned media collected from APP transgenic cortical neurons as the source of oligomeric Aβ. Unlike synthetic Aβ, which generates oligomers and fibrils within minutes to hours, naturally secreted Aβ peptides mainly assemble into low molecular weight species from dimers to tetramers. We demonstrated that, when oAβ was acutely applied to the cortical surface of the healthy mouse brain after cranial window implantation, the resting calcium levels were dramatically increased in all cellular compartments including neuronal soma, processes and dendritic spines. While it is conceivable that the surgical procedure itself sensitizes neurons towards Aβ neurotoxicity, the calcium rise could not be attributed solely to the experimental approach itself. Indeed, removal of Aβ from the conditioned media or, alternatively, acute application of conditioned media from wild type neurons, abolished this effect. Aβ-induced elevation of resting calcium was significant 1 h after application but could no longer be detected in the same brains after 5 h, suggesting clearance of the peptide assemblies, and/or recovery via intracellular buffering mechanisms. Interestingly, the relatively fast increase of intraneuronal calcium levels after exposure to Aβ leads to long-lasting morphological alterations with a significantly decreased spine density detected only 24 h after treatment with TgCM while no change could be detected at 1 h. The extent of oAβ-induced spine loss is similar to what has been reported in the immediate vicinity of amyloid plaques, where high concentrations of oAβ are thought to exist [8, 45]. The difference in kinetics between oAβ-dependent calcium overload and synaptic collapse strongly argues in favor of a primary neuronal dysfunction that precedes morphological changes at the synapse, perhaps via activation of calcineurin or other calcium dependent signaling pathways [5, 15, 27]. This is of particular interest considering that spine loss is the parameter that correlates best with cognitive impairment in AD patients [46, 47].

Understanding the source of the calcium entry in the presence of oAβ and the channels involved is important as calcium influx through different channels may trigger various signaling cascades which independently impact gene transcription and neuronal homeostasis [48]. The role of extracellular calcium and its influx through the activation of NMDA receptors was demonstrated in vivo, as oAβ-dependent calcium rise was prevented by incubation with MK-801. Indeed, Aβ has been shown to reduce long term potentiation (LTP) and facilitate long term depression (LTD), processes that involved trafficking of glutamate receptors [49, 50]. In addition, prefibrillar amyloid and Aβ oligomers have been shown to directly interact with glutamatergic receptors, activate NMDAR and result in calcium increase in primary neurons [51–53]. While those in vitro studies have established a direct association between oAβ and NMDAR, our results do not exclude the possibility that intermediate steps also participate in the rise of intraneuronal calcium levels. For example, pathologically elevated levels of Aβ have been shown to block glutamate uptake at the synaptic cleft, leading to increased glutamate levels, which could also activate synaptic NMDA receptors [54]. Whether or not the activation of NMDAR is a direct or indirect effect of extracellular oAβ, our data strongly suggest that the rise in intracellular calcium via NMDAR may impair synaptic plasticity and spine density, and thus represent the initial steps in the pathological changes that occur in AD.

ER calcium stores have been suggested to play a role in regulation of Aβ production [55, 56] and calcium release from the ER via ryanodine and IP_3 receptors has also been implicated in calcium dyshomeostasis in AD [11, 57, 58]. Specifically, chronic treatment with the ryanodine receptor antagonist, dantrolene, was shown to normalize ER calcium responses, improve cognitive deficits and modulate the amyloid pathology in mouse models of AD [59]. Conversely, our data suggest that oAβ initially facilitates calcium entry from extracellular pools, at least largely via NMDA receptors, whereas ryanodine receptors do not appear to play a role primarily. It is possible that the ER pools are involved in a second step in calcium-dependent calcium release from the ER, resulting in further rise in cytosolic calcium levels. In the brains of AD mouse models chronically exposed to Aβ oligomers and fibrils, the sustained increase in resting calcium [18] may result from a concomitant dysregulation of extracellular calcium entry or intracellular calcium buffering systems that further induce downstream events such as synapse loss and alterations in APP processing. This may not be the case in the healthy brain in which calcium is highly regulated, explaining why the effect of oAβ on $[Ca^{2+}]_i$ is not abolished by blocking RyR, as the initial rise in calcium is not dependent on ER stores.

Finally, we cannot exclude that exposure of the cortical surface to oAβ impacts intraneuronal calcium homeostasis via non-cell autonomous mechanisms, eventually involving the participation of astroglial cells as well [60]. The effect of oAβ on cultured astrocytes has indeed been investigated over the past [61, 62], showing in particular that oligomerized Aβ can induce astrocytic glutamate release in an α7nAChR-dependent manner, activate extrasynaptic NMDAR and lead to synaptic loss. In vivo studies in AD mice have revealed that calcium transients in astrocytes were more frequent and synchronously coordinated in transgenic animals as compared with controls [63, 64], an effect potentially mediated by paracrine purinergic signaling that could be blocked by P2Y receptors inhibitors [65]. However, most of the work conducted in animals has been done using transgenic mouse models, so the sole effect of oAβ on astrocytic calcium homeostasis remains to be elucidated. Additionally, studying the respective impact of oligomeric amyloid species concomitantly on neurons and astrocytes will give further information about the initial molecular mechanisms in play.

In light of these observations, it is clear that therapeutic strategies aimed at reducing or inhibiting calcium influx into cells through NMDAR may be of importance. In parallel, efforts to prevent or reduce the levels of soluble oAβ levels will likely lead to treatments that effectively delay or restore neuronal dysfunction in AD.

Conclusions

The present study demonstrates that low-molecular weight species of Amyloid β can acutely disrupt neuronal calcium homeostasis in non-transgenic animals through the activation of NMDA receptors. Interestingly, although calcium levels are rapidly restored to baseline, decreased spine density is detected 24 h after exposure to oAβ, suggesting that calcium dyshomeostasis precedes synaptic morphological changes. This work implicates small oAβ species in the deleterious effects that occur during degenerative processes at the synapse.

Additional files

Additional file 1: Figure S1. Biochemical characterization of Aβ oligomers present in Tg conditioned media (TgCM). **a** Representative profile showing the amount of Aβ40 detected by ELISA in each fraction after separation of the different oligomeric species present in TgCM (red bars) by size-exclusion chromatography (SEC, Superdex 75 SEC columns). The molecular weight markers (kDa) that ran at the same conditions are indicated above (arrowheads). **b** Measurements of oligomeric Aβ within each SEC fraction show that most of oAβ is of low molecular weight (fractions 12–18).. A smaller peak of high-molecular weight species was also detected in TgCM (fractions 2–6 in both ELISAs).

Additional file 2: Figure S2. Time course of oAβ-induced increase in resting calcium levels after acute exposure with TgCM on a healthy brain. C57BL/6 mice were injected with AAV-CBA-YC3.6 into the somatosensory cortex and acutely exposed to TgCM containing oAβ. The changes in YFP/CFP ratios in the neurites were measured at baseline before treatment and 30 min, 1 h and 5 h after topical application of TgCM. A progressive increase in the levels of resting calcium (YFP/CFP ratio and the actual calcium levels on the lower and upper x-axis, respectively) was detected that reached a peak after 1 h (20.6% of overloaded neurites), before returning to baseline levels after 5 h (1.7% overloaded neurites).

Acknowledgements
Not applicable.

Funding
This work was funded by NIH EB000768, S10 RR025645, Alzheimer Association IIRG-11-205935, NIH-MARC U*STAR 5T34GMO92711-04 and NIA R01 AG044263.

Authors' contributions
MAO and EH designed the experiments, collected and analyzed data and wrote the manuscript. JRB performed the in vitro experiments in primary neurons and analyzed data. TH and ST performed the SEC analysis of WtCM and TgCM. KVK and SH wrote the ImageJ and Matlab macros in order to calculate the YC ratios and generate the illustrative pseudocolored images. CRL, AMB, NS and PBT helped with the image analyses. AM and RAB performed the statistical analyses. BTH and BJB oversaw the experimental design, discussed the data and edited the manuscript. All authors read and approved the final manuscript.

Authors' information
Not applicable.

Competing interests
The authors declare that they have no competing interests.

Author details
[1]Alzheimer Research Unit, Department of Neurology, Massachusetts General Hospital and Harvard Medical School, 114, 16th St., Charlestown, MA 02129, USA. [2]Department of Neuropathology, The University of Tokyo, Tokyo, Japan. [3]Skirball Institute, NYU School of Medicine, New York, NY 10016, USA. [4]Department of Biostatistics, Harvard School of Public Health, 50 Staniford Street, Boston, MA, USA.

References

1. Spires TL, Meyer-Luehmann M, Stern EA, McLean PJ, Skoch J, Nguyen PT, Bacskai BJ, Hyman BT. Dendritic spine abnormalities in amyloid precursor protein transgenic mice demonstrated by gene transfer and intravital multiphoton microscopy. J Neurosci. 2005;25:7278–87.
2. Knowles RB, Wyart C, Buldyrev SV, Cruz L, Urbanc B, Hasselmo ME, Stanley HE, Hyman BT. Plaque-induced neurite abnormalities: implications for disruption of neural networks in Alzheimer's disease. Proc Natl Acad Sci U S A. 1999;96:5274–9.
3. Selkoe DJ. Soluble oligomers of the amyloid beta-protein impair synaptic plasticity and behavior. Behav Brain Res. 2008;192:106–13.
4. Shankar GM, Li S, Mehta TH, Garcia-Munoz A, Shepardson NE, Smith I, Brett FM, Farrell MA, Rowan MJ, Lemere CA, et al. Amyloid-beta protein dimers isolated directly from Alzheimer's brains impair synaptic plasticity and memory. Nat Med. 2008;14:837–42.
5. Wu HY, Hudry E, Hashimoto T, Kuchibhotla K, Rozkalne A, Fan Z, Spires-Jones T, Xie H, Arbel-Ornath M, Grosskreutz CL, et al. Amyloid beta induces the morphological neurodegenerative triad of spine loss, dendritic simplification, and neuritic dystrophies through calcineurin activation. J Neurosci. 2010;30:2636–49.
6. Busche MA, Chen X, Henning HA, Reichwald J, Staufenbiel M, Sakmann B, Konnerth A. Critical role of soluble amyloid-beta for early hippocampal hyperactivity in a mouse model of Alzheimer's disease. Proc Natl Acad Sci U S A. 2012;109:8740–5.
7. Viola KL, Velasco PT, Klein WL. Why Alzheimer's is a disease of memory: the attack on synapses by A beta oligomers (ADDLs). J Nutr Health Aging. 2008;12:51S–7S.
8. Koffie RM, Meyer-Luehmann M, Hashimoto T, Adams KW, Mielke ML, Garcia-Alloza M, Micheva KD, Smith SJ, Kim ML, Lee VM, et al. Oligomeric amyloid beta associates with postsynaptic densities and correlates with excitatory synapse loss near senile plaques. Proc Natl Acad Sci U S A. 2009;106:4012–7.
9. Disterhoft JF, Moyer Jr JR, Thompson LT. The calcium rationale in aging and Alzheimer's disease. Evidence from an animal model of normal aging. Ann N Y Acad Sci. 1994;747:382–406.
10. Khachaturian ZS. Calcium hypothesis of Alzheimer's disease and brain aging. Ann N Y Acad Sci. 1994;747:1–11.
11. Chakroborty S, Stutzmann GE. Calcium channelopathies and Alzheimer's disease: Insight into therapeutic success and failures. Eur J Pharmacol. 2013.
12. Mattson MP. Calcium and neurodegeneration. Aging Cell. 2007;6:337–50.
13. Smith IF, Green KN, LaFerla FM. Calcium dysregulation in Alzheimer's disease: recent advances gained from genetically modified animals. Cell Calcium. 2005;38:427–37.
14. Reese LC, Laezza F, Woltjer R, Taglialatela G. Dysregulated phosphorylation of Ca(2+)/calmodulin-dependent protein kinase II-alpha in the hippocampus of subjects with mild cognitive impairment and Alzheimer's disease. J Neurochem. 2011;119:791–804.
15. Hudry E, Wu HY, Arbel-Ornath M, Hashimoto T, Matsouaka R, Fan Z, Spires-Jones TL, Betensky RA, Bacskai BJ, Hyman BT. Inhibition of the NFAT pathway alleviates amyloid beta neurotoxicity in a mouse model of Alzheimer's disease. J Neurosci. 2012;32:3176–92.
16. Malleret G, Haditsch U, Genoux D, Jones MW, Bliss TV, Vanhoose AM, Weitlauf C, Kandel ER, Winder DG, Mansuy IM. Inducible and reversible enhancement of learning, memory, and long-term potentiation by genetic inhibition of calcineurin. Cell. 2001;104:675–86.
17. Kayyali US, Zhang W, Yee AG, Seidman JG, Potter H. Cytoskeletal changes in the brains of mice lacking calcineurin A alpha. J Neurochem. 1997;68:1668–78.
18. Kuchibhotla KV, Goldman ST, Lattarulo CR, Wu HY, Hyman BT, Bacskai BJ. Abeta plaques lead to aberrant regulation of calcium homeostasis in vivo resulting in structural and functional disruption of neuronal networks. Neuron. 2008;59:214–25.
19. Busche MA, Eichhoff G, Adelsberger H, Abramowski D, Wiederhold KH, Haass C, Staufenbiel M, Konnerth A, Garaschuk O. Clusters of hyperactive neurons near amyloid plaques in a mouse model of Alzheimer's disease. Science. 2008;321:1686–9.
20. Grienberger C, Rochefort NL, Adelsberger H, Henning HA, Hill DN, Reichwald J, Staufenbiel M, Konnerth A. Staged decline of neuronal function in vivo in an animal model of Alzheimer's disease. Nat Commun. 2012;3:774.
21. Rudinskiy N, Hawkes JM, Betensky RA, Eguchi M, Yamaguchi S, Spires-Jones TL, Hyman BT. Orchestrated experience-driven Arc responses are disrupted in a mouse model of Alzheimer's disease. Nat Neurosci. 2012;15:1422–9.
22. Stern EA, Bacskai BJ, Hickey GA, Attenello FJ, Lombardo JA, Hyman BT. Cortical synaptic integration in vivo is disrupted by amyloid-beta plaques. J Neurosci. 2004;24:4535–40.
23. Santacruz K, Lewis J, Spires T, Paulson J, Kotilinek L, Ingelsson M, Guimaraes A, DeTure M, Ramsden M, McGowan E, et al. Tau suppression in a neurodegenerative mouse model improves memory function. Science. 2005;309:476–81.
24. Skoch J, Hickey GA, Kajdasz ST, Hyman BT, Bacskai BJ. In vivo imaging of amyloid-beta deposits in mouse brain with multiphoton microscopy. Methods Mol Biol. 2005;299:349–63.
25. Grynkiewicz G, Poenie M, Tsien RY. A new generation of Ca2+ indicators with greatly improved fluorescence properties. J Biol Chem. 1985;260:3440–50.
26. Palmer AE, Tsien RY. Measuring calcium signaling using genetically targetable fluorescent indicators. Nat Protoc. 2006;1:1057–65.
27. Wu HY, Hudry E, Hashimoto T, Uemura K, Fan ZY, Berezovska O, Grosskreutz CL, Bacskai BJ, Hyman BT. Distinct dendritic spine and nuclear phases of calcineurin activation after exposure to amyloid-beta revealed by a novel fluorescence resonance energy transfer assay. J Neurosci. 2012;32:5298–309.
28. Mehta PD, Pirttila T, Mehta SP, Sersen EA, Aisen PS, Wisniewski HM. Plasma and cerebrospinal fluid levels of amyloid beta proteins 1–40 and 1–42 in Alzheimer disease. Arch Neurol. 2000;57:100–5.
29. Nagai T, Yamada S, Tominaga T, Ichikawa M, Miyawaki A. Expanded dynamic range of fluorescent indicators for Ca(2+) by circularly permuted yellow fluorescent proteins. Proc Natl Acad Sci U S A. 2004;101:10554–9.
30. Mattson MP, Magnus T. Ageing and neuronal vulnerability. Nat Rev Neurosci. 2006;7:278–94.
31. Tesli M, Skatun KC, Ousdal OT, Brown AA, Thoresen C, Agartz I, Melle I, Djurovic S, Jensen J, Andreassen OA. CACNA1C risk variant and amygdala activity in bipolar disorder, schizophrenia and healthy controls. PLoS ONE. 2013;8, e56970.
32. Green EK, Grozeva D, Jones I, Jones L, Kirov G, Caesar S, Gordon-Smith K, Fraser C, Forty L, Russell E, et al. The bipolar disorder risk allele at CACNA1C also confers risk of recurrent major depression and of schizophrenia. Mol Psychiatry. 2010;15:1016–22.
33. Lu AT, Dai X, Martinez-Agosto JA, Cantor RM. Support for calcium channel gene defects in autism spectrum disorders. Mol Autism. 2012;3:18.
34. Schapira AH. Calcium dysregulation in Parkinson's disease. Brain. 2013;136:2015–6.
35. Ilijic E, Guzman JN, Surmeier DJ. The L-type channel antagonist isradipine is neuroprotective in a mouse model of Parkinson's disease. Neurobiol Dis. 2011;43:364–71.
36. Bezprozvanny I. Role of inositol 1,4,5-trisphosphate receptors in pathogenesis of Huntington's disease and spinocerebellar ataxias. Neurochem Res. 2011;36:1186–97.
37. Bezprozvanny I, Mattson MP. Neuronal calcium mishandling and the pathogenesis of Alzheimer's disease. Trends Neurosci. 2008;31:454–63.
38. Bojarski L, Herms J, Kuznicki J. Calcium dysregulation in Alzheimer's disease. Neurochem Int. 2008;52:621–33.
39. Green KN. Calcium in the initiation, progression and as an effector of Alzheimer's disease pathology. J Cell Mol Med. 2009;13:2787–99.
40. Kopeikina KJ, Wegmann S, Pitstick R, Carlson GA, Bacskai BJ, Betensky RA, Hyman BT, Spires-Jones TL. Tau causes synapse loss without disrupting calcium homeostasis in the rTg4510 model of tauopathy. PLoS ONE. 2013;8, e80834.
41. Kuchibhotla KV, Wegmann S, Kopeikina KJ, Hawkes J, Rudinskiy N, Andermann ML, Spires-Jones TL, Bacskai BJ, Hyman BT. Neurofibrillary tangle-bearing neurons are functionally integrated in cortical circuits in vivo. Proc Natl Acad Sci U S A. 2014;111:510–4.
42. Shankar GM, Bloodgood BL, Townsend M, Walsh DM, Selkoe DJ, Sabatini BL. Natural oligomers of the Alzheimer amyloid-beta protein induce reversible synapse loss by modulating an NMDA-type glutamate receptor-dependent signaling pathway. J Neurosci. 2007;27:2866–75.
43. Walsh DM, Selkoe DJ. A beta oligomers - a decade of discovery. J Neurochem. 2007;101:1172–84.
44. Cheng IH, Scearce-Levie K, Legleiter J, Palop JJ, Gerstein H, Bien-Ly N, Puolivali J, Lesne S, Ashe KH, Muchowski PJ, Mucke L. Accelerating amyloid-beta fibrillization reduces oligomer levels and functional deficits in Alzheimer disease mouse models. J Biol Chem. 2007;282:23818–28.
45. Howlett DR, Bowler K, Soden PE, Riddell D, Davis JB, Richardson JC, Burbidge SA, Gonzalez MI, Irving EA, Lawman A, et al. Abeta deposition and related pathology in an APP x PS1 transgenic mouse model of Alzheimer's disease. Histol Histopathol. 2008;23:67–76.

46. Terry RD, Masliah E, Salmon DP, Butters N, DeTeresa R, Hill R, Hansen LA, Katzman R. Physical basis of cognitive alterations in Alzheimer's disease: synapse loss is the major correlate of cognitive impairment. Ann Neurol. 1991;30:572–80.
47. DeKosky ST, Scheff SW, Styren SD. Structural correlates of cognition in dementia: quantification and assessment of synapse change. Neurodegeneration : a journal for neurodegenerative disorders, neuroprotection, and neuroregeneration. 1996;5:417–21.
48. West AE, Griffith EC, Greenberg ME. Regulation of transcription factors by neuronal activity. Nat Rev Neurosci. 2002;3:921–31.
49. Selkoe DJ. Alzheimer's disease is a synaptic failure. Science. 2002;298:789–91.
50. Kim JH, Anwyl R, Suh YH, Djamgoz MB, Rowan MJ. Use-dependent effects of amyloidogenic fragments of (beta)-amyloid precursor protein on synaptic plasticity in rat hippocampus in vivo. J Neurosci. 2001;21:1327–33.
51. Texido L, Martin-Satue M, Alberdi E, Solsona C, Matute C. Amyloid beta peptide oligomers directly activate NMDA receptors. Cell Calcium. 2011;49:184–90.
52. Pellistri F, Bucciantini M, Relini A, Nosi D, Gliozzi A, Robello M, Stefani M. Nonspecific interaction of prefibrillar amyloid aggregates with glutamatergic receptors results in Ca2+ increase in primary neuronal cells. J Biol Chem. 2008;283:29950–60.
53. Snyder EM, Nong Y, Almeida CG, Paul S, Moran T, Choi EY, Nairn AC, Salter MW, Lombroso PJ, Gouras GK, Greengard P. Regulation of NMDA receptor trafficking by amyloid-beta. Nat Neurosci. 2005;8:1051–8.
54. Li S, Hong S, Shepardson NE, Walsh DM, Shankar GM, Selkoe D. Soluble oligomers of amyloid Beta protein facilitate hippocampal long-term depression by disrupting neuronal glutamate uptake. Neuron. 2009;62:788–801.
55. Green KN, Demuro A, Akbari Y, Hitt BD, Smith IF, Parker I, LaFerla FM. SERCA pump activity is physiologically regulated by presenilin and regulates amyloid beta production. J Cell Biol. 2008;181:1107–16.
56. Cheung KH, Shineman D, Muller M, Cardenas C, Mei L, Yang J, Tomita T, Iwatsubo T, Lee VM, Foskett JK. Mechanism of Ca2+ disruption in Alzheimer's disease by presenilin regulation of InsP3 receptor channel gating. Neuron. 2008;58:871–83.
57. Christensen RA, Shtifman A, Allen PD, Lopez JR, Querfurth HW. Calcium dyshomeostasis in beta-amyloid and tau-bearing skeletal myotubes. J Biol Chem. 2004;279:53524–32.
58. Demuro A, Parker I. Cytotoxicity of intracellular abeta42 amyloid oligomers involves Ca2+ release from the endoplasmic reticulum by stimulated production of inositol trisphosphate. J Neurosci. 2013;33:3824–33.
59. Peng J, Liang G, Inan S, Wu Z, Joseph DJ, Meng Q, Peng Y, Eckenhoff MF, Wei H. Dantrolene ameliorates cognitive decline and neuropathology in Alzheimer triple transgenic mice. Neurosci Lett. 2012;516:274–9.
60. Osborn LM, Kamphuis W, Wadman WJ, Hol EM. Astrogliosis: An integral player in the pathogenesis of Alzheimer's disease. Prog Neurobiol. 2016;144:121–41.
61. Drews A, Flint J, Shivji N, Jonsson P, Wirthensohn D, De Genst E, Vincke C, Muyldermans S, Dobson C, Klenerman D. Individual aggregates of amyloid beta induce temporary calcium influx through the cell membrane of neuronal cells. Sci Rep. 2016;6:31910.
62. Talantova M, Sanz-Blasco S, Zhang X, Xia P, Akhtar MW, Okamoto S, Dziewczapolski G, Nakamura T, Cao G, Pratt AE, et al. Abeta induces astrocytic glutamate release, extrasynaptic NMDA receptor activation, and synaptic loss. Proc Natl Acad Sci U S A. 2013;110:E2518–27.
63. Kuchibhotla KV, Lattarulo CR, Hyman BT, Bacskai BJ. Synchronous hyperactivity and intercellular calcium waves in astrocytes in Alzheimer mice. Science. 2009;323:1211–5.
64. Takano T, Han X, Deane R, Zlokovic B, Nedergaard M. Two-photon imaging of astrocytic Ca2+ signaling and the microvasculature in experimental mice models of Alzheimer's disease. Ann N Y Acad Sci. 2007;1097:40–50.
65. Delekate A, Fuchtemeier M, Schumacher T, Ulbrich C, Foddis M, Petzold GC. Metabotropic P2Y1 receptor signalling mediates astrocytic hyperactivity in vivo in an Alzheimer's disease mouse model. Nat Commun. 2014;5:5422.

The NLRP3 and NLRP1 inflammasomes are activated in Alzheimer's disease

Marina Saresella[1*†], Francesca La Rosa[1†], Federica Piancone[1], Martina Zoppis[1], Ivana Marventano[1], Elena Calabrese[1], Veronica Rainone[2], Raffaello Nemni[1,3], Roberta Mancuso[1] and Mario Clerici[1,3]

Abstract

Background: Interleukin-1 beta (IL-1β) and its key regulator, the inflammasome, are suspected to play a role in the neuroinflammation observed in Alzheimer's disease (AD); no conclusive data are nevertheless available in AD patients.

Results: mRNA for inflammasome components (NLRP1, NLRP3, PYCARD, caspase 1, 5 and 8) and downstream effectors (IL-1β, IL-18) was up-regulated in severe and MILD AD. Monocytes co-expressing NLRP3 with caspase 1 or caspase 8 were significantly increased in severe AD alone, whereas those co-expressing NLRP1 and NLRP3 with PYCARD were augmented in both severe and MILD AD. Activation of the NLRP1 and NLRP3 inflammasomes in AD was confirmed by confocal microscopy proteins co-localization and by the significantly higher amounts of the pro-inflammatory cytokines IL-1β and IL-18 being produced by monocytes. In MCI, the expression of NLRP3, but not the one of PYCARD or caspase 1 was increased, indicating that functional inflammasomes are not assembled in these individuals: this was confirmed by lack of co-localization and of proinflammatory cytokines production.

Conclusions: The activation of at least two different inflammasome complexes explains AD-associated neuroinflammation. Strategies targeting inflammasome activation could be useful in the therapy of AD.

Keywords: Alzheimer's disease, Neuroinflammation, Inflammasome, Beta amyloid, Mild cognitive impairment

Background

Alzheimer's disease (AD) is a devastating neurodegenerative condition characterized by neuronal cell death and progressive dementia. It is widely accepted that the extracellular accumulation of amyloid-β (Aβ) in senile plaques and the formation of neurofibrillary tangles (NFT) inside neurons as a result of the abnormal phosphorylation of the microtubules-associated tau protein are the main event in the pathogenesis of AD, but the cellular events leading to plaque-induced neuronal dysfunction are less clear [1]. Inflammatory mediators play an essential role in the neuroinflammation observed in AD. In particular interleukin IL-1β is increased in this condition, and the activation of its key regulator, the inflammasome, is suspected to be involved in the pathogenesis of the disease.

The inflammasomes are multiprotein complexes mainly expressed in myeloid cells that are required for the activation of caspase 1 protease and the downstream secretion of two of its substrates, the proinflammatory cytokines IL-1β and IL-18 [2]. Inflammasome-dependent innate immune responses are initiated by Nod-like receptors (NLRs), cytoplasmic pattern recognition receptors that detect invading pathogens. NLRs are activated by bacterial, fungal, or viral molecules that contain pathogen-associated molecular patterns (PAMPs) or by non-microbial danger signals (DAMPs) released by damaged cells [3, 4]. NLR activation leads to their oligomerization to form multiprotein inflammasome complexes that serve as platforms for the recruitment, cleavage, and activation of inflammatory caspases. Four inflammasome complexes (NLRP1, NLRP3, IPAF, and AIM2) have been identified. These complexes contain either a specific NLR family protein or AIM2, as well as the PYCARD and/or Cardinal adaptor proteins and pro-caspases-1, 5 and 8 [5, 6]. NLRP3 is the best-characterized inflammasome; its formation requires multiple steps. In a priming step, transcriptionally active signalling receptors induce the NF-kB-dependent induction of NLRP3 itself as

* Correspondence: msaresella@dongnocchi.it
†Equal contributors
[1]Don C. Gnocchi Foundation, IRCCS, Piazza Morandi, 3, 20121 Milan, Italy
Full list of author information is available at the end of the article

well as that of the caspase 1 substrates of the pro-IL-1β family [7, 8]. The NLRP3 is, at this stage, in a signalling incompetent conformation; this is modified upon a second signal, that will induce the assembly of a multimolecular complex with PYCARD and caspase 1. Multiple signals, which are potentially provided in combination, thus trigger the formation of an active inflammasome, which, in turn, will stimulate the cleavage and the release of bioactive cytokines including IL-1β and IL-18 [8–18]. Although these cytokines have a beneficial role in promoting inflammation and eliminating infectious pathogens, mutations that result in constitutive inflammasome activation and overproduction of IL-1β and IL-18 have been linked to inflammatory and autoimmune disorders [19–21].

The NLRP3 inflammasome complex is suspected to play a role in AD, as its activation in the microglia by Aβ triggers neuroinflammation [14, 22, 23]. Notably, NLRP3 inflammasome deficiency favours the differentiation of microglia cells to an M2 (anti-inflammatory) phenotype and results in a decreased deposition of amyloid-β in the APP/PSI model of AD; these results reinforce the suggestion that the NLRP3 inflammasome is involved in the pathogenesis of the disease [24]. No conclusive data are nevertheless available in patients. To better investigate the involvement of the inflammasome in AD we performed in-depth analyses of the expression of genes and proteins that are part of the inflammasome complex in individuals with a diagnosis of either AD or mild cognitive impairment (MCI). Results indicated that two different inflammasomes, NLRP3 and NLRP1, are activated in AD but not in individuals with a diangnosis of mild cognitive impairment (MCI).

Results

Up-regulation of inflammasome genes in LPS-primed and $A\beta_{42}$-stimulated-monocytes of AD patients

mRNA expression of 84 genes involved in the assembly, the activation, and the down-stream signalling of inflammosomes was quantified by qPCR in all patients and controls. Data are expressed as the fold change (nFold) between the results obtained in unstimulated cells and those obtained upon stimulations of cells with either LPS, Aβ42 or LPS and Aβ42. In this initial set of experiments, pools of cells from donors with the same clinical diagnosis (MCI; MILD AD; severe AD) as well as from HC were created. Data obtained in LPS-primed and $A\beta_{42}$-stimulated-monocytes, showed the presence of a significant up-regulation involving genes, that codify for the proteins that form the inflammasome in MILD and severe AD, as well as in MCI. In cells of MCI individuals, though, not all the genes that are necessary for the assembly of a fully functional inflammasome complex were up-regulated. To summarize: 1) the expression of NLRP1, NLRP3 and caspase 8 was greatly increased in all groups of patients (nFold >10) compared to HC, with no detectable differences being observed between individuals with a diagnosis of AD or MCI; and 2) PYCARD, caspase 1 and caspase 5 expression was increased in AD (nFold ≥10) but not in MCI individuals. Only minor differences were seen between patients and controls in the expression of these genes in monocytes-stimulated with either LPS or $A\beta_{42}$ alone; both stimuli induced IL-1β and IL-6 up-regulation in HC (nFold >10) (Fig. 1).

RT-PCR performed on each individual specimen was used next to verify the expression of NLRP1, NLRP3, PYCARD, caspase 1, caspase 5 and caspase 8 in LPS and $A\beta_{42}$-stimulated monocytes of patients and HC. Results of mRNA expression confirmed that: 1) NLRP1, NLRP3 and caspase 8 are significantly increased in AD and MCI individuals compared to HC ($p < 0.05$), with the highest values observed in severe AD, and 2) PYCARD, caspase 1 and caspase 5 are significantly increased in AD compared to MCI and HC ($p < 0.05$) (Fig. 2a).

Up-regulation of inflammasome-related cytokines in LPS-primed and $A\beta_{42}$-stimulated- monocytes of AD patients

Stimulation of monocytes with either LPS or $A\beta_{42}$- alone resulted in the moderate increase of IL-1β and IL-6 expression; notably LPS or $A\beta_{42}$- alone were not sufficient to trigger inflammasome assembly, as no differences were detect in these conditions either in NLRP3 or IL-18 mRNA (Fig. 1). Once cells were activated with LPS and $A\beta_{42}$, nevertheless, both IL-1β (nFold >10) and IL-18 (nFold ≥10) mRNA was significantly increased in severe and MILD AD compared to MCI and HC (Fig. 1). Results obtained by single-PCR confirmed that in these experimental conditions IL-1β and IL-18 mRNA ($p < 0.05$ vs. all other groups) is significantly increased in severe and MILD AD, with the highest values in severe AD (Fig. 2b).

IL-33 and IL-37, two relatively novel cytokines that are members of the IL-1 family, were analyzed as well in the study. We found that IL-33 gene expression was greatly increased in MCI (nFold >10) compared to AD and HC; no significant differences, on the other hand, were observed in IL-37 gene expression among groups analyzed (Fig. 1). Single RT-PCR confirmed these results (Fig. 2c).

NLRP3 protein is significantly augmented in LPS-primed and $A\beta_{42}$-stimulated- monocytes of AD and MCI patients

The expression of NLRP3 protein, the best-characterized protein within the inflammasome complex, was investigated next by Western Blot analyses in LPS-primed and Aβ42-stimulated-monocytes of all patients and controls. Different NLRP3 isoforms are known: the long form (118 KDa) is prevalent in cell lines (THP1 or Jurkat) while the short one (NLRP3s 75 KDa) is seen in primary immune cells [25]. Results of analyses performed on whole-cell lysates confirmed that NLRP3s expression is

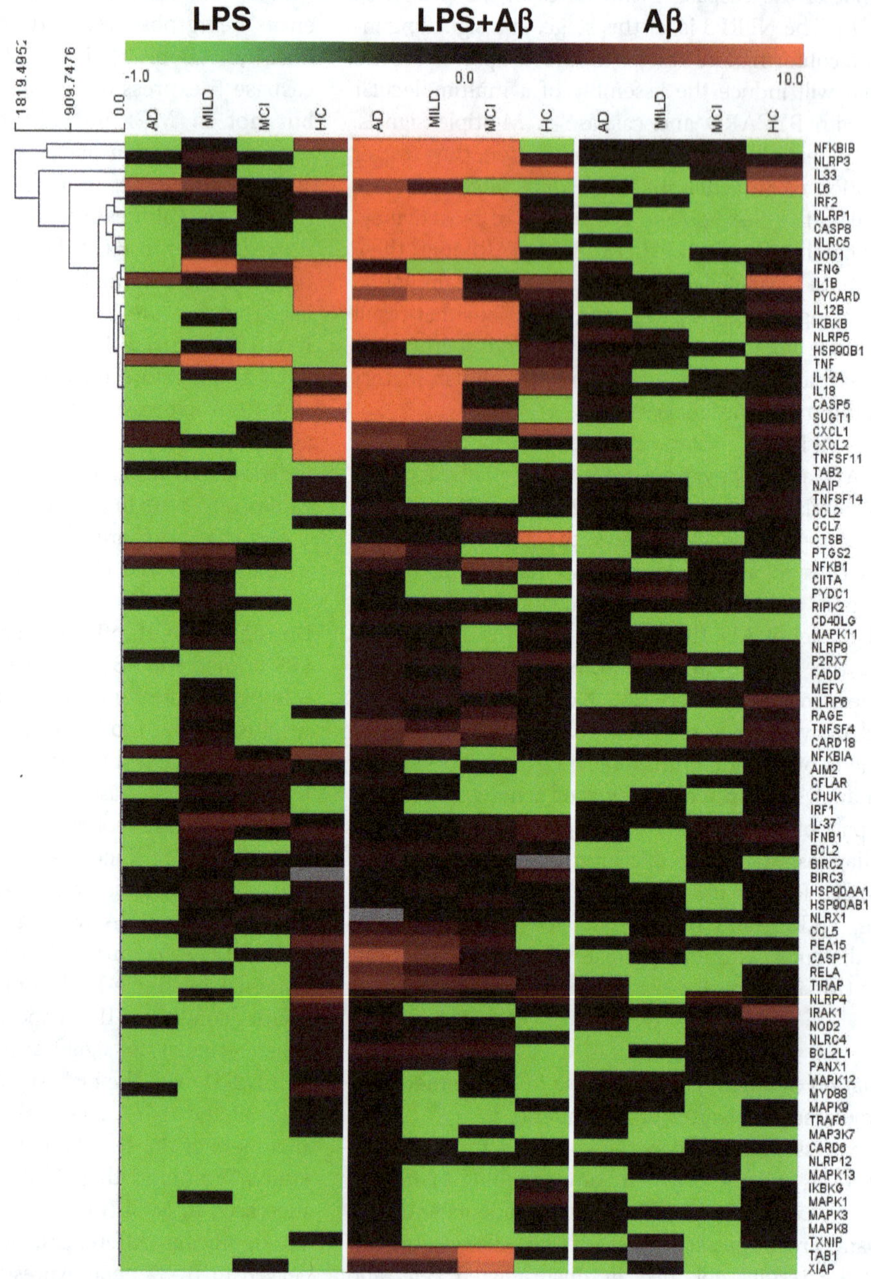

nFold ≥ 10	LPS+Aβ			
Genes	**AD**	**MILD**	**MCI**	**HC**
NLRP1	437,2	385,2	119,3	2,3
NLRP3	1334,4	1007,1	309,7	2,9
PYCARD	28,0	19,0	3,0	2,0
CASP1	20,0	15,0	4,0	6,0
CASP5	16,0	17,0	1,2	-1,2
CASP 8	138,3	129,7	275,9	1,0
IL1β	37,0	19,0	1,0	5,9
IL18	20,0	10,0	3,0	6,0
IL33	365,9	404,3	1259,0	42,6

Fig. 1 (See legend on next page.)

(See figure on previous page.)
Fig. 1 Messenger RNA expression levels of genes within the inflammasome pathway. Expression of 84 genes involved in the inflammasome pathway assessed by real-time quantitative RT-PCR-array in monocytes of individuals with a diagnosis of either severe Alzheimer's disease (AD), moderate Alzheimer's disease (MILD) or Mild Cognitive Impairment (MCI) and of age- and sex-matched Healthy Controls (HC). Heat maps of Log_2 Fold changes are presented. Results obtained upon stimulating cells with LPS or $A\beta_{42}$ alone, or upon LPS-priming followed by $A\beta_{42}$ stimulation are presented. Fold-changes >10 in the expression of LPS + $A\beta_{42}$ stimulated genes of importance are summarized in the Table

significantly increased in severe (mean ± S.E.M.: 2.29 ± 0.35 AU), and MILD AD (1.32 ± 0.42 AU) compared to healthy controls (0.1 ± 0.06 AU)($p = 0.023$ vs. severe AD; $p = 0.0362$ vs. MILD AD). NLRP3s expression was also increased when MCI individuals (0.78 ± 0.24 AU) were compared to HC, even if this difference did not reach statistical significance ($p = 0.081$) (Fig. 3).

LPS-primed and $A\beta_{42}$-stimulated monocytes that express inflammasome proteins are significantly augmented in AD

Peripheral CD14+ monocytes that express NLRP3 or co-express NLRP3 and PYCARD, NLRP3 and caspase 1, or NLRP3 and caspase 8 were augmented in LPS-primed and $A\beta_{42}$-stimulated-cells of both groups of AD patients compared to MCI individuals and HC. The Fluorochrome Inhibitor of Caspases (FLICA) kit was used to analyze the presence in cells of active caspases; in this method, once inside the cell, the FLICA inhibitor probe binds covalently to active caspases (p20) alone. Staining of active caspase 1 and caspase 8 inhibitors was performed using the green fluorescent probe FAM-YVAD-FMK and FAM-LETD-FMK respectively. Results showed that 1) CD14+/NLRP3+, CD14+/NLRP3+/caspase1+, and CD14+/NLRP3+/Caspase8+ immune cells were significantly increased in severe AD patients alone compared to MCI and HC ($p < 0.05$) and 2) CD14+/NLRP3+/PYCARD +, cells were augmented both in severe and MILD AD compared to MCI and HC (MCI and HC vs. moderate AD $p < 0.05$; vs. severe AD $p < 0.01$)(Fig. 4a).

LPS-primed and $A\beta_{42}$-stimulated NLRP1-expressing CD14 cells were significantly increased as well in both groups of AD patients compared to MCI and HC ($p < 0.05$), while CD14+/NLRP1+/PYCARD + and CD14+/NLRP1+/caspase1+ immune cells were augmented, although not significantly, in AD patients compared to other two groups. Finally, no differences could be observed in CD14+/NLRP1+/caspase 5+ cells (Fig. 4b). These results confirm those obtained in PCR analyses and indicate that, even if some inflammasome components are up regulated in MCI, fully functional inflammasomes are not assembled in this situation.

Co-localization of inflammasome proteins in LPS-primed and $A\beta_{42}$-stimulated monocytes by confocal microscopy analyses

Aggregation and activation of inflammasome complexes was further analyzed by evaluating the co-localization of NLRP3 and NLRP1 with PYCARD, caspase 1 or caspase 8 by confocal microscopy. Co-localization efficiency was calculated using the Pearson co-localization coefficient (PCC). Results showed a clear co-localization of NLRP3 with PYCARD, caspase 1 and caspase 8 in LPS-primed and $A\beta_{42}$-stimulated monocytes of AD patients alone; no co-localization could be detected in untreated cells (data not shown). In particular: 1) NLRP3/PYCARD, NLRP1/PYCARD and NLRP3/caspase1 co-localization was increased in both groups of AD patients compared to HC and MCI; 2), NLRP3/caspase8 and NLRP1/caspase5 co-localization was increased in severe AD alone; and 3) NLRP1/caspase1 co-localization was seen only in cells of MILD AD individuals. In all cases, with the exception of the NLRP1-caspase 1 complex, the highest PCC values were detected in cells of patients with severe AD disease (Fig. 5 and Table 1).

Inflammasome-related cytokines production in LPS-primed and $A\beta_{42}$-stimulated - monocytes of AD patients

Aggregation of the inflammasome results in the downstream production of pro-inflammatory cytokines. Because FACS and confocal microscopy data indicated that the different subunits that compose the inflammasome do aggregate in LPS-primed and $A\beta_{42}$-stimulated- monocytes of AD patients, and PCR analyses showed that mRNA for these cytokines is increased in monocytes of AD patients, IL-1β, IL-18, IL-33 and IL-37 were next measured. Results showed that the concentration of IL-1β, IL-18 in supernatants was significantly increased in both groups of AD patients compared to MCI and HC (IL-1β $p < 0.05$; IL-18 $p < 0.01$)(Fig. 6a and b). CD14+/IL-1β+ cells were significantly increased as well in MILD and severe AD compared to MCI and HC ($p < 0.05$)(Fig. 6a), whereas lack of proper reagents prevented IL18-expressing cells to be analyzed by FACS. The fact that IL-1β+ and IL-18 were not increased in MCI is not surprising considering that in this condition NLRPs but not PYCARD expression was augmented, thus preventing the assembly of a functional inflammasome; these data confirm the findings obtained with FACS and confocal analyses.

IL-33 could not be quantified in supernatants (data not shown), probably because the inflammatory mature form of this cytokines is not cleaved and secreted. Results obtained by flow-cytometry, nevertheless showed that CD14+/IL-33+ cells were increased in MCI and in MILD AD, with the lowest percentages of these cells

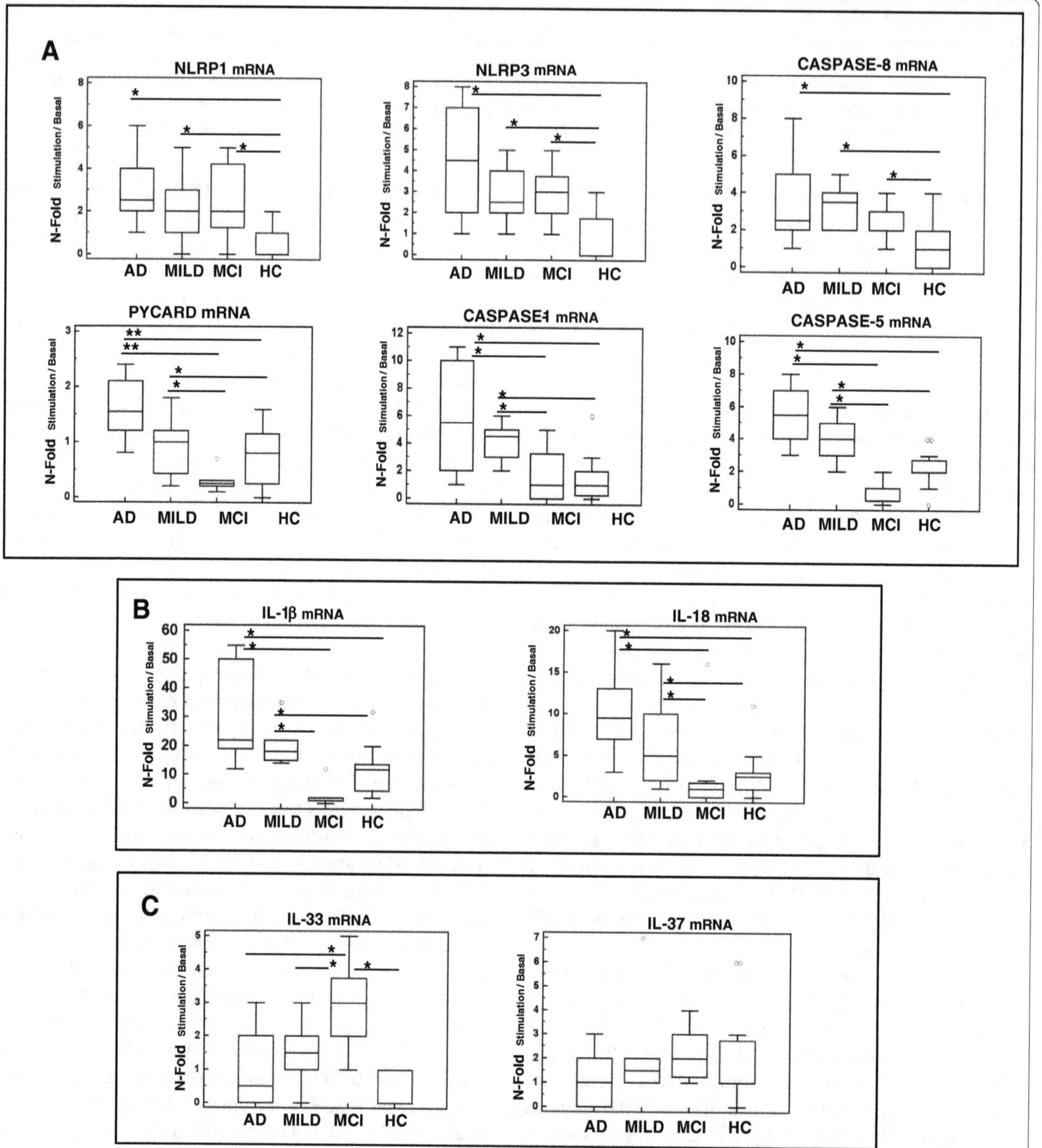

Fig. 2 mRNA expression by Real-Time PCR. Single Real-Time PCR results obtained in LPS and $A\beta_{42}$ -stimulated monocytes of individuals with a diagnosis of either severe Alzheimer's disease (AD), moderate Alzheimer's disease (MILD) or Mild Cognitive Impairment (MCI) and of age- and sex-matched Healthy Controls (HC). **a** NLRP1, NLRP3, caspase 8, PYCARD, caspase 1 and caspase 5 are shown in panel **a**; IL-1β and IL-18 in panel **b** and IL-33 and IL-37 in panel **c**. The results are shown as fold-change expression from the un-stimulated samples. Gene expression was calculated relative to GAPDH housekeeping gene. Summary results are shown in the bar graphs. The boxes stretch from the 25 to the 75 percentile; the line across the boxes indicates the median values; the lines stretching from the boxes indicate extreme values. Outside values are displayed as separate points. Statistical significance is shown *(p <0.05), **(p <0.01)

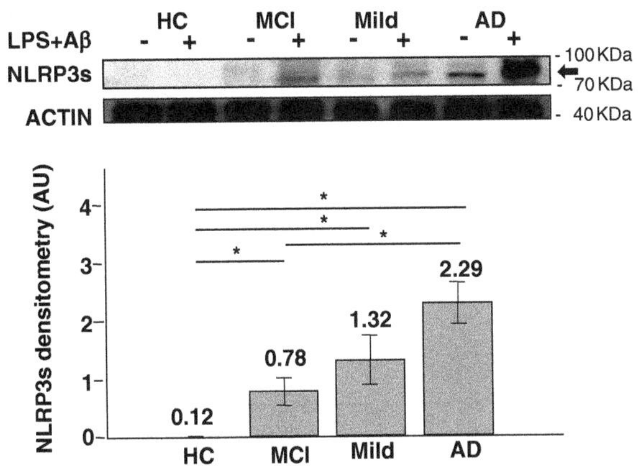

Fig. 3 NLRP3s expression in Monocyte by Western blot: NLRP3s protein expression assessed by western blotting in monocyte of individuals with a diagnosis of either severe Alzheimer's disease (AD), moderate Alzheimer's disease (MILD) or Mild Cognitive Impairment (MCI) and of age- and sex-matched Healthy Controls (HC). The same protein concentration of whole-cells lysates was loaded into the gel, as confirmed by actin. Representative results obtained in un-stimulated or in LPS-primed and $A\beta_{42}$-stimulated monocytes are presented in the *upper panel*. Quantitative evaluation (arbitrary unit, AU) of NLRP3s expression obtained comparing band density (normalized to actin) in un-stimulated or in LPS-primed Aβ42-stimulated monocytes is shown in the *lower panel*. ($N = 5$, mean ± s.e.m., *T* test, $^*p < 0.05$). ($N = 5$/group, mean ± S.E.M and statistical significance are shown. $^*(p < 0.05)$

seen in severe AD ($p < 0.01$)(Fig. 6c). Notably this cytokine was shown to have a multifaceted protective role against AD and to negatively modulate NF-kB activity, dampening inflammation. Finally, CD14+/IL-37+ cells were marginally increased in AD compared to MCI and HC (Fig. 6d).

Discussion

Inflammasomes are intracellular complexes formed by the assembly of multiple subunits that regulate the maturation and the secretion of pro-inflammatory cytokines [2]. At least four different inflammasomes are known; the NLRP3, in particular, is suspected to play a role in the pathogenesis of AD. Thus, in the APP/PSI animal model of AD, NLRP3 up regulation induces the production of IFN1β by microglia [14]; and, on the other hand, its deficiency results in a decreased deposition of amyloid-β [24, 26–29]. We have previously shown that peripheral monocytes of AD individuals are characterized by an inflammatory profile and a higher surface density of TLR molecules [30]. Further analyses performed in these same individuals allowed us to demonstrate that these cells also express binary complexes formed by Aβ peptides and MHC-molecules, possibly initiating Aβ-specific acquired immune reponses [31]. Herein we investigate the role of the inflammasome in the neuroinflammation that accompanies AD by analyzing peripheral immune cells of patients with MCI or AD. Results obtained using molecular, confocal and cytofluorimetic analyses indicated that the NLRP3 and NLRP1 inflammasomes are indeed activated in AD. The assembly of functional inflammasomes in AD was confirmed by the significantly increased amount of the proinflammatory cytokines IL-1β and IL-18 that were produced by LPS-primed and $A\beta_{42-}$-stimulated- monocytes of AD patients.

Notably, NLRP1, NLRP3 and caspase 8, but not PYCARD were increased in individuals with a diagnosis of MCI, a condition that is often but not always prodromic to the development of AD. In this situation the assembly of a functional inflammasome is not possible. Consequently, neither a significant co-localization of inflammasome subunits nor increased amount of IL-1β and IL-18 were detected in these individuals. It is interesting to observe that in MCI a partial, initial up regulation of inflammasome proteins limited to NLRP proteins is observed. Only a percentage of MCI progresses to AD; these results thus allow the speculation that the inflammasome is somehow "primed" to be activated in all individuals with a diagnosis of MCI. An increased transcription of the other inflammasome components, the assembly of the functional complex, and the production of proinflammatory cytokines, occurs only in some cases, possibly because of still unknown "triggering" events that act on an "NLRP-primed" background.

NLRP3 and caspase 8 mRNA were up regulated in cells of severe AD patients; CD14+/NLRP3+/caspase8+ cells were increased as well in these individuals in whom the co-localization of caspase 8 with NLRP3 was also detected. Recent data showed that caspase 8 is not only an inducer of cell apoptosis but, together with the Fas-Associated protein with Death Domain (FADD), it interacts with NLRP3. Such interaction is required for caspase 1 activation, as well as for IL-1β and IL-18 secretion [5]. Confocal analyses confirmed that caspase 8 is present in the NLRP3 inflammasome complex, where it is involved in the cleavage of pro caspase 1 and IL-1β. These results support a direct role for caspase 8 in the processing of caspase 1 [6]. Our data confirm these findings, as well as recent results indicating that caspase 8 contributes to both NF-kB–dependent priming and post-translational activation of the NLRP3 inflammasome [5]. Increased NLRP1 and caspase 5 mRNA levels were also detected in cells of individuals with a diagnosis of severe AD. NLRP1 and caspase 5 colocalized in CD14 cells, and higher percentages of CD14+/NLRP1+/caspase 5+ immune cells were also seen in these patients. These data indicate that the NLRP1 inflammasome complex is also activated in severe AD; notably, recent results indicate that SNPs in the NLRP1 gene are associated with AD [32].

Inflammasome assembly leads to the production of proinflammatory cytokines; IL-1β and IL-18 mRNA and

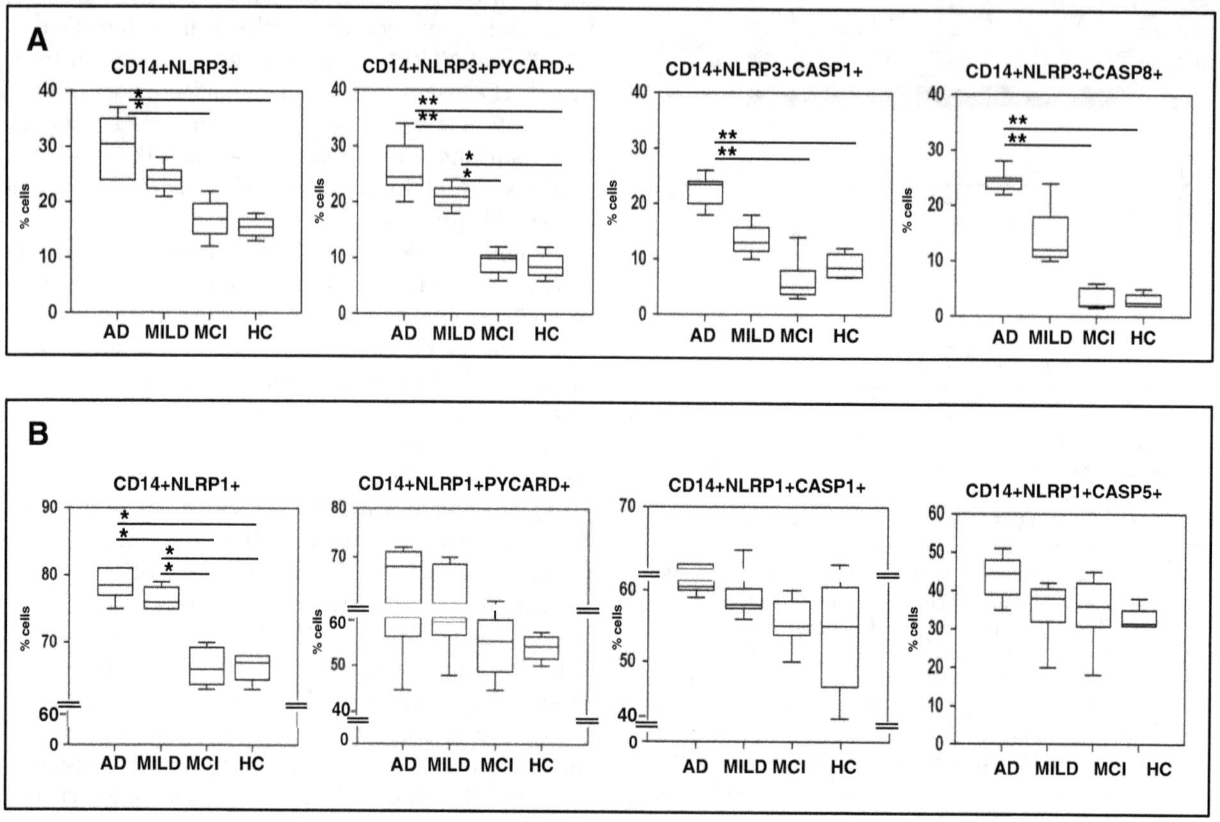

Fig. 4 FACS analyses: co-expression of inflammasome proteins in CD14+ cells. Co-expression of inflammasome proteins in LPS-primed and Aβ_{42}-stimulated CD14+ of individuals with a diagnosis of either severe Alzheimer's disease (AD), moderate Alzheimer's disease (MILD) or Mild Cognitive Impairment (MCI) and of age- and sex-matched Healthy Controls (HC). Two-hundred-thousand cells were acquired and gated on CD14 expression and side scatter properties. CD14+ cells co-expressing NLRP3-associated inflammasome components are shown in panel **a**; CD14+ cells co-expressing NLRP1-associated inflammasome components are shown in panel **b**. Summary results are shown in the bar graphs. The boxes stretch from the 25° to the 75°percentile; the line across the boxes indicates the median values; the lines stretching from the boxes indicate extreme values. Statistical significance is shown *(p <0.05), **(p <0.01)

secretion were indeed significantly increased in AD. Interestingly, incubation of cells with Aβ_{42} was sufficient to induce IL-1β mRNA expression, but a significantly increased production of IL-1β and IL-18 was seen in LPS-primed and Aβ_{42}-stimulated cells of AD patients alone. These findings indicate that such experimental conditions result in the assembly of fully functional inflammasomes only in cells of AD patients. Notably, transfection of human PBMC with siRNA specific for NLRP3 and PYCARD greatly reduced IL-1β production, confirming that the production of this cytokine is dependent on inflammasome assembly [33]. That IL-1β plays a role in the pathogenesis of AD has been repeatedly shown. To summarize: this cytokine induces a loss of phagocytic activity by the microglia [34], stimulates the hyperphosphorylation of tau protein [35] and affects synaptic plasticity. As a consequence of these effects, IL-1β can impair learning and memory processes [36, 37]. IL-18 has been involved in AD as well, even if fewer data are available. Thus, increased amounts of IL-18 were detected in the brain [38], plasma [39], and peripheral blood lymphocytes of AD [40], and the expression of the IL-18R complex is greatly augmented in peripheral blood cells of MCI and AD individuals [41]. Finally, recent data indicate that IL-18 directly stimulates Aβ production by human neuron-like cells, suggesting a key role for this cytokine in the pathogenesis of AD [42].

Two other novel cytokines, IL-33 and IL-37 were analyzed as well in this study; these cytokines are members of the IL-1β family and are produced upon activation of the inflammasome. Whereas no significant differences were seen in IL-37, mRNA levels of IL-33 were increased in both MILD AD and MCI compared to the values observed in severe AD. Analysis of peripheral CD14+/IL-33+ cells confirmed this observation, as these cells were increased both in MCI and MILD AD compared to severe AD and HC. IL-33 and IL-37 are dual function proteins with both intra and extra-cellular mechanisms of action as, besides being able to bind to their cognate receptors on target cells, they can act

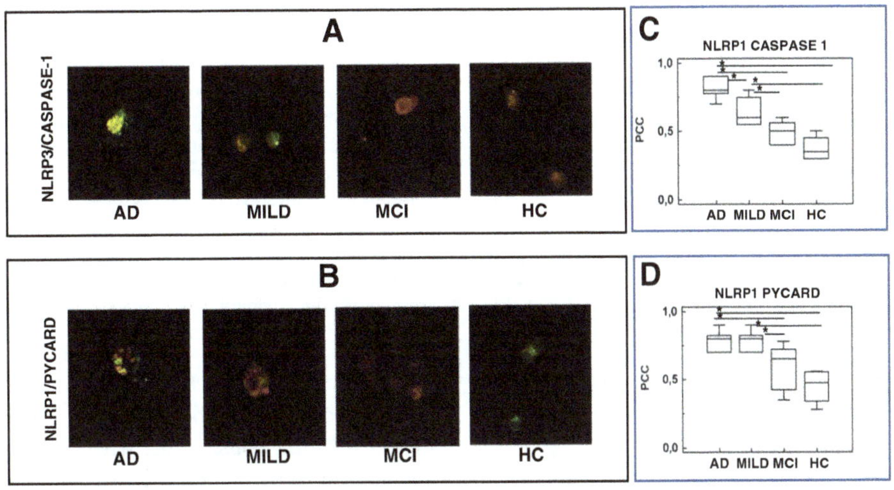

Fig. 5 Confocal microscopy: co-localization of inflammasome proteins in CD14+ cells. Representative confocal fluorescence images (63× magnification) of experiments (N = 5) showing the effect of LPS-priming and $A\beta_{42}$-stimulation on NLRP3/PYCARD (**a**) and NLRP1/caspase 1 (**b**) co-localization in monocytes of individuals with a diagnosis of either severe Alzheimer's disease (AD), moderate Alzheimer's disease (MILD) or Mild Cognitive Impairment (MCI) and of age- and sex-matched Healthy Controls (HC). Summary results of NLRP3/PYCARD and NLRP1/caspase-1 PCC (Pearson co-localization efficiency) are presented in (**c**) and (**d**), respectively. The boxes stretch from the 25 to the 75 percentile; the line across the boxes indicates the median values; the lines stretching from the boxes indicate extreme values. Statistical significance is shown *(p <0.05), **(p <0.01)

intracellularly as nuclear factor. IL-33 is reduced in AD brains [43]. This cytokine is believed to have a neuroprotective role secondary to the reduction of Aβ peptides secretion [44] and the activation of the phagocytosis of amyloid-β peptide by the microglia [45]. IL-33 also interacts intracellularly with the NF-kB p65 subunit [44]; the resulting IL-33/NF-kB p65 complex interferes with NF-kB–dependent transcription by impeding p65-mediated transactivation. This causes a negative modulation of NF-kB activity, with a dampening effect on inflammation [46]. The increase of IL-33 production in MCI and in MILD AD could thus be seen as an attempt of the immune response to reduce neuroinflammation. On the other hand, the observation that the levels of IL-33 seen in severe AD are comparable to those observed in elderly healthy individuals suggest that the IL33-dependent anti-inflammatory effects do not need to be activated in the absence of the pathological alterations present in AD.

Results herein stem from immunological analyses performed in peripheral blood immune cells; a number of data nevertheless provide evidence that the brain is invaded by peripherally derived monocytes/macrophages [47]. In murine models of Alzheimer's disease, mice brains are infiltrated by bone marrow-derived macrophages that associate with amyloid plaques and clear Aβ deposits from the brain [48]. Our data indicate that the CD14+ cells that are likely present in the CNS of AD

Table 1 Co-localization coefficient of inflammasome proteins. Pearson's co-localization coefficient (PCC) of NLRP1 and NLRP3 with PYCARD, caspase-1, caspase-5 and caspase-8, in LPS-primed and $A\beta_{42}$-stimulated CD14+ monocyte of patients with a diagnosis of either severe or moderate (MILD) Alzheimer's Disease (AD) and mild cognitive impairment (MCI). Result obtained in and in age-and sex-matched healthy controls (HC) are also shown. Index reference values: PC range= −1 and +1

PCC	severe AD	MILD AD	MCI	HC
NLRP1+ PYCARD +	0.8[ac] (0.7-0.82)	0.8 [de] (0.7-0.82)	0.5[ad] (0.3-0.6)	0.4[ce] (0.3–0.5)
NLRP1+ CASPASE-1+	0.6 (0.4-0.7)	0.8 (0.7-0.84)	0.6 (0.4-0.65)	0.5 (0.5-0.7)
NLRP1+ CASPASE-5+	0.7[bac] (0.5–0.8)	0.4[b] (0.23-0.5)	0.3[a] (0.1-0.32)	0.3[c] (0.2-0.5)
NLRP3+ PYCARD +	0.8[ac] (0.6-0.82)	0.8 [de] (0.7-0.82)	0.6[ad] (0.5-0.7)	0.5[ce] (0.4-0.6)
NLRP3+ CASPASE-1+	0.9[bac] (0.8-0.9)	0.8[bde] (0.5-0.8)	0.5[ad] (0.4-0.56)	0.3[ce] (0.3-0.4)
NLRP3+ CASPASE-8+	0.8[ac] (0.7-0.85)	0.6 (0.5-0.72)	0.5[a] (0.3-0.55)	0.5[c] (0.3-0.6)

Median values, interquartile range and statistical significances are presented (p <0.05)
[a]AD vs. MCI
[b]AD vs. MILD AD
[c]AD vs. HC
[d]MILD AD vs. MCI
[e]MILD AD vs. HC

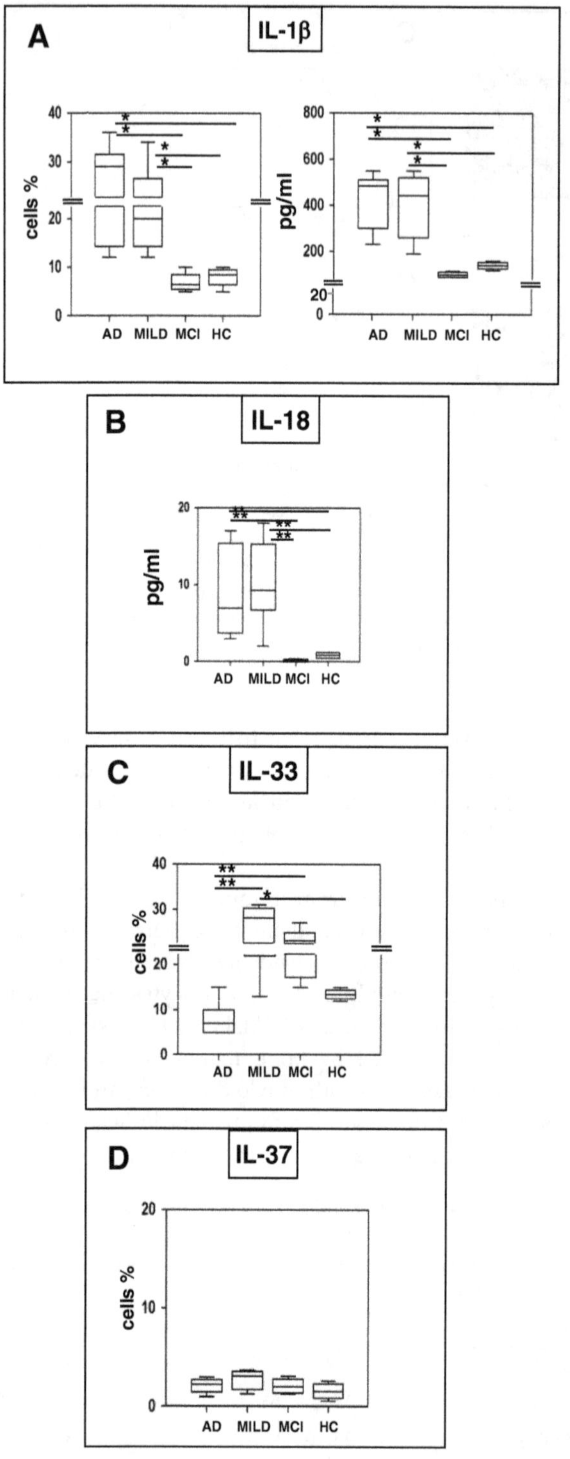

Fig. 6 IL-1β, IL-18, IL-33 and IL-37 production. IL-1β, (panel **a**), IL-18 (panel **b**), IL-33 (panel **c**) and IL-37 (panel **d**). Interleukin-1β and IL-18 production was assessed by multiplex ELISA in supernatants. CD14+/IL-1β+, CD14+/IL-33 and CD14+/IL-37+ cells were analyzed by flow-cytometry. In both cases, LPS-primed and Aβ_{42}-stimulated monocytes of individuals with a diagnosis of either severe Alzheimer's disease (AD), moderate Alzheimer's disease (MILD) or Mild Cognitive Impairment (MCI) and of age- and sex-matched Healthy Controls (HC) were analyzed. Summary results are shown in the bar graphs. The boxes stretch from the 25° to the 75°percentile; the line across the boxes indicates the median values; the lines stretching from the boxes indicate extreme values. Statistical significance is shown *(p <0.05), **(p <0.01)

patients can carry active inflammasome complexes. It also has to be remembered that the role of inflammation in AD is ambiguous. Thus, whether this phenomenon is considered to be responsible for AD-associated neurodegeneration, an alternate hypothesis sees it as a monocyte/macrophages-mediated attempt to slow down the accumulation of Aβ plaques in the brain. Longitudinal studies and analyses performed in animal models will be needed to clarify this issue.

Conclusions

NLRP3 up regulation in mice or human microglia cell line or in brain of AD patients has been previously reported [14, 24, 49], these are nevertheless the first data showing NLRP3 and NLRP1 inflammasome activation in Aβ stimulated peripheral monocytes of individuals with a diagnosis of AD. It will be interesting to verify whether these data could have a prognostic and/or diagnostic value in the clinical setting. In particular, the observation that some (NLRP1, NLRP3) but not not all (PYCARD, caspase 1) of the genes necessary for the assembly of an inflammosome complex genes are upregulated in MCI suggests that monitoring the transcription rate of, e.g. PYCARD in MCI could offer an early diagnostic tool for AD development. Migration of peripheral monocyte across the blood-brain barrier is likely an important factor in the neuroinflammation that accompanies Alzheimer's disease. Very recent results showed that nucleoside reverse transcriptase inhibitors inhibit the activation of the inflammasome [50]. If neuroinflammation is deleterious in AD, these drugs could be an interesting tool in the treatment of this disease.

Methods

Patients and controls

Twenty individuals with a diagnosis of mild cognitive impairment (MCI) and a Mini- Mental State Examination (MMSE) score >24, 21 patients with moderate Alzheimer's disease (MMSE score 19–23), 19 patients with severe Alzheimer's disease (MMSE score <19) and 40 age-and sex-matched healthy controls (HC) were enrolled in the study. The clinical diagnosis of Alzheimer's disease was performed according to the NINCDS-ADRDA work group criteria [51] and the DMS IV-R [52]. All Alzheimer's disease patients underwent complete medical and neurological evaluation, as well as laboratory analysis, and CT scan or MRI. Additional investigations (e.g., EEG, SPECT scan, CSF examination, etc.) were performed in some cases to exclude reversible causes of dementia. Neuropsychological evaluation and psychometric assessment were performed with a neuropsychological battery that included the MMSE [53], Digit Span Forward and Backward, Logical Memory and Paired Associated Words Tests, Token Test, supra Span Corsi Block Tapping Test, Verbal Fluency Tasks, Raven Colored Matrices, the Rey Complex Figure, Clinical Dementia Rating Scale (CDR) [54], and the Hachinski Ischemic Scale. Individuals with a diagnosis of MCI were selected among subjects seen at our Memory Disorders Outpatients Service for the diagnostic evaluation of memory complaints without difficulties in daily activities. MCI diagnosis was based on Petersen's criteria [55] as follows: 1) reported cognitive decline, 2) impaired cognitive function, 3) essentially normal functional activities, and 4) exclusion of dementia. The healthy controls were selected according to the SENIEUR protocol for immunogerontological studies of European Community's Control Action Program on Aging [56, 57]. The cognitive status of HC was assessed by administration of MMSE (score for inclusion as normal control subjects >28). Written consent was obtained and ethical approval was granted by the Ethics Committee of the Don C Gnocchi Foundation in Milano, Italy.

Blood sample collection and cell separation

Fifty ml of whole blood were collected in vacutainer tubes containing ethylenediaminetetraacetic acid (EDTA) (Becton Dickinson & Co., Rutherford, NJ, USA). Peripheral blood mononuclear cells (PBMC) were separated on lympholyte separation medium (Cedarlane, Hornby, Ontario, CA) and washed twice in PBS at 1500 RPM for 10 min; viable leukocytes were determined using a Scepter 2.0 Handheld Automated Cell Counter (Millipore, Billerica, MA).

Cell cultures

PBMC (1×10^6/ml) were cultured in 12 well cell culture plate (Greiner Bio-One GmbH Frickenhausen Germany) with RPMI 1640 supplemented with 10 % human serum, 2 mM L-glutamine, and 1 % penicillin (Invitrogen Ltd, Paisley, UK) for 2 h at 37 °C in a humidified 5 % CO_2 atmosphere [58]. Non adhering PBMC were then washed away and monocytes were either resuspended in medium alone (medium), or were stimulated with: 1) 2 g/ml Lipopolysaccharide (LPS) for 2 h (Sigma-Aldrich, St. Luis, MO, USA), 2) 10 g/ml of 1–42 amyloid-beta peptide oligomer ($A\beta_{42}$)(Sigma-Aldrich) for 24 h, or 3) primed with LPS (2 g/ml) for 2 h before stimulation with 10 g/ml of $A\beta_{42}$ peptide oligomer for 24 h. In all cases cells were incubated at 37 °C in a humidified 5 % CO_2 atmosphere. As it has been repeatedly shown, LPS pre-incubation is necessary to induce the intracellular accumulation of NLRP3 and pro-IL-1β, thus allowing the assembly of fully functional inflammasome complexes [13, 14, 59, 60]. For confocal microscopy analyses PBMC were cultured on chamber slide (Lab Tek Nalge Nunc Intern. Naperville IL USA) for 2 h at 37 °C in a humidified 5 % CO_2 atmosphere [58]. Non adhering PBMC were then washed away and monocytes were either resuspended in medium alone or were stimulated with 1) 2 g/ml LPS for 2 h (Sigma-Aldrich), 2) 10 g/ml of $A\beta_{42}$oligomer (Sigma-Aldrich) for 24 h, or 3) primed with LPS (2 g/ml) for 2 h before stimulation with 10 g/ml of $A\beta_{42}$ peptide oligomer for 24 h. In all cases cells were incubated at 37 °C in a humidified 5 % CO_2 atmosphere. Finally monocytes on chamber slide were fixed in 4 % paraformaldehyde in PBS for 15 min.

RNA extraction and reverse transcription

RNA was extracted from unstimulated, LPS- or $A\beta_{42}$-primed, or LPS-primed and $A\beta_{42}$-stimulated-monocytes using the acid guanidium thiocyanate–phenol–chloroform method. RNA was dissolved in RNase-free water and purified from genomic DNA with RNase-free DNase (RQ1 DNase; Promega, Madison, WI). One microgram of RNA was reverse transcribed into first-strand cDNA in a 20 l final volume containing 1 M random hexanucleotide primers, 1 M oligo dT and 200 U Moloney murine leukemia virus reverse transcriptase (Clontech, Palo Alto, CA). cDNA were evaluated for GAPDH expression by Real Time PCR to test RNA quality.

Inflammasome signalling pathway

The human Inflammasomes RT^2 Profiler PCR Array (Qiagen PAHS-097Z) was used to analyze gene expression of inflammasome components and signalling pathways. In this array a set of optimized primer assays allows the detection of mRNA transcripts of 84 genes as well as five housekeeping genes in a 96-well plate by real-time PCR. Individual specimens were pooled according to MMSE scores (severe AD, MILD AD, MCI, HC). cDNA from unstimulated cells and from cells stimulated with either LPS or $A\beta_{42}$ alone or, finally, that had been LPS-primed and $A\beta_{42}$ stimulated were grouped in different pools for PCR arrays. Data were analyzed by the comparative Ct method using GAPDH as the reference gene. Results are expressed as the fold changes between LPS or $A\beta_{42}$ or LPS-primed and $A\beta_{42}$ stimulated pools from each disease state and unstimulated condition. Heat maps were generated and genes hierarchically clustered by Euclidean distance and single linkage using TIGR MultiExperiment Viewer (MeV) v4.9 [61].

Real time quantitative reverse transcription

Real Time quantitative Reverse Transcription PCR (RQPCR) was performed on a ABI Prism 7000 instrument (PE Applied Biosystems, Foster City, CA, USA) with gene specific primers and the SybrGreen chemistry to confirm the gene expression changes observed by arrays. All primers were cDNA specific and were purchased from Qiagen (Venlo, PB Venlo, The Netherlands). Specific PCR products amplification was detected using the RT2 SYBR Green Fluor with a 25 l final volume of 12.5 l RT2 qPCR Mastermix (Qiagen) 10.5 l H2O, 1.0 l of either diluted template or 1.0 l RT2 qPCR Primer Assay. Results were expressed as ΔΔCt and presented as ratios between the target gene and the GAPDH housekeeping mRNA. Experiments were run on each subject included in the study.

Western blotting

Unstimulated and LPS-primed and $A\beta_{42}$ stimulated-monocytes were washed and lysed with M-PER Mammalian Protein Extraction Reagent with phosphatase and protease inhibitors (10 l/ml, Halt™ Protease and Phosphatase Inhibitor Cocktail, Thermo Scientific Inc, Rockford, IL, USA). After protein estimation using the Bradford Assay reagent (Bio-Rad) 20 g of cell lysate was resolved by electrophoresis on a 10 % SDS-polyacrylamide gel under reducing conditions. Proteins were then transferred to PVDF membrane by electrophoretic blotting and blocked for 1 h in blocking buffer (Blocker BLOTTO Blocking Buffer, Thermo Scientific). Membranes were then incubated overnight with sheep anti-recombinant NALP3 (AF6789, R&D Systems) or for 1 h with sheep anti beta-actin antibody (AF4000, R&D Systems), then diluted 1:1000 in blocking buffer followed by HRP-conjugated anti-sheep IgG (HAF016, R&D Systems). Bound antibodies were visualized with a chemiluminescence development reagent (LiteAblot TURBO, Euroclone, Italy) according to the manufacturer's instructions. Bands were imaged in a Gel-Doc Cabinet and the density of the image was measured. The density of each band was normalized with beta-actin (as housekeeping protein) and for each sample an arbitrary units (AU) value was calculated as follows: normalized density of NLRP3 band obtained from stimulated (LPS-primed+Aβ) monocytes/normalized density of NLRP3 band obtained from unstimulated monocytes.

Flow cytometry immunofluorescent staining

Unstimulated and LPS-primed and $A\beta_{42}$-stimulated-monocytes were stained with anti-CD14-PC7 (clone RMO52, isotype mouse IgG_{2a}, Beckman Coulter, CA USA) mAb for 30 min at 4°. Cells were then washed, treated with FIX and PERM Cell kit (eBioscience, San Diego, CA, USA), and stained with anti- NLRP3-PE (clone 768319; isotype rat IgG_{2a} R&D Systems Inc. Minneapolis MN, USA), –NLRP1-APC (isotype rabbit polyclonal IgG Proteintech, Chicago, IL, USA), –caspase 5-FITC (isotype rabbit polyclonal; LifeSpan BioSciences,Inc, Seattle, WA USA), – PYCARD-FITC (clone HASC-71; isotype mouseIgG$_{1k}$, eBioLegend San Diego CA,USA), IL-1β FITC(-clone 8516; isotype mouse IgG_1; R&D) IL-33-APC (clone 39412 isotype rat IgG_{2B} R&D), or IL-37-PE (clone 6A6, isotype mouse IgG_{1k} LSBioSciences, Inc) mAb for 30 min at 4°. The Fluorochrome Inhibitor of Caspases (FLICA) kit was used to analyze caspases. This kit uses a novel approach to detect active caspases. Once inside the cell, the FLICA inhibitor probe binds covalently to the active caspase (p20) alone. Staining of active caspase 1 and caspase 8 inhibitors was performed using the green fluorescent probe FAM-YVAD-FMK and FAM-LETD-FMK respectively, following the procedures suggested by the manufacturer (AM-FLICA, Immunochemistry, Bloomington, IN, USA). NLRP1, caspase 5 and PYCARD were conjugated using the Lightning-Link APC or FITC conjugation kit (Innova Biosciences, Cambridge, UK). Cells were finally analyzed using a Beckman-Coulter GALLIOS flow cytometer equipped with a single 15 mW argon ion laser operating at 488 nm and interfaced with CXP Software 2.1. 200,000 cells were acquired and gated on CD14 expression and side scatter properties. Isotype control or single fluorochrome-stained preparations were used for color compensation.

Confocal microscopy analysis

Unstimulated, LPS- or $A\beta_{42}$- primed, or LPS-primed and $A\beta_{42}$-stimulated-PBMC were cultured on chamber slide (Lab Tek Nalge Nunc Intern. Naperville IL USA) for 24 h at 37 °C. Non-adherent cells were then washed away and monocytes were grown on chamber slides, fixed in 4 % paraformaldehyde in PBS for 15 min, and treated for 1 h at room temperature with FLICA staining of active caspase 1 or caspase 8 using green fluorescent FAM-YVAD-FMK probes, following the procedures suggested by the manufacturer (AM-FLICA). Cells were then treated with FIX and PERM Cell kit (eBioscience), and stained with PE or APC or FITC conjugated -mAbs specific for NLRP3 or NLRP1 and PYCARD or caspase 5 for 24 h at 4 °C. Finally cells were fixed with paraformaldehyde 1 % for 15 min, washed and mounted on slides using the Vectashield Mounting Medium (Vector Laboratories, Inc, Burlingame, CA, USA). Fluorescent images were acquired on a Leica TCS DMRE spectral laser-scanning confocal microscope (Leica Microsystems, Wetzlar, Germany) with the appropriate filters and laser (488, 633) and a 63× objective lens. Image analysis was performed using the Leica Confocal Software and co-localization index with ImageJ Software. Co-localization indexes were calculated using the plug in JACoP (Justo Another Co-localization Plugin) [62]. The summarized co-localization efficiency data was expressed as Pearson correlation coefficient (PCC) as previously described [63–65]. Briefly this coefficient measures the significance of true co-localization. The significance test evaluates the probability that the measured value of r obtained from the two colours is significantly greater than values of r that would be calculated if there were only random overlap. The test is performed by randomly scrambling the blocks of pixels (instead of individual pixels, because each pixel's intensity is correlated with its neighbouring pixels) in one image, and then measuring the correlation of this image with the other (unscrambled) image (Costes et al.) The test produces values in the range −1 + 1, 0 indicating that there is no discernible correlation and −1 and +1 meaning strong negative and positive correlations, respectively.

Cytokines in supernatants

Supernatants of unstimulated, LPS- or $A\beta_{42}$- primed, or LPS-primed and $A\beta_{42}$-stimulated-PBMC were analyzed. Interleukin-1β, IL-18 and IL-33 concentration were measured using the Human IL-1 β (Quantikine ELISA Kit DLB50; R&D Systems), Human IL-33 (Quantikine ELISA KitD3300; R&D Systems), and Human IL-18 (ELISA Kit -LS-F118-1; LifeSpan BioSciences, Inc.) according to the manufacturer's recommendations.

Statistical analyses

Quantitative data were not normally distributed (Shapiro–Wilk test) and are thus summarized as median and Interquartile Range (IQR) (25° and 75° percentile). Comparisons between groups were analyzed used a Kruskal-Wallis ANOVA for each variable. Comparisons among the different groups were made using a 2-tailed Mann-Whitney *U* test performed for independent samples. Western Blot data were normally distributed, and were summarized as mean ± standard error. In this case, comparisons were performed using ANOVA and unpaired Student's *t* test. Data analysis was performed using the MedCalc statistical package (MedCalc Software bvba, Mariakerke, Belgium).

Abbreviations

IL: interleukin; Aβ: amyloid-β; MCI: mild cognitive impairment; AD: Alzheimer's disease; HC: healthy controls; NLRs: Nod-like receptors; PAMPs: pathogen-associated molecular patterns; DAMPs: damage-associated molecular pattern molecules; ROS: reactive oxygen species; FADD: Fas-Associated protein with death domain; LTP: long-term potentiation; MMSE: mini- mental state examination; PBMC: peripheral blood mononuclear cell; FACS: fluorescence-activated cell sorting.

Competing interest

The authors declare that they have no competing interest.

Authors' contributions

MS carried out the immunophenotypic studies, performed the statistical analysis, coordinated the lab work and drafted the manuscript. FLR and FP carried out the molecular biology studies and drafted the manuscript. MZ and VR took care of the immunoassays and drafted the manuscript. IM took care of confocal microscopy and helped to draft the manuscript. RM carried out the Western Blotting analyses and drafted the manuscript. EC and RN were responsible for the selection of patients and controls participated in the sequence alignment and helped to revise the manuscript. MC conceived the study, participated in its design and coordination and helped to draft the manuscript. All authors read and approved the final manuscript.

Authors' information

MS: senior researcher, laboratory coordinator, expertise in basic laboratory research, flow cytometry analyses, and in clinical immunology. FLR: PhD, expertise in molecular biology analyses. FP: PhD, expertise in molecular biology.MZ: young researcher, expertise in immunoassay analyses. VR: PhD, expertise in immunoassay analyses. IM, technician, expertise in confocal microscopy analyses. RM: senior researcher, expertise in basic laboratory research, W.B. analyses. EC: MD, Neurologist, patient selection and characterization. RN: MD, Associated Professor in neurology, clinical studies coordinator. MC: MD, Full Professor of immunology, Scientific Director and laboratory chief, researchers coordinator.

Acknowledgments

This research work was supported by grants from Ricerca Corrente 2013–2014 (Italian Ministry of Health).

Author details

[1]Don C. Gnocchi Foundation, IRCCS, Piazza Morandi, 3, 20121 Milan, Italy. [2]Departments of Biomedical and Clinical Sciences "Luigi Sacco", University of Milano, 20100 Milan, Italy. [3]Departments of Physiopathology and Transplants, University of Milano, 20100 Milan, Italy.

References

1. Hardy J, Selkoe DJ. The amyloid hypothesis of Alzheimer's disease: progress and problems on the road to therapeutics. Science. 2002;19:353–6.
2. Schroder K, Tschopp J. The inflammosomes. Cell. 2010;140(6):821–32.
3. Jin C, Flavell RA. Molecular mechanism of NLRP3 inflammasome activation. J Clin Immunol. 2010;30(5):628–31.
4. Lamkanfi M. Emerging inflammasome effector mechanisms. Nat Rev Immunol. 2011;11(3):213–20.
5. Gurung P, Anand PK, Malireddi RK, Vande Walle L, Van Opdenbosch N, Dillon CP, Weinlich R, Green DR, Lamkanfi M, Kanneganti TD. FADD and caspase-8 mediate priming and activation of the canonical and noncanonical Nlrp3 inflammasomes. J Immunol. 2014;192(4):1835–46.
6. Gurung P, Kanneganti TD. Novel roles for caspase-8 in IL-1β and inflammasome regulation. Am J Pathol. 2015;185(1):17–25.
7. Bauernfeind FG, Horvath G, Stutz A, Alnemri ES, MacDonald K, Speert D, Fernandes-Alnemri T, Wu J, Monks BG, Fitzgerald KA, Hornung V, Latz E. Cutting edge: NF-kappaB activating pattern recognition and cytokine receptors license NLRP3 inflammasome activation by regulating NLRP3 expression. J Immunol. 2009;183(2):787–91.
8. Martinon F, Mayor A, Tschopp J. The inflammasomes: guardians of the body. Annu Rev Immunol. 2009;27:229–65.
9. Agostini L, Martinon F, Burns K, McDermott MF, Hawkins PN, Tschopp J. NALP3 forms an IL-1beta-processing inflammasome with increased activity in Muckle-Wells autoinflammatory disorder. Immunity. 2004;20(3):319–25.
10. Martinon F, Agostini L, Meylan E, Tschopp J. Identification of bacterial muramyl dipeptide as activator of the NALP3/cryopyrin inflammasome. Curr Biol. 2004a;14(21):1929–34.
11. Martinon F, Tschopp J. Inflammatory caspases: linking an intracellular innate immune system to autoinflammatory diseases. Cell. 2004b;117(5):561–74.
12. Kanneganti TD, Body-Malapel M, Amer A, Park JH, Whitfield J, Franchi L, Taraporewala ZF, Miller D, Patton JT, Inohara N, Núñez G. Critical role for Cryopyrin/Nalp3 in activation of caspase-1 in response to viral infection and double-stranded RNA. J Biol Chem. 2006;281(48):36560–8.
13. Mariathasan S, Weiss DS, Newton K, McBride J, O'Rourke K, Roose-Girma M, Dixit VM. Cryopyrin activates the inflammasomein response to toxins and ATP. Nature. 2006;440(7081):228–32.
14. Halle A, Hornung V, Petzold GC, Stewart CR, Monks BG, Reinheckel T, Fitzgerald KA, Latz E, Moore KJ, Golenbock DT. The NALP3 inflammasome is

involved in the innate immune response to amyloid-beta. Nat Immunol. 2008;9(8):857–65.

15. Bryant C, Fitzgerald KA. Molecular mechanisms involved in inflammasome activation. Trends Cell Biol. 2009;19(9):455–64.
16. Horvath GL, Schrum JE, De Nardo CM, Latz E. Intracellular sensing of microbes and danger signals by the inflammasomes. Immunol Rev. 2011; 243(1):119–35.
17. Wen H, Miao EA, Ting JP. Mechanisms of NOD-like receptor-associated inflammasome activation. Immunity. 2013;39(3):432–41.
18. Lamkanfi M, Dixit VM. Mechanisms and functions of inflammasomes. Cell. 2014;157(5):1013–22.
19. Rubartelli A. Redox control of NLRP3 inflammasome activation in health and disease. J Leukoc Biol. 2012;92(5):951–8.
20. Master SL. Specific inflammasomes in complex diseases. Clin Immunol. 2013; 143:223–8.
21. Pollard KM, Kono DH. Requirements for innate immune pathways in environmentally induced autoimmunity. BMC Med. 2013;11:100.
22. Salminen A, Ojala J, Suuronen T, Kaarniranta K, Kauppinen A. Amyloid-beta oligomers set fire to inflammasomes and induce Alzheimer's pathology. J Cell Mol Med. 2008;12(6A):2255–62.
23. Masters SL, O'Neill LA. Disease-associated amyloid and misfolded protein aggregates activate the inflammasome. Trends Mol Med. 2011;17(5):276–82.
24. Heneka MT, Kummer MP, Stutz A, Delekate A, Schwartz S, Vieira-Saecker A, Griep A, Axt D, Remus A, Tzeng TC, Gelpi E, Halle A, Korte M, Latz E, Golenbock DT. NLRP3 is activated in Alzheimer's disease and contributes to pathology in APP/PS1 mice. Nature. 2013;493(7434):674–8.
25. Kummer JA, Broekhuizen R, Everett H, Agostini L, Kuijk L, Martinon F, van Bruggen R, Tschopp J. Inflammasome components NALP 1 and 3 show distinct but separate expression profiles in human tissues suggesting a site-specific role in the inflammatory response. J Histochem Cytochem. 2007;55(5):443–52. PubMed PMID: 17164409, Epub 2006 Dec 12.
26. Heneka MT, Kummer MP, Latz E. Innate immune activation in neurodegenerative disease. Nat Rev Immunol. 2014;14(7):463–77.
27. Heneka MT, Carson MJ, Khoury J, Landreth GE, Brosseron F, Feinstein DL, Jacobs AH, Wyss-Coray T, Vitorica J, Ransohoff RM, Herrup K, Frautschy SA, Finsen B, Brown GC, Verkhratsky A, Yamanaka K, Koistinaho J, Latz E, Halle A, Petzold GC, Town T, Morgan D, Shinohara ML, Perry VH, Holmes C, Bazan NG, Brooks DJ, Hunot S, Joseph B, Deigendesch N, Garaschuk O, Boddeke E, Dinarello CA, Breitner JC, Cole GM, Golenbock DT, Kummer MP. Neuroinflammation in Alzheimer's disease. Lancet Neurol. 2015a;14:388–405.
28. Heneka MT, Golenbock DT, Latz E. Innate immunity in Alzheimer's disease. Nat Immunol. 2015b;16:229–36.
29. Tan MS, Yu JT, Jiang T, Zhu XC, Tan L. The NLRP3 inflammasome in Alzheimer's disease. Mol Neurobiol. 2013;48(3):875–82.
30. Saresella M, Calabrese E, Marventano I, Piancone F, Gatti A, Alberoni M, Nemni R, Clerici M. Increased activity of Th-17 and Th-9 lymphocytes and a skewing of the post-thymic differentiation pathway are seen in Alzheimer's disease. Brain Behav Immun. 2011;25(3):539–47.
31. Saresella M, Marventano I, Calabrese E, Piancone F, Rainone V, Gatti A, Alberoni M, Nemni R, Clerici M. A complex proinflammatory role for peripheral monocytes in Alzheimer's disease. J Alzheimers Dis. 2014;38(2):403–13.
32. Pontillo A, Catamo E, Arosio B, Mari D, Crovella S. NALP1/NLRP1 genetic variants are associated with Alzheimer disease. Alzheimer Dis Assoc Disord. 2012;26(3):277–81.
33. Darisipudi MN(1), Thomasova D, Mulay SR, Brech D, Noessner E, Liapis H, Anders HJ. Uromodulin triggers IL-1β-dependent innate immunity via the NLRP3 inflammasome. J Am Soc Nephrol. 2012;23(11):1783–9.
34. Ni J, Wang P, Zhang J, Chen W, Gu L. Silencing of the P2X7 receptor enhances amyloid-b phagocytosis by microglia biochemical and biophysical research. Communications. 2013;434:363–9.
35. Griffin WS, Liu L, Li Y, Mrak RE, Barger SW. Interleukin-1 mediates Alzheimer and Lewy body pathologies. J Neuroinflammation. 2006;3:5–9.
36. Pickering M, O'Connor JJ. Pro-inflammatory cytokines and their effects in the dentate gyrus. Prog Brain Res. 2007;163:339–54.
37. Murray CA, Lynch MA. Evidence that increased hippocampal expression of the cytokine interleukin-1 beta is a common trigger for age- and stress-induced impairments in long-term potentiation. J Neurosci Off J Soc Neurosci. 1998;18(8): 2974–81.
38. Ojala J, Alafuzoff I, Herukka SK, van Groen T, Tanila H, Pirttila T. Expression of interleukin-18 is increased in the brains of Alzheimer's disease patients. Neurobiol Aging. 2009;30(2):198–209.
39. Malaguarnera L, Motta M, Di Rosa M, Anzaldi M, Malaguarnera M. Interleukin-18 and transforming growth factor-beta 1 plasma levels in Alzheimer's disease and vascular dementia. Neuropathology. 2006;26(4):307–12.
40. Bossù P, Ciaramella A, Salani F, Vanni D, Palladino I, Caltagirone C, Scapigliati G. Interleukin-18, from neuroinflammation to Alzheimer's disease. Curr Pharm Des. 2010;16(38):4213–24.
41. Salani F, Ciaramella A, Bizzoni F, Assogna F, Caltagirone C, Spalletta G, Bossù P. Increased expression of interleukin-18 receptor in blood cells of subjects with mild cognitive impairment and Alzheimer's disease. Cytokine. 2013;61(2):360–3.
42. Sutinen EM, Pirttilä T, Anderson G, Salminen A, Ojala JO. Pro-inflammatory interleukin-18 increases Alzheimer's disease-associated amyloid-β production in human neuron-like cells. J Neuroinflammation. 2012;9:199.
43. Chapuis J, Hot D, Hansmannel F, Kerdraon O, Ferreira S, Hubans C, Maurage CA, Huot L, Bensemain F, Laumet G, Ayral AM, Fievet N, Hauw JJ, DeKosky ST, Lemoine Y, Iwatsubo T, Wavrant-Devrièze F, Dartigues JF, Tzourio C, Buée L, Pasquier F, Berr C, Mann D, Lendon C, Alpérovitch A, Kamboh MI, Amouyel P, Lambert JC. Transcriptomic and genetic studies identify IL-33 as a candidate gene for Alzheimer's disease. Mol Psychiatry. 2009;14:1004–16.
44. Fryer JD, Taylor JW, DeMattos RB, Bales KR, Paul SM, Parsadanian M, Holtzman DM. Apolipoprotein E markedly facilitates age-dependent cerebral amyloid angiopathy and spontaneous hemorrhage in amyloid precursor protein transgenic mice. J Neurosci. 2003;23:7889–96.
45. Lee DCY, Landreth GE. The role of microglia in amyloid clearance from the AD brain. J Neural Transm. 2010;117:949–60.
46. Ali S, Mohs A, Thomas M, Klare J, Ross R, Schmitz ML, Martin MU. The dual function cytokine IL-33 interacts with the transcription factor NF- B to dampen NF- B-stimulated gene transcription. J Immunol. 2011;187:1609–16.
47. Rezai-Zadeh K, Gate D, Town T. CNS infiltration of peripheral immune cells: D-Day for neurodegenerative disease? J Neuroimmune Pharmacol. 2009;4: 462–75.
48. Cameron B, Landreth GE. Inflammation, microglia, and Alzheimer's disease. Neurobiol Dis. 2010;37(3):503–9.
49. Pan XD, Zhu YG, Lin N, Zhang J, Ye QY, Huang HP, Chen XC. Microglial phagocytosis induced by fibrillar b-amyloid is attenuated by oligomeric b-amyloid: implications for Alzheimer's disease. Mol Neurodegener. 2011;6:45.
50. Fowler BJ, Gelfand BD, Kim Y, Kerur NM, Tarallo V, Hirano Y, Amarnath S, Fowler DH, Radwan M, Young MT, Pittman K, Kubes P, Agarwal HK, Parang K, Hinton DR, Bastos-Carvalho A, Li S, Yasuma T, Mizutani T, Yasuma R, Wright C, Ambati J. Nucleoside reverse transcriptase inhibitors possess intrinsic anti-inflammatory activity. Science. 2014;346:1000–3.
51. McKhann G, Drachman D, Folstein M, Katzman R, Price D, Stadlan EM. Clinical diagnosis of Alzheimer's Disease: report of the NINCDS-ADRDA Work Group under the auspices of Department of Health and Human Service Task Force on Alzheimer's Disease. Neurology. 1984;34(7):939–44.
52. American Psychiatric Association. Diagnostic and statistical manual of mental disorders DSM-IV-R. 1994.
53. Folstein MF, Folstein SE, McHugh PR. Mini-mental state. A practical method for grading the cognitive state of patients for the clinicians. J Psychiat Res. 1975;12(3):189–98.
54. Hughes CP, Berg L, Danziger WL, Coben LA, Martin RL. A new clinical scale for staging of dementia. Br J Psychiatry. 1982;140:566–72.
55. Petersen RC. Mild cognitive impairment as a diagnostic entity. J Intern Med. 2004;256(3):183–94.
56. Ligthart GJ, Corberand JX, Fournier C, Galanaud P, Hijmans W, Kennes B, Müller-Hermelink HK, Steinmann GG. Admission criteria for immunogerontological studies in man: the SENIEUR protocol. Mech Ageing Dev. 1984;28(1):47–55.
57. Speciale L, Calabrese E, Saresella M, Tinelli C, Mariani C, Sanvito L, Longhi R, Ferrante P. Lymphocyte subset patterns and cytokines production in Alzheimer's disease patients. Neurbiol Aging. 2007;28(8):1163–9.
58. Delirezh N, Shojaeefar E, Parvin P, Asadi B. Comparison the effects of two monocyte isolation methods, plastic adherence and magnetic activated cell sorting methods, on phagocytic activity of generated dendritic cells. Cell J. 2013;15:218–23.
59. Martinon F, Petrilli V, Mayor A, Tardivel A, Tschopp J. Gout-associated uric acid crystals activate the NALP3 inflammasome. Nature. 2006;440:237–41.
60. Dostert C, Pétrilli V, Van Bruggen R, Steele C, Mossman BT, Tschopp J. Innate immune activation through Nalp3 inflammasome sensing of asbestos and silica. Science. 2008;320:674–7.
61. Saeed AI, Sharov V, White J, Li J, Liang W, Bhagabati N, Braisted J, Klapa M, Currier T, Thiagarajan M, Sturn A, Snuffin M, Rezantsev A, Popov D, Ryltsov

A,Kostukovich E, Borisovsky I, Liu Z, Vinsavich A, Trush V, Quackenbush J. TM4: a free, open-source system for microarray data management and analysis. Biotechniques. 2003;34:374-8.
62. Bolte S, Cordelières FP. A guided tour into subcellular colocalization analysis in light microscopy. J Microsc. 2006;224:213-232.
63. Manders EMM. Chromatic shift in multicolour confocal microscopy. J Microsc. 1997;185:321-28.
64. French AP, Mills S, Swarup R, Bennet MJ, Pridmore TP. Colocalization of fluorescent markers in confocal microscope images of plant cells, Nat Protoc. 2008;4:619-28.
65. Xiang Li, Zhang Y, Xia M, Gulbins E, Boini KM, Li PL. Activation of Nlrp3 Inflammasomes Enhances Macrophage Lipid-Deposition and Migration: Implicationof a Novel Role of Inflammasome in Atherogenesis. PLOS ONE. 2014;9(1):e87552.

Permissions

All chapters in this book were first published in MN, by BioMed Central; hereby published with permission under the Creative Commons Attribution License or equivalent. Every chapter published in this book has been scrutinized by our experts. Their significance has been extensively debated. The topics covered herein carry significant findings which will fuel the growth of the discipline. They may even be implemented as practical applications or may be referred to as a beginning point for another development.

The contributors of this book come from diverse backgrounds, making this book a truly international effort. This book will bring forth new frontiers with its revolutionizing research information and detailed analysis of the nascent developments around the world.

We would like to thank all the contributing authors for lending their expertise to make the book truly unique. They have played a crucial role in the development of this book. Without their invaluable contributions this book wouldn't have been possible. They have made vital efforts to compile up to date information on the varied aspects of this subject to make this book a valuable addition to the collection of many professionals and students.

This book was conceptualized with the vision of imparting up-to-date information and advanced data in this field. To ensure the same, a matchless editorial board was set up. Every individual on the board went through rigorous rounds of assessment to prove their worth. After which they invested a large part of their time researching and compiling the most relevant data for our readers.

The editorial board has been involved in producing this book since its inception. They have spent rigorous hours researching and exploring the diverse topics which have resulted in the successful publishing of this book. They have passed on their knowledge of decades through this book. To expedite this challenging task, the publisher supported the team at every step. A small team of assistant editors was also appointed to further simplify the editing procedure and attain best results for the readers.

Apart from the editorial board, the designing team has also invested a significant amount of their time in understanding the subject and creating the most relevant covers. They scrutinized every image to scout for the most suitable representation of the subject and create an appropriate cover for the book.

The publishing team has been an ardent support to the editorial, designing and production team. Their endless efforts to recruit the best for this project, has resulted in the accomplishment of this book. They are a veteran in the field of academics and their pool of knowledge is as vast as their experience in printing. Their expertise and guidance has proved useful at every step. Their uncompromising quality standards have made this book an exceptional effort. Their encouragement from time to time has been an inspiration for everyone.

The publisher and the editorial board hope that this book will prove to be a valuable piece of knowledge for researchers, students, practitioners and scholars across the globe.

List of Contributors

Yue Wang, Zheng Wu, Yu-Ting Bai and Gong Chen
Department of Biology, Huck Institutes of Life Sciences, Pennsylvania State University, University park, PA 16802, USA

Gang-Yi Wu
Department of Biology, Huck Institutes of Life Sciences, Pennsylvania State University, University park, PA 16802, USA
School of Life Science, South China Normal University, Guangzhou 510631, China

Peter Pytel
Department of Pathology, The University of Chicago, Chicago, IL 60637, USA

Michal Arbel-Ornath, Eloise Hudry, Josiah R. Boivin, Shuko Takeda, Steven Hou, Carli R. Lattarulo, Arianna M. Belcher, Naomi Shakerdge, Pariss B. Trujillo, Bradley T. Hyman and Brian J. Bacskai
Alzheimer Research Unit, Department of Neurology, Massachusetts General Hospital and Harvard Medical School, 114, 16th St., Charlestown, MA 02129, USA

Tadafumi Hashimoto
Alzheimer Research Unit, Department of Neurology, Massachusetts General Hospital and Harvard Medical School, 114, 16th St., Charlestown, MA 02129, USA
Department of Neuropathology, The University of Tokyo, Tokyo, Japan

Kishore V. Kuchibhotla
Alzheimer Research Unit, Department of Neurology, Massachusetts General Hospital and Harvard Medical School, 114, 16th St., Charlestown, MA 02129, USA
Skirball Institute, NYU School of Medicine, New York, NY 10016, USA

Alona Muzikansky and Rebecca A. Betensky
Department of Biostatistics, Harvard School of Public Health, 50 Staniford Street, Boston, MA, USA

Yi-Ling Liu, Yu-Yi Lin and Po-Hung Lu
Institute of Brain Science, National Yang-Ming University, Taipei, Taiwan

Wei-Ting Chen
Brain Research Center, National Yang-Ming University, Taipei, Taiwan

Irene Han-Juo Cheng
Institute of Brain Science, National Yang-Ming University, Taipei, Taiwan
Brain Research Center, National Yang-Ming University, Taipei, Taiwan
Infection and Immunity Research Center, National Yang-Ming University, Taipei, Taiwan

Shie-Liang Hsieh
Genomics Research Center, Academia Sinica, Taipei, Taiwan
Institute of Clinical Medicine, School of Medicine, National Yang-Ming University, Taipei, Taiwan
Institute of Microbiology and Immunology, National Yang-Ming University, Taipei, Taiwan
Department of Medical Research and Education, Taipei Veterans General Hospital, Taipei, Taiwan

Hunter S. Futch, Cara L. Croft, Van Q. Truong and Todd E. Golde
Department of Neuroscience, University of Florida, Gainesville, FL 32610, USA
Center for Translational Research in Neurodegenerative Disease, University of Florida, Gainesville, FL 32610, USA
McKnight Brain Institute, University of Florida, 1149 Newell Drive, Gainesville, FL 32610, USA

Eric G. Krause
Department of Pharmacodynamics, College of Pharmacy, University of Florida, Gainesville, USA
McKnight Brain Institute, University of Florida, 1149 Newell Drive, Gainesville, FL 32610, USA

Takashi Kasai, Takuma Ohmichi and Masaki Kondo
Department of Neurology, Kyoto Prefectural University of Medicine, Kyoto 602-0841, Japan

Harutsugu Tatebe
Department of Neurology, Kyoto Prefectural University of Medicine, Kyoto 602-0841, Japan
Department of Zaitaku (Homecare) Medicine, Kyoto Prefectural University of Medicine, Kyoto 602-0841, Japan

Yusuke Kishi and Tomoshi Kakeya
Strategic Marketing Division, SCRUM Inc, Tokyo 130-0021, Japan

Masaaki Waragai
Department of Neurology, Higashi Matsudo Municipal Hospital, Matsudo 270-2222, Japan

David Allsop
Division of Biomedical and Life Sciences, Faculty of Health and Medicine, Lancaster University, Lancaster LA1 4YQ, UK

Takahiko Tokuda
Department of Neurology, Kyoto Prefectural University of Medicine, Kyoto 602-0841, Japan
Department of Molecular Pathobiology of Brain Diseases, Kyoto Prefectural University of Medicine, Kyoto 602-0841, Japan

Sookja Kim Chung
Research Center of Heart, Brain, Hormone and Healthy Aging, LKS Faculty of Medicine, The University of Hong Kong, Hong Kong, Special Administrative Region, China
Hong Kong University Alzheimer's Disease Research Network, LKS Faculty of Medicine, The University of Hong Kong, Hong Kong, Special Administrative Region, China
School of Biomedical Sciences, LKS Faculty of Medicine, The University of Hong Kong, Hong Kong, Special Administrative Region, China

Joanna L. Jankowsky
Department of Neuroscience, Baylor College of Medicine, Houston, TX 77030, USA
Department of Neurology, Baylor College of Medicine, Houston, TX 77030, USA
Department of Neurosurgery, Baylor College of Medicine, Houston, TX 77030, USA
Department of Molecular and Cellular Biology, Baylor College of Medicine, Houston, TX 77030, USA
Huffington Center on Aging, Baylor College of Medicine, Houston, TX 77030, USA

Hui Zheng
Department of Neuroscience, Baylor College of Medicine, Houston, TX 77030, USA
Department of Molecular and Cellular Biology, Baylor College of Medicine, Houston, TX 77030, USA
Huffington Center on Aging, Baylor College of Medicine, Houston, TX 77030, USA
Department of Molecular and Human Genetics, Baylor College of Medicine, Houston, TX 77030, USA

Justyna Sosna, Stephan Philipp, Ricardo Albay III and Jorge Mauricio Reyes-Ruiz
Department of Molecular Biology and Biochemistry, University of California, Irvine, USA

Charles G. Glabe
Department of Molecular Biology and Biochemistry, University of California, Irvine, USA
Biochemistry Department, Faculty of Science and Experimental Biochemistry Unit, King Fahd Medical Research Center, King Abdulaziz University, Jeddah 21589, Saudi Arabia

David Baglietto-Vargas and Frank M. LaFerla
Institute for Memory Impairments and Neurological Disorders (UCIMIND), University of California, Irvine, USA

Wei Cao and Hui Zheng
Department of Molecular and Human Genetics, Baylor College of Medicine, Huffington Center on Aging, Houston, TX 77030, USA

Jiqing Cao and Dongming Cai
James J Peters VA Medical Center, Research & Development, Bronx, NY 10468, USA
Department of Neurology, Alzheimer Disease Research Center, Icahn School of Medicine at Mount Sinai, New York, NY 10029, USA
The Central Hospital of The Hua Zhong University of Science and Technology, Wuhan, China

Jianwei Hou
James J Peters VA Medical Center, Research & Development, Bronx, NY 10468, USA
Department of Neurology, Alzheimer Disease Research Center, Icahn School of Medicine at Mount Sinai, New York, NY 10029, USA

Jing Ping
The Central Hospital of The Hua Zhong University of Science and Technology, Wuhan, China

Anna K. Engstrom and Zhengui Xia
Toxicology Program, Department of Environmental and Occupational Health Sciences, University of Washington, Seattle, WA 98195, USA

Jessica M. Snyder
Department of Comparative Medicine, School of Medicine, University of Washington, Seattle, WA 98195, USA

Nobuyo Maeda
Department of Pathology and Laboratory Medicine, University of North Carolina, Chapel Hill, NC 27599, USA

Pierre De Rossi, Virginie Buggia-Prévot, Robert J. Andrew, Ruben Lesnick, Alexandra Botté, Carole Deyts, Someya Salem, Eshaan Rao, Richard C. Rice and Angèle Parent
Department of Neurobiology, The University of Chicago, JFK R212, 924 East 57th Street, Chicago, IL 60637, USA

Gopal Thinakaran
Department of Neurobiology, The University of Chicago, JFK R212, 924 East 57th Street, Chicago, IL 60637, USA
Department of Neurology, The University of Chicago, Chicago, IL 60637, USA
Department of Pathology, The University of Chicago, Chicago, IL 60637, USA

Benjamin L. L. Clayton and Brian Popko
Department of Neurology, The University of Chicago, Chicago, IL 60637, USA

Jared B. Vasquez, Carson van Sanford and Steven Estus
Sanders-Brown Center on Aging and Department of Physiology, University of Kentucky, Lexington, KY 40536, USA

Satyabrata Kar
Centre for prions and protein folding diseases, University of Alberta, Edmonton, AB T6G 2B7, Canada

Min Jian
Department of Medicine, LKS Faculty of Medicine, The University of Hong Kong, Hong Kong, Special Administrative Region, China

Patrick Ka Kit Yeung and Lena Lei Zhou
School of Biomedical Sciences, LKS Faculty of Medicine, The University of Hong Kong, Hong Kong, Special Administrative Region, China

Philip Wing-Lok Ho, Kenneth King-Yip Cheng, Ruby Lai-Chong Hoo and Aimin Xu
Department of Medicine, LKS Faculty of Medicine, The University of Hong Kong, Hong Kong, Special Administrative Region, China
Research Center of Heart, Brain, Hormone and Healthy Aging, LKS Faculty of Medicine, The University of Hong Kong, Hong Kong, Special Administrative Region, China

Koon Ho Chan
Department of Medicine, LKS Faculty of Medicine, The University of Hong Kong, Hong Kong, Special Administrative Region, China
Research Center of Heart, Brain, Hormone and Healthy Aging, LKS Faculty of Medicine, The University of Hong Kong, Hong Kong, Special Administrative Region, China
Hong Kong University Alzheimer's Disease Research Network, LKS Faculty of Medicine, The University of Hong Kong, Hong Kong, Special Administrative Region, China
Neuroimmunology and Neuroinflammation Research Laboratory, LKS Faculty of Medicine, The University of Hong Kong, Hong Kong, Special Administrative Region, China
LKS Faculty of Medicine, The University of Hong Kong, Hong Kong, HKSAR, 8/F Department of Medicine, 21 Sassoon Road, Pofulam, China

Roy Chun-Laam Ng, On-Yin Cheng and Jason Shing-Cheong Kwan
Department of Medicine, LKS Faculty of Medicine, The University of Hong Kong, Hong Kong, Special Administrative Region, China
Neuroimmunology and Neuroinflammation Research Laboratory, LKS Faculty of Medicine, The University of Hong Kong, Hong Kong, Special Administrative Region, China

Song Li and Cheng Cheng
Center for Translational Research on Neurological Diseases, the First Affiliated Hospital, Dalian Medical University, 116021 Dalian, China

Juan Yang
Key Laboratory of Stem Cell Biology, Institute of Health Sciences, Shanghai Institutes for Biological Sciences, Chinese Academy of Sciences/Shanghai Jiao Tong University School of Medicine, 200031 Shanghai, China

Karen Siu-Ling. Lam
Department of Medicine, LKS Faculty of Medicine, The University of Hong Kong, Hong Kong, Special Administrative Region, China
Research Center of Heart, Brain, Hormone and Healthy Aging, LKS Faculty of Medicine, The University of Hong Kong, Hong Kong, Special Administrative Region, China
Hong Kong University Alzheimer's Disease Research Network, LKS Faculty of Medicine, The University of Hong Kong, Hong Kong, Special Administrative Region, China
LKS Faculty of Medicine, The University of Hong Kong, Hong Kong, HKSAR, 8/F Department of Medicine, 21 Sassoon Road, Pofulam, China

Weidong Le
Center for Translational Research on Neurological Diseases, the First Affiliated Hospital, Dalian Medical University, 116021 Dalian, China
Key Laboratory of Stem Cell Biology, Institute of Health Sciences, Shanghai Institutes for Biological Sciences, Chinese Academy of Sciences/Shanghai Jiao Tong University School of Medicine, 200031 Shanghai, China
Collaborative Innovation Center for Brain Science, the First Affiliated Hospital, Dalian Medical University, 116011 Dalian, China

Xi-Biao He
Shanghai University of Medicine and Health Sciences, Shanghai 201318, China

Marina Saresella, Francesca La Rosa, Federica Piancone, Martina Zoppis, Ivana Marventano, Elena Calabrese and Roberta Mancuso
Don C. Gnocchi Foundation, IRCCS, Piazza Morandi, 3, 20121 Milan, Italy

Veronica Rainone
Departments of Biomedical and Clinical Sciences "Luigi Sacco", University of Milano, 20100 Milan, Italy

Raffaello Nemni and Mario Clerici
Don C. Gnocchi Foundation, IRCCS, Piazza Morandi, 3, 20121 Milan, Italy
Departments of Physiopathology and Transplants, University of Milano, 20100 Milan, Italy

Index

www.ingramcontent.com/pod-product-compliance
Lightning Source LLC
LaVergne TN
LVHW080700210926
848485LV00003B/400